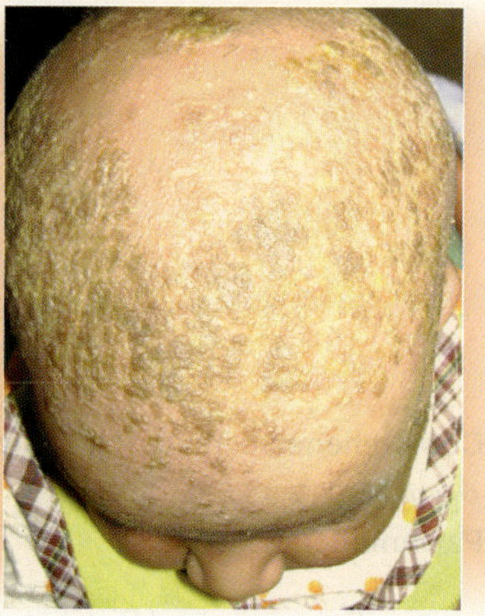

Comprehensive Textbook of DERMATOLOGY

VIJAY K GARG
MD, MNAMS
Professor and Head
Department of Dermatology and STD
Maulana Azad Medical College and Lok Nayak Hospital, New Delhi

KABIR SARDANA
MD, DNB, MNAMS
Associate Professor
Department of Dermatology and Venereology
Maulana Azad Medical College and Lok Nayak Hospital, New Delhi

PEEPEE
PUBLISHERS AND DISTRIBUTORS (P) LTD.

Comprehensive Textbook of Dermatology

Published by
Pawaninder P. Vij

Peepee Publishers and Distributors (P) Ltd.
Head Office:
160, Shakti Vihar, Pitam Pura
Delhi-110034 (India)

Correspondence Address:
7/31, First Floor, Ansari Road, Daryaganj
New Delhi-110002 (India), Post Box-7243

Ph: 65195868, 9811156083, 23246245

e-mail: peepee160@yahoo.co.in

e-mail: peepee160@rediffmail.com

e-mail: peepee160@gmail.com

www.peepeepub.com

First Edition: **2010**

ISBN: 81-8445-066-4

Printed at
Paras Offset Pvt. Ltd., New Delhi-28

The book is dedicated to
our students, parents, wife and
children and above all to
our patients!

—Editors

I dedicate this book to my father General Sardana who taught me honesty and discipline!

My mother Amba Sardana for being God fearing and conscientious.

My wife Dr Supriya who is the "wind beneath my wings".

And my daughter Zoya who is the joy of our life.

And lastly to the motto of Karamdharma!

—Dr Kabir Sardana

"Gayatri Mantra"

गायत्री मंत्र

ॐ भूर्भुवः स्वः
तत्सवितुर्वरेण्यम्
भर्गो देवस्य धीमहि
धियो यो नः प्रचोदयात्।

"OM BHUR, OM BHUVAHA, OM SWAHA, OM MAHAHA, OM JANAHA, OM TAPAHA, OM SATYAM, OM TAT SAVITUR VARENYAM BHARGHO DEVASYA DHIMAHI DHIYO YONAHA PRACHODAYAT."

"O God, You are the giver of life, the remover of pain and sorrow, the bestower of happiness; O Creator of the Universe, may we receive Your supreme sin-destroying light; may You guide our intellect in the right direction."

KARAMDHARMA

Bhagavad-gita (4.17-18)

Bhagavad-gita (4.17-18) says: "The intricacies of action are very hard to understand. Therefore one should know properly what action is, what forbidden action is, and what inaction is. One who sees inaction in action, and action in inaction, is intelligent among men, and he is in the transcendental position, although engaged in all sorts of activities."

Endowed with wisdom, giving up the fruits resulting from actions, attaining self-realization and freed from the bondage of birth, verily they go to that abode which is free from evil.

Established in yoga, O Dhananjaya (Arjuna), perform actions, giving up attachment, and unconcerned as to the success or failure.

To work alone you have the right, but never claim its results. Let not the result of actions be your motive, nor be attached to inaction.

Not by mere abstaining from action does a man reach the state of actionlessness, nor by mere renunciation does he arrive at perfection.

The wise man should not unsettle the faith of the ignorant who are attached to work. He should make them devoted to all work, performing action himself intently.

He whose actions are free from the hankering for desires, whose actions have been burnt by the fire of knowledge, him the wise call a sage.

Verily no one becomes a yogi without renouncing desire for the fruit of action.

PREFACE

The genesis of this book was to bridge the gap between a textbook basic enough for those pursuing MBBS with a focus on what is now crucial to getting an MD, that is entrance exam which are based on MCQs.

A problem with most books is that they are written totally divorced from the basic need to cover topics focusing on MCQs asked in various exams. Also references used are not mentioned thus students are forced to refer to expensive and sometimes inaccurate source of information in form of esoteric books written mostly by non experts.

So we have written text around the needs of *MBBS students*, with a focus on MCQs asked in exams with references. **The important topics for MCQs use are marked in bold text throughout the book.**

The book has chapters of varying levels of knowledge with the majority sufficiently endowed for *Postgraduate* in MD, Diploma and DNB to help in quick revision of the course. References from standard dermatology, leprosy and STD textbooks with national and international guidelines add to the authenticity of the book. We have desisted from mentioning personal views to ensure unbiased transfer of knowledge.

The photographs will also help the *General Practitioner /Physician /Pediatrician* to learn the basics of dermatology.

Lastly, the therapeutic recommendations have been gleaned from a multitude of sources that will help the *busy practitioner* to use it as a ready reference.

We hope the primary and secondary reader will be equally benefited from the book.

We thank the contributors which include our faculty and senior residents for their effort. We also thank Dr Surabhi Sinha and Dr Shikha Chugh for proof-reading of the book.

Lastly, we thank Mr. Pawaninder P Vij and his team who have tirelessly pursued the aim of publishing this book specially Pawan Sharma for his assistance.

CONTRIBUTORS

Garg Vijay Kumar
MD, MNAMS
Prof and Head
Maulana Azad Medical College and Lok Nayak Hospital
New Delhi
Editing

Sardana Kabir
MD, DNB, MNAMS
Associate Professor
Maulana Azad Medical College and Lok Nayak Hospital
New Delhi
Editing
(Chapters 1, 2, 4-13, 15, 16-21, 22-24)

Arora Pooja
Senior Resident
Maulana Azad Medical College and Lok Nayak Hospital
New Delhi
(Chapter 2)

Barman Krishna Deb
MD
Associate Professor
Maulana Azad Medical College and Lok Nayak Hospital
New Delhi
(Chapter 11)

Bansal Shikha
MD
Specialist (Grade 2)
VMMC and Safdarjung Hospital
New Delhi
(Chapter 24)

Chugh Shikha
MD
Senior Resident
Maulana Azad Medical College and Lok Nayak Hospital
New Delhi
Proof Reading
(Chapter 19)

Kochhar Atul M
MD, DNB, MNAMS
Specialist (Grade 1)
Maulana Azad Medical College and Lok Nayak Hospital
New Delhi
(Chapter 1)

Mahajan Supriya
MD
Consultant Dermatologist
Kailash Hospital Gr Noida
Metro Hospital Noida
(Chapters 4, 9)

Nair Vivek
MD
Senior Resident
Maulana Azad Medical College and Lok Nayak Hospital
New Delhi
(Chapters 19, 22)

Relhan Vineet
MD
Senior Medical Officer
Maulana Azad Medical College and Lok Nayak Hospital
Delhi
(Chapters 3, 22)

Sarkar Rashmi
MD, MNAMS
Associate Professor
Maulana Azad Medical College and Lok Nayak Hospital
New Delhi
(Chapter 11)

Sinha Surabhi
MD
Senior Resident
Maulana Azad Medical College and Lok Nayak Hospital
New Delhi
Proof Reading
(Chapter 14)

Sharma Sudhanshu
Senior Resident
Maulana Azad Medical College and Lok Nayak Hospital
New Delhi
(Chapter 24)

REFERENCES USED FROM MAIN TEXTBOOKS

DERMATOLOGY

1. **Rook's Textbook of Dermatology** D. A. Burns , S. M. Breathnach , Neil Cox , Christopher E. Griffiths 7th edn 2004
2. **Fitzpatrick's Dermatology in General Medicine** 6th edn 2003
3. **Thieme's Pocket Dermatology 2006** by Wolfram Sterry , Walter Burgdorf , Ralf Paus
4. **Andrews' Diseases of the Skin: Clinical Dermatology** by William D. James, Timothy Berger, Dirk Elston 2005
5. **Therapeutic Strategies in Dermatology** Timothy G. Berger, M.D. Bruce U. Wintroub, M.D.
6. **A Clinical Atlas of 101 Common Skin Diseases** A. Bernard Ackerman, M.D. 2000
7. **Dermatological Signs of Internal Disease** 3rd edn Vol 1, Callen and Lorizzo

LEPROSY

1. **Hand Book of Leprosy,** Ridley Jopling 2004
2. **Textbook of Leprosy,** Hastings 1998
3. **Leprosy** SJ Yawalkar 1992
4. **A New Atlas of Leprosy** by AC McDougall and Yo Yuasa (2000)
5. **An Atlas of Leprosy** Guinto RS, Abalos Am, Celona AV, Fajardo T.T. Sasakawa Memorial Health Foudation 1983
6. **How to Diagnose and Treat Leprosy** ILEP
7. **How to Recognize and Manage Leprosy Reactions ILEP**
8. Report of the **Eighth Meeting of the WHO Technical Advisory Group on Leprosy Control Aberdeen,** Scotland 21st April 2006 WHO
9. **NLEP,** Government of India
10. **WHO Recomendations**

STD

1. **Sexually Transmitted Diseases,** Holmes May 2007 McGraw-Hill
2. **Venereal Diseases,** King A, Nicol C, Rodin P., 4th edn ELBS 1980; 251
3. **Sexually Transmitted Diseases Treatment Guidelines, 2006** CDC
4. Flow Charts on the **Syndromic Management of Sexually Transmitted Infections** NACO Aug 2007
5. **WHO and NACO Guidelines on HIV**

HISTOLOGY

1. **Histologic Diagnosis of Inflammatory Skin Diseases. An Algorithmic Method Based on Pattern Analysis,** 3rd edn A. Bernard Ackerman, MD, Almut Böer, MD, Bruce Bennin, MD and Geoffrey J. Gottlieb, MD 2005
2. **Lever's Histopathology of the Skin** by David E Elder, Rosalie Elenitsas, Bernett L Johnson, George F Murphy 9th edn 2004

JOURNALS

- **British Journal of Dermatology.**
- **Dermatology Clinics of North America.**
- **International Journal of Dermatology.**
- **Journal American Academy Dermatology.**
- **Lancet.**
- **Medical Clinics of North America.**

CONTENTS

Section 1

Section 2

Section 3

Section 4

Section 5

Section 6

Section 7

Section 8

Section 9

Section 10

CHAPTER 1

INTRODUCTION OF SKIN DISEASES

Structure and Function of Skin

The skin consists of three compartments: (1) epidermis and epithelial structures of adnexa continuous with it; (2) dermis and nonepithelial structures of adnexa lodged in it; and (3) subcutis.

The epidermis thickness varies from approximately **0.03 mm on the eyelids to 1.5 mm on** the palms of a young adult; the average thickness of epidermis is **about 0.4 mm**.

The **dermis**, depending on the anatomical site, is **15 to 40 times** thicker than the epidermis, but its metabolic requirements are far less. Cells of various kinds in variable numbers are scattered throughout the mature dermis, these being fibrocytes, dermal dendrocytes, histiocytes, **langerhans' cells** and mast cells. Within the dermis are housed nerves, blood vessels, lymph vessels, smooth muscles and **epithelial structures of adnexa**.

A fully formed **dermis** is divisible into two distinct compartments: (1) a thin zone immediately beneath the epidermis (papillary dermis) and around adnexa (periadnexal dermis); and (2) a thick zone (reticular dermis) that extends from the base of the papillary dermis to the surface of the subcutaneous fat (Fig. 1.1).

The combination of **papillary and periadnexal dermis** has been termed as **adventitial dermis**.

The reticular dermis is formed mostly of thick bundles of collagen arranged in orthogonal pattern. Elastic fibers course among these bundles. Proportionally fewer fibrocytes and blood vessels and less ground substance are present in the thick reticular dermis than in the thin adventitial dermis.

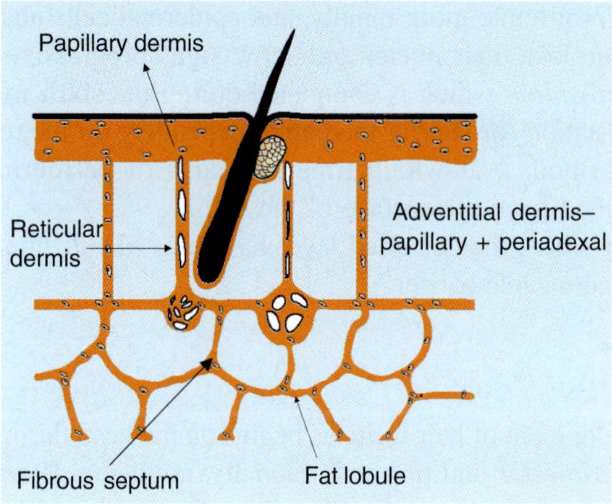

Fig. 1.1: Structure of dermis

EMBRYOLOGY

All constituents of human skin are derived from either **ectoderm or mesoderm**. The epithelial structures, i.e., the epidermis (surface and infundibular), apocrine units, sebaceous units, hair follicles, eccrine units and nail units come from **ectoderm.**

Melanocytes, nerves and specialized sensory receptors develop from **neuroectoderm.**

The other elements in skin, i.e., Langerhans' cells, macrophages, mast cells, fibrocytes, blood vessels, lymph vessels, muscles and adipocytes originate from **mesoderm.**

In a **3-week-old embryo**, the primordial epidermis consists of a single layer of flattened epithelial cells (Fig. 1.2).

By 4 weeks (Fig. 1.3) the epithelium develops into a basal germinative layer made up of cuboidal cells and an outer layer of slightly flattened cells that possess microvilli and cytoplasmic blebs along the border that faces the amniotic fluid.

Near the end of the first trimester (Fig. 1.4), several layers of large cells rich in glycogen appear in the middle of a still-developing epidermis. Unlike cells of the periderm, these intermediate cells contain clumps of cytoplasmic *tonofilaments* that at intercellular junctions connect with specialized contacts called *desmosomes.*

After the fifth month, *keratohyaline* granules appear in the upper part of the intermediate zone. Basal germinative cells proliferate more rapidly, and epidermal cells near the surface lose their nuclei and show signs progressively of *cornification,* which is completed during the **sixth month** of gestation (or shortly thereafter, depending on the region of the body), at which time remnants of periderm are sloughed from the surface of the skin.

By term, the cornified layer has come to function as a semipermeable barrier.

HAIR

Development of hair follicles begins on the head during the ***first trimester*** and proceeds caudally, not being detectable on the trunk until the fourth month. These dramatic series of changes culminates by approximately the ***28th week of gestation*** in the formation of an entire *infundibuloapocrine-sebaceous-follicular unit*. The infundibulum, a funnel-shaped epithelial structure that is continuous above with surface epidermis and below with the isthmus of the hair follicle, actually is not a part of the folliculosebaceous unit.

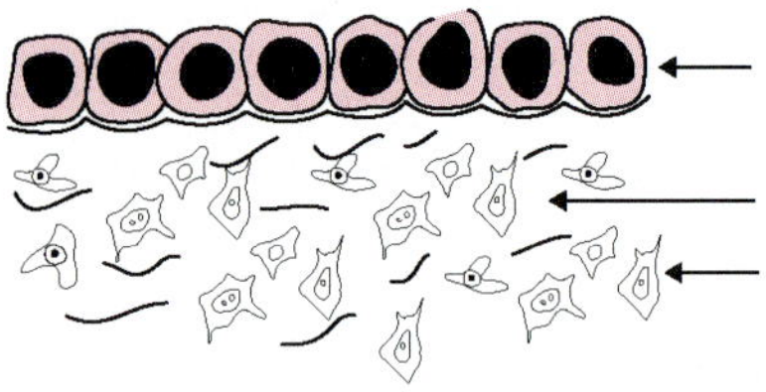

Fig. 1.2

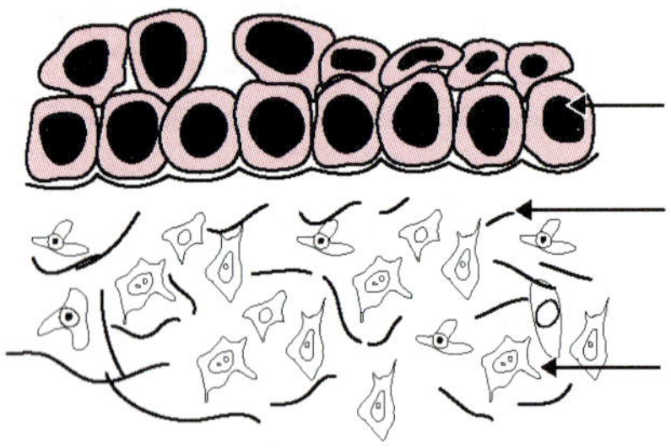

Fig. 1.3

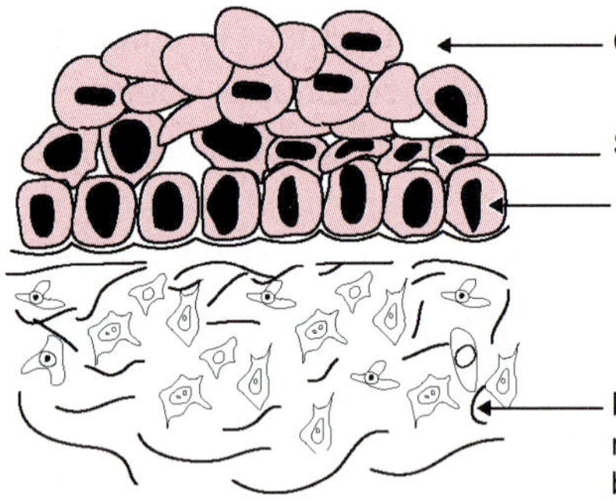

Fig. 1.4: Embryology of epidermis

CONSTITUENTS OF COMPONENT OF SKIN

Epidermis

Keratinocytes are cells that synthesize keratins. They represent the site for synthesis of a class of soluble molecules, namely, cytokines that are important in the regulation of contiguous epithelial cells of the epidermis, as well as of cells in the dermis. Epidermal keratinocytes undergo characteristic alterations during a short trip of about two weeks in which they are transformed from undifferentiated basal cells to fully differentiated cornified cells. Four continuous cellular "layers", namely, basal, spinous, granular and cornified layers are part of successive stages of maturation of germinative keratinocytes to fully cornified ones (Fig. 1.5).

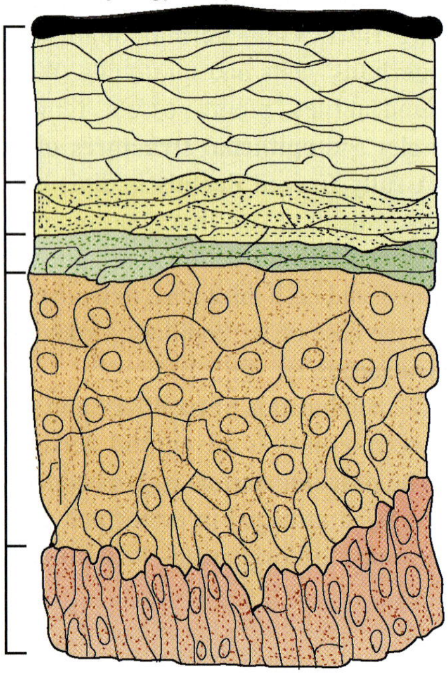

Fig. 1.5: Layers of epidermis

The **process of cornification involves** (1) synthesis of *lamellar granules* and distinctive *proteins*, e.g., differentiation-specific keratins, filaggrin, loricrin, involucrin, and desmosomal proteins that are cross-linked by transglutaminases, and (2) changes progressively of nuclei, cytoplasmic organelles, plasma membranes, and desmosomes.

Basal Layer

The **basal row** of keratinocytes consists of cuboidal or low columnar cells that contains larger oval nuclei and more basophilic cytoplasm than the more mature keratinocytes above them.

- This deepest layer of the epidermis is made up of a single layer of columnar cells which have a basophilic cytoplasm and an oval nucleus.
- These cells are firmly attached to the *lamina densa* of the basement membrane with the help of *hemidesmosomes.*
- The distribution of keratins (K) in the various layers of epidermis is as follows:
  Basal cell layer—K5/K14
  Spinous—K1/K10, K5/K14
  Granular—K2/K11
- The basal cells contain melanin – the amount of melanin present in the basal cells is reflected as the skin colour.
- In the light skinned the melanin granules, *melanosomes* are barely visible while in the dark skinned there are innumerable distinct granules predominantly forming supra nuclear caps.

Spinous or Prickle Layer

- This layer, which lies above the basal layer, is made up of polygonal cells forming a mosaic of 5-10 layers; they are attached to each other by interlocking cytoplasmic processes, numerous *desmosomes* (attachment plaques) and the *intercellular cement* (of glycoproteins).
- It is the presence of desmosomes which gives the cells of this layer an appearance of prickles (under the light microscope).
- Under the electron – microscope, these cells are filled with *tonofilaments*.
- The cells of the upper part of this layer are filled with *odland* or *lamellar bodies.*

Granular Layer

- The granular layer is made up of 1-3 layers.
- The cytoplasm of granular cells is filled with *tonofilaments* and basophilic *keratohyaline* granules – these two structures gradually merge during keratinisation.
- The lysosomal enzymes of the granular cells destroy the cell nuclei and intracytoplasmic organelles, as the granular layer cells become horny cells.

The spinous zone merges with horizontally oriented diamond-shaped cells filled with coarse, basophilic keratohyaline granules, i.e., cells of the granular zone. Keratohyaline granules are made up of profilaggrin, an electron-dense protein, loricrin, and keratin intermediate filaments.

Near the top of the spinous zone, **lamellar granules** (also referred to as Odland bodies) appear near the Golgi apparatus, navigate the cytoplasm, and fuse with the plasma membrane, where their contents are discharged from keratinocytes into intercellular spaces. These granules contain free sterols, polar lipids, e.g., phospholipids and glucosylceramides (the precursors of ceramides), and several hydrolytic enzymes, e.g., lipases, glycosidases, and acid phosphatase. After contents of lamellar granules are released into intercellular spaces, they are restructured into lamellae that provide the basic structure for an effective epidermal barrier to permeability.

Desmosomes (Fig. 1.6)

Desmosomes consist of a number of proteins, among them being desmoglein 1 and 3, desmoplakin, plakoglobin and desmosomal cadherins. When the function of desmosomes is impaired, keratinocytes tend to become detached from one another and, in the process, assume a *round shape*.

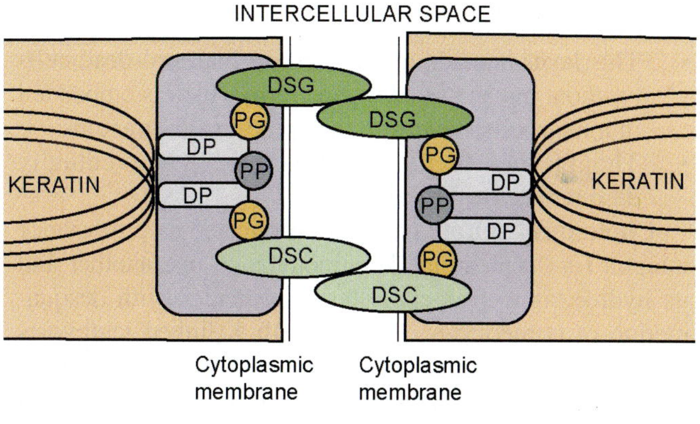

Fig. 1.6: Desmosome

DP=Desmoplakin
PG=Plakoglobin
PP=Periplakin
DSG= Desmoglein
DSC=Desmocollin

The phenomenon occurs in conditions as disparate as **pemphigus vulgaris** (autoantibodies against desmoglein 3), **pemphigus foliaceus** (autoantibodies against desmoglein 1), and **staphylococcal scalded skin syndrome** in which exfoliatins produced by the Gram-positive cocci compromise desmosomes severely.

The assembly of desmosomes is dependent on calcium and phosphorylation, calcium acting as a major signal for keratinocyte maturation, desmosome formation and for enzyme activation like transglutaminase. Both extracellular calcium and 1,25 dihydroxyvitamin D are necessary for enabling keratinocytes to mature. Within hours of the "calcium switch" having been turned on, keratinocytes shift from making basal keratins, namely, Keratin 5 and Keratin 14, and begin producing Keratin 1 and Keratin 10, followed soon thereafter by an increase in levels of profilaggrin, involucrin and loricrin. Molecular defects in transportation of calcium are thought to be responsible for skin diseases in which the structural integrity of keratinocytes is impaired, as is the case in conditions characterized by acantholysis, e.g., **Hailey-Hailey disease and Darier's disease.**

The Stratum Lucidum

It is a thin, clear layer of dead skin cells in the epidermis, and is named for its translucent appearance. It contains a clear substance called eludin, which eventually becomes keratin.

This layer is only found on the *soles and palms*.

The cells of the stratum lucidum are flattened and contain an oily substance that is thought to be the result of lysosome disintegration. It is this substance that gives the stratum lucidum its waterproof properties and thus, it is also called the *barrier* layer of the skin.

Stratum Corneum

- This layer is made up of piled up flattened dead cells (without nuclei) filled with keratin which is embedded in a matrix derived from the keratohyalin granules.
- Though these cells stick together, they eventually desquamate at the surface.

Cholesterol sulfate has been implicated as a substance integral for "cementing" keratinocytes to one another and its hydrolysis to free cholesterol, coincides with desquamation of corneocytes. Patients with X-linked ichthyosis lack steroid sulfatase, **the absence of which prevents, shedding of corneocytes,** resulting in hyperkeratosis that is reflected clinically as plate-like scales.

CELL KINETICS

Epidermal Cell Proliferation

There remains a balance in the number of cells produced and shed by the epidermis.

***Cell cycle*:** The basal cell passes through a definite cycle as it multiplies. A newly formed cell is in the G_1 phase of the cycle. It synthesizes proteins, RNA and attains a definite size. It is then triggered to enter the *S Phase* or the phase of DNA synthesis. The cell next enters the G_2 or *post-synthetic phase* and finally divides in the *M phase.* One of the daughter cells moves up to become a keratinocyte, while the other enters the G_1 *phase* (sometimes the G_0 or *resting stage*). Various factors control the epidermal cell proliferation (*epidermopoiesis*). Cytokines, growth factors and hormones influence the rate of epidermopoiesis.

- Normal *cell cycle time 311 hours (60-450 hours).*
- Time required for basal cell to reach stratum corneum—*53 days.*
- Time required for cell to be shed off from stratum corneum—*14 days.*
- Total cell proliferation time–52-75 days.*

HAIR FOLLICLES

During its lifetime, a particular follicle may generate all three types of hair. A follicle on the scalp may produce a **lanugo hair** initially, a **terminal hair** later, and a **vellus hair** in baldness.

Parts of a Hair

A hair follicle is continuous with an infundibulum, the funnel-shaped component of epidermis that reaches from the ostium at the surface of the skin above to the uppermost part of the follicle, i.e., the isthmus, below. In a longitudinal section, a mature follicle may be divided histologically (Fig. 1.7) into (1) an upper segment constituted of a single part, i.e., the ***isthmus*** that extends from the base of the infundibulum above to the place where corneocytes of the inner root sheath desquamates below, and (2) a ***lower***

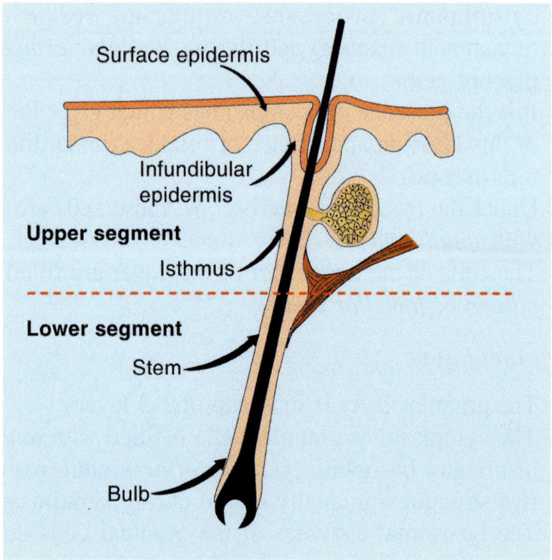

Fig. 1.7: Structure of pilosebaceous unit

* Rook's Textbook of Dermatology.

segment that consists of two parts, i.e., the **stem**, which stretches from the base of the isthmus to the end of the keratogenous zone at Adamson's fringe, and the **bulb**, which is the part of a follicle that resides below Adamson's fringe. (**Adamson's fringe** is the boundary between nucleated cells of a hair in the bulb of a follicle and anucleate cells of a hair in the stem of a follicle).

Histology of Hair

From outside in (Fig. 1.8), the follicle at the bulb consists of:

1. *Pale* and *clear cells* of the **outer root sheath**,
2. *Trichohyalin-containing cells* of the **inner root sheath**, and
3. *Nucleated corneocytes* of the future hair.

It is at the "Adamson's fringe" where cornification of viable keratinocytes is recognizable first.

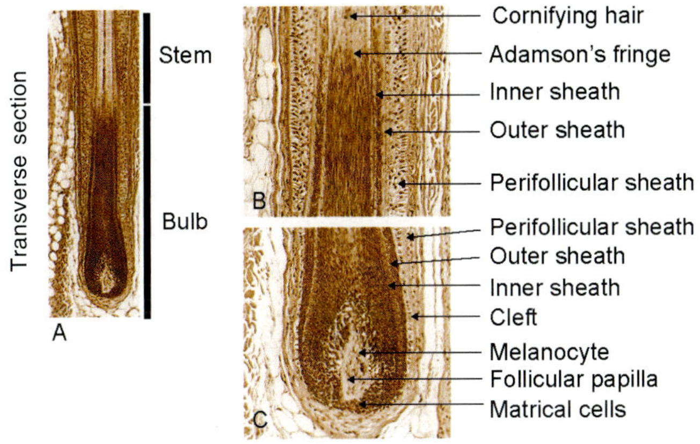

Fig. 1.8: Histological structure of hair

Growth of Hair

The growth of hair is cyclical (Fig.1.9). The three phases of the cycle are:

1. Growing (anagen).
2. Involuting (catagen), and
3. Resting (telogen).

The follicle beneath the isthmus, i.e., the bulb and the stem, is transitory, as it disappears during the involutional phase (catagen) of the follicular cycle and re-forms during the growth phase (anagen). In contrast, the part of the follicle that is stationary, i.e., the isthmus, is not involved in the follicular cycle. If a follicle can be divided histologically into an **isthmus (upper segment)**, stem and bulb *(lower segment)*, it can also be conceived of functionally, as

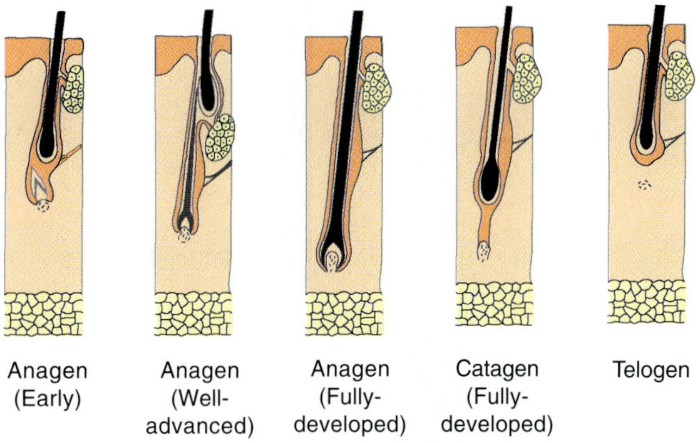

Fig. 1.9: Phases of hair cycle

consisting of an upper fixed isthmus and a lower mobile stem and bulb. The isthmus, which histologically is an integral component of the outer root sheath, does not join the rest of the outer root sheath during the follicular cycle in a to-and-fro migration along a fibrous track, but is a mere bystander of movements that take place below it.

The **"bulge-activation hypothesis"** states that the bulge of a follicle, which serves as a site for attachment of a muscle of hair erection, also serves as a reservoir for stem cells that, at the outset of anagen, gives rise to a new inferior segment of a follicle.

Unlike certain animals whose coat of hair is shed in synchronous waves, hairs in human *are normally lost randomly and inconspicuously* because adjacent follicles are in different phases of the follicular cycle, most of them being in anagen. An intriguing feature of the follicular cycle is differences in interval of time among the growing, involuting and the resting phases.

Scalp hair, for example, grow for about 3 to 10 years, involute over a period of approximately 3 to 4 weeks, and rest for nearly 3 to 4 months. In healthy young adults, at least **85%** of all follicles on a scalp, at any point of time, are in **anagen.** Of the approximately 100,000 follicles present on an average on the scalp, at least *70 to 100 telogen hair are shed normally each day*. As a rule, the growing phase of follicles (and, therefore, of hair) on the eyebrows, trunk, and extremities does not exceed 6 months, and the duration of the resting phase is roughly half that period of time. When hair are extracted with force manually, the root of an anagen hair is noted to be deeply pigmented, whereas the bulbous tip of a telogen hair is unpigmented (Fig. 1.10).

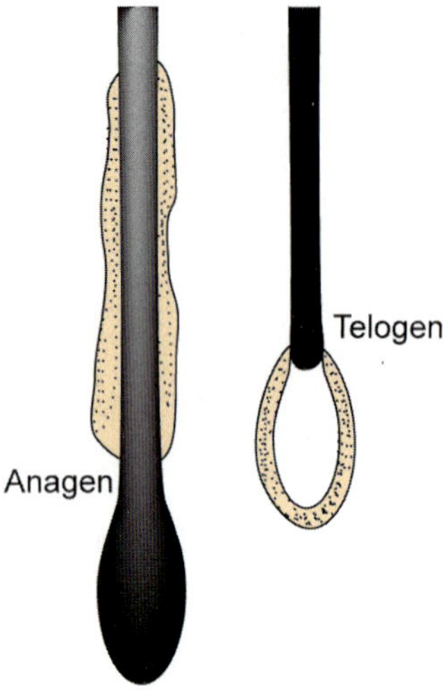

Fig. 1.10: Types of hair

The clubbed appearance of such a hair is the result of thickening at the base consequent to adherence of the inner sheath to the hair itself.

GLANDS

Sebaceous Units

Sebaceous gland, a lipid-producing epithelial structure, develops in the **fourth month** of fetal life from a protuberance of epithelium that lies between the uppermost protrusion, which represents the future apocrine unit, and the lower bulge, which represents the site for future attachment of muscles of hair erection. *With the exception of the palms, soles, and dorsa of the feet,* sebaceous glands of various sizes are distributed over the entire skin surface. They are most populous and most productive on the scalp and face, and are largest on the forehead, nose and upper part of the back.

Nearly all sebaceous glands are connected by a duct to the infundibular epidermis, the entry of the duct being at the junction of infundibulum and isthmus (Fig. 1.11).

Modified Glands

At certain sites, *sebaceous glands are joined to infundibula in the absence of follicles; no isthmus, stem, or bulb is present* e.g. in the buccal mucosa and vermilion of the lip **(Fordyce's spots),** areolae of women **(Montgomery's tubercles),** labia minora and glans **(Tyson's glands),** eyelids **(Meibomian glands).**

When the widely dilated ostia of the infundibula affiliated with sebaceous follicles are plugged by the corneocytes, the result is comedones, important lesions of **acne vulgaris.**

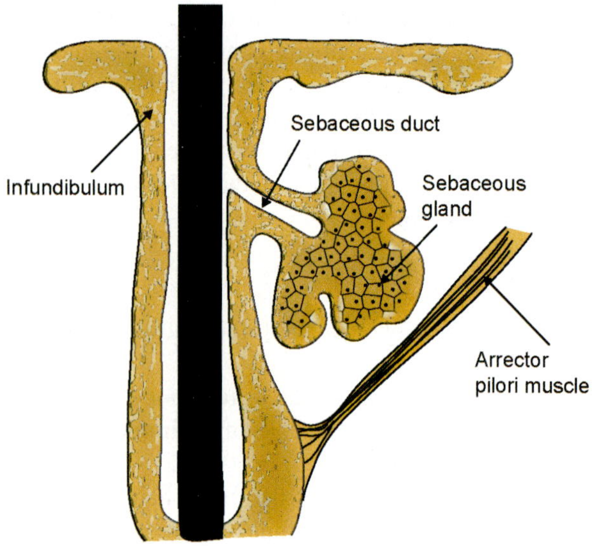

Fig. 1.11: Pilosebaceous unit

APOCRINE UNITS

Apocrine units in humans are found in the axillae, areolae, periumbilical region, perineal and circumanal areas, prepuce, scrotum, mons pubis, labia minora, and *external auditory canals (ceruminous glands), and on the eyelids (Moll's glands).*

Parts of the Gland

An apocrine unit consists of:

1. A coiled secretory portion, i.e., the gland itself, situated in the lower part of the reticular dermis or in the subcutaneous fat.
2. A straight duct that empties into an infundibulum at a level above the entrance of a sebaceous duct.
3. A duct that spirals through infundibular epidermis, i.e., the apocrine acrosyringium (Fig. 1.12).

Histology

In cross section, the diameter of an apocrine gland is about 10 times greater than that of an eccrine gland.

The lumen of an apocrine gland is lined by a *single row of columnar cells* with abundant eosinophilic cytoplasm and a round nucleus situated near the base.

The convex apical border of the secretory cells projects to variable extent into the lumen, depending on the particular stage in the secretory cycle. The apical portion of glandular cells shows changes specific for apocrine secretion, namely, the appearance of being decapitated or pinched off

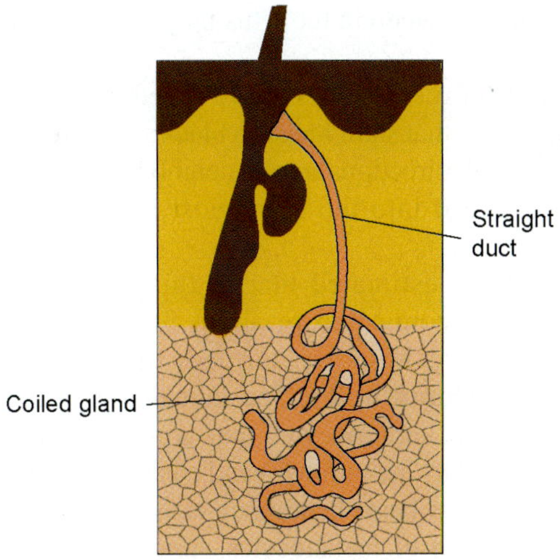

Fig. 1.12: Apocrine gland

(Fig. 1.12). "*Decapitation secretion*", "pinching-off secretion", and "apocrine secretion" are synonyms.

Surrounding the secretory cells are (1) a layer of contractile *myoepithelial cells;* (2) a *basement membrane*; and (3) *collagen bundles* and elastic fibers of the periadnexal dermis.

Disorders

Apocrine units do not play an important role in inflammatory diseases of the skin. Even **Fox-Fordyce disease,** referred to often as "apocrine miliaria", is not analogous to true eccrine miliaria (rubra); it seems to result from a plug of corneocytes in contiguous infundibula that reside in "apocrine regions", i.e., axillae and pubis, and, therefore, is really an abnormality of epidermis rather than a malady of apocrine units *per se*.

Hidradenitis suppurativa also is a misnomer; it is a suppurative infundibulitis that affects apocrine units only secondarily.

ECCRINE UNITS

The eccrine gland is the *only true sweat gland* in humans. Eccrine sweat is a hypotonic solution that flows from the gland to the surface of the skin where it cools the body by evaporation. Approximately *3 million* eccrine sweat units are present at birth, and no additional ones are formed thereafter.

Parts of the Gland

The eccrine unit can be divided into: (Fig. 1.13)

1. A **coiled secretory gland** proximally.
2. A **coiled dermal duct** that leads from the secretory gland.
3. A **straight duct** that passes through the length of the dermis, and

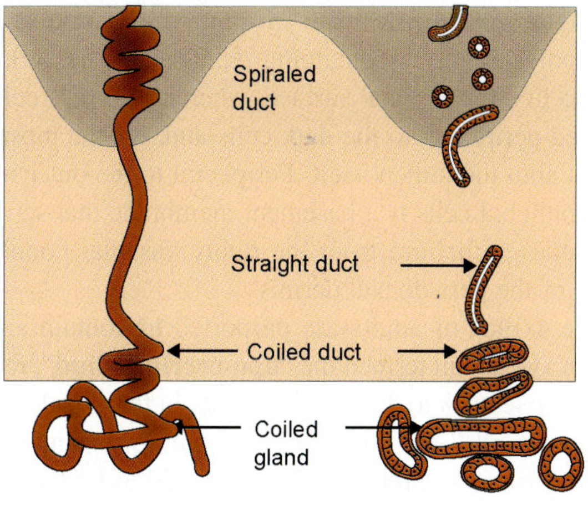

Fig. 1.13: Eccrine gland

4. **A spiralled intraepidermal** duct known also as acrosyringium.

Histology

The coiled gland is formed of two rows of cells (Fig. 1.14), namely:

1. A discontinuous outer row of spindle-shaped, contractile **myoepithelial cells,** and
2. An inner row of **pyramidal, secretory** epithelial cells.

The single inner row of **secretory cells** that lines the lumen of a gland consists of two types (Fig. 1.15), large

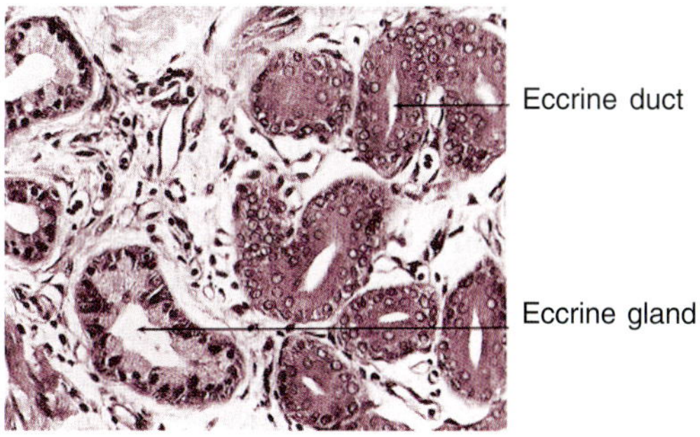

Fig. 1.14: Histology of eccrine gland

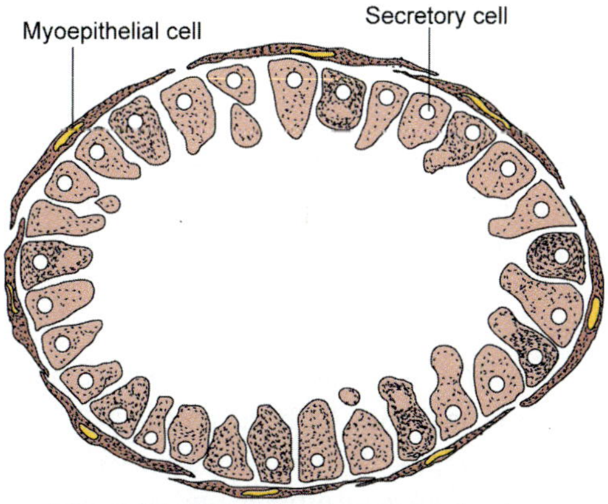

Fig. 1.15: Histology of eccrine gland

glycogen-containing *pale or clear cells* and smaller mucopolysaccharide-containing *dark cells*. The dark cells tend to line the luminal surface, whereas the pale cells are situated peripheral to the dark cells and, for the most part, do not abut the lumen itself. Peripheral to the outer row of myoepithelial cells is a basement membrane that separates glandular epithelium from the richly vascular connective tissue of the periadnexal dermis.

The axillae of adults are purported to contain another type of sweat unit termed the **"apo-eccrine gland**", reputed to comprise 10% to 45% of all glands in that locale. "Apo-eccrine glands" are supposed to develop during puberty from eccrine-like precursors and are said to be larger than typical eccrine glands, but smaller than typical apocrine glands. The epithelial lining of the dilated glandular segment of an "apo-eccrine gland" is said to resemble an apocrine gland, whereas the epithelial lining of the undilated segment resembles an eccrine gland.

Disorders of Eccrine Glands

Eccrine glands on the palms, soles, axillae and forehead unlike those on the rest of the body, respond predominantly to *emotional rather than thermal* stimuli. This produces a pattern of sweating visible easily in individuals who are experiencing pain, anger or fear.

Hyperhidrosis itself may be a source of considerable anxiety in social circumstances. Another deleterious effect of sweating occurs when allergic contact sensitizers are leached from jewellery or clothing by salts present in sweat. This enhances induction of allergic contact dermatitis in susceptible persons.

Miliaria rubra, known colloquially as "heat rash" and "prickly heat", is a spongiotic inflammatory process thought to be centered in acrosyringia and related somehow to obstruction in flow of sweat through intraepidermal ducts.

SPECIAL CELLS

Melanocytes

Melanocytes synthesize melanin. From the precursors in the neural crest, melanocytes migrate normally to the epidermis, the bulb of hair follicles, epithelia of various mucous membranes, leptomeninges, inner ear, and a few other tissues. Primitive melanocytes first appear in the skin during the *eighth week* of fetal life, but at that time they produce little melanin. Only in postnatal life do normal melanocytes begin to function fully, except in certain cutaneous loci, such as nipples and genitalia, and in the bulb of follicles, wherein the fetus they synthesize melanin in abundance.

Dendrites of melanocytes are revealed more effectively with silver salts that stain melanin black; they are then seen to arborize in all directions among neighboring keratinocytes and even extend into the uppermost part of the dermis (Fig. 1.16).

It has been estimated that in this manner a single melanocyte is connected to about 36 keratinocytes, a relationship that has been termed, **imprecisely, "the epidermal melanin unit"**. The unit really consists of a melanocyte and keratinocytes that are supplied by it. In sections stained by hematoxylin and eosin, the average ratio of melanocytes to basal keratinocytes is about 1 to 10, but the concentration of melanocytes varies according to the region of the body, being more numerous in the skin of the face (up to 2,900 melanocytes per mm^2) than on the trunk (up to 1,250 melanocytes per mm^2).

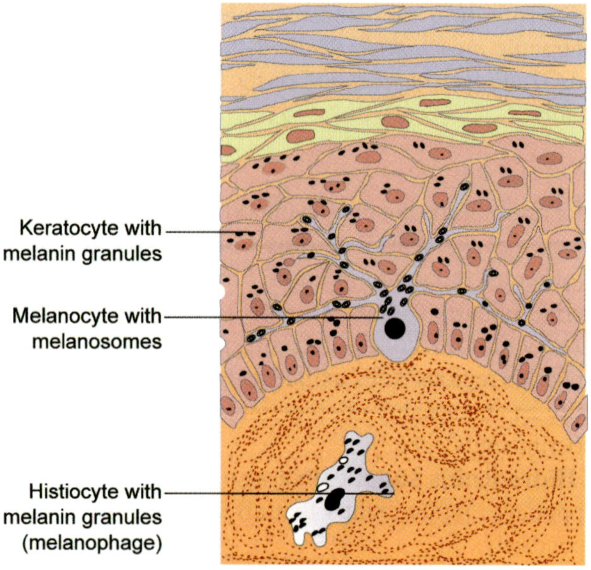

Fig. 1.16: Distribution of melanocyte

LANGERHANS' CELLS

Langerhans' cells, named after Paul Langerhans who, while a medical student in Berlin in 1868, was the first to describe them, are dendritic cells that reside just above the middle of the spinous zone of the epidermis. They make their appearance there by the *14th week* of fetal life.

The most reliable means for identification of Langerhans' cells is electron microscopy, which reveals within the cytoplasm the characteristic granules that display a hemispherical bleb at one end of a linear platelike structure. The appearance in vertical section of these granules has been likened to that of a tennis racquet. Cells identical in all respects to Langerhans' cells, except for lack of **Birbeck's granules**, have been termed indeterminate cells. A calcium-dependent lectin with specificity for binding mannose, namely langerin, is thought to induce formation of Birbeck's granules.

MERKEL CELLS

Merkel cells migrate from neural crest. Most numerous on digital pads, lips, oral cavity, and hair follicles, they are involved in sensation. They act as mechanoreceptors and contain neurotransmitter materials.

DERMOEPITHELIAL INTERFACE

The basement membrane was defined first by conventional microscopy as a thin band situated immediately beneath basal keratinocytes, a strip that was stained magenta by the Periodic Acid-Schiff method (Fig. 1.17). In time, with the aid of electron microscopy, it came to be recognized as a specialized structure that formed at the junction of epithelial cells and connective tissue adjacent to them.

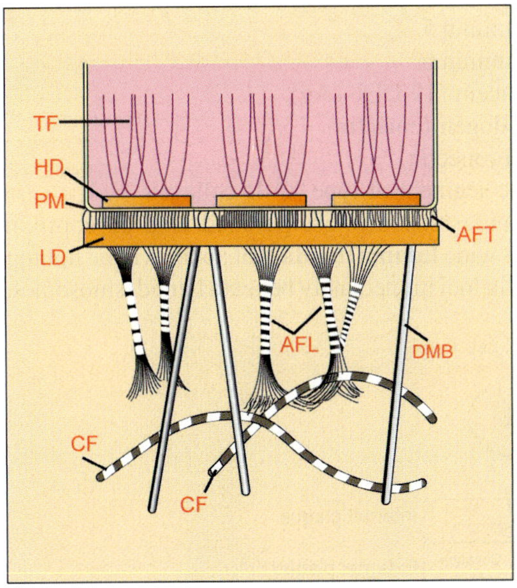

Fig. 1.17: Dermoepithelial interface

TF= Tonofilament
HD= Hemidesmosome
PM= Plasma Membrane
LD=Lamina Densa
AFT= Anchoring Filaments
AFL= Anchoring Fibrils
CF=Collagen

The junction between epidermis and dermis nears maturity by the *12th week* of gestation. Based on findings by examination ultrastructurally, the dermoepidermal interface has been divided, by convention, into four zones:

1. The cytoskeleton, that is, **hemidesmosomes and plasma membrane** of *basal keratinocytes* that constitute the upper boundary of the interface.
2. The **lamina lucida,** an electron-lucent region that lies beneath basal keratinocytes.
3. The **lamina densa,** an electron-dense plate situated below the lamina lucida and above the papillary dermis; and
4. The **sub-lamina densa** seated immediately below the lamina densa and consisting of the uppermost portion of the papillary dermis.

The plasma membrane of basal keratinocytes forms the roof of the structurally integrated unit known as **the dermoepidermal junction**.

1. Hemidesmosomes (Fig. 1.18)

- **Plaque proteins** involved in IF anchorage—BPAG1, Plectin.
- **Transmembrane proteins** mediating cell matrix adhesion—BPAG2, $\alpha6\beta4$ integrin.
- Additional proteins – IFAP300, p200.

Hemidesmosomes, stationed at intervals along the plasma membrane, are formed of both intracellular and extracellular components. On the cytoplasmic side of the plasma membrane, a hemidesmosome consists of an electron-dense *attachment plaque*. **Tonofilaments** of keratin housed within the cytoplasm of basal cells converge on the *attachment plaque.*

Proteins in hemidesmosomes are plectin, **bullous pemphigoid antigen 1 (BPAg1), bullous pemphigoid antigen 2 (BPAg2)**, integrin subunit $\alpha6$, and integrin subunit $\beta4$. Destruction of hemidesmosomes leads inevitably to development of a subepidermal blister as occurs, for example, in **bullous pemphigoid**. Patients with bullous pemphigoid synthesize antibodies to two of the antigens in a hemidesmosome. Bullous pemphigoid antigen 2, a 180-KDa/Type XVII collagen, is targeted by autoantibodies in patients with bullous pemphigoid and herpes gestationis, as well as in some with linear IgA bullous dermatosis, and cicatricial pemphigoid.

Plectin, a 500-KDa protein and a constituent of the intracellular component of hemidesmosomes, attaches intermediate filaments to both hemidesmosomes and plasma

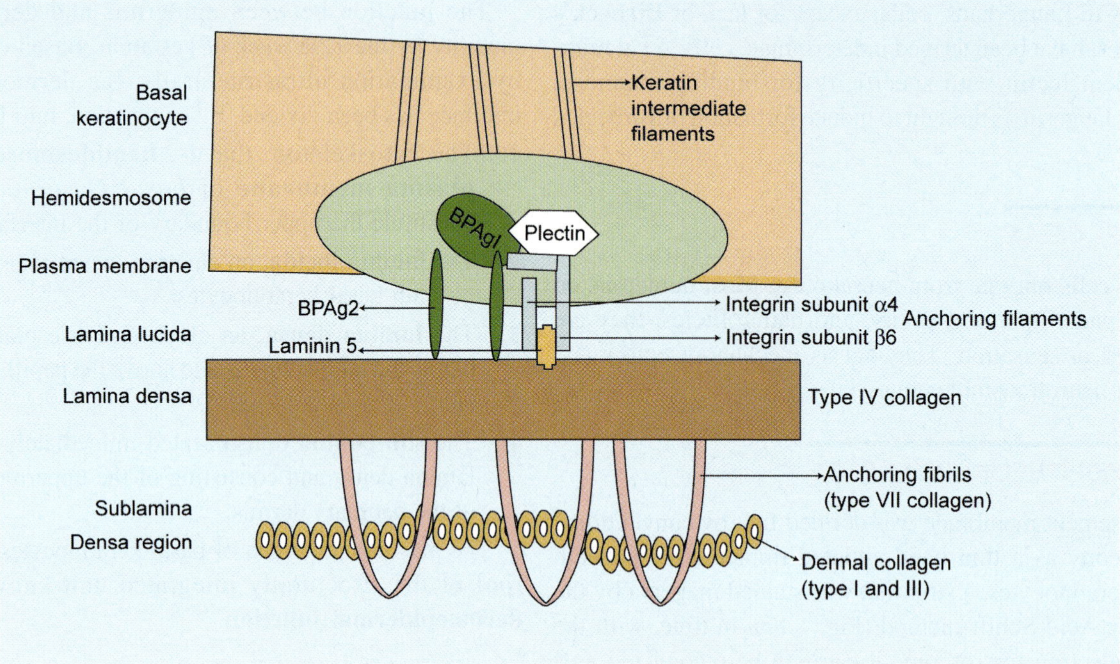

Fig. 1.18: Detailed constituents of hemidesmosome

membranes of basal keratinocytes. Mutations in the gene that encodes plectin are responsible for **epidermolysis bullosa simplex.**

2. Lamina Lucida—Site for Salt Split Technique (Fig. 1.19)

- Weakest link in the DEJ and separates easily.
- Distributed throughout lamina lucida are ANCHORING FILAMENTS.

Constituents

- Laminin 5.
- Laminin 6.
- Uncein (19 DEJ-1Ag).
- Nidogen (entactin).
- Fibronectin.
- E/c segment of type XVII collagen.

Hemidesmosomes are perched atop an approximately 50-nm–wide **lamina lucida** that appears to be homogenous, except in loci immediately beneath hemidesmosomes. These

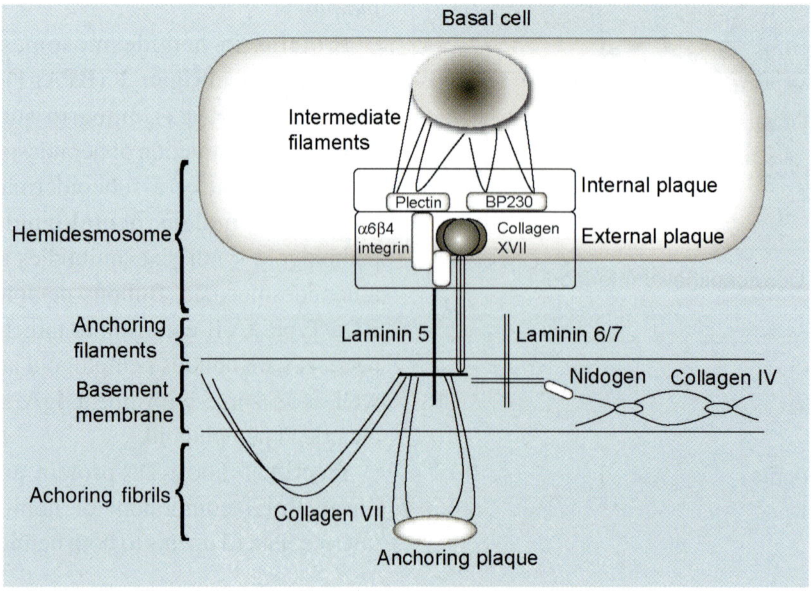

Fig. 1.19: Structure of lamina lucida

thin filaments, called **anchoring filaments**, extend from the basal plasma membrane across the lamina lucida through the sub-basal dense plaque and end on the **lamina densa**.

Laminins are a family of at least 14 heterotrimeric glycoproteins. They are most abundant of the structural noncollagenous glycoproteins in the basement membrane. Laminins 5, 6 and 10 are present in the epidermal basement membrane. Laminin 5 plays an essential part in adhesion of the epidermis to the dermis, being localized to the interface of the lamina lucida and the lamina densa where it is thought to form a critical link between hemidesmososme anchoring filament complexes, lamina densa and anchoring fibrils. Inherited or targeted disruptions in gene-encoding **laminin 5 units (LAMA3, LAMC2)** result in a phenotype characterized by formation of a subepidermal blister, detachment of the epidermis, and, ultimately, death, and occur, for example, in **junctional epidermolysis bullosa of the Herlitz type**.

3. Lamina Densa (Figs. 1.17 and 1.18)

- Lies just beneath lamina lucida and rests on underlying dermal connective tissue.
- **Type IV collagen** is the primary component of lamina densa.
  (It is a non-banded network forming collagen synthesized by keratinocytes that provides support and flexibility to this layer).
  The antigenic components are:
- Laminin 1.
- Nidogen.
- Perlecan.
- Heparan sulfate.
- Chondroitin sulfate.

Type IV collagen is the major constituent of the lamina densa, a structure that appears magenta when exposed to the Periodic Acid-Schiff stain. Other components of the lamina densa are laminin 5, 6 and 10, heparin sulfate proteoglycan and nidogen (entactin). **Anchoring fibrils** emanate from the lamina densa and assume a crosshatched configuration.Genetic defects in some patients with recessive and *dominant dystrophic kinds of epidermolysis bullosa* are responsible for an abnormality in Type VII collagen and immunologic damage to Type VII collagen is the cause of acquired *epidermolysis bullosa and bullous lupus erythematosus.*

4. Lamina Fibroreticularis

- The major constituent of this layer are ANCHORING FIBRILS which are composed of Type VII collagen.
- These are curved structures with an irregularly spaced central cross banding that insert into LAMINA DENSA and extend into upper part of dermis.
- They may also insert into amorphous bodies in superficial dermis known as ANCHORING PLAQUES, or more typically curve back to have a second insertion in LAMINA DENSA.
- They vary widely in individuals and vary in density in different regions of body.
- The antigenic components of lamina fibroreticularis are:
  - EBA Ag (in Type VII collagen).
  - 285 kDa protein (some cases of LINEAR IgA BULLOUS DERMATOSIS).

Table 1.1: Basement membrane antigens

Constituents	*Location*	*Genodermatosis*	*Autoimmune bullous disease*
Keratins 5 and 14	Basal keratinocyte	EB simplex	None
$\alpha_6\beta_4$ integrin	DEJ	JEB-pyloric atresia	None
BP180	DEJ	GABEB	BP, CP, HG, LPP
Plectin	Hemidesmosome	EBS-MD	BP
BP230	Hemidesmosome		BP
Laminin 5	Lamina lucida	Junctional EB	CP
Type VII collagen	Sublamina densa	Dystrophic EB	EBA, BSLE, LAD

BP—Bullous Pemphigoid
CP—Cicatrical Pemphigoid
HG—Herpes Gestationis
LPP—Lichen Planus Pemphigoides
EBA—Epidermolysis Bullosa Acquisita
BSLE—Bullous SLE
LAD—Linear IgA Dermatosis

Table 1.2: Autoimmune bullous diseases—Target antigens

Disease	*Target Ag (M wt in kDa)*	*Site of Ag*
P.foliaceous	Desmoglein 1 (160)	Desmosomes of upper epidermis
IgA Pemphigus	Desmocollin 1	Desmosomes (transmembrane)
P.vulgaris	Desmoglein 3 (130)	Desmosomes of lower epidermis
EBA	Type VII collagen (290)	Anchoring fibrils
Paraneoplastic pemphigus	Desmoplakin 1 (250)	Cytoplasmic plaques
Bullous pemphigoid	BPAg1(230) BPAg2 (180)	Hemidesmosome transmembrane protein
Pemphigoid gestationis	BPAg2 (180)	
DH	Transglutaminase 2	Unknown structure most likely keratin
Linear IgA disease	LAD –1 ladinin (97) 285 kDa	Anchoring filament Sublamina densa
Ocular CP	Not named	Conjunctiva
Cicatricial pemphigoid	BPAg2 (180) Epiligrin	Against 3 subunit of laminin 5
—	—	—

NERVES AND RECEPTORS OF THE SKIN (Fig. 1.20)

The innervation of the skin recapitulates the blood flow: large, myelinated, cutaneous branches of the musculocutaneous nerves branch in the subcutaneous tissue to form a deep nerve plexus in the reticular dermis. Nerve fibers from the deep plexus ascend to form a superficial subpapillary plexus. Nerves from these plexuses innervate the skin as free nerve endings which function as important sensory receptors. They transmit touch, pain, temperature, itch, and mechanical stimuli. These exist in the papillary dermis as individual fibers surrounded by Schwann cells.

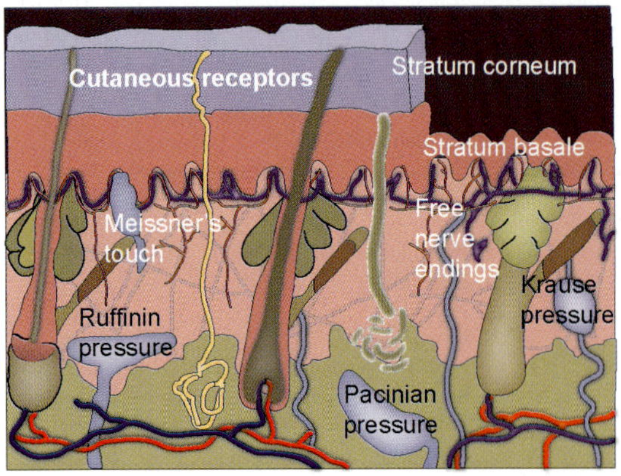

Fig. 1.20: Arrangement of cutaneous receptors

SKIN IS RICHLY SUPPLIED BY BOTH SENSORY AND AUTONOMIC NERVES (Fig. 1.20)

Types of sensory receptors:

i. **Free nerve endings:** Nerve terminal loses its myelin sheath at the epidermal/dermal junction and pass into the epidermis, ending in the stratum granulosum. They sense *pain and temperature*.
ii. **Hair follicle receptors:** Axon loses myelin sheath and the bare axon coils around the shaft within the external root sheath; senses air motion and its direction.
iii. **Merkel cell endings:** Axon loses its myelin and forms a disc like structure with the Merkel cell at the base of the epidermis (stratum basale); **senses edges, corners and curvature (pins and needles), slowly-adapting type response** (readily de-activated).
iv. **Meissner's corpuscle:** Encapsulated nerve ending in the dermal papilla; sense dynamic deformation of skin with high sensitivity but poor special resolution, **rapidly adapting type response (readily de-activate), sense slip of surface over skin (tools)**.
v. **Krause's end bulb:** Axon loses myelin and passes into a capsule then branches within it, found in the papillary layer of the dermis of skin and in the epidermis of oral mucosa and tongue, **senses tension (force), slowly-adapting response**.
vi. **Pacinian corpuscle:** Axon loses myelin and passes into a capsule and a single process continues into the core of the corpuscle, corpuscle is multilayered with a thin sheet of cells separated by a gelatinous material, found deep in the dermis and in the hypodermis, senses high frequency, **low amplitude displacements (10 nm displacement at 200 Hz, vibrations) with poor spatial resolution (tools again), rapidly adapting response.**
vii. **Ruffini endings:** Axon loses myelin and penetrates an oblong, thinly capsulated structure and branches profusely within it, found in the deep dermis and in the hypodermis especially in the **plantar glabrous skin,** corpuscle is oriented with the long axis of collagen fibers and is attached to them, sense displacement/tension in collagen fibers in the dermis/hypodermis, **slowly adapting type response.**

VASCULATURE OF THE SKIN

- The dermal vasculature is composed of a superficial and deep plexus of arterioles and venules that are interconnected by communicating vessels.
- The incoming blood flow to the superficial capillary plexus in the upper dermis can be decreased by increased smooth muscle tone in the ascending arterioles, or it can be shunted directly from the arterioles to the venous channels in the deeper plexus systems via glomus bodies, which are modified arterioles surrounded by multiple layers of muscle cells.
- During cold temperatures, decreased papillary blood flow to the papillary dermis, in essence, shunts the blood away from the skin surface and decreases heat loss from the body.
- Body temperature is regulated, in part, through control of dermal blood flow. Lowering body temperature is accomplished through increased blood flow in the vascular plexus in the high papillary dermis, allowing heat to be removed through radiation from the skin.

THE SUBCUTANEOUS LAYER

- The subcutis, or subcutaneous fat, is arranged into distinct fat lobules which are divided by fibrous septae composed primarily of collagen.
- Blood vessels, nerves and lymphatics are also found in the fibrous septae.
- In addition to its role as a caloric reserve, the subcutaneous fat serves as a heat insulator and shock absorber.

FUNCTIONS OF SKIN

- Barrier functions.
- Physical barrier and percutaneous absorption—in epidermis—mainly in stratum corneum.

- Chemical—antimicrobial peptides (AMP's).
- Barrier against UVR.
- Temperature regulation.
- Mechanical function—mainly dermis.
- Immunological barrier.
- Sensory and autonomic function.
- Melanogenesis and role of melanocytes.
- Glands of skin.
- Role of subcutaneous fat layer.

STRUCTURE OF SKIN BARRIER

Brick and Mortar (Fig. 1.21)

- Corneocyte – brick.
- Envelope of corneocyte – linker.
- Extracellular matrix – mortar.
- Drawback – barrier is not a static structure.

The "Bricks and Mortar of the Stratum Corneum"

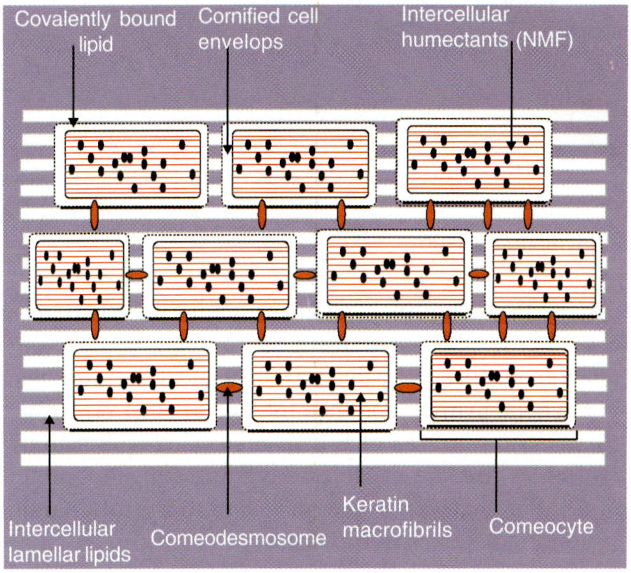

Fig. 1.21: Brick and mortar model

Constituents of Skin Barrier

- Cornified envelope – each corneocyte is 1 micron thick with 10 nm thick tough protein envelope. It is made of structural proteins – INVOLUCRINS and LORICRINS which are cross-linked by sulfhydryl oxidases and transglutaminases. Internally, the envelope is linked to bundles of keratin filaments inside the cell.
- Lipid envelope – on external surface of cornified envelope, a covalently bound layer of very long chain doxyceramides which are ester linked to the involucrin amino acids.
- Lipid envelope is formed by lipids secreted by lamellar body.

IMMUNOLOGICAL BARRIER (Fig. 1.22)

Skin Associated Lymphoid Tissue (SALT)

- **SALT –** an integrated system in which (1) resident keratinocytes and Langerhans cells; (2) migrant epidermotropic lymphocytes; and (3) draining lymph nodes work in concert to provide the skin with immunological protection against external environment toxins, infections and development of cutaneous neoplasms. Also these cells act as vast reservoir of soluble biological response modifiers called cytokines.

Resident Cells

- LANGERHANS CELLS.
- Make up 2-4% of epidermis – mostly suprabasal.
- With long dendritic processes – make an immunological net in epidermis trapping antigens efficiently.
- In normal non-inflamed skin, they are the only cells expressing class II MHC antigens (HLA – DP, DQ & DR) in humans.
- Present antigens to naïve T cells and also to memory T cells (Fig. 1.22).
- **Primary response:** Antigen bearing Langerhans cells– undergo phenotypic changes – migrate through dermal lymphatics – to regional lymph nodes – where they become like dendritic cells of lymph nodes – stimulate specific naïve T cells to proliferate and differentiate.
- **Secondary response:** The memory T cells which are already primed – Antigen recognition occurs entirely within the skin – faster and boosted response.
- Langerhans cells express ICAM-1 and lymphocyte function associated antigen (LFA-3) which are ligands for LFA-1 and CD2/LFA2 respectively on T lymphocytes.

  They also secrete IL-1b to promote immune response.

Keratinocytes

- Make up >90% epidermal cells.
- Constitutively synthesize IL-1a and also 1b – when activated by other cytokines – may secrete these too. Thus serve as vast reservoir of this proinflammatory cytokine.
- Also express class II MHC when skin is inflamed due to secretion of IFN-gamma by activated T lymphocytes which in turn activates keratinocytes to transiently express HLA-DR. IFN-gamma also induces expression of ICAM-1 on them so T cells may adhere by LFA-1.

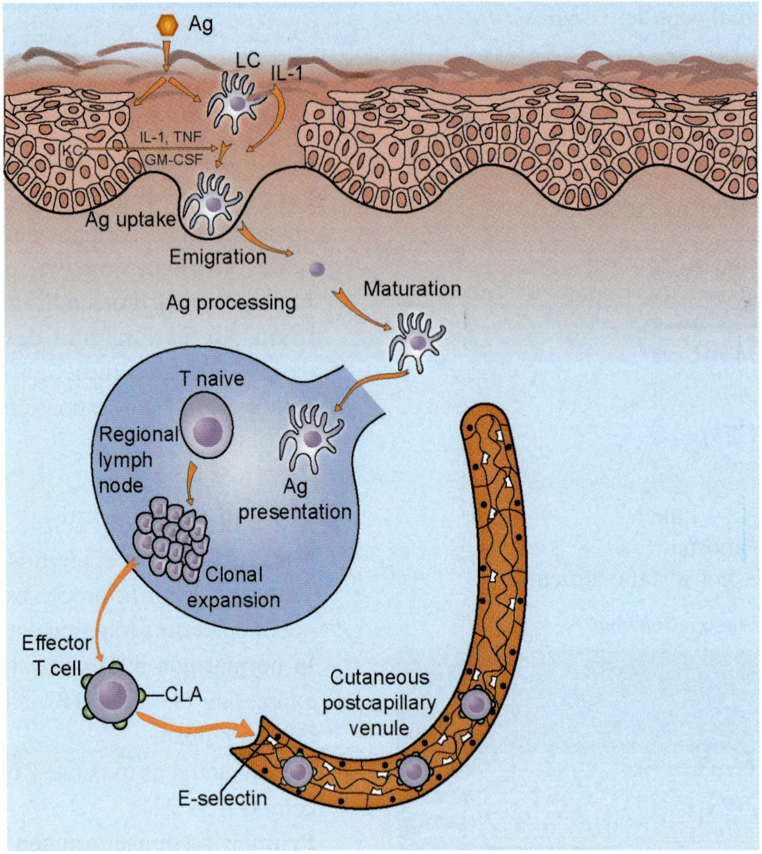

Fig. 1.22: Skin associated lymphoid tissue

Migrant Cells

- Epidermotropic T lymphocytes.
- 90% cutaneous T cells – perivascular or periadnexal.
- Approximately equal number of CD_4 and CD_8 cytotoxic and suppressor.
- <2% T cells are in epidermis– make up 0.16% epidermal cells.
- Virtually all intraepidermal T cells are CD_2+ CD_3+ CD_8+ suppressor – cytotoxic T cells.
- Adhere to both endothelial cells and keratinocytes by ICAM-1 – LFA-1 conjugate formation.

Immune Cell Response

The immune system is made up of two components. The most primitive arm of the immune system is referred to as "innate" immunity. **Innate immunity** mainly involves the action of cells like macrophages, as well as serum proteins, which control infection in a non-specific fashion. For example, macrophages efficiently engulf bacteria, protozoans, viruses and particulate substances that they encounter in the body.

Upon engulfment, macrophages will try to destroy the pathogen (Fig. 1.23A). The other component of the immune system, the "**adaptive**" immune system, contains B and T cells that respond to challenge by foreign particles in a much more specific manner. Both B and T cells originate in the bone marrow and then migrate to other organs and tissues. The surfaces of B cells are coated with antibody molecules that are capable of binding antigens (protein molecules that can induce a response by the immune system) in a very specific fashion.

Once stimulated, the B cells will release the antibody molecules into blood, which allows them to counteract the antigens (Fig. 1.23B). T cells are divided into two subpopulations, CD_8 and CD_4 cells. CD_8 T cells are known as killer cells.

For example, if a skin cell presents a viral protein as a result of its infection by a virus, the CD_8 T cell will recognize this cell as abnormal and proceed to destroy it (Fig. 1.23C). CD_4 T cells, or helper cells, are intimately involved in regulating antibody production and activate CD_8 T cells so that they can become better killers. CD_4 T cells are also critical in enhancing or subduing inflammation, which they do by secreting proteins called cytokines that control cell function (Fig. 1.23D). CD_4 T cells are instrumental in facilitating many autoimmune diseases like

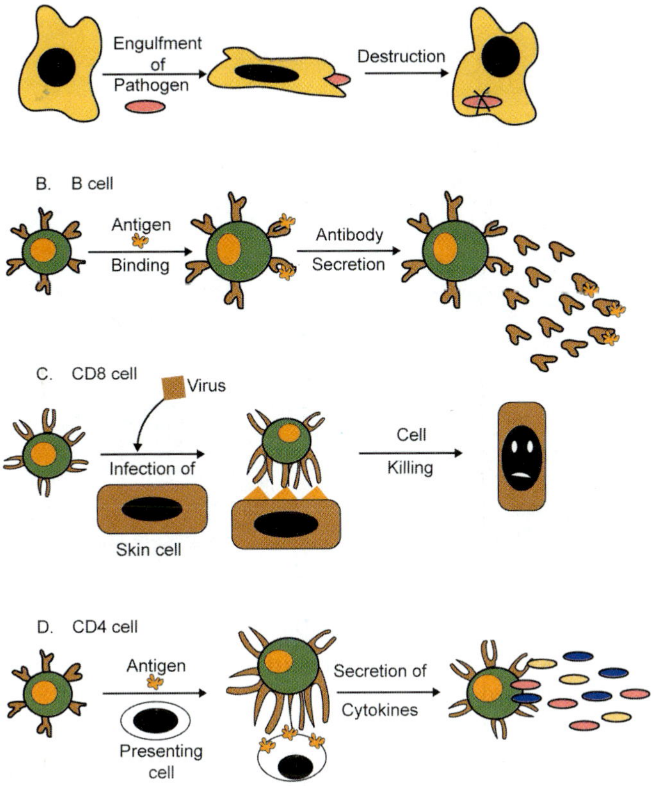

Figs. 1.23A to 1.23D: Immune cell response

PSORIASIS AND LICHEN PLANUS, in which the immune system responds abnormally to the body's own molecules (called "self antigens"). It is now clear that CD_4 T cells are also a main target for the human immunodeficiency virus (HIV) that causes AIDS. Understanding how to control CD_4 T cells will allow us to develop better vaccines, abolish many forms of autoimmunity, and control allergies.

REFERENCES

- L.P. Gartner and J.L. Hiatt: Color Textbook of Histology, 3rd edn., Elsevier, 2007, p 331-336.
- Junqueria and Carneiro: Basic Histology Text and Atlas, 11th edn., McGraw-Hill, 2005, p 361.
- Histologic Diagnosis of Inflammatory Skin Diseases. An Algorithmic Method Based on Pattern Analysis, 3rd edn. *A. Bernard Ackerman, MD, Almut Böer, MD, Bruce Bennin, MD and Geoffrey J. Gottlieb, MD* 2005.
- Rook's Textbook of Dermatology; D. A. Burns , S. M. Breathnach, Neil Cox, Christopher E, Griffith's 7th edn 2004.
- Fitzpatrick's Dermatology in General Medicine, 6th edn 2003.
- Lever's Histopathology of the Skin by David E Elder, Rosalie Elenitsas, Bernett L Johnson, George F Murphy, 9th edn. 2004.
- Thieme's Pocket Dermatology 2006 by Wolfram Sterry, Walter Burgdorf, Ralf Paus.
- Veedon Textbook of Histopathology.
- Ackerman Textbook of Histopathology.
- Morschella Textbook of Dermatology.

Essentials of Histopathology

DEFINITIONS OF HISTOLOGICAL TERMS

1. Abscess

Definition:

- Neutrophils are joined by products of necrosis and degeneration.

Example:

- Munro's microabscess and spongiform pustule of Kogoj-Psoriasis.

2. Acantholysis

A process whereby epithelial cells, as a consequence of loss of connections (desmosomes) between them, separate from one another.

Cause

- Immunoglobulins.
- Neutrophils on keratocytes in the lower part of the epidermis.
- Vesicants.

Primary

- Pemphigus vulgaris.
- Hailey Hailey disease.
- Squamous cell carcinoma.
- Warty dyskeratoma (acantholytic dyskeratotic acanthoma).
- Epidermal nevus typified by foci of acantholytic dyskeratosis.
- Darier's disease.

Secondary

- Dermatitis herpetiformis.
- Linear IgA dermatosis.
- Bullous lupus erythematosus.
- Impetigo.
- Majocchi's "granuloma".
- Herpes.

3. Acanthosis

- Increase in number of spinous cells—psoriasis.
- Size of spinous cells—lichen planus.
- Number and size of spinous cells—lichen simplex chronicus.

4. Dyskeratosis (Fig. 1.24)

- Dyskeratotic cells have pyknotic nuclei and eosinophilic cytoplasm.
- Filaments of keratin in perinuclear aggregation.

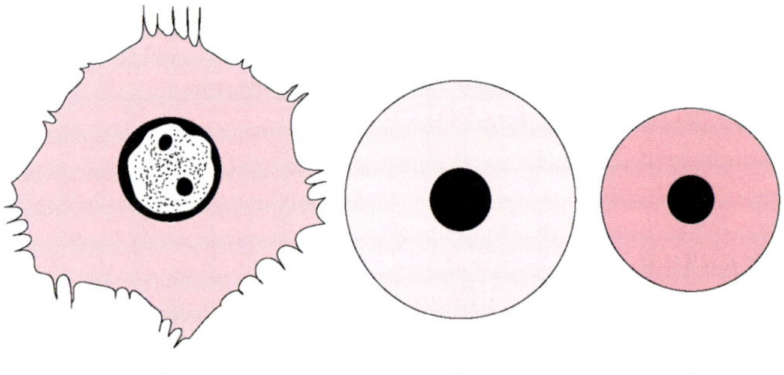

Fig. 1.24: Progression from (Normal) keratinocyte to dyskeratosis

- Grover's disease.
- Verrucous stage of Incontinentia pigmenti.
- Neoplastic diseases–Bowen's disease and subungual keratoacanthoma.
- Genodermatoses–Darier's disease.
- Cystic conditions such as warty dyskeratoma.

5. Granuloma (Fig. 1.25)

A collection of histiocytes, usually epithelioid ones:

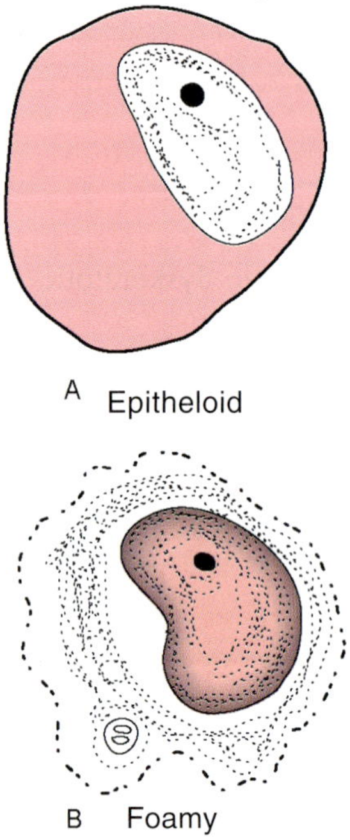

Figs. 1.25A and 1.25B

- Epithelioid histiocytes–TT/BT (Fig 1.25A).
- Foamy histiocytes–Lepromatous leprosy, xanthogranulomas (Fig. 1.25B).
- Multinucleate histiocytes (Langhans', Touton and foreign body).

Types of Tubercle (Fig. 1.26)

Epithelioid Cells are the Basic Requisite for all Granuloma

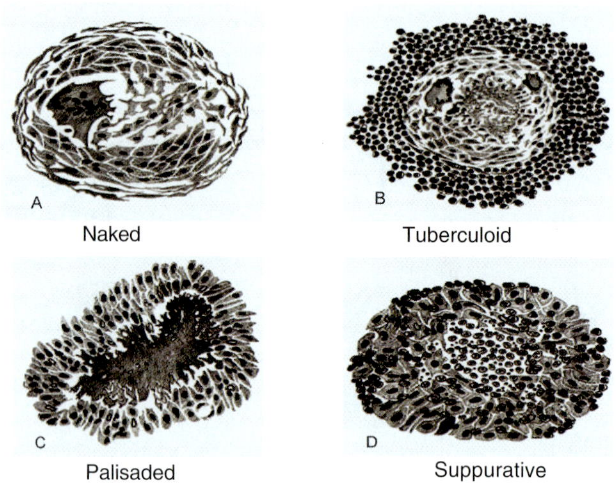

Fig. 1.26

A. "Naked" tubercle-sarcoidal: A granuloma not surrounded by any lymphocytes (Sarcoidosis, MRSA, Foreign body, L scrofulosorum).

B. Tuberculoid granulomas: A classic granuloma where there is central caseation, Langhans Giant cell and surrounded by Lymphocytes (TB, LMDF, Cryptococcosis, Histoplasmosis).

C. Palisaded: A granuloma composed of alternating bands on mucin, collagen and epithelioid cells (interstitial Garnuloma annulare).

D. Suppurative: A granuloma composed of neutrophils.

6. Hypergranulosis

- *Increased thickness of the granular zone of an epidermis.*

Examples:

- Lichen planus.
- Lichen simplex chronicus.
- Bullous congenital ichthyosiform erythroderma.

7. Hyperkeratosis

- Increase in the layers of stratum corneum – seen in psoriasis and other psoriasiform disorders.

Basket-Weave Orthokeratosis (Fig. 1.27)

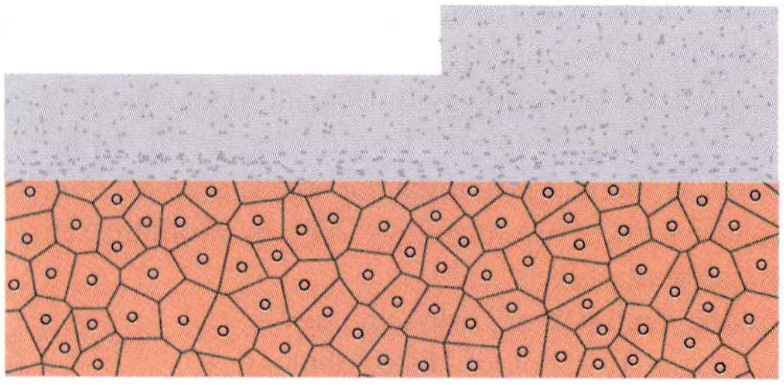

Fig. 1.27

- This alludes to the pattern of Hyperkeratosis which occasionally is because of an artifact due to processing.

***Examples*:** Tinea versicolor, verruca plana.

Compact Orthokeratosis (Fig. 1.28)

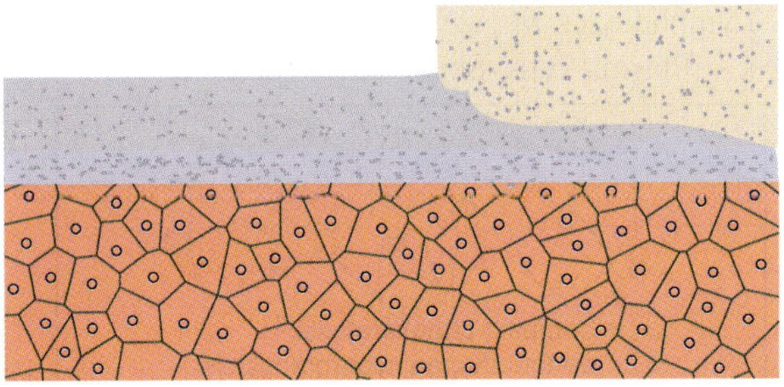

Fig. 1.28

Increased layers which are closely set.

Examples: Lichen simplex chronicus, lichen planus.

Laminated Orthokeratosis (Fig. 1.29)

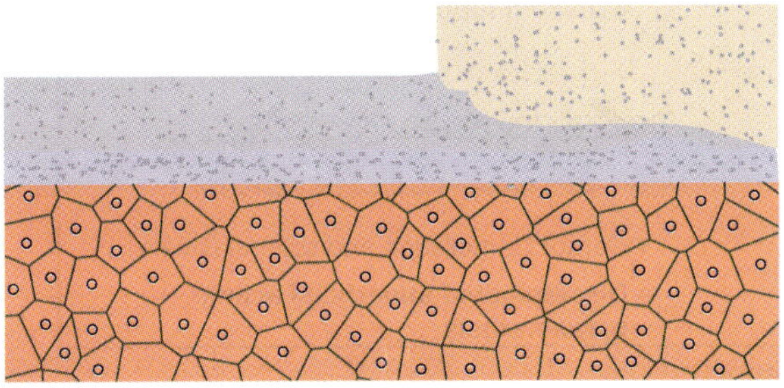

Fig. 1.29

Characterized by discrete layers of stratum corneum.

Examples: Ichthyosis vulgaris and X-linked ichthyosis.

Infundibular Hyperkeratosis

In this the hyperkeratosis is localized to the follicular opening.

Examples: Keratosis pilaris, lichen spinulosus, pityriasis rubra pilaris, lichen planopilaris, and discoid lupus erythematosus.

8. Parakeratosis (Fig. 1.30)

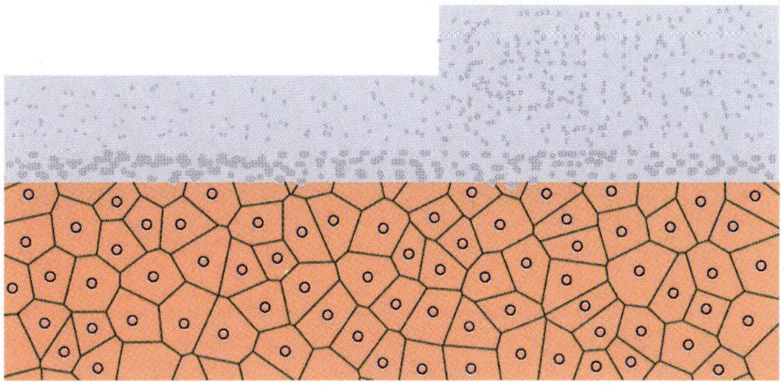

Fig. 1.30

Presence of nuclei in the stratum corneum seen in hyperproliferative disorders like psoriasis.

9. Hypogranulosis

A decrease in the stratum granulosum which is almost always seen in disorders with increase proliferation which cause parakeratosis.

Examples:

- Ichthyosis vulgaris.
- Psoriasis.
- Inflammatory linear verrucous epidermal nevus.
- Solar keratosis.

PERIVASCULAR DERMATITIS

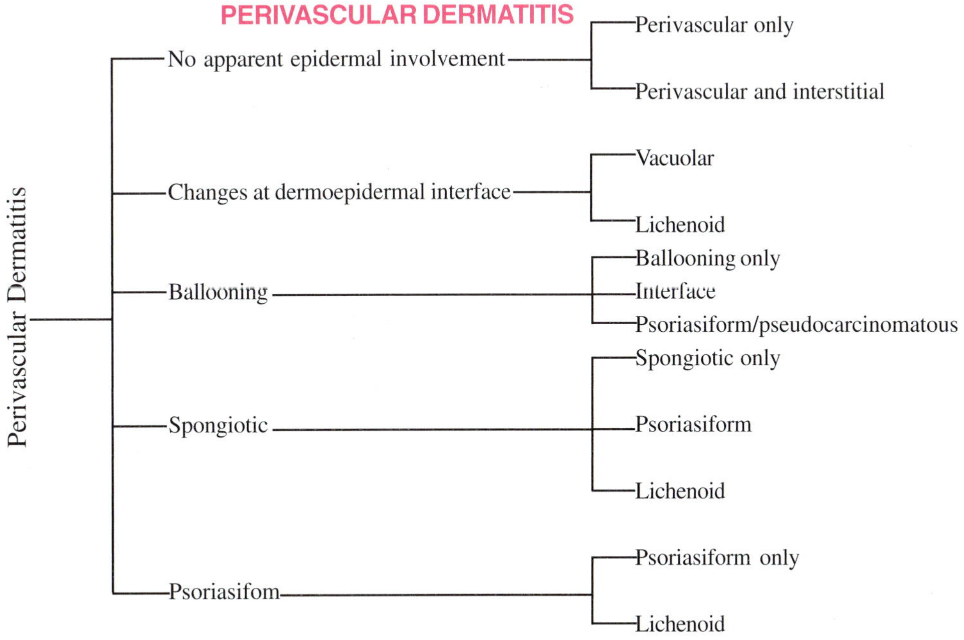

10. Superficial Perivascular Dermatitis Important Patterns (Figs. 1.31-1.33)

Sup Perivascular Psoriasiform

- Lymphocytes–Chronic Atopic Dermatitis.
- Plasma cells–Secondary Syphilis.
- Eosinophil–Chronic ACD.
- Neutrophil– Psoriasis Vulgaris.

Sup Perivascular-Lichenoid

- Lymphocytes–Lichen planus.
  Lymphocytes *plus*.
  i. Plasma cells–Secondary syphilis.

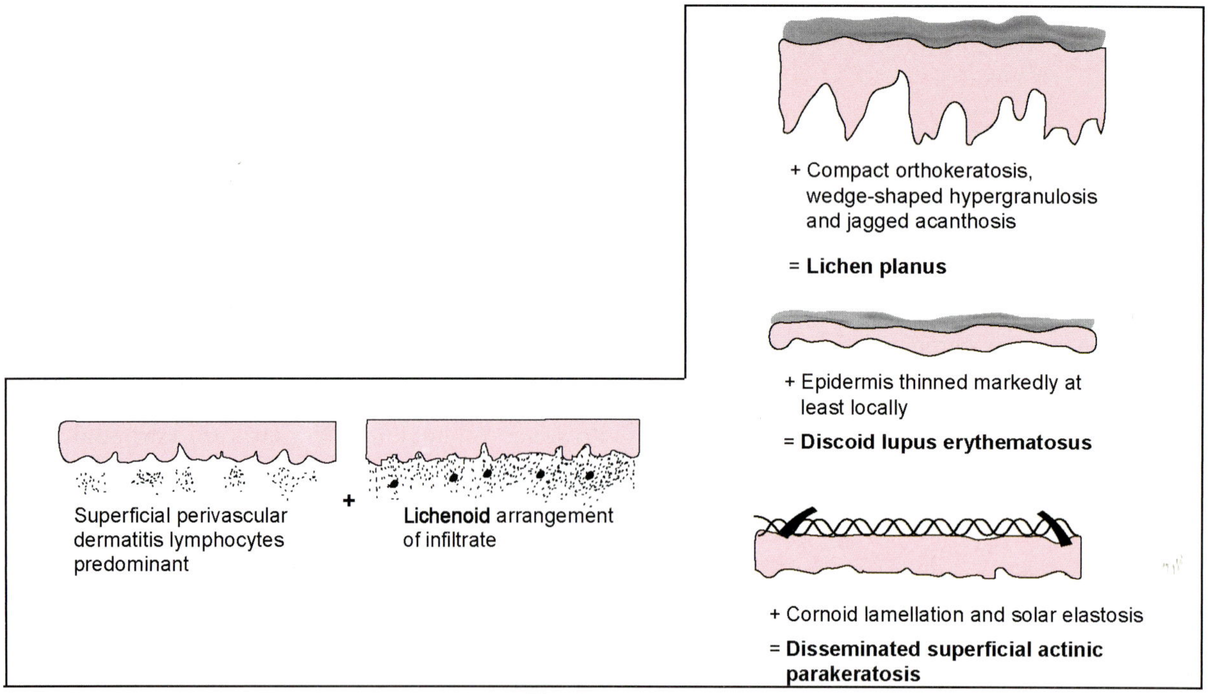

Fig. 1.31: Lichenoid

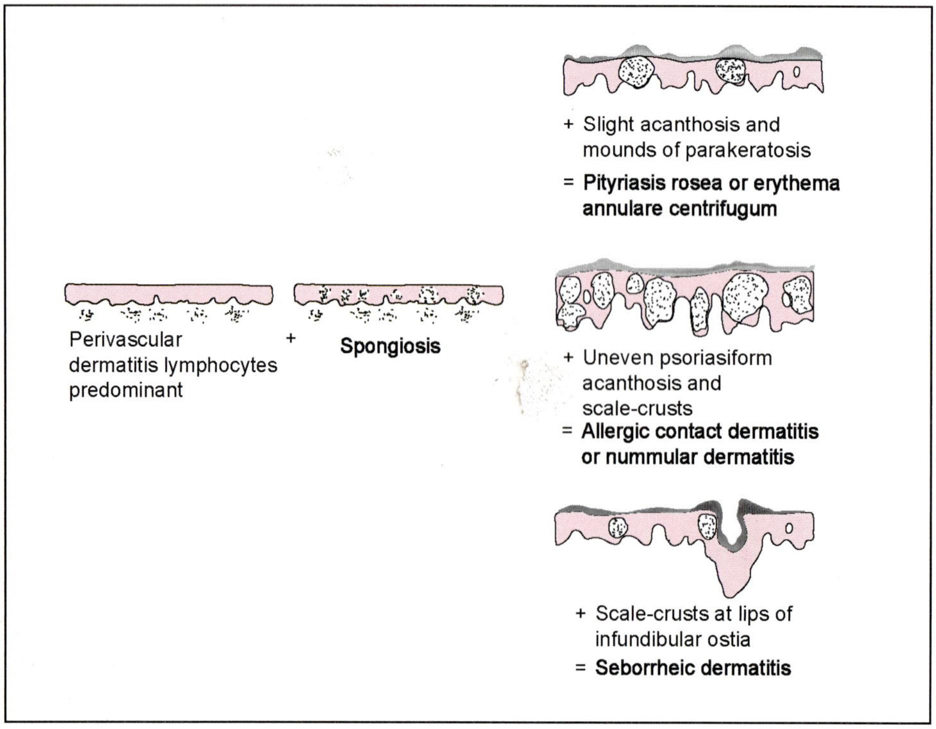

Fig. 1.32: Spongiotic

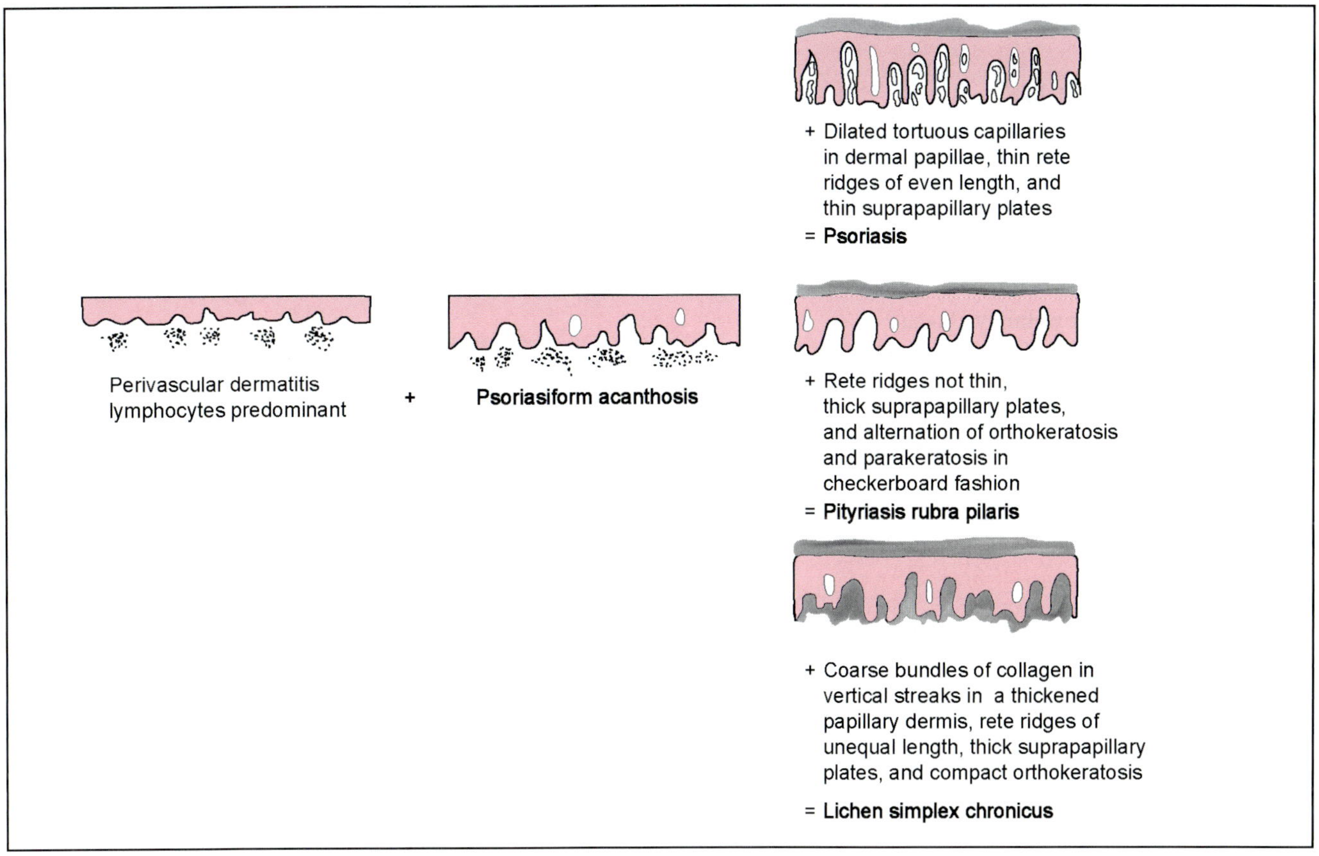

Fig. 1.33: Psoriasiform

ii. Eosinophil–Drug eruption.
iii. Melanocyte–Post inflammatory hyperpigmentation.
iv. Histiocytes–L nitidus.
v. Mast cells–Urticaria pigmentosa.

11. Interface Dermatitis

- **"Vacuolar"** (a sprinkling of inflammatory cells, usually lymphocytes, in conjunction with vacuolar alteration along that interface).
- **"Lichenoid"** (a bandlike infiltrate of inflammatory cells, usually lymphocytes, that, in association with vacuolar alteration, tends to obscure the interface).

Examples:

- Apoptic cells–Erythema multiforme.
- Minimal apotopsis–Dermatomyosistis.
- Variable–drug eruption.
- BMZ thickening–LE.

12. Vesicular Dermatitis

a. *The level of split*

i. Intraepidermal (Fig. 1.34)
ii. Subepidermal (Fig. 1.35)
Scant Cells=Porphyria Cutanea Tarda
Lymphocyte= Lichen Planus
Eosinophil = Bullous Pemphigoid
Neutrophil = Dermatitis Herpetiformis
Mast cell = Urticaria Pigmentosa

iii. Intra- and Subepidermal (Fig. 1.36)

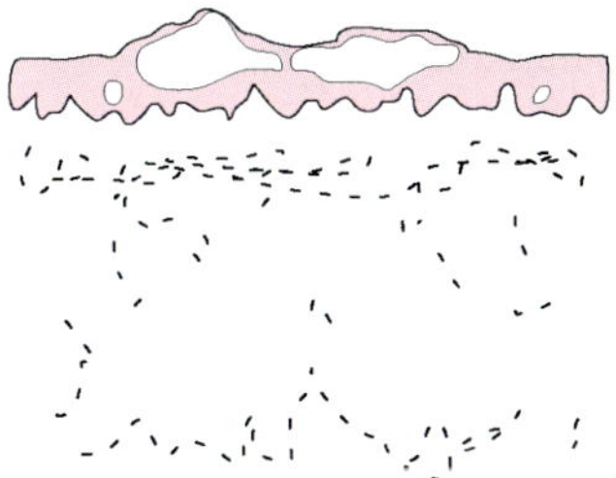

Fig. 1.34: Intraepidermal

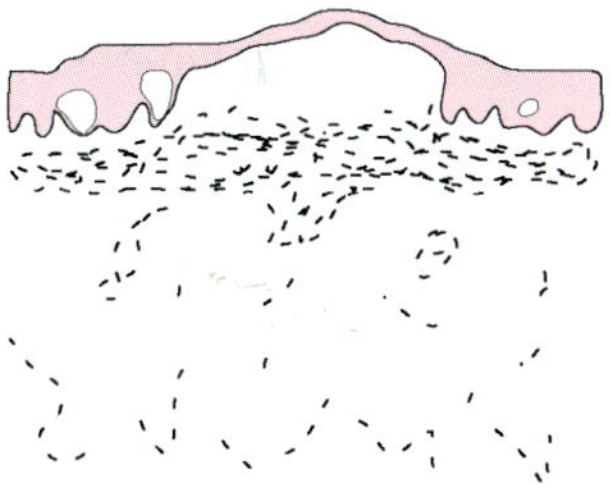

Fig. 1.35: Subepidermal

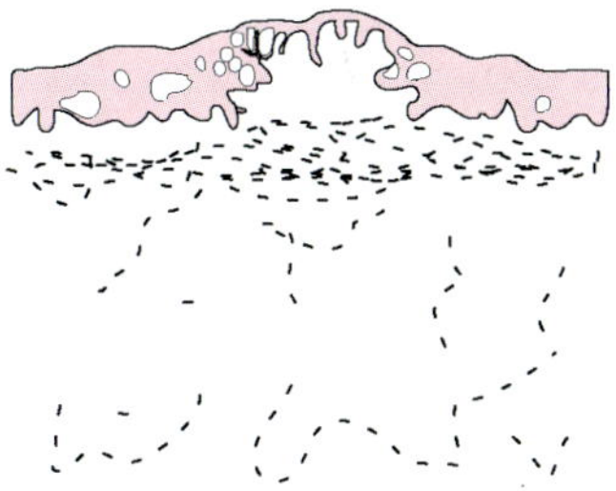

Fig. 1.36: Intra and Subepidermal

b. *Position of a vesicle within an epidermis (Intraepidermal)*

i. Suprabasal (Fig. 1.37)
- Scant cells – Grover's disease
- Lymphocyte + Plasma cells= Seborrheic keratosis
- Lymphocytes + Eosinophils= Pemphigus vulgaris

ii. Intraspinous (Fig. 1.38)
Spongiosis—Miliria rubra, ACD, pustular psoriasis
Acantholytic
Scanty cells=Hailey Hailey Disease
Lymphocyte=Herpes Simplex
Eosinophil=P. Vegetans

iii. Subcorneal (Fig. 1.39)
- Staphylococcal scalded skin syndrome.
- Impetigo.
- ETN (Erythoma Toxicum Neonatorum).

c. *Mechanism of formation of a vesicle*

i. **Spongiosis:** Classic of eczema due to vascular dilatation with extravasation of fluid causing space between the keratinocytes (Fig. 1.40).
ii. **Ballooning:** Characteristic of viral infection with a characteristic net like (festooning) (Fig. 1.41).
iii. **Acantholysis:** Seen in pemphigus (Fig. 1.42).

13. Panniculitis

a. ***Panniculitis (with vasculitis)***
- PAN, nodular **Vasculitis,** Churg-Strauss Syndrome.
- Mixed.
  Traumatic, histiocytic cytophagic type.

b. ***Panniculitis (without vasculitis)***
   i. *Septal*
   - Erythema Nodosum,
   - S/C Granuloma Annulare, scleroderma.

   ii. *Lobular*
   - Lymphocytes=lupus
   - Eosinophils=eosinophilic fascitis
   - Histiocytes=cytophagic histiocytic panniculitis
   - Foam cells=Weber Christian disease.

A summary of the stains used in dermatology are given below for quick reference:

Table 1.3: Common special stains

Stain	*Used to identify*
Hematoxylin-eosin	(Routine)
Alcian blue	Mucin
Congo red	Amloid
Fite Faraco	Mycobacteria
Fontana-Masson	Melanin
Giemsa	Mast cells
Hale (colloidal iron)	Mucin
Masson trichrome	Collagen

Contd.

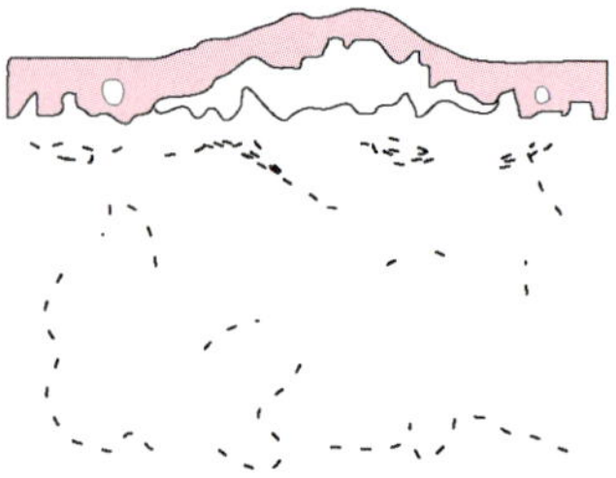

Fig. 1.37: Suprabasal

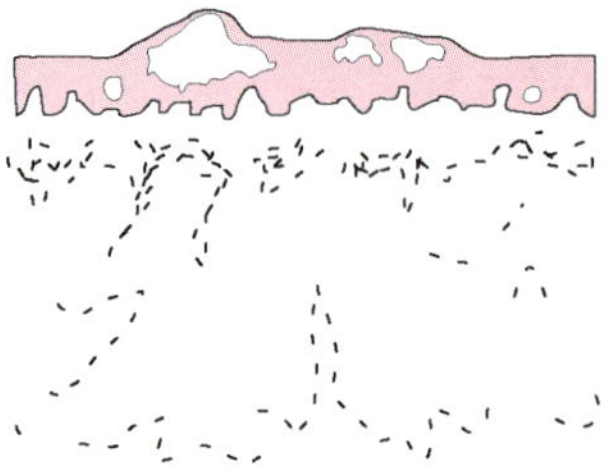

Fig. 1.38: Intraspinous

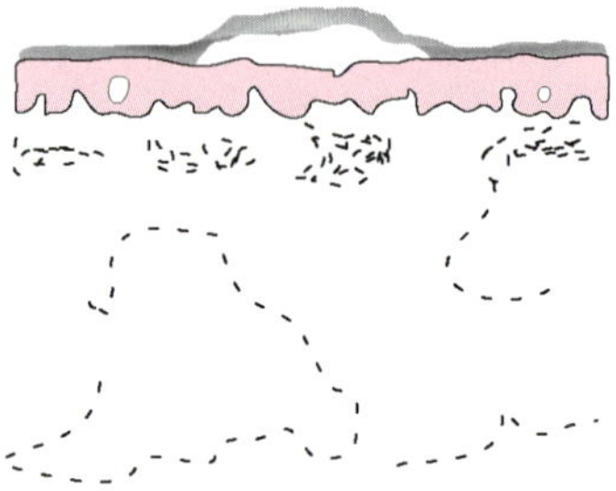

Fig. 1.39: Subcorneal

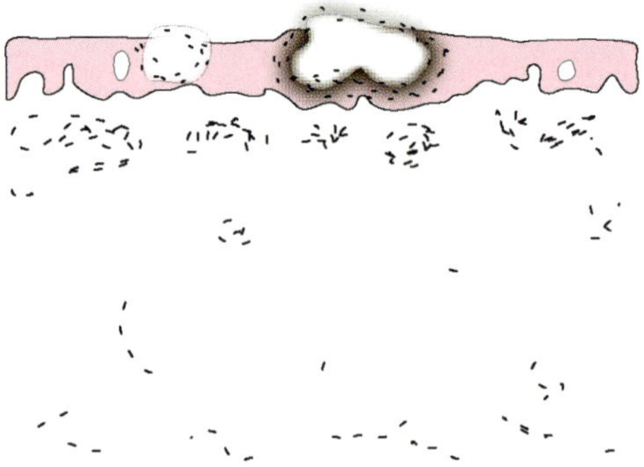

Fig. 1.40: Spongiosis

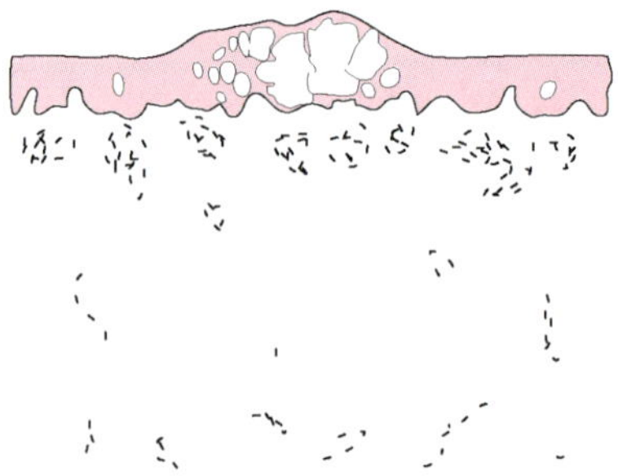

Fig. 1.41: Ballooning degeneration

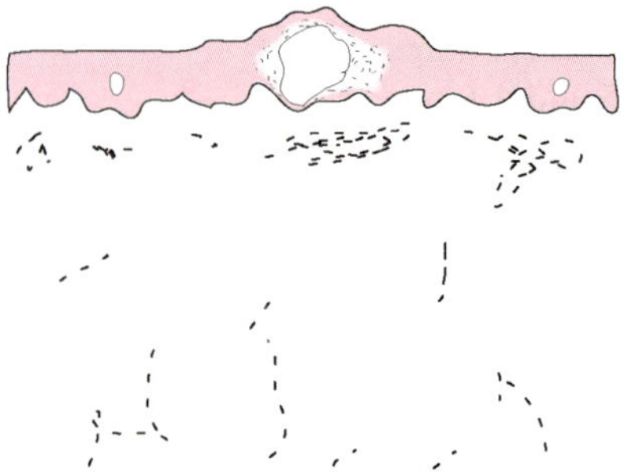

Fig. 1.42: Acantholysis

Contd.

Methenamine silver	Fungi, basement membrane
Periodic Acid-Schiff (PAS)	Fungi, glycogen, basement membrane
Silver nitrate	Melanin
Toluidine blue	Mucin
Von Kossa	Calcium
Verhoeff-van Gieson	Elastic fibers
Warthin-Starry	Spirochetes

Table 1.4

Stain	*Identifies*
Bcl2	Follicular B-cell lymphoma (negative in primary cutaneous follicular center lymphoma)
Bcl6	Follicular B-cell lymphoma
Carcinoembryonic antigen (CEA)	Eccrine, apocrine glands, Paget disease
CD 3	T-cells (T-cell receptor)
CD 8	Cytotoxic T-cells
CD 10	B-cell and T-cell precursors
CD 20	B-cells
CD 34	Stem cells, dermatofibrosarcoma protuberans
CD 35	Follicular dendritic cells
CD 45 RO	Effector and memory T-cells
CD 68	Macrophages
CD 79a	B-cells
CD 117	Mast cells
Cytokeratins	Epidermis, appendages, and related tumors
Desmin	Smooth and skeletal muscle
Epithelial membrane antigen (EMA)	Eccrine, apocrine, sebaceous glands and their tumors
Factor VIII	Endothelial cells, vascular tumors
Factor XIIIa	Dermal dendrocytes, dermatofibromas
HMB-45	Melanocytes, more often in melanoma than nevi
Ki-67	Proliferation marker
Leukocyte common antigen (LCA)	Leukocytes
Melan A	Melanocytes nevi, melanomas
S-100	Melanocytes, neural cells, many others
Smooth muscle actin	Smooth muscle cells and myofibroblasts

REFERENCES

- Histologic Diagnosis of Inflammatory Skin Diseases. An Algorithmic Method Based on Pattern Analysis, 3rd edn. *A. Bernard Ackerman, MD, Almut Böer, MD, Bruce Bennin, MD and Geoffrey J. Gottlieb, MD* 2005.
- Rook's Textbook of Dermatology D. A. Burns, S. M. Breathnach, Neil Cox, Christopher E, Griffith's 7th edn. 2004.
- Lever's Histopathology of the Skin by David E Elder, Rosalie Elenitsas, Bernett L Johnson, George F Murphy 9th edn. 2004.
- Thieme's Pocket Dermatology 2006 by Wolfram Sterry, Walter Burgdorf, Ralf Paus.

Fundamentals of Diagnosis

The diagnosis and treatment of skin diseases is basically the recognition of basic and sequential lesions of the skin, and their patterns in which they occur in a large variety of diseases and syndromes. The visibility and accessibility of the skin are at the root of the challenge and satisfaction of dermatological diagnosis.

Individual skin lesions are analogous to the letters of the alphabet, and groups of lesions can be analogous to words or phrases. Once the component of the skin affected by a pathologic process is determined to the extent possible by clinical examination, the lesion or lesions should be assessed in terms of their type, shape, arrangement and distribution. A definitive diagnosis may require the information provided by a complete history, physical examination, laboratory tests, and histopathologic analysis.

Based on three important points, dermatologists often prefer to examine the patient before obtaining the history.

- The diagnostic accuracy may be higher when visual examination is approached without preconceived ideas.
- The preconceived ideas have the power to limit thinking and eliminate important considerations from differential diagnosis.
- The dermatologic lesions and eruptions are so distinctive that a history is not required to make a diagnosis.

But the history, in turn, should provide direction for a subsequent and refined reexamination and includes following:

- **Identifying data:** Age, sex and race.
- History of present illness, with particular regard to onset, evolution and precipitating factors.
- **Past medical history:** Illnesses, operations, hospital admissions, pregnancies, allergies (especially drug sensitivities), hazardous exposures, habits and diet. In all cases, the presence or history of *atopic disorders* (asthma, hay fever, allergic rhinitis, atopic eczema) should be specifically asked about and recorded.
- Present or recent medications (prescribed and non-prescribed); illicit drug use.
- **Social history:** Birthplace, residence, travel, employment, hobbies, emotional status, pets.
- Sexual history with particular attention to risk factors for sexually transmitted diseases.
- **Family history:** Skin diseases, allergies, atopic disorders diabetes, hypertension, bleeding disorders, anemia, and neurologic, muscular, intellectual, or

emotional disturbances. In pruritic patients, it is especially helpful to determine whether anyone at home, or with whom the patient has close physical contact, is also itching.

- **Review of systems:** Constitutional symptoms.

Approach to the Patient

History taking is of extreme importance. In dermatology the 'Sandwich Appproach' of 'Examination – History – examination' is ideal. It is best, when the patient comes, to have a quick examination and then go in for a detailed and thorough history tailor made to patients' complaints. This history can again be followed by a detailed examination.

In the history taking, the following points should be carefully recorded:

History of Skin Lesions

- When did it start?
- Does it itch, burn, or hurt?
- Where on the body did it start?
- How has it spread? (Pattern of spread)
- How have individual lesions changed? (Evolution)
- Provocative factors.
- Previous treatment(s).

Constitutional and Prodromal Symptoms

- Acute illness syndrome (fever, sweats, chills, headache, nausea, vomiting, etc.)?
- Chronic illness syndrome (fatigue, anorexia, weight loss, malaise)?
- Arthralgias, Raynaud's phenomenon, sicca symptoms.

The Past History is equally important but should be taken with special reference to certain dermatological conditions.

Past Medical History

- Operations.
- Illnesses.
- Allergies, especially drug allergies.
- Medications (present and past).

Personal History

- Habits (smoking, alcohol intake, drug abuse).
- Atopic history (asthma, hay fever, eczema).
- *Social history,* with particular reference to occupation, hobbies, exposures, travel.
- *Sexual history.*

The examination should commence with general features of the skin:

- Color.
- Moisture.
- Texture.
- Temperature.
- General Features of the Hair and Nails.

Physical Examination

- *Type of lesion:* Macule, papule, nodule, vesicle, etc.
- *Shape of individual lesions:* Annular, iris, arciform, linear, round, oval, umbilicated.
- *Arrangement of multiple lesions:* Isolated, scattered, grouped, herpetiform, zosteriform, annular, arciform, linear, reticular, etc.
- *Distribution* (be sure to examine scalp, mouth, palms, and soles).
- *Extent of involvement:* Circumscribed, regional, generalized, universal. What percentage of the body surface is involved (the palm is roughly equivalent to 1%).
- *Pattern:* Symmetry, exposed areas, sites of pressure, intertriginous areas.
- *Characteristic location:* Flexural, extensor, intertriginous, glabrous, palms and soles, dermatomal, trunk, lower extremities.

PRIMARY SKIN LESIONS

Macule (Fig. 1.43)

Change in the *colour of an area* of skin without any change in its consistency which can be seen and cannot be differentiated from the surrounding skin by palpation.

- Erythematous macule: Red coloured due to vasodilatation or extravasation of blood.
- Hyperpigmented macule: Due to excessive formation of melanin or some other black pigment.
- Depigmented macule: White due to complete loss of melanin.
- Hypopigmented macule: When the loss of melanin is only partial.

- The shape of the macule may be circular, oval or irregular and its margin may be well demarcated or ill-defined.

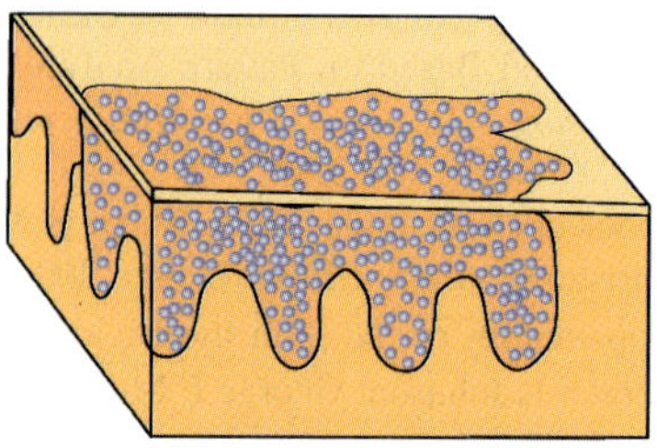

Fig. 1.43: Macule

Papule (Fig. 1.44)

A lesion, which is smaller than **5 mm** in diameter raised above the surface of skin and formed either by proliferation of the tissue cells or by infiltration of the area by inflammatory cells. Lichen nitidus is characterized by very small papules which are only 1-2 mm in diameter and are called *micropapules. Lesions that are larger than 5 mm* with depth are called **nodules**, while *those larger than 10 mm* are called **tumours**.

- Red papule—insect bites.
- Skin coloured—verruca plana.
- Brownish coloured—verruca vulgaris.
- Yellow coloured—xanthoma.
- Black—pigmented mole or have normal skin colour.
- *Violaceous—papules of lichen planus.*
- *Pearly white—molluscum contagiosum.*

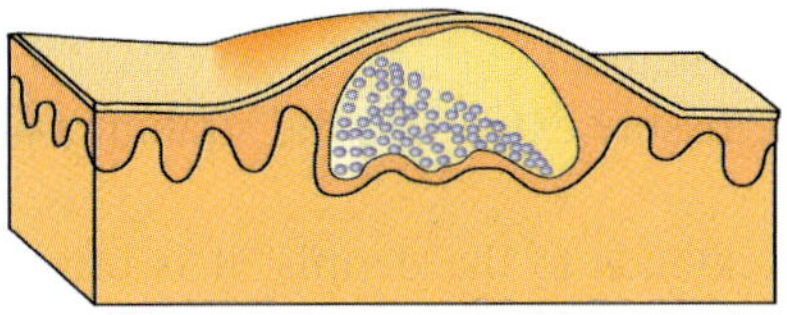

Fig. 1.44: Papule

The shape of the papule varies in different diseases:

- Acuminate papules—scabies and insect bites have a broad base and pointed top.
- Hemispheral papules—pigmented moles and new growths.
- Round; flat topped—lichen planus.
- Flat surface—plane warts.
- Filiform papules—warts.
- Pedunculated papules—neurofibroma.
- Follicular papules or follicules—pityriasis rubra pilaris and phrynoderma.

Vesicle (Fig. 1.45)

- A raised lesion like a papule, but contains fluid (Fig. 1.46).

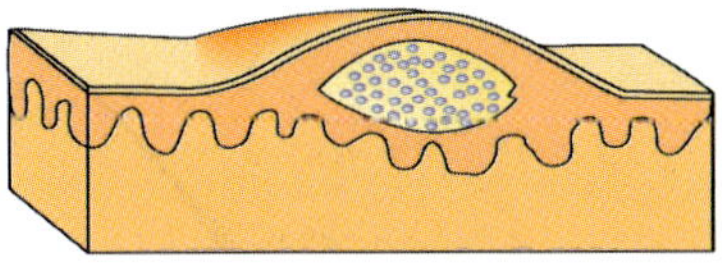

Fig. 1.45: Vesicle

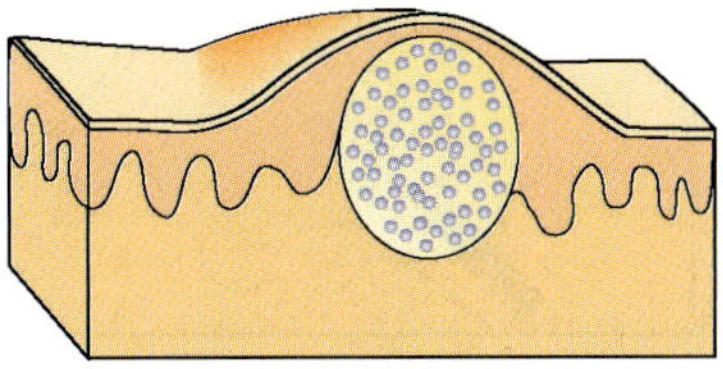

Fig. 1.46: Bulle

- Lesion larger than 5 mm is called a bulla or a *blister*.
- A bulla may be *flaccid as in pemphigus*, or *tense* as in *dermatitis herpetiformis*.
- Large and flaccid bullae can be irregular in shape, but vesicles are always tense.
- Vesicles or bullae may be surrounded by a zone of erythema as in erythema multiforme or may be situated on apparently normal skin as in pemphigus vulgaris.
- Vesicles of small pox occur singly and are diffusely scattered.
- Herpes zoster occur in groups.
- Sometimes vesicles may be overlapping each other and are called "over-riding" vesicles.

Pustule (Fig. 1.47)

- It is like a vesicle, but it contains pus instead of serous fluid.
- It is formed when the inflammatory exudates, rich in degenerated polymorphonuclear leucocytes collects in or under a localized area of the epidermis.
- A pustule may be surrounded by a zone of erythema and induration as in boils, or it may be located on apparently healthy skin.

Wheal (Fig. 1.48)

- A lesion characteristic of *urticaria* and is formed when there is sudden extravasation of fluid without the formation of any definite space.
- Due to the pressure of the exuded fluid, the area of the wheal may become pale, but a variable zone of erythema always surrounds it.
- The size may vary from a small lesion resembling a papule to several centimeters in diameter.
- Wheals are very evanescent and almost always disappear within ½ to 24 hours.
- The shape of a small wheal tends to be circular, while larger lesions are more often irregular in shape.
- Some wheals have pseudopodia.

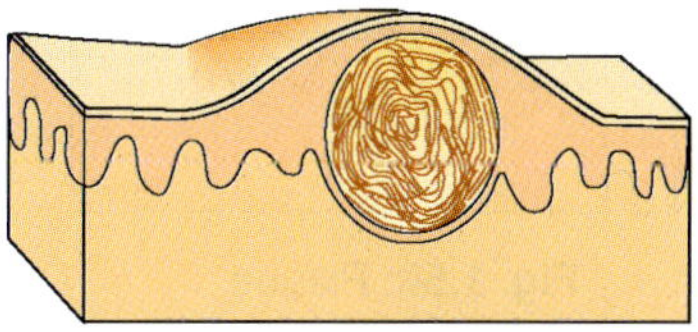

Fig. 1.47: Pustule

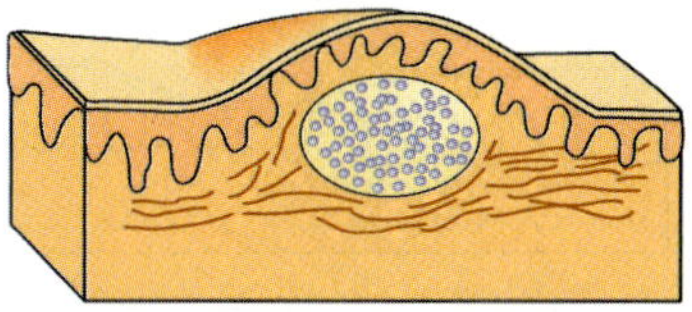

Fig. 1.48: Wheal

Scale (Fig. 1.49)

- A flake like lesion, which represents visible shedding of the skin.
- Scales can be very and *fine and powdery* seen in pityriasis versicolor, pityriasis rosea and seborrhea capitis, to very large in ichthyosis vulgaris.
- Scales of psoriasis are *small and silvery*.
- The scales of seborrhea capitis are *yellowish and greasy*.
- Ichthyosis vulgaris have large, *brownish and angulated* scales.

Plaque (Fig. 1.50)

- A large flat area which is either raised or depressed below the surface of the skin and width is more than the height.
- Annular plaque is depressed in the center and raised at the periphery.
- Some plaques are ulcerated and crusted in certain areas as in lupus vulgaris.

Atrophy (Fig. 1.51)

- It can occur either in the epidermis or in the dermis.
- In epidermis, that area of skin looks shiny and shows fine wrinkles on pressing the skin between a finger and the thumb. This is due to reduction in the thickness of the epidermis and flattening of the dermo-epidermal junction, because of the loss of epidermal ridges and dermal papillae. This type of atrophy may accompany an underlying inflammatory process such as leprosy or it may occur when the skin gets stretched over rapidly enlarging swellings.
- Atrophy of the dermis manifests as an area of depression in the skin surface without any induration as in atrophoderma.

Fissure (Fig. 1.52)

- A crack in the continuity of skin surface.
- Sites involved are folds of skin such as the groins, axillae, inframammary clefts of the hands and feet.
- An inflammatory process in such areas makes the tissue very fragile and liable to cracking under the effect of routine movements.
- The fissure is completely asymptomatic limited to the stratum corneum.
- When the fissure extends to the stratum malpighi, it is painful.
- When it extends to the dermis, it is often associated with bleeding.

Comedone (Fig. 1.53)

- Black-head or an open comedone is a small papule through the top of which is visible a black plug made up of keratin, sebaceous secretion and bacteria.
- Frequently seen in patients suffering from acne vulgaris, but also in old individuals (senile comodones).

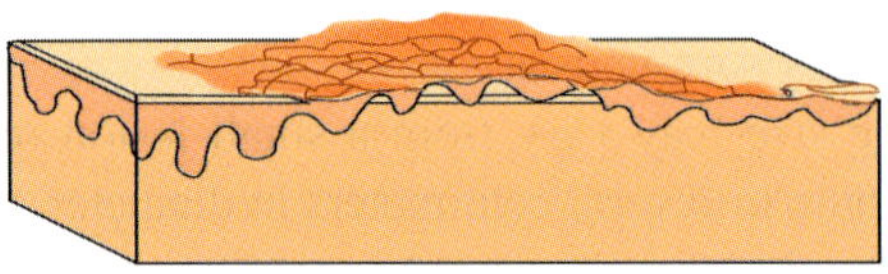

Fig. 1.49: Scale

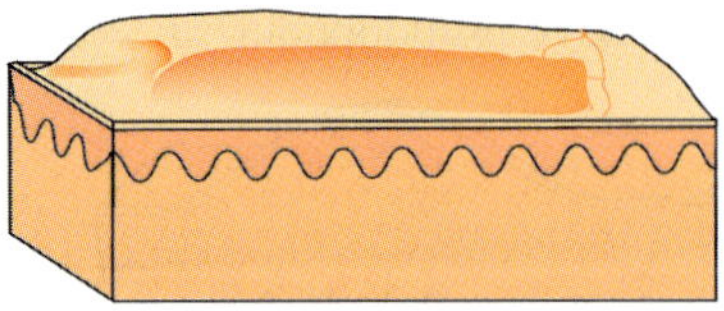

Fig. 1.50: Plaque

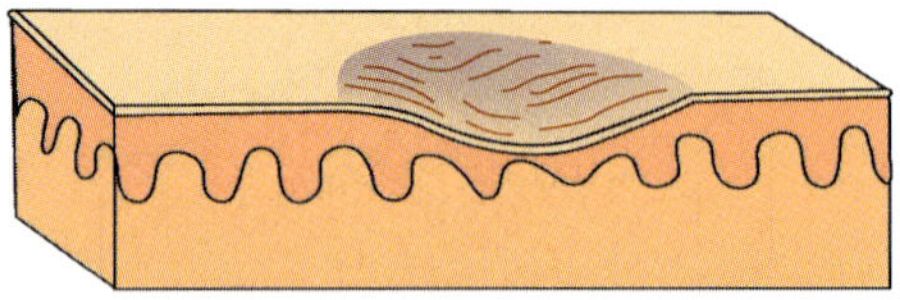

Fig. 1.51: Atrophy

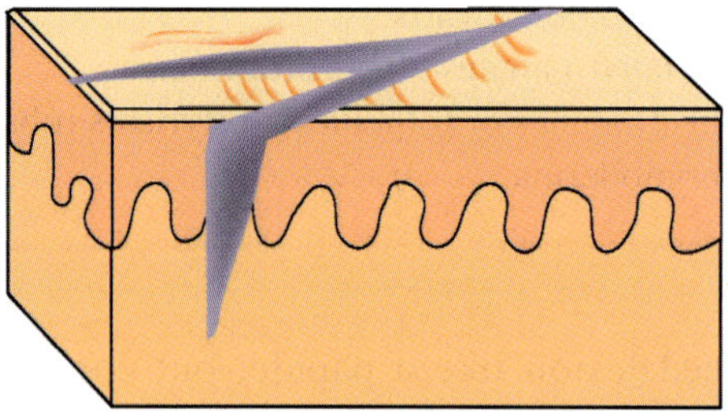

Fig. 1.52: Fissure

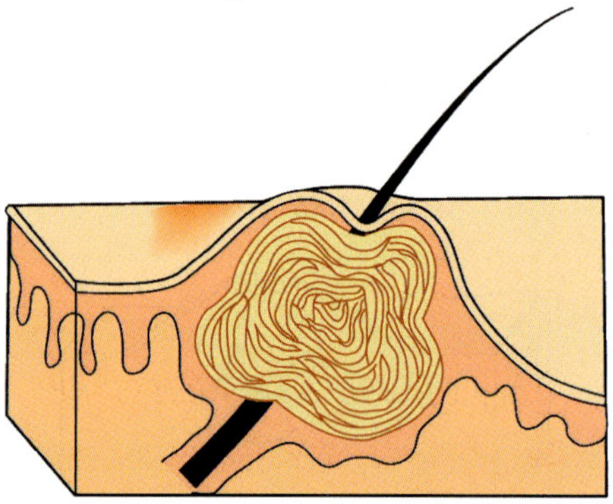

Fig. 1.53: Comedone

- Closed comedone is a lesion which on the surface looks like an ordinary acuminate papule but it contains a similar keratinous plug inside and is paler in colour and occur only in acne.

Burrow (Fig. 1.54)

- A lesion specific of scabies and is produced when a gravid female acarus penetrates the stratum corneum obliquely for some length.
- Such lesions are commonly found on the wrists, interdigital clefts, shaft of penis and abdomen.

Hyperkeratosis

- A histopathological term, but can be used clinically also when the lesion consists almost entirely of a thickening of the stratum corneum.
- It occurs mainly on the palms and soles and may involve the entire surface of palms or soles as in tylosis or occur only in localized areas as in punctate keratoderma and corns.

SECONDARY CHANGES

Excoriation (Fig. 1.55)

- Linear dapression in the stratum corneum.
- Papular lesions associated with severe itching can get excoriated.
- Excoriations can also occur without any lesions when the patient has severely scratched his pruritic skin and may occur in lines corresponding to the direction of scratching.

Lichenification (Fig. 1.56)

- It is a diffuse thickening of skin with the formation of papules and *hyperkeratosis*, **along with *hyperpigmentation severe itching*, and increase skin marking**.
- It occurs in the lesions of some diseases such as dermatophytosis, lichen simplex chronicus and atopic dermatitis.

Umbilication

- This change, most frequently seen in molluscum contagiosum, is due to necrosis and loss of material from the center of the papule.

Maceration

- Some inflammatory lesions associated with hyperkeratosis or scaling develop a whitish deposit on their surface called maceration.
- This change occurs mainly in the folds of skin where the moisture cannot evaporate easily and thus leads to soddening of the stratum corneum.

Ulceration (Fig. 1.57)

- An area of skin from which the surface layers upto reticular dermis have been lost is called an ulcer.

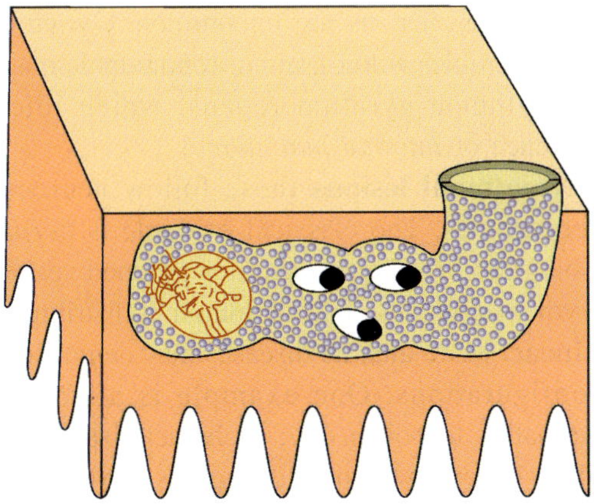

Fig. 1.54: Burrow

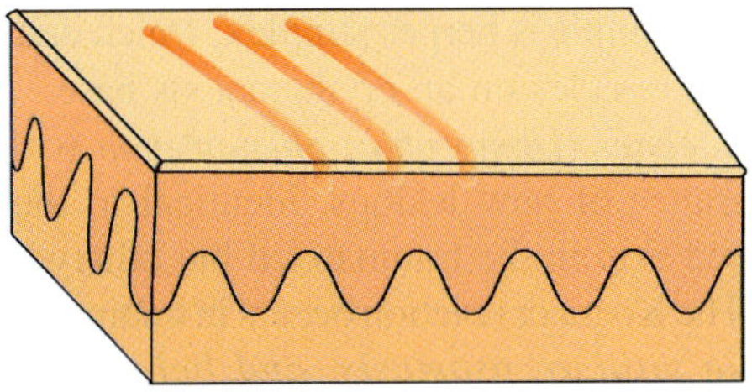

Fig. 1.55: Excoriation

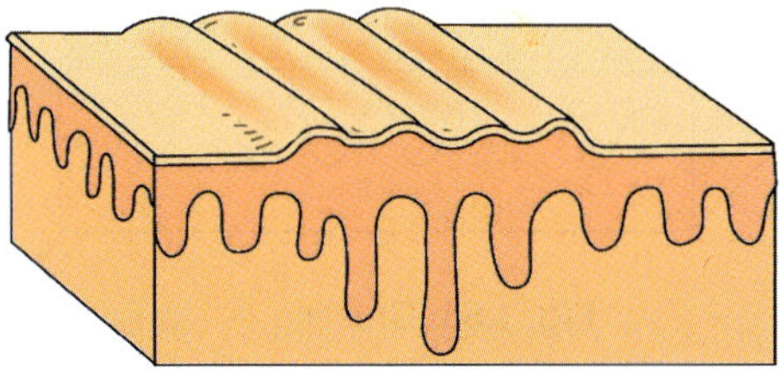

Fig. 1.56: Lichenification

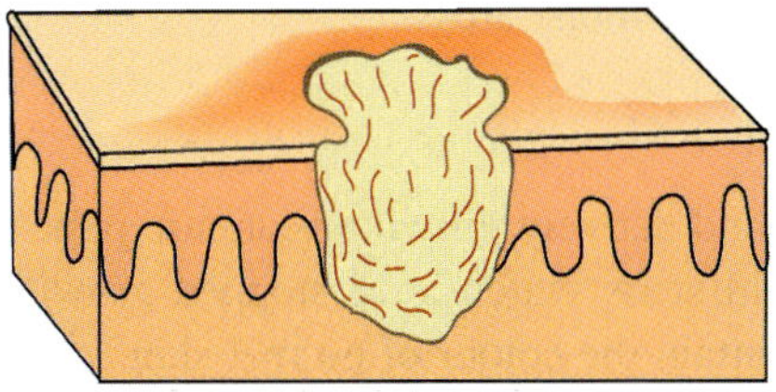

Fig. 1.57: Ulceration

- The rupture of the roof of a blister generally forms superficial ulcers, while deep are formed by necrosis and loss of tissue.
- The margin of a superficial ulcer is like a collar because the ruminants of the roof of the blister form it.
- In deep ulcers, the margin may be overhanging as in a tubercular sinus, punched out as in a gumma, irregular as in a non-specific ulcer.

Crusting (Fig. 1.58)

- A crust can be differentiated from a scale by the fact that scaling occurs in dry lesions while a crust is associated with some sort of an exudate.
- In the late healing stage however, there may be no exudation.
- A crust can be removed *en masse* and is fragile, while scales may separate from each other and are not fragile.
- The colour of a fresh crust can give some clue to the type of exudates from which the crust has formed.
- Serous exudates produces a dirty white or cream coloured crust, pus gives rise to a yellow crust, while blood stained discharge results in a dark brown or black crust.
- A crust may be firmly attached to the base or it may be poorly formed and loose.
- Loose crusts are likely to have a lake of pus underneath, which impedes healing.
- A crust can also form when a necrosed tissue dries up.

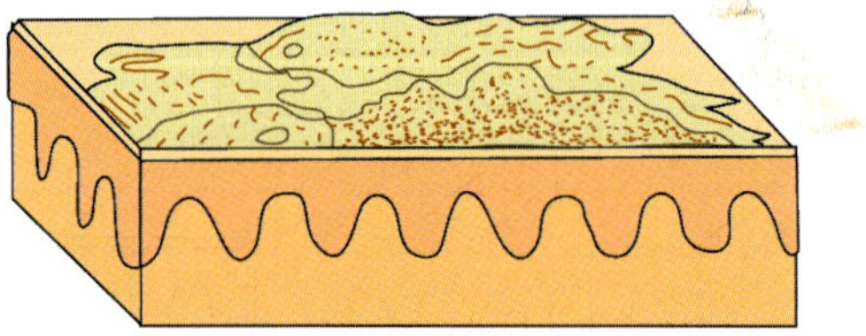

Fig. 1.58: Crusting

Vegetations

- In some superficial ulcers, the epidermal cells forming the base of the ulcer, start proliferating at a very fast rate resulting in an aggregate of nodular lesions lying very close to each other and are situated in the folds of skin or other moist areas.

Scarring (Fig. 1.59)

- Recent and actively growing scars are pink in colour, while old scars which have stopped growing further tend to attain the colour of normal skin.
- The size and shape of the scar depend upon the original lesion.

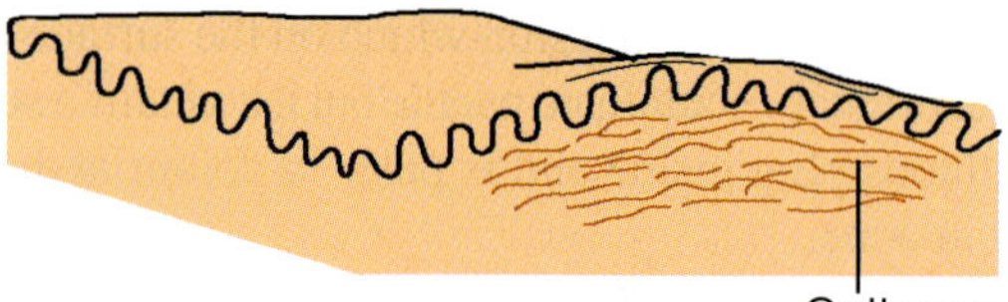

Fig. 1.59: Scarring

- Scars of small pox are small and circular, while those of acne vulgaris are small but irregular.
- Scars of syphilitic gumma are characteristically large, but thin and paper-like.
- A *hypertrophic scar* is produced when the amount of fibrous tissue formed is more than the tissue destroyed. Such a scar is raised above the skin surface, but it does not grow beyond the limits of the original lesion.
- A *keloid* in contrast, continues to grow beyond the limits of the original lesion.

SHAPE AND ARRANGEMENT AND CONFIGURATION OF LESIONS

A single lesion may assume a linear shape, or a number of lesions may be arranged in a linear pattern. Some but not all cutaneous diseases demonstrate characteristic arrangements or configurations of lesions.

- **Annular lesions** are ring-shaped. Annular plaques are seen in *granuloma annulare, tinea corporis, and erythema marginatum.*
- **Gyrate** which means "to turn around in a circle". Gyrate skin lesions are uncommon. Gyrate erythema that resembles wood-grain or topographic maps is seen in erythema gyratum repens, which idicates the presence of *internal malignancy.*
- **Dermatomal lesions** those follow neurocutaneous dermatomes. The classical example is *herpes zoster* (shingles), which demonstrates grouped vesicles on an erythematous base in a dermatomal distribution.
- **Linear:** More than 20 diseases may demonstrate linear configurations. One example is allergic contact dermatitis to poison ivy; it characteristically demonstrates linear erythematous papules or vesicles.
- **Grouped:** Papules, pustules, or blisters (vesicles or bullae) may demonstrate grouped configurations. A typical example is herpes simplex, which demonstrates grouped vesicles on an erythematous base.
- The *Koebner (isomorphic) phenomenon* is defined as appearance of new lesions, identical to those in the diseased skin in the traumatized but otherwise normal skin. The Koebner reaction occurs in traumatized normal skin *in vitiligo, psoriasis, and lichen planus(true)* among other conditions. The Koebner phenomenon may

occur in recent scars or at pressure points. In case of *pseudo Koebners* an infectious etiology is incriminated (*Warts, Molluscum, Herpes*).

Distribution of Skin Lesions

- Seborrheic dermatitis characteristically occurs on the scalp, nasolabial folds, retroauricular areas, eyelids, eyebrows, and presternal areas; it tends to spare the extremities.
- Psoriasis may resemble seborrheic dermatitis, but it characteristically demonstrates a different distribution, usually involving the extremities (elbows, knees), intergluteal fold, scalp and nails.

LINEAR LESIONS AND LINEAR ARRANGEMENT NODULES

- Superficial thrombophlebitis.
- Temporal arteritis or polyarteritis nodosa.
- Deep mycoses (sporotrichosis and coccidioidomycosis).
- Epidermal nevi.
- Factitial dermatosis, ulcers, atrophy, scars, or all three, frequently occur in a linear pattern.
- Linear scleroderma (*coup de sabre*).

Vesicles

- **Herpes zoster**

CLINICAL TESTS

1. *Dimple sign* is application of lateral pressure with the thumb and index finger results in the formation of a depression (dimple) in a *dermatofibroma*.
2. *Nikolsky's sign* refers to the sheetlike removal of epidermis by gentle traction and observed in pemphigus *vulgaris and toxic epidermal necrolysis*.
3. *Darier's sign* is an urticarial wheal in the lesions of *urticaria pigmentosa* (a brown macule or a slightly elevated papule) after they are rubbed with the rounded end of a pen. The wheal, which is strictly confined to the borders of the lesion, may not appear for 5 to 10 min.
4. *Auspitz's sign* is the appearance of pinpoint dots of blood at the tops of ruptured capillaries when scale is forcibly removed from *psoriatic* plaques.
5. *Patch testing* to diagnose *Allergic* contact dermatitis.
6. **Magnification** with hand lens is important to note the fine details of skin lesions: Magnification is essential to examine follicular plugging in lupus erythematosus, **Wickham's striae in lichen planus,** telangiectasia and translucence in basal cell carcinoma, changes in colour in malignant melanoma comedourea of acne.
7. **Diascopy** consists of pressing a transparent slide or plastic spatula over a skin lesion. Examiner will find this of special value to distinguish erythema and purpura. It is useful to detect the glassy yellow-brown appearance of papules in *sarcoidosis, tuberculosis and other granuloma.*

AIDS TO DERMATOLOGIC DIAGNOSIS

- Special procedures.
- Biopsy.
- Electron microscopy.
- Immunofluorescence.
- Bacterial and fungal cultures.
- Gram's stain of crusts, scales, or exudates.
- KOH prep for yeast or fungi.
- Tzanck smear.
- Bacteriologic, viral, and fungal cultures as indicated.
- Wood's lamp examination of urine for porphyrins and of hair and skin for fluorescence, and for changes in pigmentation.
- Scraping for scabies mite.
- Patch tests.
- General: Hematology, chemistry, urinalysis, serologic tests (e.g., STS, ANA), stool examination, and imaging studies.

KOH EXAMINATION

Scrapings are taken from the affected area with a #15 blade. The moist scales are transferred from the blade to a glass slide. One or two-drops of KOH (10-20%) are added, and the specimen is cover-slipped. The KOH preparation is gently warmed, but not boiled, and then examined under the microscope. It is important to focus back and forth through the material so that the refractile hyphae can be found. Cylindrical shapes with branching and presence of septae can recognize fungal hyphae. Older lesions may demonstrate numerous rounded spores called arthrospores.

Fungal Culture

The diagnosis can also be proved by fungal cultures. The easily broken, infected hairs are embedded in the media. A new toothbrush can also be "brushed" through the affected area of the scalp and then applied to the media. Sabouraud's dextrose agar is a standard in mycology laboratories. It consists of dextrose (energy source), peptone (protein source), and agar (for a firm surface). Antibiotics are added to suppress contaminants, and cyclohexamide is added to suppress yeasts and nondermatophytes. Plain Sabouraud's agar is a good culture medium for *Candida albicans.*

WOOD'S LAMP EXAMINATION

A Wood's light produces invisible long-wave ultraviolet radiation, or "black light", at 360 nm. In a dark room, when this light strikes the surface of the skin or urine, fluorescence is produced in certain conditions.

Uses of Wood's Lamp

- Tinea capitis *(Microsporum* spp. Fluoresce—green (colour).
- Tinea versicolor (dull **yellow** fluorescence) (colour).
- Erythrasma (coral red fluorescence) (colour).
- *Pseudomonas* infections of the skin (green fluorescence).
- Porphyria cutanea tarda, in which the urine fluoresces red.

Vitiligo lesion appears more white and ashleaf macule in **Tuberous sclerosis** is more apparent.

Tzanck Smear

A Tzanck smear is a standard technique for the rapid diagnosis of herpes simplex virus (HSV) or varicella-zoster virus (VZV) infections. It cannot distinguish between these two agents, nor can it distinguish between HSV subtypes (HSV type 1 or 2). It is performed by scraping the base of a fresh blister with a scalpel blade and then spreading the adhering cells and material on a glass slide. The slide is then stained with Giemsa, Wright's, or Sedi stain. The typical multinucleated giant cells or atypical keratinocytes with large nuclei are then sought under the microscope (Tzanck Cell) which have a jigsaw-puzzle like appearance.

Demonstration of Mite

The best method is to scrape a burrow and demonstrate the parasite inside it. A classic burrow appears as an irregular, linear, slightly elevated lesion, best found on the flexor wrists, finger webs and genitalia. Eighty-five percent of adult male patients with scabies will have mites on the hands or wrists. Occasionally, the mite can be seen with the naked eye as a small dot at one end of the burrow. A sample is collected with a number 15 scalpel blade. Following the application of mineral oil on either the blade or skin, the burrow is scraped vigorously, but not so vigorously as to draw blood. The mineral oil is collected from the skin and transferred to a glass slide, which is then examined under the microscope. The diagnosis is established by identifying either the fecal pellets (scybala), eggs, or mite.

Darkfield Examination

Darkfield examination of the chancre is the most specific test for the diagnosis of syphilis. This test is typically positive unless" the patient has applied or ingested antibiotics. In addition to primary syphilis, darkfield microscopy can also be used to diagnose all the mucocutaneous lesions of secondary syphilis. It is less reliable for examining specimens from the mouth or rectum because of the high prevalence of commensal, nonpathogenic treponemes in these locations that may be mistaken for *Treponema pallidum,* the agent of syphilis. The best specimens for darkfield examination are serous fluid expressed from the bases of the chancre following cleaning with sterile saline and clean gauze. The specimen then should be immediately evaluated for the organism's characteristic corkscrew morphology and flexing, hairpin motility. If a patient is suspected of having a syphilitic chancre and a darkfield is negative, it should be repeated at least once before the diagnosis is excluded. A darkfield examination offers immediate results and is a cheap test. However, it is often not available.

Gram Stain

A Gram stain of a urethral discharge in symptomatic males is an excellent method of diagnosing gonorrhea. A positive Gram stain showing multiple neutrophils, some containing clusters of gram-negative diplococci with the sides flattened toward one another.

Patch Test

The suspected allergen is usually placed in an appropriate vehicle in an appropriate concentration. The patch test allergens are usually purchased in prepared forms, but less common allergens can be prepared individually. The allergens are placed in special wells that are then taped against the skin of the back for 48 hours and then removed. This skin area is then examined 24-72 hours after the patch is removed for a reading. A strong positive reaction has erythema, infiltration, papules and vesicles. A bullous reaction is extremely positive.

This tests the type IV hypersensitivity reaction and it is a confirmatory test for allergic contact dermatitis.

Standard patch test is used to screen and confirm allergic contact dermatitis. Further breakdown of the test may require patch test with different series e.g. fragrance series. The test materials are applied to the back under aluminium discs with occlusion. The sites are inspected at 48 hours and test materials removed. The sites are re-inspected **at 96 hours for delayed reaction**. The grading of the reaction will be as follows:

No reaction:	0
Doubtful:	+/-
Weak (erythema, non-vesicular):	+
Strong (vesicular or edematous):	++
Extreme (with ulceration):	+++
Irritant reaction:	IR
Not tested:	NT

Skin Biopsy

A skin biopsy with routine hematoxylin-eosin staining is the best diagnostic technique for many cutaneous neoplasms that cannot be diagnosed visually. It is also helpful in many inflammatory skin disorders, especially those in which a specific diagnosis cannot be made from clinical examination, blood tests, and scrapings of the skin.

IMMUNOFLUORESCENCE

Direct immunofluorescence (DIF) of the skin is a histologic stain for antibodies or other tissue proteins in skin biopsy specimens. The specific immunoreactants present, and the pattern and intensity of staining, are used to determine the diseases most likely to be associated with the DIF findings. Many of the immunobullous diseases have specific DIF findings, including bullous pemphigoid, herpes gestationis, cicatricial pemphigoid, epidermolysis bullosa acquisita, dermatitis herpetiformis, linear IgA bullous dermatosis, and the various types of pemphigus. In addition, DIF may be helpful in evaluating cutaneous and systemic lupus erythematosus, other collagen vascular diseases, types of vasculitis such as Henoch-Schönlein purpura, and certain porphyrias.

OTHER TESTS

Prick testing is much less helpful in dermatology. Multiple positive skin tests to commercially prepared diluted antigens may only imply the atopic tendency of the tested subject. It is the interpretation of the wet smear which may require some experience. (**ACETOWHITENING**) Acetic acid test on genital or cervical papules facilitates detection of subclinical condylomata acuminata. Gauze saturated with 5% acetic acid is wrapped around area for 5 to 10 minutes and the use of colposcope or magnifying hand lens to detect the lesional white papules.

REFERENCES

- Rook's Textbook of Dermatology; D. A. Burns, S. M. Breathnach, Neil Cox, Christopher E., Griffith's 7th edn 2004.
- Fitzpatrick's Dermatology in General Medicine, 6th edn 2003.

CHAPTER 2

INFECTIONS

Viral

A virus particle or virion, consists of a length of nucleic acid, either RNA or DNA within a protein shell, the capsid. It requires host cell ribosomes for translation of proteins involved in viral replication. This absolute dependence on the host is the characteristic feature of viruses.

A classification of viruses causing disease in humans is shown in Table 2.1.

Table 2.1: Classification of viruses causing disease

Nucleic	*Family*	*Virus*	*Disease*
ds-DNA	Poxviridae	Variola, vaccinia	Vesicular eruption
		Orf	Cutaneous tumors (benign)
	Herpes viridae	Herpes simplex	Vesicles/encephalitis
		Varicella	Chickenpox/ Shingles
		Cytomegalovirus	Congenital/ immunocompromised patients
		EBV	Infectious mononucleosis
		Human herpes:	
		virus 6	Roseola infantum
		virus 7	Macular eruption
		virus 8	Kaposi sarcoma
	Papillomas Virus	HPV types	Warts cervical cancer
ssDNA	Parvoviridae	Human parovirus B_{19}	Erythema infectiosum
ssRNA	Retroviridae	Lentivirus HIV 1,2	AIDS
	Togaviridae	Rubella	German measles
	Flaviviridae	Dengue	Febrile illness
	Picornaviridae	Foot and mouth	Foot and mouth disease
		Coxsackie A	
		Coxsackie B	Meningitis
		Echovirus	
	Paramyxoviridae	Measles	Measles

HERPES VIRUSES

- Consists of large DNA viruses.
- Replication is intranuclear→produce intranuclear inclusions.
- Subgrouped according to genome into:
  - Herpes virus hominis HSV 1 and 2.
  - Herpes virus 3, (varicella VZ virus).
  - Cytomegalovirus.
  - EBV.
  - Human herpes virus 6, 7, 8.
- Characteristic feature of herpes virus infection→ absence of virus elimination following clinical recovery→leading to latent infection in cells.

Herpes Simplex

Aetiology

Two major antigenic types:

Type 1 associated with facial infections; and type 2, which is typically genital.

Primary Type 1 infections occur mainly in infant and young children, often subclinical.

Type 2 infections occur mainly after puberty and are often transmitted sexually. Primary HSV-2 infection is more commonly symptomatic.

Mode of infection is by direct contact with, or droplets from, infected secretions. Trauma facilitates transfer of the virus to fully keratinized skin. Source may be endogenous (auto-inoculation), or exogenous inoculation.

i. **Primary infection:** Acquisition of HSV infection in a previously seronegative individual.
ii. **Non-primary first episode:** Acquisition of HSV at a new site in a patient previously infected at a different site, and/or in a seropositive patient.
iii. **Recurrent infection**.

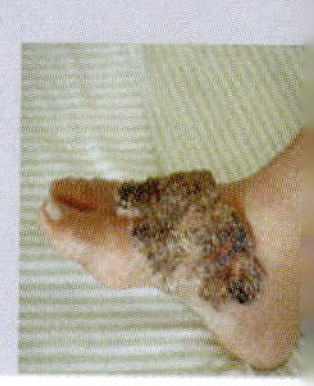

Clinical Features

Primary Infections

- Often subclinical.
- When clinical lesions develop, the severity is generally greater than in recurrences.

1. Herpetic gingivostomatitis

- Most common clinical manifestation of primary infection by HSV-1.
- Occurs in children between 1 and 5 years of age.
- Incubation period: 5 days.
- Begins with fever, malaise, restlessness, dribbling of saliva, foul breath, swollen gums, may bleed.
  ↓
- Vesicles—white plaques—ulcers with yellowish pseudomembrane.
- **Site:** Tongue, pharynx, palate, buccal mucosa. Enlargement of regional lymph nodes, recovery in 2 weeks.

2. Herpes genitalis

- Sexually transmitted.
- HSV-2 etiology.
- Increasing frequency of HSV-1 infection due to orogenital contact.
- Painful erosions—glans, prepuce and shaft of penis.
- Recovery in 2 to 3 weeks—with marked erythema and oedema.
- Male homosexual—perianal area.
- In female—painful vulvo-vaginitis, cervicitis, urethritis, and cystitis with burning and dysuria.

3. Keratoconjunctivitis

- Purulent conjunctivitis with opacity.
- Superficial ulceration of cornea.
- Enlargement of pre-auricular gland.

4. Herpetic Whitlow

- Inoculation of the herpes virus onto the fingertips—in which painful deep vesicles coalesce to produce ulcer.

Complications of Herpes Virus Infection

- **Eczema herpeticum**→cutaneous viral infection in a patient with pre-existing skin disease e.g. atopic dermatitis.
  - **Pharyngitis.**
  - **Radiculoneuropathy.**
  - **Disseminated/systemic infection.**
  - **Headache and meningism.**
  - **Encephalitis.**
  - **Hepatitis.**
  - **Lower respiratory tract infection.**
  - **Arthritis.**

Recurrent Infections

Recurrence Rate:

- 30-50% in cases of oral herpes.
- 95% in gential HSV-2 infection triggered by minor trauma, other infections, UV radiation, surgeries, premenstrual period, emotional stress.
- Recurrent lesion: Smaller size of vesicles, no constitutional symptoms.
- Recurrences occur in the same region but not always on the identical site.
- Complications rare with recurrent herpes.

Diagnosis

1. Direct examination of stained smear (cytodiagnosis by **Tzanck** smears or pap smears)—**multinucleated giant cells**, secondary acantholysis (Fig. 2.1).
2. Tissue culture of the virus from vesicle fluid most reliable method but expensive.
3. **Serodiagnosis**
   - Limited value.
   - Primary infection can be distinguished by seroconversion or rise in antibody titre.
   - Recurrences tend to produce little change in antibody titre.
4. **Detection of viral antigen**
   - Immunofluorescence—in scrapings from lesions.
   - Electron microscopy.
   - Detection in CSF by PCR.

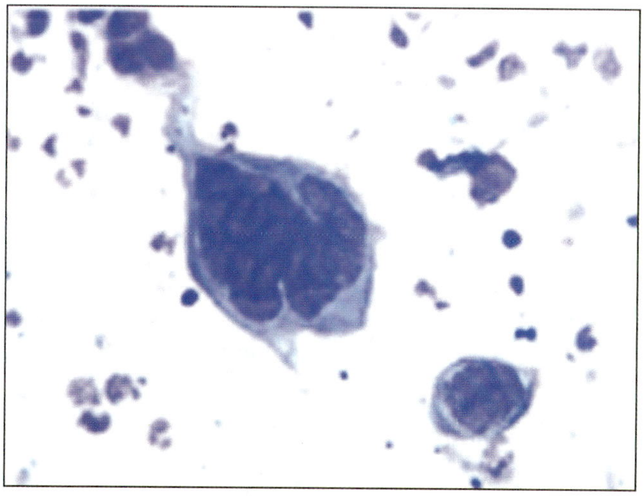

Fig. 2.1: Large giant cells with a jigsaw puzzle pattern of nuclei

Treatment

General measures

- Lesions should be cleaned with soap and water.
- Occlusive dressings and topical steroids avoided.
- Topical antibacterial agents→prevent 2° infection.
- Supportive therapy—antipyretics, antihistaminics.

Antiviral agent

a. **Acyclovir:** 200 mg 5 times/day OR 400 tds × 7-10 days
   Suppressive therapy > 6 recurrences/year
   Acyclovir 400 mg BD × 6 months or more.

b. **Valacyclovir:** Greater oral bioavailability
   1 gm BD × 10 days
   500 mg BD × 5 days (Recurrent episode)
   500 mg OD for prophylaxis.

c. **Famciclovir:** 250 mg tds × 5-7 days.

d. **Other antiviral agents:**

Idoxuridine Trifluridine Vidarabine	Ophthalmic preparations used for herpetic keratitis and keratoconjunctivitis.

Immunocompromised patients—IV **acycylovir can be used.**

Chickenpox Varicella and Zoster (Shingles)

Etiology

Varicella and zoster are caused by the same virus, herpes virus varicellae (varicella-zoster virus).

Varicella is the primary infection with a viremic stage, after which the virus persists in nerve ganglion cells, usually sensory. Zoster is the result of reactivation of this residual latent virus.

Varicella (Fig. 2.2)

- Incubation period: 14 to 17 days.

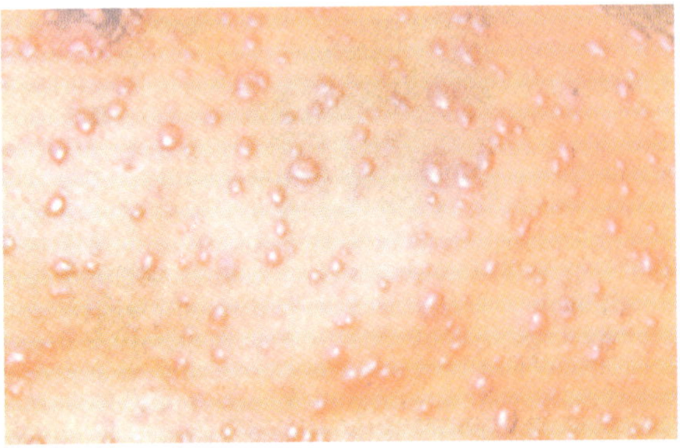

Fig. 2.2: Vesicles on an erythematosus base resembling a dew drop on a rose petal

- Mode of infection: Droplet infection from nasopharynx.
- Period of infectivity: 2 days before to 5 days after onset of rash, dry scabs—not infectious.
- Age 2-10 years.

Clinical Features

Fever and malaise (May be absent in children)
↓ (1-2 days)
Morbilliform erythema
↓
Papules
↓
Become tense, clear unilocular vesicles
↓
Contents become turbid
Pustules surrounded by red areola
↓ 2-4 days
Dry crust
↓
Separates
↓
May heal with superficial scars.

Site: Centripetal distribution.
Characteristic feature: Pleomorphic rash.
Oral mucosal involvement common with vesicles on the palate, conjunctival and anal mucosa may be involved.
Fever: variable in severity.
constitutional disturbances.
Adult→Severe involvement with constitutional disturbances.

Complications

Rare in healthy children, common in immunosuppressed.

- Encephalitis.
- Varicella pneumonia and hepatitis (Reye's syndrome).
- Secondary infection.
- Thrombocytopenic purpura.
- Arthritis.

Diagnosis

- Clinically.
- Tzanck smear.
- Viral culture.

Prevention

- Pre-exposure prophylaxis.
- Post-exposure prophylaxis.
- Antiviral prophylaxis.

Pre-exposure Prophylaxis

- Live attenuated vaccine—reduces incidence and severity of varicella 2 doses given 3 months apart.
- Duration of immunity—10 years.

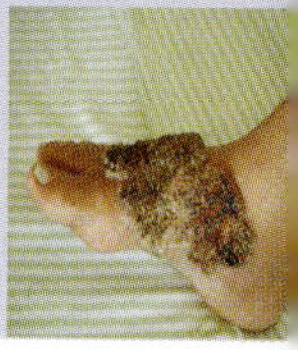

Post-exposure Prophylaxis

- Zoster immunoglobulin administered within 10 days of contact reduces severity of varicella, though it does not prevent it, given for immunocompromised children and adults, and for neonates (with maternal varicella).

Antiviral Prophylaxis

Acyclovir given from about 9 hours after exposure for 1 week appears to be effective in reducing severity or aborting chickenpox.

Treatment

- Calamine lotion for local application.
- Antihistamines.
- Oral antibiotics for secondary infection.
- In adults and severe cases:
  T. acyclovir 800 mg 5 times/day × 7 days.
  T famciclovir 500 mg tablets TDS × 7 days.
  Valacyclovir 1 gm TDS × 7 days.

Shingles/Herpes Zoster

'Zoster'means girdle.

- Usually occurs in adults.
- Burning, tingling pain precedes the eruption.
- Starts as painful grouped erytematous papulovesicles along a dermatome confined to one side of the body. Vesicles enlarge in size and may become pustular (Fig. 2.3).

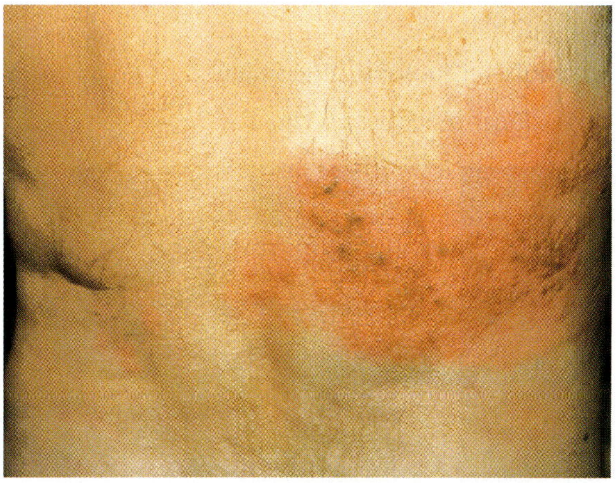

Fig. 2.3: Linear band of vesicles on the chest

- Most common—thoracic dermatomes.
- Lesions on the nose—indicate eye involvement (Hutchinson's rule).
- In immunocompromised patients—dissemination/ multiple dermatome involvement—haemorrhagic and deep ulcerated lesions.
- Recovery in 2-3 weeks.
- Pain and paresthesia—persist for long time (12 months).

Complications

1. Post herpetic neuralgia most common sequelae which increases with age.
2. Ophthalmic complications: Corneal ulcers, scarring.
3. Bell's palsy, meningitis, paralysis of limbs.
4. Herpes zoster **oticus**, with VIIth palsy (Ramsay Hunt Syndrome).
5. Secondary infection.
6. Guillain-Barré syndrome, transverse myelitis.

Treatment

Mild Cases: Symptomatic treatment.
- Calamine lotion.
- Analgesics.
- Topical antibacterial agent.

Severe Cases/Elderly:
- Oral acyclovir 800 mg 5 times × 7 days.
- Valaciclovir Igm TDS × 7 days.
- Famciclovir 500 mg TDS × 7 to 10 days.
- Given within 2-3 days of onset of lesions.
- Immunocompromised patient—IV acyclovir.
- Impending Bell's palsy—oral prednisolone in addition to antivirals.

Post herpetic neuralgia:
- Carbamazepine.
- Phenytoin.
- Amitryptiline.
- Gabapentin.
- Pregabalin.

WARTS (VERRUCAE) (Table 2.2)

Caused by human papilloma viruses (HPV) that are double stranded DNA viruses. Various clinical types of wart are caused by particular antigenic types.

Table 2.2: Clinical presentation and HPV tyre

Clinical presentation	*Common HPV types*
Common warts	1,2,4,26-29
Plantar warts	1,2,4,63
Flat warts	3,10,26-29, 41
Butcher's warts	7
Epidermodysplasia verruciformis	5,8,9,12,14,15,17,19-25, 36,38, 46
Anogenital warts	6,11,1,18,30-21
Laryngeal papilloma	6,11

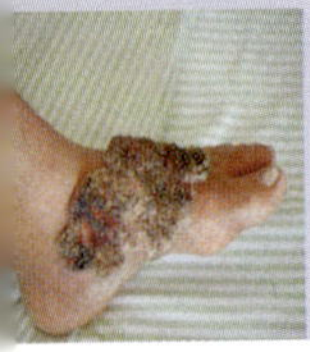

Mode of infection: HPV infects squamous epithelia of both keratinizing and non-keratinizing surfaces by direct inoculation with infected material. Genital warts are usually caused by venereal contact. Perianal warts may be transmitted by homosexual contact.

Most Common Antigenic Types

• Verruca vulgaris	2,4
• Myrmecia warts	1
• Plane warts	3, 10
• Mosaic warts	2
• Epidermodysplasia verruciformis	5, 8
• Genital warts	6, 11
• Laryngeal papilloma	6, 11

Verruca vulgaris (Fig. 2.4)

- Asymptomatic keratotic papules of varying sizes.
- Single/multiple.
- Sites: Back of hands and fingers, feet and legs.
- Koebner's phenomenon occurs.
- Periungeal wart/subungual warts→resistant to treatment.
- Usually disappear spontaneously.

Plane warts (Fig. 2.5)

- Smooth, flat/mildly elevated round papules.
- Size 1-5 mm.
- Common in children.
- Sites: Face, dorsum of hands and feet.

Filiform/Digitate warts

- Finger like projections 2-10 mm in length.
- Site: Face of young males, scalp.

Plantar warts (Fig. 2.6)

- Pressure points of forefoot/heel usually affected.
- Keratotic papules/plaques.
- Multiple.
- **Mosaic warts**—Plaques of closely grouped warts.
- **Myrmecia warts**—Deep, painful, dome shaped, single.

  DD: Corns/callosities.

Genital: Condyloma acuminatum

Sexually tran-smitted, moist cauliflower like lesions over anogenital areas, usually multiple.

Treatment (Table 2.3)

- Regress spontaneously.
- Treatment may be required to reduce transmission.

Topical

1. Salicylic acid ointment/paint for plantar warts 5-40%.
2. Trichloroacetic acid.
3. Cytotoxics—Podophyllin/5-FU weekly application.
4. Tretinoin 0.025-0.05%.
5. Antivirals —Cidofovir, imiquimod.
6. Intralesional IFN, bleomycin.

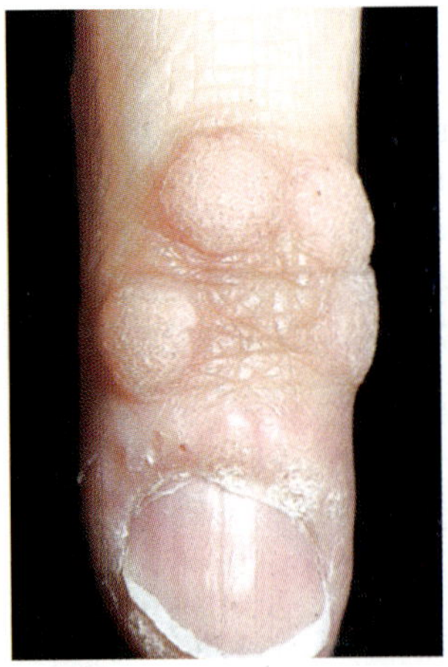

Fig. 2.4: Raised verrucous papules of common warts

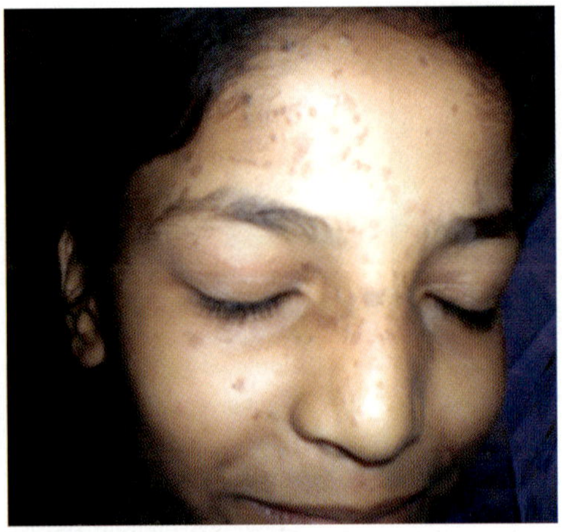

Fig. 2.5: Flat pigmented papule of plane warts

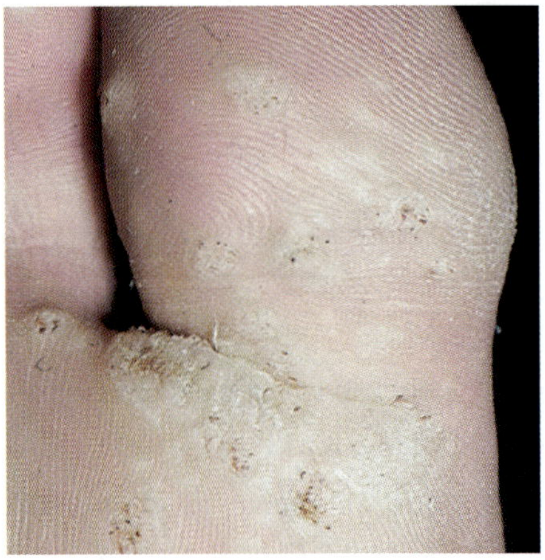

Fig. 2.6: Multiple areas of plantar warts

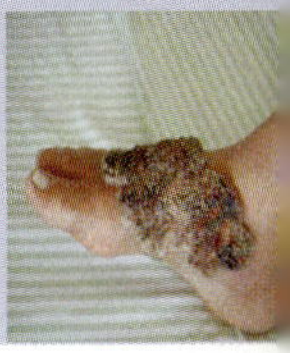

Table 2.3: Treatment of warts

Chemotherapy
- Salicylic acid
- Lactic acid
- Monochloroacetic, Bichloroacetic, Trichloroacetic acid
- Formalin

Glutaraldehyde
Cantharidin
Podophyllin /podophyllotoxin*
Tretinoin (topical)*
Bleomycin (intralesional)*
Cryotherapy
Surgery
- Excision
- Curettage
- Electrosurgery
- Laser therapy

Immunotherapy
- Imiquimod
- Oral zinc
- Cimetidine (oral)*
- Interferon*
- Diphencyprone (DPCP)*
- Tape occlusion
- Neglect due to benign nature

*Not recommended during pregnancy

Surgical and Physical Methods

- Electrodesiccation.
- Cryotherapy.
- Curettage.
- Excision.
- CO_2 laser.

MOLLUSCUM CONTAGIOSUM

- Caused by DNA containing pox virus.
- Transmission:
  - Skin to skin contact, rarely fomite transmission.
  - Sexual transmission in adults.
  - Autoinoculation.

Incubation period: 2 weeks-6 months.
Clinical features: Shiny, pearly white, hemispherical umbilicated papule, which may show a central depression (Fig. 2.7).

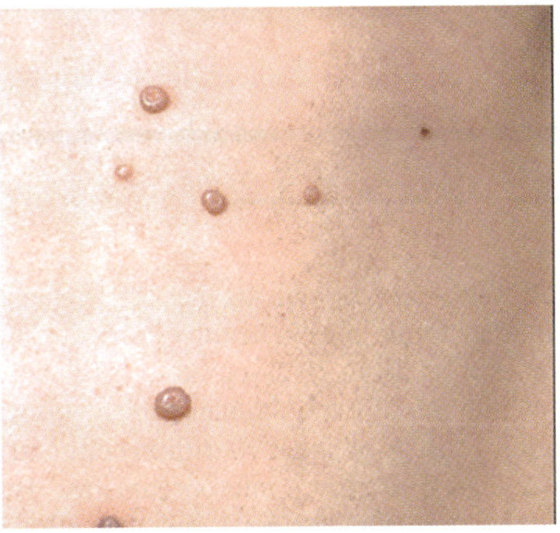

Fig. 2.7: White umbilicated papules

- Heal without scarring
  - Most cases—self limiting (6-9 m).
  - **Site**—Children→limbs.
    —Adults→Neck/trunk/face.

Other common sites: Eyelids, scalp.

Diagnosis

Clinical

- Giemsa's/Gram's stain—from smear of the cheesy material from the lesions. Shows—intracytoplasmic inclusion bodies that are eosinophilic, smooth, ovoid and homogenous within epithelial cells.

Treatment

In persistent cases to prevent spread of infection.
Basis: to induce epidermal damage.
- Chemical cautery.
- TCA (Trichloroacetic acid).
- Liquid phenol.
- Salicylic and lactic acid paint, silver nitrate.
- Curettage.
- Cryotherapy.
- Electrodessication.
- Topical IFN, imiquimod.

Systemic

- Levamisole.

REFERENCE

- Andrews' Diseases of the Skin: Clinical Dermatology by William D. James, Timothy Berger, Dirk Elston 2005.

Bacterial

NORMAL FLORA OF THE SKIN

Term used to describe organisms that are frequently found in particular anatomic sites in healthy individuals.

This microbial flora is associated with the skin and mucous membrane of every human shortly after birth.The healthy adult consists of about 10 trillion cells and routinely harbours at least 100 trillion microorganisms. In health, a balance exists between the host and that allows for the mutual survival and coexistence of both. This balance is best maintained when humans have operative Host Defense mechanism: i.e.

1. Intact skin.
2. A functional group of phagocytic cells consisting principally of RES; and
3. The ability to produce a humoral immune response.

Defects in any one, combination or all of these host defense mechanisms may shift the balance and predispose the host to the risk of developing an infectious process.

The normal flora is classified into the following:

1. **Resident Flora** are organisms that live on the skin and are relatively stable in number and composition at particular sites. Increase in their numbers results from multiplication of those already present and not due to addition from outside.
   e.g.: *Staph. epidermidis.*
2. **Transient Flora** are organisms that lie free on the skin surface without attachment and are derived from exogenous sources. They are unable to multiply on skin. They disappear from skin within a short time.
   e.g.: Gram (- ve) bacilli in perianal area and perineum (get contaminated from GIT).
   e.g.: *Staph. saprophyticus*-periurethral area.
3. **Temporary/Transient Residents or Associate Flora:** They colonize the skin of a small percentage of subjects in modest numbers for a somewhat longer time.
   e.g.: *Staph. aureus* in nose.

NORMAL FLORA OF THE SKIN

i. Bacteria

Aerobic

Gram +ve: *Cocci:* Staphylococci (*Staph. epidermidis Staph. hominis, Staph. capitis, Staph. saprophyticus) Micrococci (M. luteus, M varians, M lyrac*).

Bacilli: Corynebacteria (C. bovis, C. minutissimum, C. xerosus, C. hofmanni) Brevibacterium epidermidis, Propionibacteria (some species).

Gram –ve: Acinetobacter.

Anaerobic

Propionibacteria (*P. acnes, P. granulosum, P. avidum*).

II. Yeasts (Fungi)—Lipophilic

Malassezia furfur, *M. obtuse, M. pachydermatis, M. restricta.*

THE FLORA OF SPECIALISED AREAS

1. **The Nasal Vestibule:** 25-30% of healthy adults in the community harbor *S. aureus* in their anterior nares at any given time; 15% permanently and 15% transiently.
2. **External Auditory Canal:** Coagulase –ve staph., coryneforms, proteus, *E. coli, Neisseria catarrhalis* have been isolated in small but significant numbers from normal ears.
   Fungi include Aspergillus, Alternaria, Penicillium and Candida.
3. **Axilla:** Coryneforms, *P. acnes* is usually transient and *P. avidum* is often found.
4. **Toe Clefts:** Toe cleft is hyperhydrated and the skin macerated in shoe wearers. Brevibacterium sp., Acinetobacter, coliform and other organism of intestinal orgin.
5. **Umbilicus** of the newborn is frequently colonised by *Staph. aureus* shortly after birth. It may also be colonised by *Strep. pyogenes.*
6. **Perineum and Groin:** Coagulase -ve staph, Aerobic coliforms, Acinetobacter.
7. **Vulva:** Coag. –ve staph., Coliforms.
8. **Vagina:** Gram +ve bacillus–Doderleins bacillus which acts on the glycogen in the vaginal epithelial cells to produce lactic acids—responsible for acidity of the vaginal mucosa.

ADVANTAGES OF NORMAL FLORA

1. **Prevention of colonisation by potential pathogens.**
2. **Bacterial Interference**
   - Skin bacteria produce fatty acids which discourage other species from invading.
   - *P. acnes* and gram +ve cocci are capable of hydrolysing lipids of sebum to produce FFA.
   - Vaginal lactobacilli maintain an acid environment, with suppresses growth of other bacteria.
   - Adhere to epithelial binding site, thereby preventing the attatchment to that receptor site by a potential microbial pathogen.

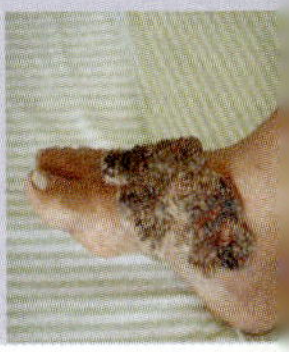

CLASSIFICATION OF PYODERMAS

Primary

- Impetigo.
- Ecthyma.
- Folliculitis
  - Superficial.
  - Deep.
- Furuncle, carbuncle.
- Erysipelas, cellulitis.
- Necrotising fascitis.

Secondary

- Secondary infection of preexisting dermatoses ***e.g.*** Eczema, Infestations, Ulcers.

Cutaneous Disease Due to Effects of Bacterial Toxins

- Staphylococcal scalded skin syndrome (SSS).
- Toxic shock syndrome.
- Scarlet fever.

SUSPECTED ORGANISMS

- **Impetigo:** *Group A Streptococcus, Staphylococcus aureus.*
- **Folliculitis:** *Staphylococcus aureus, Pseudomonas aeruginosa.*
- **Furuncles:** *Staphylococcus aureus.*
- **Carbuncles:** *Staphylococcus aureus.*
- **Cellulitis:** *Group A Streptococcus, Staphylococcus aureus, Haemophilus influenzae.*
- **Erysipelas:** *Group A Streptococcus.*
- **Necrotizing fasciitis:** *Group A Streptococcus, Clostridium perfringens* and other species, *Bacteroides fragilis,* Enterobacteriaceae, *Pseudomonas aeruginosa.*

BACTERIAL DISEASES

The predominant primary pathogens are the group *A Streptococci or Staphylococcus aureus*. The clinical pictures vary because of the host factors and the local anatomic infections.

STAPHYLOCOCCAL INFECTIONS

1. Impetigo (Streptococci and Staphylococci)

Two clinical types of impetigo occur. The *first type* is due to *group A Streptococci or a mixture of Streptococci and Staph. aureus.* It is a disease of young children in which blisters appear on the skin around the mouth. The vesicles and pustules easily rupture, forming a thick, soft, **golden-yellow "stuck on" crust, the hallmark of impetigo** (Fig. 2.8). The skin lesions may be complicated with deep cellulitis or bacteraemia. Glomerulonephritis may follow impetigo due to Streptococcus pyogenes.

The *second type* of impetigo is **bullous impetigo**, characterized by rapid progression of vesicles to flaccid large bullae (Fig. 2.9). The bullae eventually rupture, and form thin, light brown crusts (Fig. 2.10). This infection is frequently associated with Staph. aureus of phage group II.

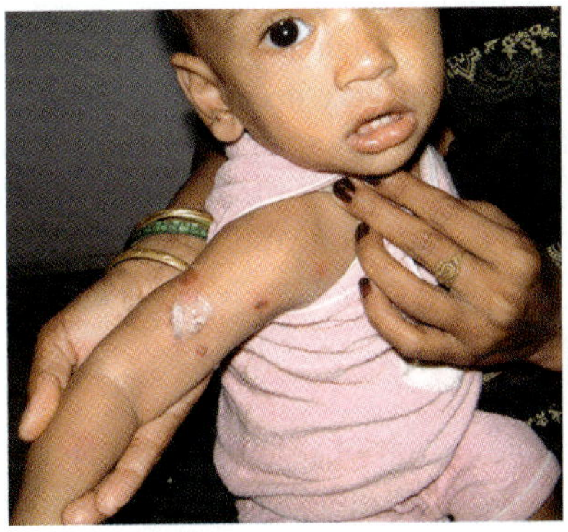

Fig. 2.8 : Yellow "stuck on" crust

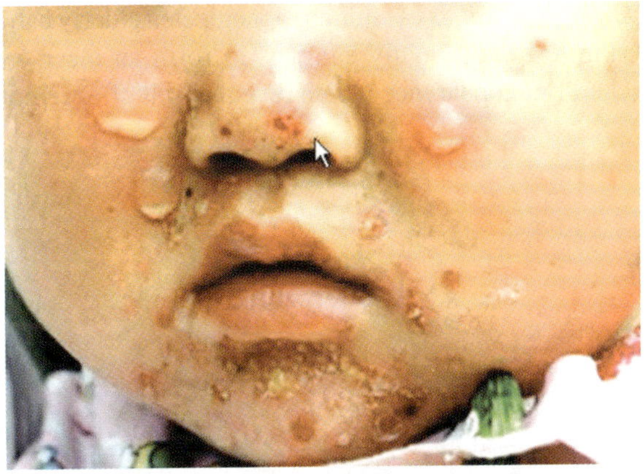

Fig. 2.9: Vesicles and bullae with yellow "stuck on" crust

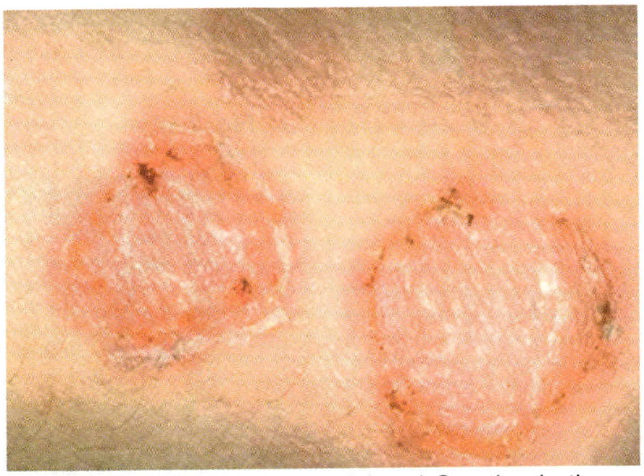

Fig. 2.10: Scaling and peripheral Crusting in the healing phase

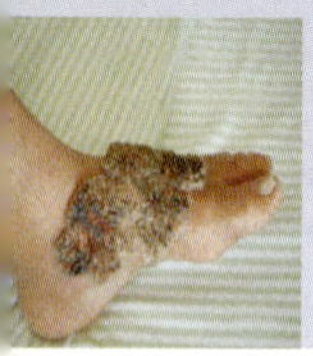

Investigation and Treatment

The diagnosis is usually made on clinical grounds. Swabs should be taken and sent to the laboratory for culture, but treatment must not be held up until the results are available.

Important:

- **ASLO** and **NADase** do not *correlate* with cutaneous *streptococcal* infection.
- **DNAase B** and **Hyaluronidase** *correlate* with streptococcal infection.

Systemic antibiotics (such as cloxacillin, erythromycin or cephalexin [cefalexin]) are needed for severe cases or if a nephritogenic strain of streptococcus is suspected (penicillin V). For minor cases the removal of crusts and a topical antibiotic such as neomycin, fusidic acid, mupirocin or bacitracin will suffice.

2. Ecthyma

It is a pyogenic infection of the skin characterized by the formation of adherent crust, beneath which an ulcer occurs.

It is caused by both streptococci and staphylococci Ecthyma initially presents as a vesicle or vesicopustule on the ***lower extremities*** of children or neglected elderly patients, the skin lesion gradually enlarges to form an ulcer with a punched-out appearance which reveals itself after removing the adherent crust (Fig. 2.11). This can heal with a **scar.** The level of involvement is deeper than impetigo (Fig. 2.12) Post-streptococcal glomerulonephritis is a known sequel.

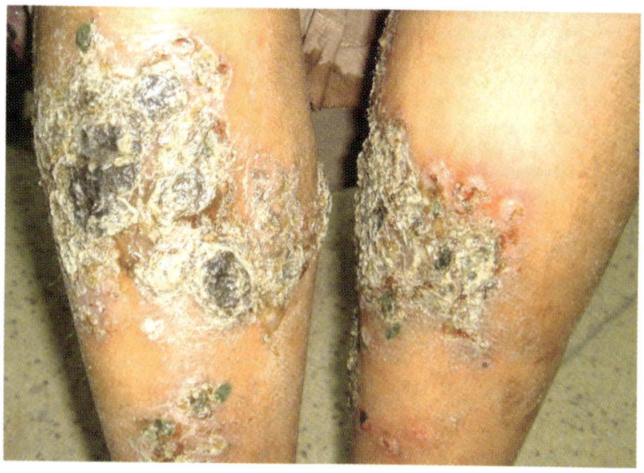

Fig. 2.11: Large plaque with adherent crust

3. Furuncles and Carbuncles

With the exception of carbuncles, these skin infections are uncomfortable and unsightly rather than serious. Furuncles or boils occur only in areas where there are hair follicles. The lesion is a deep-seated inflammatory nodule. It is tender, firm, red and fluctuant (Fig 2.13).

A carbuncle is a more extensive, deeper, infiltrated lesion and usually occurs at the nape of the neck (Fig. 2.14), the

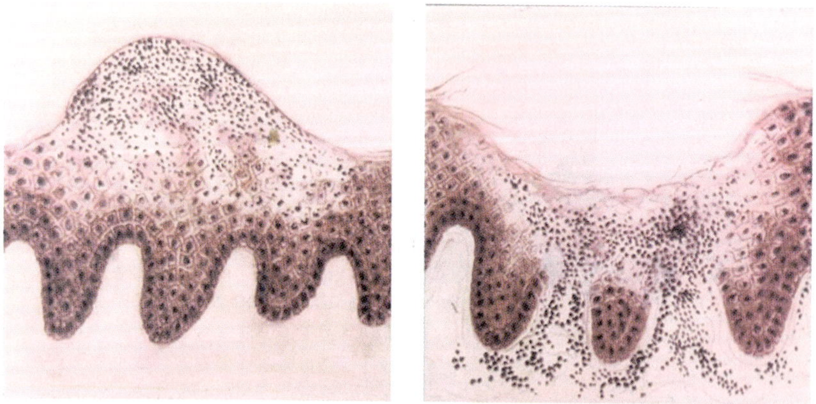

Impetigo

Ecthyma

Fig. 2.12

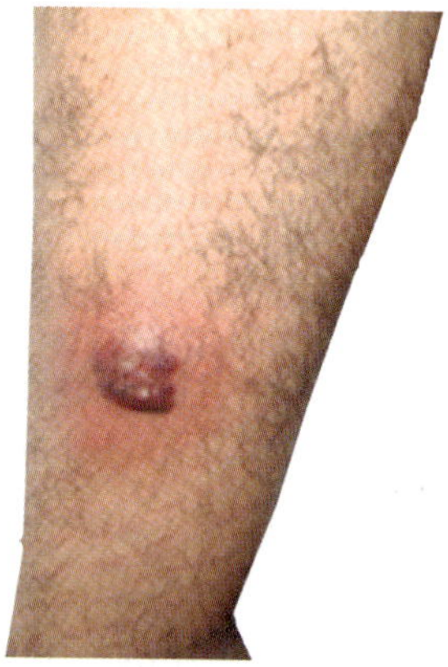

Fig. 2.13: Deep-seated inflammatory nodule (Furuncle)

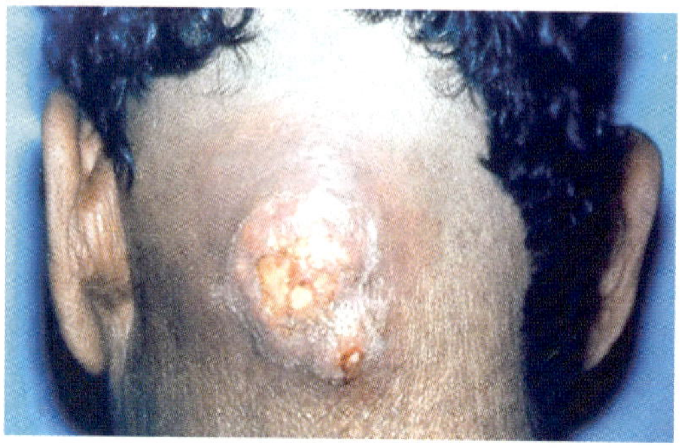

Fig. 2.14: Confluence of furuncle causes a carbuncle

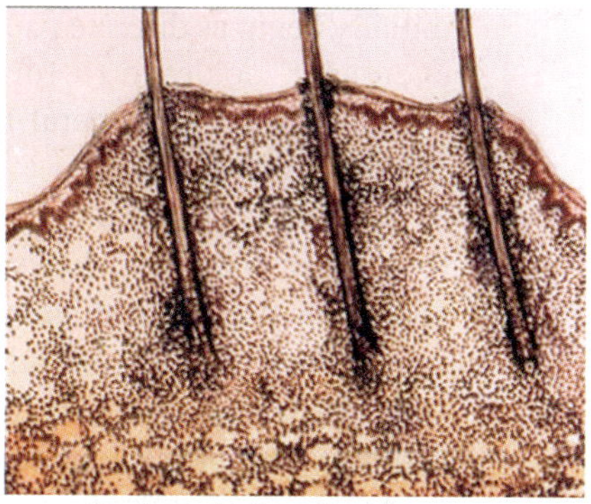

Carbuncle (coalescing of furuncle)

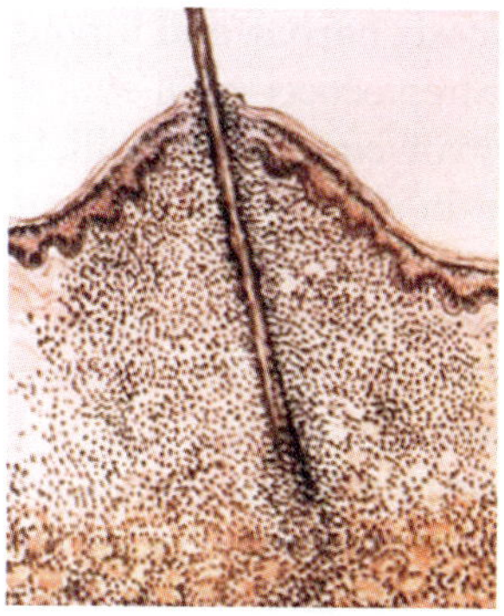

Furuncle (Follicular and perifollicular)

Fig. 2.15

back or thighs. Systemic symptoms such as fever and malaise are often present. All these lesions are caused by infection with staphylococcus aureus.

The difference between the two is that in a furuncle the involvement is follicular and perifollicular while in carbuncle multiple furuncles coalesce (Fig. 2.15).

Investigations in Chronic Furunculosis

- General examination: look for underlying skin disease (e.g. scabies, pediculosis, eczema).
- Test the urine for sugar. Full blood count.
- Culture swabs from lesions, and carrier sites (nostrils, perineum) of the patient and immediate family.
- Immunological evaluation only if the patient has recurrent or unusual internal infections too.

Treatment

Acute episodes will respond to an appropriate antibiotic; incision speeds healing. In chronic furunculosis, treat carrier sites such as the nose and perineum twice daily for 6 weeks with an appropriate topical antiseptic or antibiotic (e.g. chlorhexidine solution, mupirocin cream or clindamycin solution). Treat family carriers in the same way. Treat lesions with a topical antibiotic. In stubborn cases add 6 weeks of a systemic antibiotic chosen to cover organism's proven sensitivities.

4. Folliculitis

Infectious	*Non-infectious*
Gram positive	Pseudofolliculitis barbae
Gram negative	Acne keloidalis nuchae
Pseudomonal	Eosinophilic folliculitis
Pityrosporum	
Herpetic	

Gram Positive

This is an acute, small, painful pustular eruption of hair follicles. There are two main subtypes: **Superficial (Fig. 2.16) and deep (Fig. 2.17).**

- **Bockhart's impetigo is a superficial folliculitis**. Small, dome-shaped pustule develops at the opening of a hair follicle surrounded by erythema. It usually occurs on the limbs and the scalp.
  - Another type of superficial folliculitis caused by staphylococci is a stye, which differs in that it occurs on the eyelid.

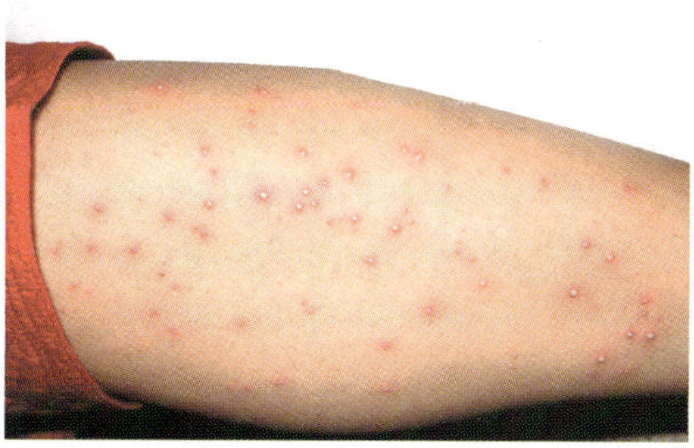

Fig. 2.16: Superficial folliculitis

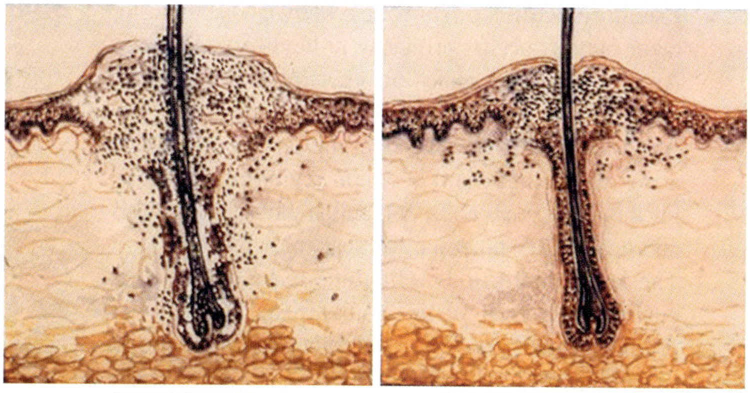

Deep folliculitis

Superficial folliculitis

Fig. 2.17: Different levels of involvement in superficial and deep folliculitis

– **Deep folliculitis include sycosis barbae and lupoid sycosis.** Staphylococcal or Streptococci are the most common pathogens. When involvement of the follicle is more extensive, resulting in a follicular centered dermal abscess, and the condition occurs on the face, it is then referred to as **sycosis barbae (vulgaris).** If the follicles are destroyed with clinically evident scarring the term **lupoid sycosis** is applied.

- **Gram-negative folliculitis** primarily occurs in patients on long-term antibiotic therapy, often those given for the treatment of acne. This type of folliculitis arises from disequilibrium of the normal skin bacteria in favor of gram-negative organisms such as *Enterobacter, Klebsiella, Escherichia, Serratia,* and *Proteus* species. These lesions manifest as multiple small pustules that are most pronounced in the perinasal region and can spread to the chin and cheeks.
- **Pseudomonal folliculitis** is another gram-negative folliculitis and is also known as hot tub (spa) folliculitis and wet suit folliculitis.
  – It is easily contracted from poorly maintained whirlpools or jacuzzis. The clinical presentation is similar to streptococcal or staphylococcal folliculitis. However, the patient may feel unwell, with a low grade fever and lymphadenopathy.
- **Pityrosporum folliculitis** is typically seen in young adults, with a slight female predominance, as intensively pruritic small uniform papules and pustules on the back, chest and shoulders.
- **Herpetic:** An uncommon form of folliculitis occurs due to an infection **with herpes viruses.** This form of folliculitis can be caused by an infection by herpes simplex viruses 1 and 2 and is found in areas adjacent to a primary cold sore, spread by shaving. These lesions appear as grouped or scattered vesicles.
- **Non-infectious:** Folliculitis can also have **a noninfectious** etiology caused by follicular trauma or occlusion or may simply be idiopathic.
  – **Pseudofolliculitis barbae**, also known as shaving or razor bumps, occurs primarily in the bearded area of African American males or other racial groups with thick, coarse, curly hair.
  – **Acne keloidalis nuchae** is a similar condition that arises on the neck and occipital region of the scalp, but this condition is both a folliculitis and peri-folliculitis and has greater potential for scarring.
  – The last noninfectious folliculitis to be discussed **is eosinophilic folliculitis**. It manifests as intensely pruritic pustules in at least 3 different clinical situations, as follows:
    ♦ The original description of eosinophilic folliculitis, also know as **Ofuji disease**, arose in Japanese males aged an average of 30 years. The lesions initially begin as discrete papules and pustules that eventually coalesce to form circinate plaques composed of a peripheral rim of pustules with central clearing.
    ♦ A second form of eosinophilic folliculitis is found to arise in patients who have **AIDS** and other conditions that result in immunosuppression. This form is seen most often in adult males with a CD_4^+ count of less than 300 cells/mL. It is persistent and does not form an annular pattern. The lesions tend to occur over the face, scalp and upper trunk.
    ♦ The last form of eosinophilic folliculitis occurs in infants, usually within the first 24 hours to first few weeks of life.

5. Ritter's Disease

Staphylococcal Scalded Skin Syndrome (SSSS)

In this condition the skin changes resemble a scald. Erythema and tenderness are followed by the loosening of large areas of overlying epidermis (Fig. 2.18).

In children the condition is usually caused by a staphylococcal infection elsewhere (e.g. impetigo or conjunctivitis) which releases toxin (exfoliatin) that causes a split to occur high in the epidermis.

This is in contrast to toxic epidermal necrolysis, which is usually drug-induced. The damage to the epidermis in toxic epidermal necrolysis is full thickness, and a skin biopsy will distinguish it from the scalded skin syndrome.

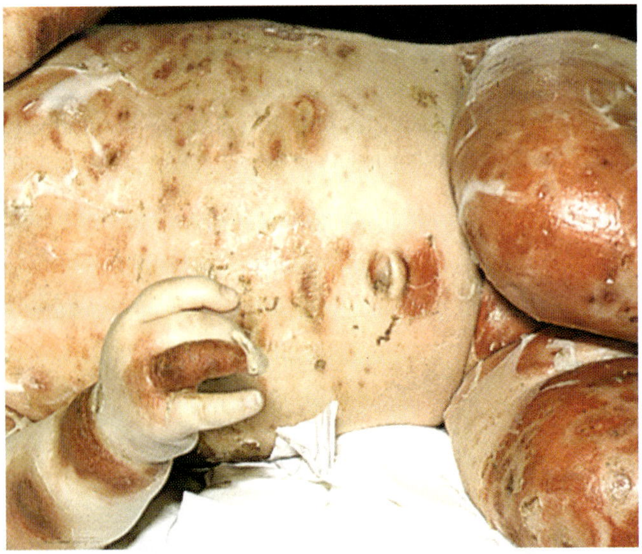

Fig. 2.18: Flaccid blisters, extensive erosions mimic an appearance of TEN (staphylococcal scalded-skin syndrome)

6. Toxic Shock Syndrome

A staphylococcal toxin **(TSST-1)** is also responsible for this condition, in which fever, a rash (that leads to a widespread erythema) and sometimes circulatory collapse are followed a week or two later by characteristic desquamation, most marked on the fingers and hands.

Many cases have followed staphylococcal overgrowth in the vagina of women using tampons.

STREPTOCOCCAL INFECTIONS

1. Erysipelas

A spreading infection most commonly due to Group A and B Streptococci presenting with a characteristic brawny, edematous, indurated and well demarcated appearance (Fig. 2.19). The patient may be acutely ill with high fever and toxaemia. Predisposing factors include alcohol abuse, diabetes mellitus, immunosuppression, venous or lymphatic obstruction.

2. Acute Cellulitis

This is an acute, spreading infection of subcutaneous tissue. There are two main bacteriological forms. The acute pyogenic cellulitis is usually due to *group A Streptococci and Staph. aureus*. It presents as a markedly red, hot, infiltrated edematous skin lesion and the borders are usually ill-defined thus differentiating it from erysipelas.

Lymphangitis and lymphadenitis involving local draining lymph glands are frequently found. The second form is the anaerobic cellulitis which is relatively rare and is usually due to a synergistic infection with both aerobic and anaerobic bacteria. The causal organisms include aerobes *(coliforms, Pseudomonas aeruginosa, staph. aureus)* and anaerobes (bacteriodes, anaerobic cocci).

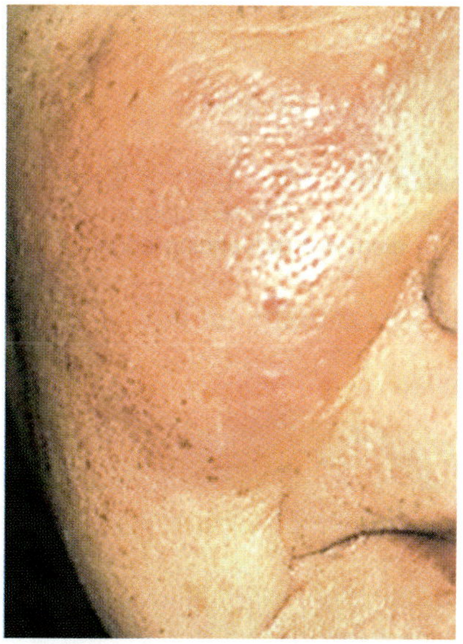

Fig. 2.19: Brawny, edematous, indurated red plaque (Erysipelas)

3. Necrotizing Fasciitis

This infection usually occurs on the lower extremities, abdominal wall, perineum and operative wounds. It is caused by streptococci and by anaerobes. The infective-ischaemic process spreads along the fascial plane causing extensive necrosis while the external appearance of the skin remains normal initially. So the damage is more extensive than the extent of the overlying skin involvement (Fig. 2.20). The involved area is swollen, red, warm and painful initially followed by infarctions and by purplish discoloration of overlying skin. Crepitus is often present. The patient is severely ill with fever and septic shock may occur.

4. Scarlet Fever

- 3 toxins A,B,C.
- **B** is more common.
- **Pastia** lines are seen on the skin folds because of petechiae. Strawberry tongue is characteristic.

MANAGEMENT OF STAPHYLOCOCCAL AND STREPTOCOCCI INFECTIONS

1. General Skin Care.

2. Local Measures

- Immobilization and elevation of the involved area to reduce local trauma.
- Cool, sterile saline dressing daily.

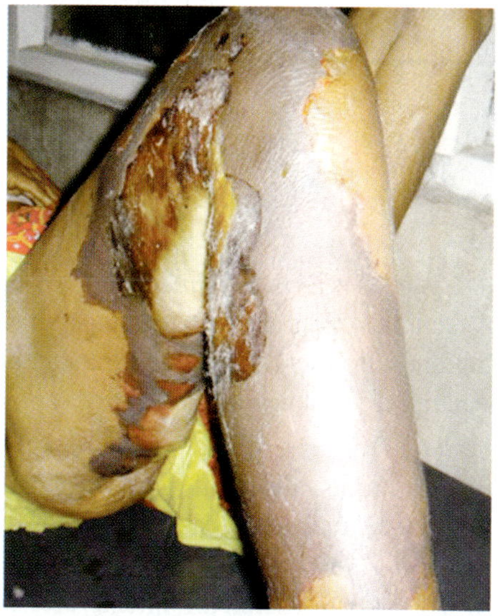

Fig. 2.20: Fascial plane involvement with necrosis

- Extensive debridement and grafting may be required for the necrotic areas.
- Mupirocin or bacitracin ointment.

3. Specific Measures

In mild cases, topical antibiotics are adequate for treatment. In widespread and severe situation, systemic antibiotics are indicated. Penicillin G, Penicillin V, and erythromycin are good antibiotics for both the streptococcal and staphylococcal infection.

Special measures should be aimed at elimination of nasal and skin carriage of *Staph. aureus*. This include the use of:

a. Local antibiotic ointment such as fusidic acid ointment in the nasal vestibule.
b. Intranasal application of mupirocin ointment.
c. Topical application of chlorhexidine or povidone iodine to eradicate *Staph. aureus* harbouring in body folds before bathing.
d. Oral antibiotics such as rifampicin.

TOXIN MEDIATED SYNDROMES

- **Streptococci pyogenes**

Pyrogen Toxin	• Scarlet Fever • Toxic Shock Syndrome

- **Staphylococcal aureus**

TSSToxin - I	Toxic Shock Syndrome
Exfoliatin Toxin	Bullous Impetigo, Staphylococcal Scalded Shock Syndrome, Scarlet fever, Recalcitrant Erythematous Desquamative Disorder (REDD).

OTHER INFECTIONS

ZOONOTIC

Erysipeloid

The causative organism is *Erysipelothrix insidiosa*. It infects a wide range of animals, birds and fish. In humans, infections are most common in butchers, fishmongers and cooks, the organisms penetrating the skin after a prick from an infected bone.

Such infections are usually mild, and localized to the area around the inoculation site. The swollen purple area spreads slowly with a clear-cut advancing edge (Fig. 2.21). With penicillin the condition clears quickly; without it, resolution takes several weeks.

Cat-Scratch Disease

The infective agent is the bacillus *Rochalimaea henselae*. A few days after a cat bite or scratch, a reddish granulomatous papule appears at the site of inoculation. Tender regional lymphadenopathy (Fig. 2.22) follows some weeks later, and lasts for several weeks, often being accompanied by a mild fever.The glands may discharge before settling spontaneously. There is no specific treatment.

Differential Diagnosis

Cat-scratch disease can be distinguished from cutaneous anthrax in the following manner:

Cat-scratch disease	*Cutaneous anthrax*
• Patient has had contact with cats • Occurrence is in fall or winter • Primary lesion is a papule or vesicle • Lymph node histopathology is characteristic of the disease	• Ulcer and eschar are surrounded by characteristic non-pitting edema

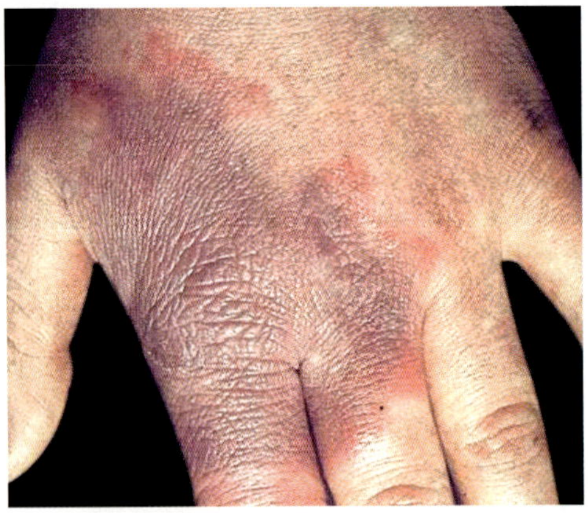

Fig. 2.21: Swollen red plaque with a clear-cut advancing edge

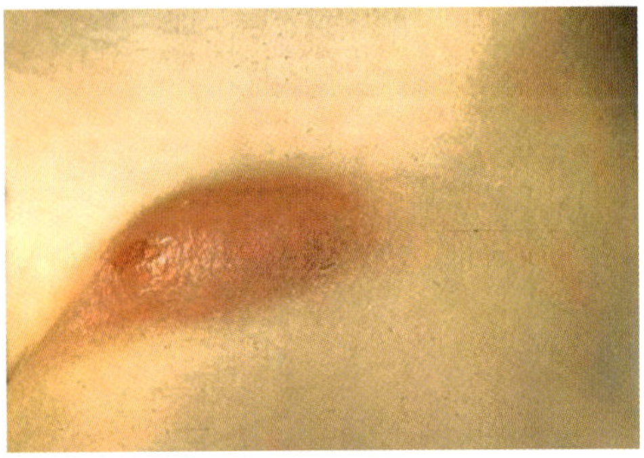

Fig. 2.22: Tender LN enlarged in the inguinal area

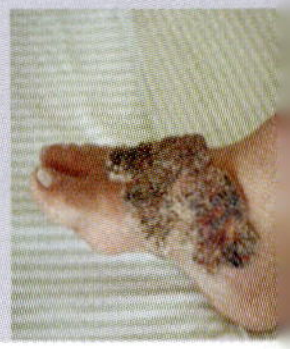

Cutaneous Anthrax

Caused by *Bacillus anthracis* a gram-positive, spore-forming bacillus that derives its name from the Greek word for coal or charcoal, *anthrakos.*

Clinical Features

In more than 95% of cases of endemic disease, spores are transmitted from infected animals or their products by means of skin abrasions (Fig. 2.23).

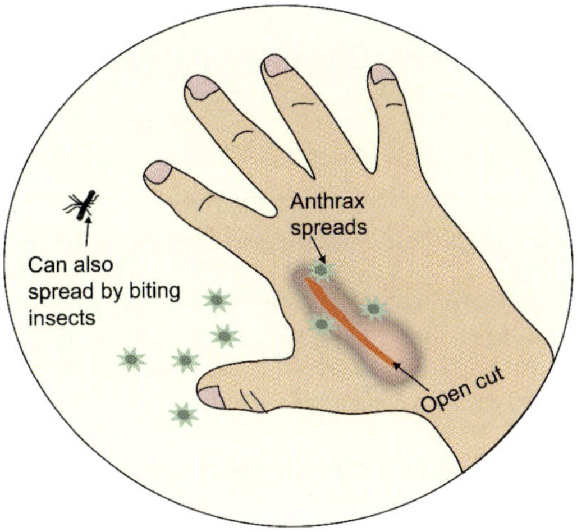

Fig. 2.23: Skin abrasions

The lesions of cutaneous anthrax have a predictable course. After a variable latency period (range, 1-12 d; mean, 5 d), a pruritic macule or papule appears at the site of inoculation. The primary lesion progresses to a vesicle or a bulla after 24-48 hours. The bulla enlarges to 1-2 cm, spontaneously ruptures, and forms an ulcer. A hemorrhagic crust develops and is often accompanied by striking edema (which is worse on the face), erythema and satellite vesicles (Fig. 2.24).The entire process is painless. Regional adenopathy, low-grade fever, and malaise often occur within 3-4 days after the primary lesion appears.

The crust develops into a thick, adherent, brown-black, painless, nontender eschar surrounded by a warm, red, edematous, indurated base. The eschar dries and detaches in 1-2 weeks (Fig. 2.25) and reportedly leaves little residual scarring. Edema and painlessness are features that help in differentiating anthrax from other diseases, such as a brown recluse spider bite or ulceroglandular tularemia.

In the absence of antibiotic treatment, 80-90% of lesions heal spontaneously, but 10-20% progress, with resultant malignant edema, septicemia, shock, renal failure and death.

The skin lesions progress despite the administration of antibiotics, which only sterilize the lesion and do not block the effects of the toxins (Table 2.4).

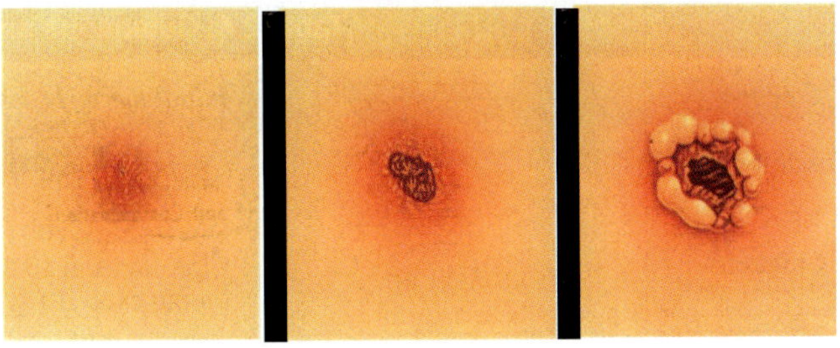

Fig. 2.24: Stages of cutaneous anthrax

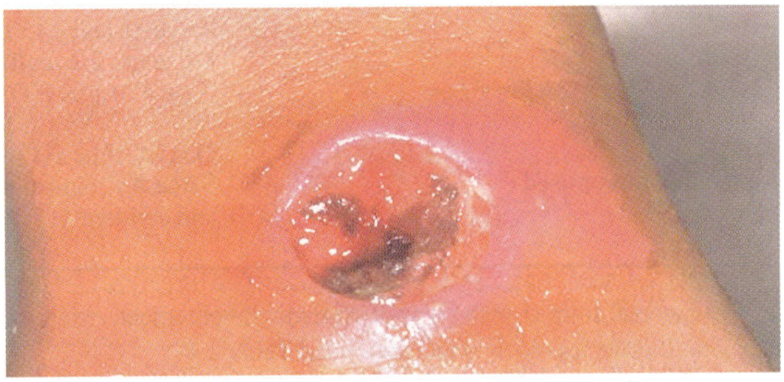

Fig. 2.25: A deep ulcer which follows removal of adherent eschar

MISCELLANEOUS BACTERIAL INFECTIONS

Ecthyma Gangrenosum

Ecthyma gangrenosum (EG) is a well-recognized cutaneous infection most commonly associated with a *Pseudomonas aeruginosa* bacteremia. EG usually occurs in patients who are critically ill and immunocompromised. The characteristic lesions of EG are hemorrhagic pustules or infarcted-appearing areas with surrounding erythema that evolve into necrotic ulcers surrounded by erythema.

Aetiopathogenesis

- EG typically occurs in patients who are immunocompromised, including patients with hematologic malignancies, immunodeficiency syndromes, severe burns, malnutrition, recent chemotherapy, immunosuppressive therapy, and diabetes mellitus.
- Breakdown of mechanical defense barriers increases susceptibility to pseudomonal or fungal infections.

Clinical Features

Primary lesions of EG initially appear as painless round erythematous macules that rapidly become pustular with surrounding erythema. A hemorrhagic focus appears in the center, forming a bulla. As the hemorrhagic bulla spreads peripherally, it evolves into a gangrenous ulcer with black/gray eschar surrounded by an erythematous halo. The

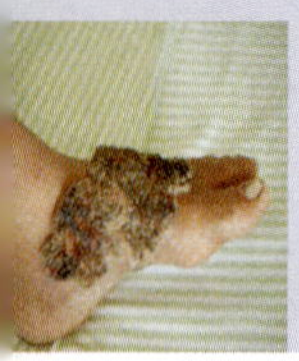

Table 2.4: Cutaneous anthrax treatment protocol*

Category	*Initial therapy (oral)**	*Duration*
Adults*	Ciprofloxacin 500 mg BID or Doxycycline 100 mg BID	60 days¥
Children*	Ciprofloxacin 10-15 mg/kg every 12 hours (not to exceed 1 g/day)† or Doxycycline: >8 years and >45 kg: 100 mg every 12 hours 8> years and <45 kg: 2.2. mg/kg every 12 hours <8 years: 2.2 mg/kg every 12 hrs	60 days¥
Pregnant women**	Ciprofloxacin 500 mg BID or Doxycycline 100 mg BID	60 days¥
Immunocompromised persons*	Same for non-immunocompromised persons and children	60 days¥

* Cutaneous anthrax with signs of systemic involvement, extensive edema, or lesions on the head or neck require intravenous therapy, and a multidrug approach is recommended Table 2.4.

† Ciprofloxacin or doxycyclin should be considered first-line therapy. Amoxicillin 500 mg po TID for adults or 80 mg/kg/day divided every 8 hours for children is an option for completion of therapy after clinical improvement. Oral amoxicillin dose is based on the need to achieve appropriate minimum inhibitory concentration levels.

¥ Previous guidelines have suggested treating cutaneous anthrax for 7-10 days, but 60 days is recommended in the setting of this, given the likelihood of exposure to aerosolized B anthracis.

** Although tetracyclines or ciprofloxacin are not recommended during pregnancy, their use may be indicated for life-threatening illness. Adverse effects on developing teeth and bones are dose related; therefore, doxycycline might be used for a short time (7-14 days) before 6 months of gestation.

transformation of an early lesion to a necrotic ulcer may occur in as little as 12 hours.

Treatment

Treatment of EG requires the use of antipseudomonal penicillins, aminoglycosides, fluoroquinolones, third-generation cephalosporins, or aztreonam. While awaiting results, an antipseudomonal penicillin (piperacillin) should be used in conjunction with an aminoglycoside (gentamicin).

Systemic antifungal coverage should be considered if fungemia is suspected, including coverage against *Aspergillus, Candida* and *Mucor* species with azole agents (e.g., voriconazole, fluconazole) and/or amphotericin B if appropriate.

CORYNEBACTERIUM UP

1. Trichomycosis Axillaris

This is a common condition, seen, if looked for, in upto one-quarter of adult males. The axillary hairs become **beaded** with concretions, usually **yellow,** made up of colonies of commensal diphtheroids (Fig. 2.26). Clothing becomes stained in the armpits. Topical antibiotic ointments, or shaving, will clear the condition.

2. Pitted Keratolysis

The combination of unusually sweaty feet and occlusive shoes encourages the growth of diphtheroid organisms that can digest keratin. The result is a **cribriform pattern** of

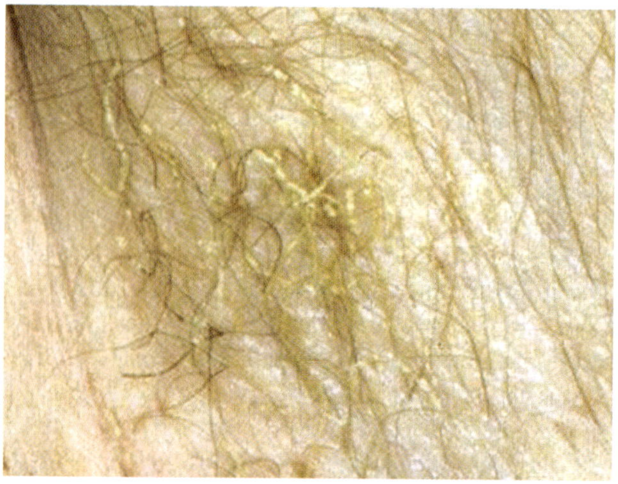

Fig. 2.26: Axillary hair with yellow concretions

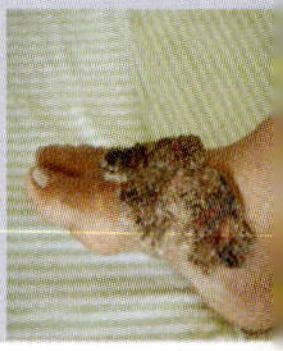

punched-out depressions on the plantar surface (Fig. 2.27), coupled with an unpleasant smell (of methanethiol). Fusidic acid, mupirocin ointment or clotrimazole are effective. Occlusive footwear should be replaced by sandals and cotton socks if possible.

3. Erythrasma

Erythrasma is a superficial bacterial skin infection due to *Corynebacterium minutissimum***.** The lesions are reddish-brown, scaly and finely wrinkled macular patches, usually involve the intertriginuous areas (Fig. 2.28). Axillary and genitocrural areas are commonly involved. The diagnosis is supported by the characteristic **"coral-red"** fluorescence under wood's light.

Treatment

1. Oral erythromycin 250 mg QID for 1 week. The lesions usually clear within several weeks.
2. Topical therapy includes aqueous clindamycin solution, Whitfield's ointment or miconazole cream.

Malakoplakia

Malakoplakia is an inflammatory condition presenting as a plaque or a nodule that usually affects the genitourinary tract but may rarely involve the skin. Malakoplakia was first described in the early 1900s as yellow soft plaques that were seen on the mucosa of the urinary bladder. Microscopically, malakoplakia is characterized by the presence of foamy histiocytes with distinctive basophilic inclusions, which are known as **Michaelis-Gutmann bodies** (Fig. 2.29).

Cutaneous malakoplakia is rare but presents in patients who are immunocompromised and have defects in macrophage function. Lesions are yellow-to-pink papules, but they can present as nodules or ulcerations and are often diagnosed only after biopsy. Cultures of the lesions can yield bacteria, most commonly *Escherichia coli*.

Progressive Bacterial Synergistic Gangrene

This infection is a gangrenous ulceration of the skin due to a mixed bacterial flora. It usually follows abdominal or thoracic infection or trauma. A small, painful, superficial ulcer develops and gradually enlarges to form a ulcer with a rim of gangrenous skin.

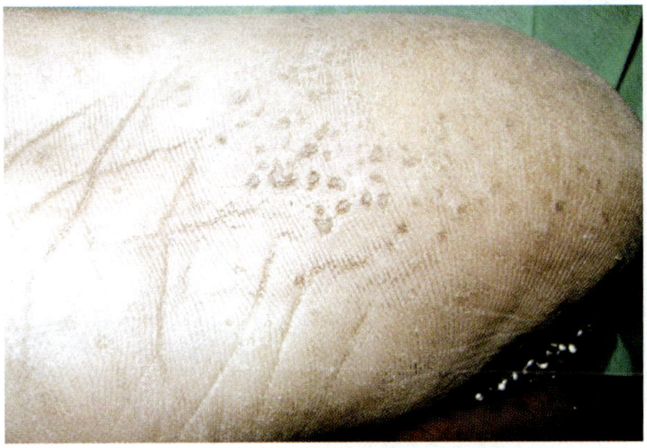

Fig. 2.27: Cribriform pattern of fine punched-out depressions on the plantar surface (Pitted keratolysis)

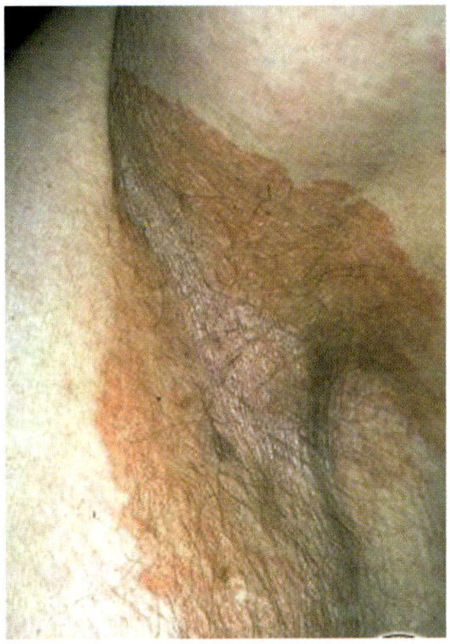

Fig. 2.28: Reddish-brown, scaly and finely wrinkled macular patches (Erythrasma)

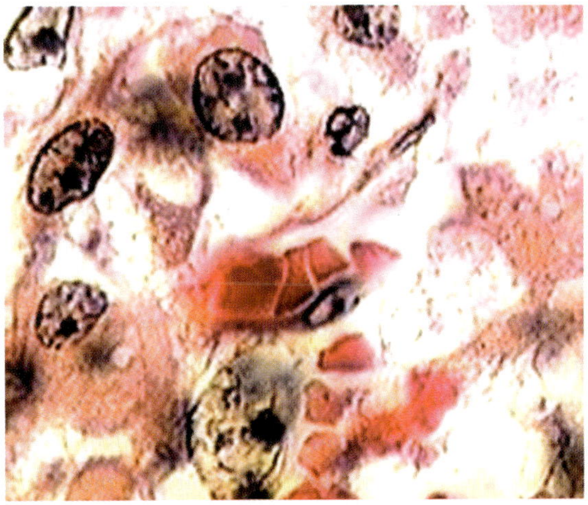

Fig. 2.29: Foamy histiocytes with distinctive basophilic inclusions (Malakoplakia)

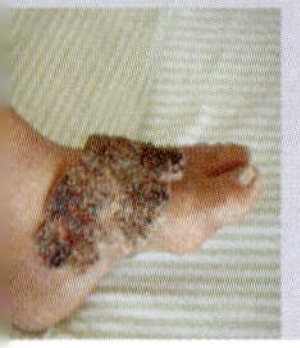

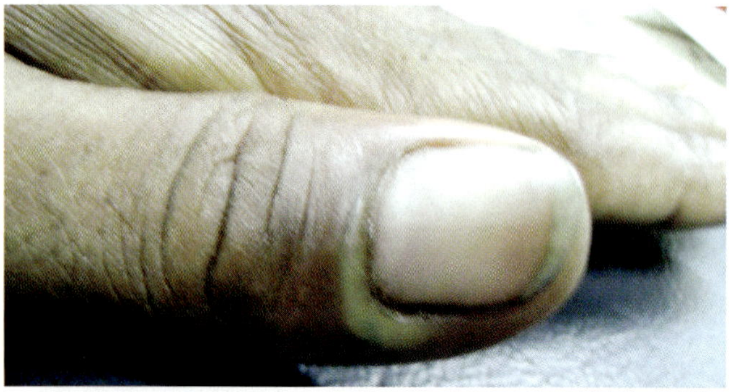

Fig. 2.30: Acute paronychia

Paronychia

Acute erythematous swelling of proximal and/or lateral nail fold which is painful and may be followed by pus formation (Fig. 2.30).

Actinomycosis

Definition: It is a subacute, chronic, cellulitic invasion of the soft tissues that causes the formation of external sinus tracts that discharge sulfur granules. This process spreads unimpeded by traditional anatomic barriers after the endogenous oral commensal organisms invade the tissues of the face and neck.

Aetiology

Usually, the disease is caused by *Actinomyces israelii,* an anaerobic gram-positive organisms that enters the tissue through a break in the mucosa.

A israelii, Actinomyces naeslundii, Actinomyces viscosus, and *Actinomyces odontolyticus*. Because of the derivative term mycosis, some believe that actinomycosis is a fungal infection, although it is not a fungal infection. Aktino referred to the radiating organism in the sulfur granule as ray fungus.

Clinical Features

- The **cervicofacial** form of actinomycetes infection is the most common presentation of actinomycosis, occurring in 55% of patients.
- GI ingestion of the organism leads to the **abdominopelvic form,** which affects approximately 20% of patients.
- Tracheobronchial aspiration of the organism from the oral cavity leads to the **pulmonothoracic** presentation, which occurs in 15% of patients.
- **Primary Cutaneous Type:** Rare.

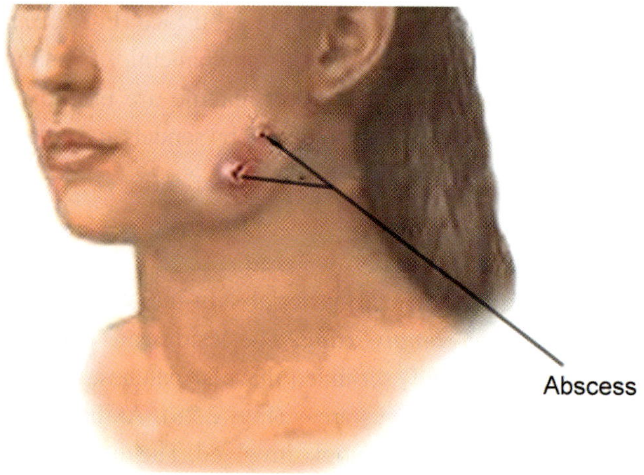

Fig. 2.31: Cervicofacial actinomycosis

The most common feature of actinomycosis infection is the presence of acute pyogenic infection in the submandibular or paramandibular area, in the angle of the mandible, in the parotid region, or in the neck (Fig. 2.31).

Treatment

- If recognized early, cervicofacial infection has an excellent prognosis with the use of antibiotics alone. In the treatment of this infection, tetracyclines are as effective as penicillin. Intravenous penicillin G (10-20 million U/d for 2-6 weeks) followed by oral penicillin (2-4 g/d for an additional 3-12 months) is the typical therapy for the most deep-seated infections.
- When tuberculosis is suspected, the effects of rifampin therapy can mask the signs of undiagnosed pulmonary actinomycosis.
- Because the bacterial species do not vary in terms of their susceptibility to first-line drugs (e.g., penicillin, tetracyclines, erythromycin, first-generation parenteral cephalosporins, clindamycin), infection with strains other than *A israelii* should also respond to adequate courses of treatment with penicillin G or any of its alternatives. Serum concentrations of sulfonamides (4-8 mg/dL) inhibit some strains of *A israelii*; therefore, proven cases of actinomycosis (that are not mistaken instances of nocardiosis) may occasionally respond to sulfonamides.

Surgical Care

Surgical management has consisted of various treatment modalities, including excision of sinus tracts, drainage of the abscess cavities, removal of the bulky infected masses, and irrigation and curettage of the osteomyelitic bony lesions.

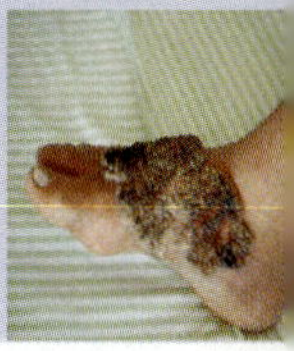

Nocardiosis

Nocardiosis is an infection caused by several species of soil-borne aerobic bacteria belonging to the genus *Nocardia*. Similar to anaerobic organisms of the genus *Actinomyces*, *Nocardia* species often form thin filaments that can resemble but are much thinner than those of true fungi (1-2 μm vs 3-5 μm in diameter).

Clinical Features

Nocardiosis can be divided into 2 broad categories, disseminated and cutaneous.

Disseminated Nocardiosis

Disseminated nocardiosis is responsible for most occurrences of nocardiosis, is most commonly caused by *Nocardia asteroides*, and typically affects immunocompromised hosts, although individuals with presumed immunocompetency also can develop the disease.

Primary Cutaneous Nocardiosis

Primary cutaneous nocardiosis, most commonly caused by *Nocardia brasiliensis*, typically affects immunocompetent individuals with a history of trauma and can be subdivided into 3 clinical entities that include (1) lymphocutaneous infection, (2) mycetoma, and (3) superficial skin infection, including ulceration, abscess and cellulitis.

Lymphocutaneous Nocardiosis

Lymphocutaneous nocardiosis is rare and often misdiagnosed as sporotrichosis (more common) because it also manifests as a primary lesion at the site of injury, followed by a proximal spread of lymphangitis and nodular lesions along the lymphatics. The lymphocutaneous or sporotrichoid form is the least common form of primary cutaneous nocardiosis.

Treatment

Most patients with primary cutaneous nocardiosis require antibiotic therapy to resolve the infection. Recommendations regarding the duration of therapy range from 2-3 months for most cutaneous infections to 1 year for chronic cutaneous and systemic infections. TMP-SMZ is used most frequently for nocardiosis.

Surgical Care

Surgical debridement or excision often is vital in the treatment of nocardiosis.

REFERENCES

- Rook's Textbook of Dermatology, 7th edition.
- Fitzpatrick's Dermatolgy in General Medicine, 6th edition.

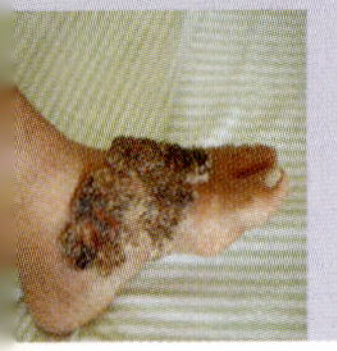

Superficial Cutaneous and Deep Mycoses

Human Fungal Infections

- **A. Superficial**
  - **Surface**
    - T. versicolor
    - T. nigra
    - Piedra
  - **Cutaneous**
    - Dermatophytosis
    - Candidiasis
    - Non-dermatophytic infection of skin and nails
- **B. Deep**
  - **Subcutaneous**
    - Mycetoma
    - Sporotrichosis
    - Chromoblastomycosis
  - **Systemic**
    - Cryptococcosis
    - Histoplasmosis
    - Candidiasis

LAB DIAGNOSIS

- **KOH**: Readily available and provides immediate diagnosis in the clinic at minimal cost.
  Hyphae: Fungal infections.
  Pseudohyphae or yeast forms: *Candida* or *Pityrosporum* infections.
- Stains may be beneficial for diagnosis (Paragon multiple stain, hematoxylin and eosin stain, Chlorazol fungal stain, Swartz lamkins fungal stain, Parker's blue ink).
- **Wood's Light** is used to rule out erythrasma or other differential diagnoses. It is inexpensive but not readily available. *Microsporum* spp. fluoresce green. Unfortunately *Trichophyton* spp. usually do not fluoresce in Wood's light.
  Blue-green fluorescence: Presence of *Microsporum audouinii and M. canis* (tinea capitis).
  Coral-red fluorescence: Presence of *Corynebacterium minutissimum* (erythrasma).
  Pale yellow fluorescence: *Malassezia furfur* (pityriasis versicolor).
- Fungal culture to identify the causative species. It is expensive, may take 2-4 weeks, and requires special fungal media to inhibit contaminants.

SURFACE INFECTIONS

1. **TINEA VERSICOLOR/PITYRIASIS VERSICOLOR**
   - Characterized by scaly hypo- or hyperpigmented irregular macules on trunk and proximal extremities.
   - **Causative agent—*Malassezia furfur.***

Treatment-Topical	- Selenium sulfide 2.5%
	- Zinc pyrithione 1%
	- Ketoconazole 2% shampoo
	- Topical imidazole, allyl amines
	- Keratolytics
	- Sodium hypo sulfite
	- Propylene glycol
	- Retinoic acid cream
Systemic	- Ketoconazole 200 mg × 7 days
	- Itraconazole 200 mg × 7-14 days
	- Fluconazole 400 mg one stat.

2. **TINEA NIGRA**
   - Asymptomatic deeply pigmented macular, non-scaly patchs over skin of palms.
     Causative agent: ***Phaeoannellomyces werneckii.***

Treatment
- Topical azoles.
- Benzoic acid ointment.
- Thiabendazole 10% suspension.

3. **PIEDRA**
   - Asymptomatic fungal infection of hair shaft (Figs. 2.33 and 2.34).
   - **Black piedra:** Caused by *Piedra hortae* characterized by presence of firmly adherent, black gritty hard nodules on hair shaft.
   - **White piedra:**
     - Capital: Caused by *Trichosporum ovoides*.
     - Crural: Caused by *T. inkin, T. asahii, T. mucoides*.

   Treatment: Shaving off the hair.
   Topical antifungal therapy.

CUTANEOUS INFECTIONS

Dermatophytosis

- Dermatophytes are moulds belonging to three asexual genera distinguished by morphology of macroconidia – Microsporum, Trichophyton, Epidermophyton.
- According to source of infection—Geophilic, Zoophilic, Anthropophilic.
- Invade only keratinized layer of epidermis, nails and hair.

Clinical Types

- Tinea capitis
- Tinea corporis
- Tinea barbae
- Tinea **facei**
- Tinea cruris
- Tinea pedis
- Tinea mannum
- Tinea unguium
- Tinea incognito (steroid modified tinea)
- Dermatophytid reactions.

TINEA CAPITIS

Classified according to clinical types and mode of infection.

Mode of Infection (Fig. 2.35)

1. Ectothrix—Hyphae are outside the hair shaft (Fig. 2.36) Wood's light green hue.

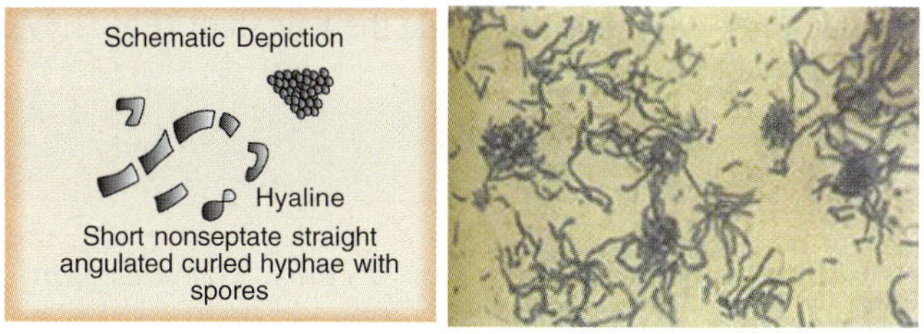

Fig. 2.32: Microscopically—spaghetti and meat ball appearance

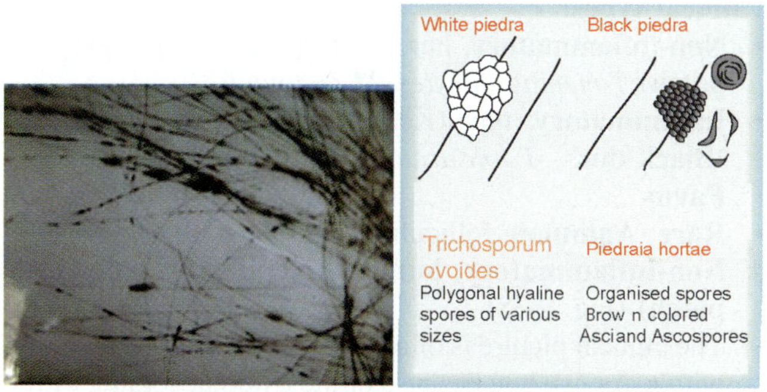
White piedra
Black piedra
Trichosporum ovoides
Polygonal hyaline spores of various sizes
Piedraia hortae
Organised spores
Brow n colored
Asci and Ascospores

Fig. 2.33: Clinical and line diagram of piedra

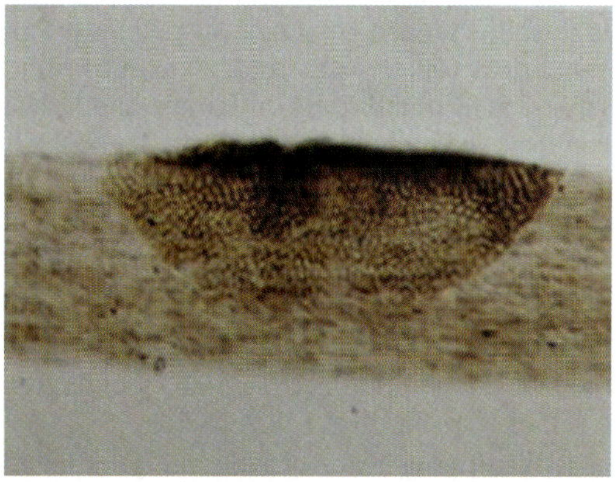

Fig. 2.34: KOH–showing spores and hyphae characteristic of piedra

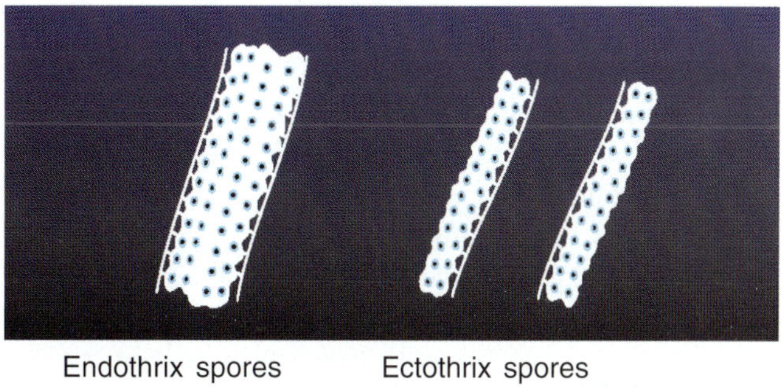

Fig. 2.35: Schematic depiction of morphology of various fungi in superficial mycosus invading the hair

2. Endothrix—Hyphae are inside the hair shaft (Fig. 2.37). Wood's light negative.
3. Favus—Special variant.

Species

- **Ectothrix–***T mentagrophytes, M canis, T verrucosum.*
- **Endothrix–***T tonsurans, T violaceum.*
- **Favus–T schoenleinii.**
- Most common type in USA—*T tonsurans.*
- Most common type in India—*T violaceum.*

Clinical types:

- **Non-inflammatory**, human or epidemic type **(grey patch)** *T mentagrophytes, M audouinii.*
- **Inflammatory** type (Kerion)—*M canis.*
- **'Black dot'**—*T tonsurans.*
- **Favus**.
- **Rare (Agminate** folliculitis).

1. **Non-inflammatory, human or epidemic type (grey patch)** (Fig. 2.38).
   The clinical picture is of an area of hair loss, with itching with a grayish hue because of the external coating of the hair shafts by spores and hyphae.
2. **Non-inflammatory (Alopecia areata type).**
3. **Inflammatory type (Kerion)**—*M canis* (Fig. 2.39).
   This is characterized by a painful nodule on the scalp with hair loss usually caused by zoophilic species.
4. **Favus—**This variant is seen in Jammu and Kashmir and is characterized by scutulae, a yellowish crust at the base of the hair, scarring alopecia (Fig. 2.40) and on KOH, air spaces in a linear fashion are seen in the hair shaft.

Treatment

- Oral antifungal agents are necessary because topical agents are not able to penetrate deeply enough into the hair follicle; griseofulvin is the first choice.
- Oral terbinafine and itraconazole are good alternatives (although more expensive).

Treatment

- Griseofulvin 10-15 mg/kg/d × 6-8 weeks.
- Terbinafine 5 mg/kg/d × 2-4 weeks.
- **Itraconazole**
  Continuous 5 mg/kg/d × 2-4 weeks.
  Pulse 5 mg/kg/d for 1 week/month × 1-3 pulses.
- **Fluconazole**
  Continuous 6 mg/kg/d × 20 days.
  Pulse 6 mg/kg/dose once per week × 8-12 weeks.
- Adjunct. therapy with antifungal shampoos.

T. CORPORIS

- Infection of non-hairy skin.
- Most common causative agents:
  – *T. rubrum.*
  – *M. canis.*
  – *T. mentagrophytes.*

Clinical Types

- **Classical annular:** Peripheral scaling and central clearing (Fig. 2.41).
- **Inflammatory:** *Trichophyton verrucosum* infection, usually from cattle, produces severe inflammatory response with uniformly round, raised lesions with moist and pustular surface, follicular pustules within hair follicles, possible secondary bacterial infection, brown hyperpigmentation, and scarring. *Trichophyton rubrum* infection produces Majocchi's granuloma, follicular papulopustules or inflammatory nodules, granulomatous nodules with necrotic areas, unusual hyphal forms, and mucinous coating.

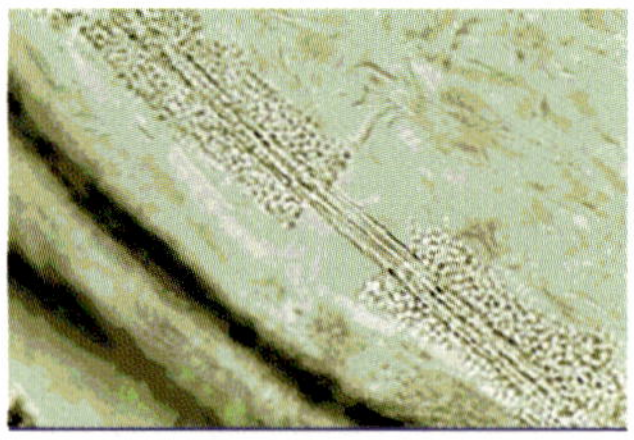

Fig. 2.36: Spores lying outside the hair shaft—ectothrix

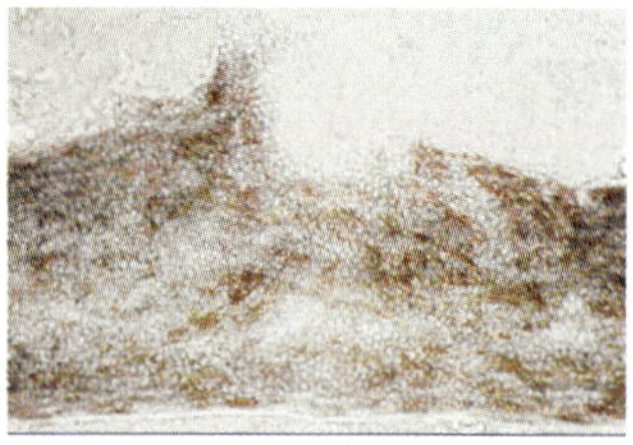

Fig. 2.37: Spores lying inside the hair shaft—endothrix

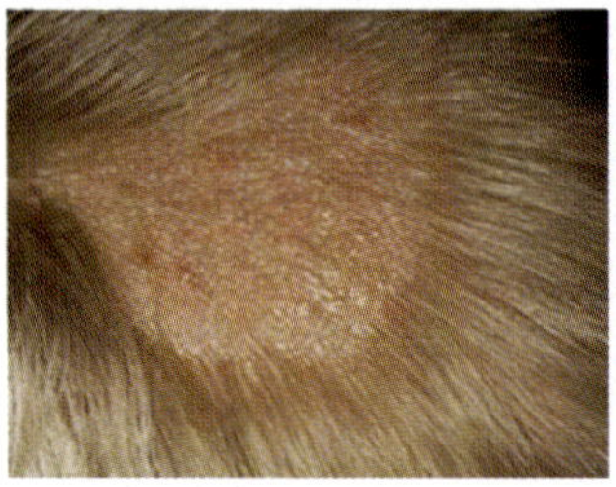

Fig. 2.38: Greyish area of alopecia–due to the coating of spores of the hair shaft (Grey patch)

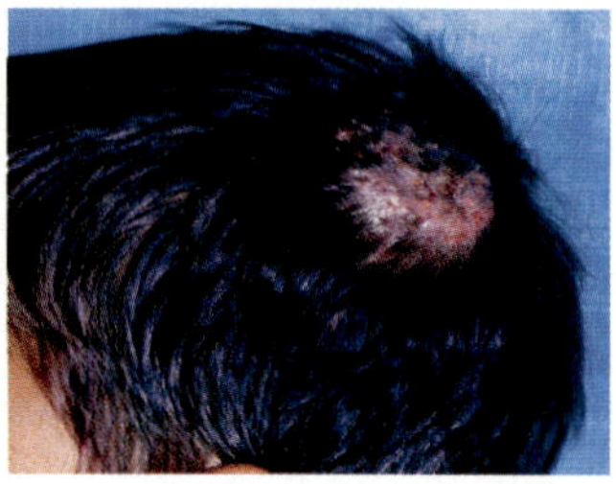

Fig. 2.39: Painful inflammatory nodule (Kerion)

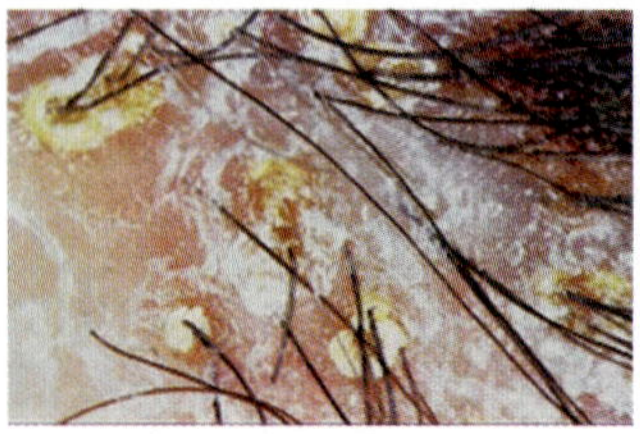

Fig. 2.40: Yellowish crust engulfing multiple hair (Favus)

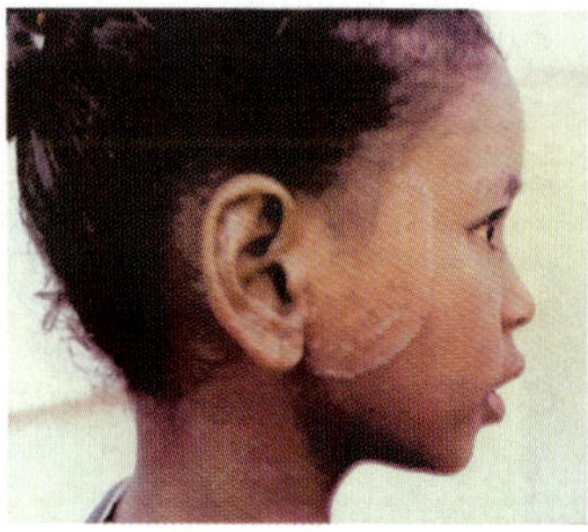

Fig. 2.41: Peripheral spread and central clearing (Tinea corporis)

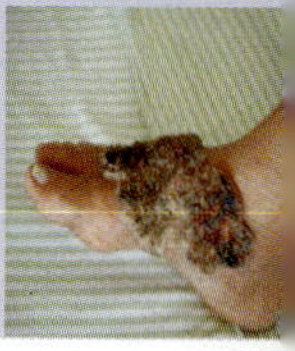

Invasive dermatophyte infection may occur in imm-uno-compromised subjects (particularly in HIV infection, or when steroids or immunosuppressive agents are administered.

- **Tinea circinata:** Annular polycyclic, concentric rings are seen (Fig. 2.42).
- **Majocchi Type:** Deep invasion of follicles and hair because of shaving with presence of nodules usually seen on the lower limb in females.

Treatment

Oral treatment is preferred unless only one or two lesions are present; terbinafine and itraconazole are equally effective.

An alternative is fluconazole 150 mg given orally once a week for upto 4 weeks.

Clotrimazole + betamethasone can be used topically, although not on the face, axilla or groin.

T. CRURIS

Infection of groin area along with infection of genitalia, pubic area, perineal and perianal skin.

Most common causative agents:

- *E. floccosum.*
- *T. rubrum.*
- *T. mentagrophytes.*

Clinical Features

- Itching of the skin.
- Bilateral lesions in crural fold (Fig. 2.43).
- Half-moon-shaped plaque progressing to definitive scaling.
- Spreading to thighs may occur as vesicular borders with red-brown centers, decreased scales, and red papules.
- Buttocks and gluteal cleft involvement may occur; scrotal involvement is indicative of *Candida.*

T. MANNUM AND T. PEDIS

Infection of hands and feet, respectively. Most common causative organisms are:

- *T. rubrum.*
- *T. mentagrophytes.*
- *E. floccosum.*
- *T. manum.*

Clinical Features

1. Scaling that is usually unilateral and involves the palmar creases (Fig. 2.44).
2. Inflammatory type with vesicles.

T. PEDIS

- **Chronic papulosquamous**: It can be unilateral, bilateral or moccasin type (Fig. 2.45) or uncommonly **hyperkeratotic** type (Fig. 2.46).
- **Chronic intertriginous**: It is associated with maceration usually seen between the 4th and 5th toe.
- **Vesicular or vesiculobullous:** Vesicle seen on bilateral feet with severe itching.
- Acute ulcerative.

Treatment

- **Topical Antifungal Agents**
  Imidazoles—Clotrimazole, ketoconazole, Econazole, Miconazole, Oxiconazole.
  Allylamines–Naftifine, Terbinafine.
  Benzyl amines—Butenafine.
- **Systemic Antifungal Agents**
  1. **Fluconazole**
     - 150 mg 1/week × 2-4 weeks for **T. corporis and cruris.**
     - 150 mg 1/week × 2-6 weeks for **T. pedis.**
  2. **Itraconazole**
     - **T. pedis/T. mannum**
       - 200 mg b.d. × 1 week or
       - 100 mg o.d. × 4 weeks or
       - 200 mg o.d. × 2 weeks
     - **T. corporis/T. cruris**
       - 200 mg o.d. × 1 week or
       - 100 mg o.d. × 2 weeks

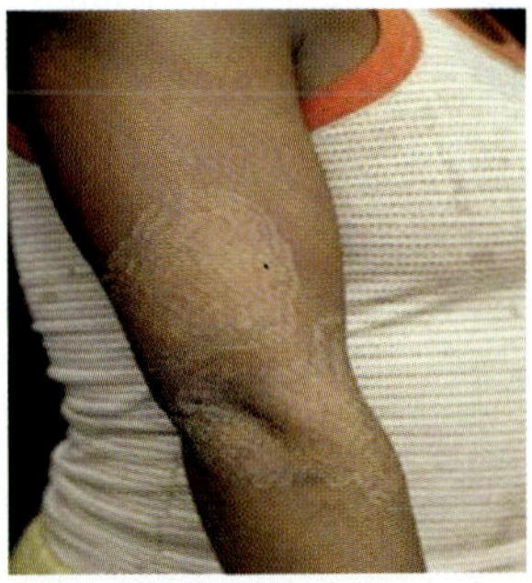

Fig. 2.42: Concentric rings with scaling (Tinea circinata)

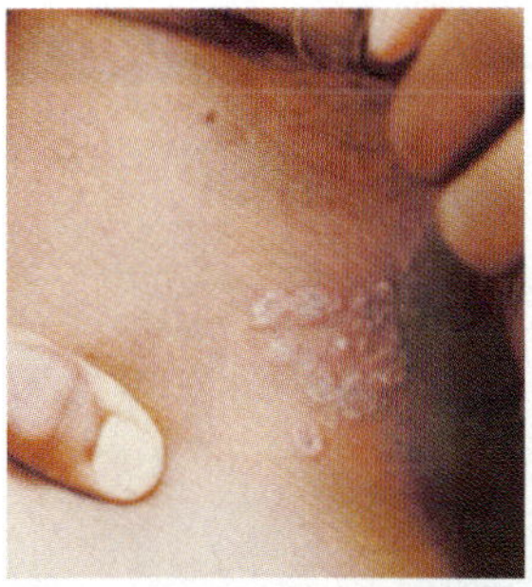

Fig. 2.43: Scaly macules on the groin (Tinea cruris)

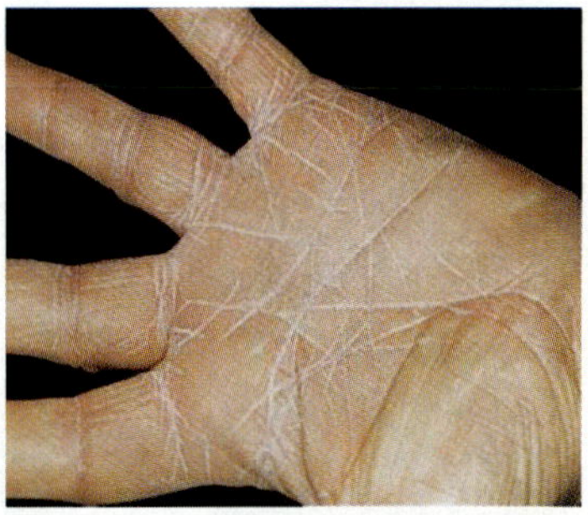

Fig. 2.44: Diffuse scaling with accentuation of palmar creases (Tinea mannum)

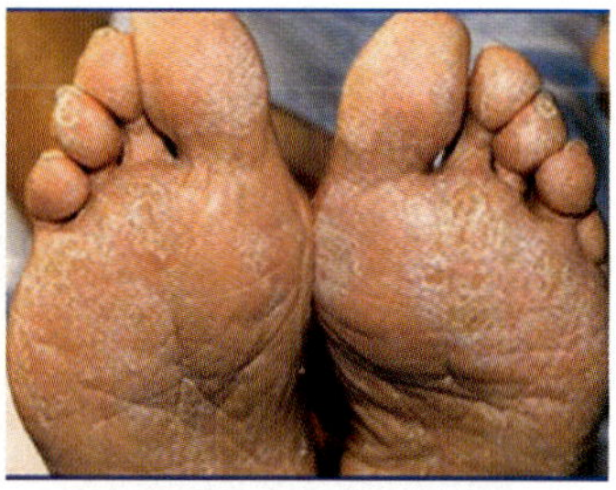

Fig. 2.45: Diffuse scaling with accentuation of plantar creases (Tinea pedis)

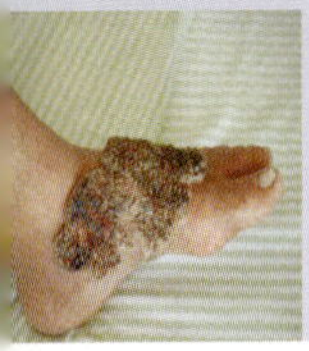

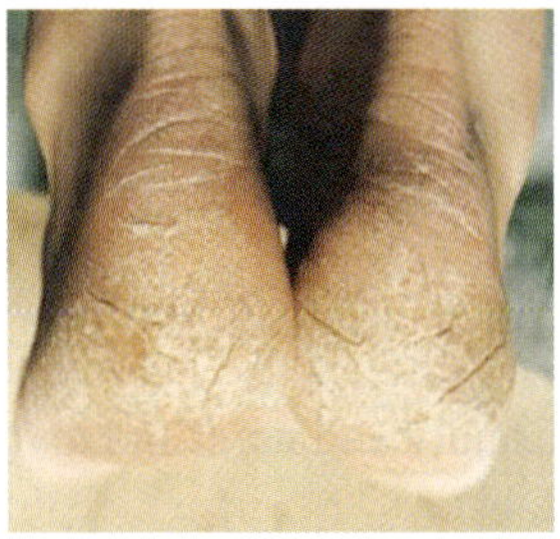

Fig. 2.46: Hyperkeratotic diffuse scaling of palmar skin

3. **Terbinafine**
   - *250 mg/day × 2-4 weeks–**T. corporis**/T. cruris.*
   - 250 mg/day × 2-6 weeks—**T. pedis.**

TINEA UNGUIUM AND ONYCHOMYCOSIS

Causative Organism

- *T. rubrum.*
- *T. mentagrophytes.*
- *E. floccosum.*
  Other–candida and moulds.

Clinical Variants

1. Distal subungual onychomycosis.
2. Proximal subungual onychomycosis.
3. White superficial onychomycosis (WSO).
4. Total dystrophic type.
5. Candidal onychomycosis.
6. Endonyx type.

Distal subungual onychomycosis (Fig. 2.47).
The most common type associated with subungual debris with associated onycholysis, most commonly caused by T. rubrum.

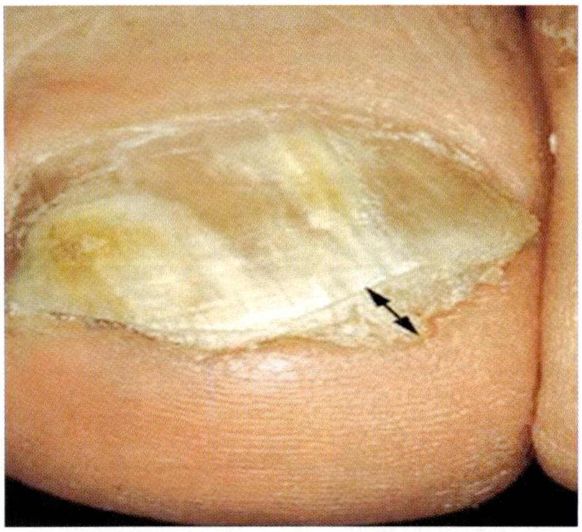

Fig. 2.47: Subungual debris with yellowish discoloration

Proximal Subungual Onychomycosis (Fig. 2.48)

The infection begins near the cuticle and invades the undersurface of the nail plate. Rarely it may extend on the nail plate resembling WSO. It affects both the toe and finger nail. It is also more common in HIV positive patients. It can be caused by *T. rubrum* or rarely by *Fusarium* species.

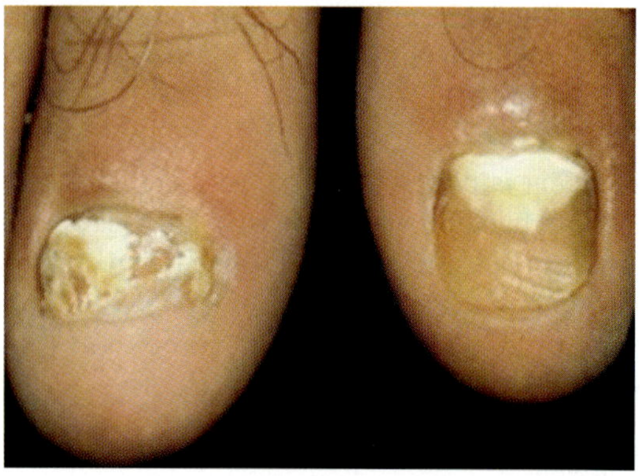

Fig. 2.48: Whitish debris on the nail plate

White Superficial Onychomycosis

It usually afflicts the dorsal nail plate of toe nail, it can be rubbed off and occasionally affects the whole nail.

It is caused by T mentagrophytes, moulds, candida and rarely T rubrum (Fig. 2.49).

Endonyx Type (Fig. 2.50)

This rare variant is identified by a milky deposit, which is composed of the fungal hyphae invading the nail plate *without* subungual debris. It is caused by *T violaceum* and *soudanese*.

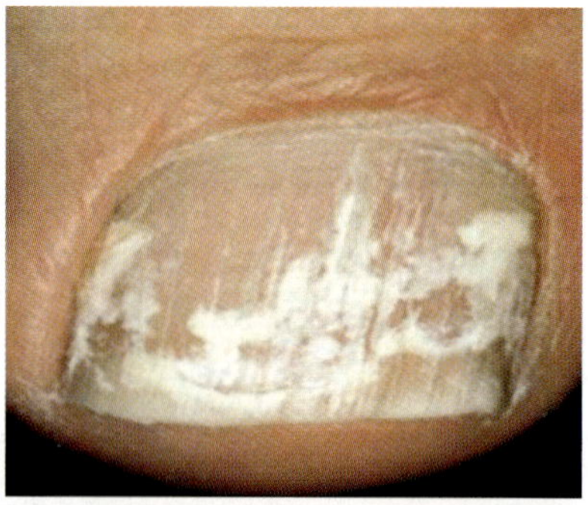

Fig. 2.49: Whitish discoloration without subungual debris

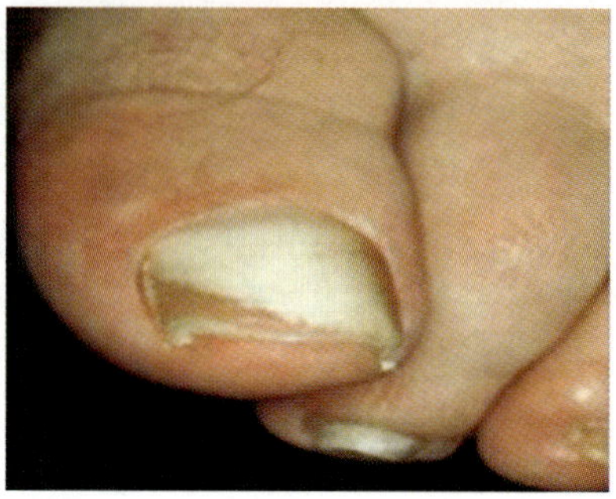

Fig. 2.50: Endonyx type

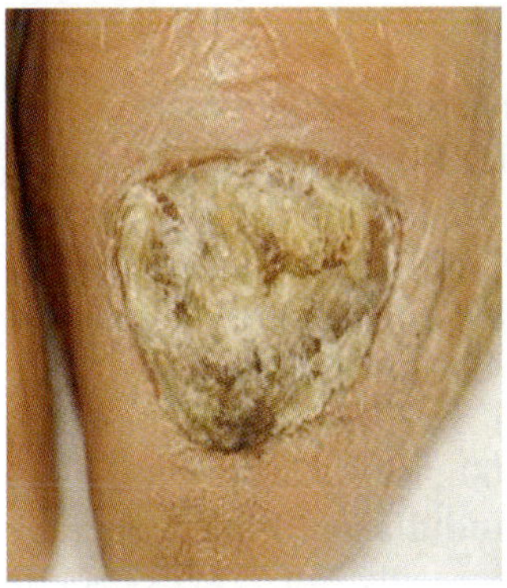

Fig. 2.51: Complete destruction of the nail

Total Dystrophic Type (Fig. 2.51)

In this there is complete and total destruction of the nail plate.

Treatment

- Topical agents are of limited benefit.
- Ciclopirox nail lacquer.
- Amorolofine nail lacquer.
- 40% urea ointment.
- Surgical nail avulsion when single nail involvement.

Systemic Therapy

1. **Griseofulvin** (10-15 mg/kg/d)
   - 4-6 months—fingernails.
   - 10-18 months—toenails.
2. **Itraconazole**
   - **Continuous**–200 mg/d × 6 weeks—fingernails
   - 200 mg/d × 12 weeks – toenails

   Pulse – 200 mg b.d. × 1 week/month
   2 pulses for fingernails
   3-4 pulses for toenails.
3. **Fluconazole**
   - 150 mg once a week–3-6 months fingernails.
   - 9-12 months toenails.
4. **Terbinafine**
   - 250 mg/day × 6 weeks—fingernails,
   - 250 mg/day × 12 weeks–toenails.

CANDIDIASIS

Most common species–*Candida albicans* (Fig. 2.52).

Factors predisposing to candidal infection:

1. Mechanical.
2. Nutritional.
3. Physiological.

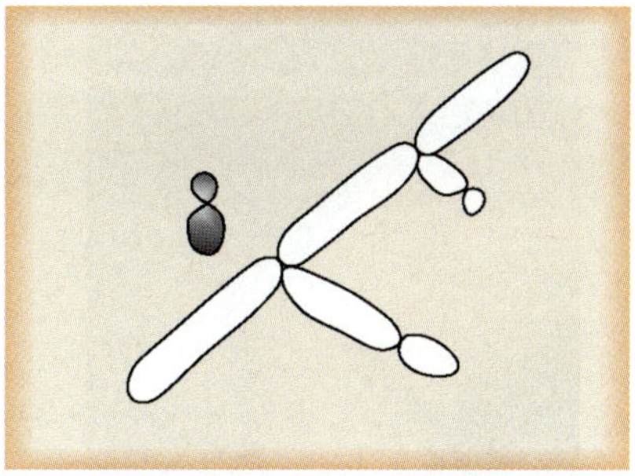

Fig. 2.52: Non-septate pseudohyphae oval spores and blastospore of candida

4. Systemic illnesses.
5. Iatrogenic causes.

Clinical Manifestations

Oral Candidiasis

- Acute pseudomembranous candidiasis (Fig. 2.53).
- Acute erythematous candidiasis.
- Chronic pseudomembranous candidiasis.
- Chronic erythematous candidiasis.
- Chronic plaque–like candidiasis.
- Chronic nodular candidiasis.
- Angular cheilitis/perleche.
- Median rhomboid glossitis.

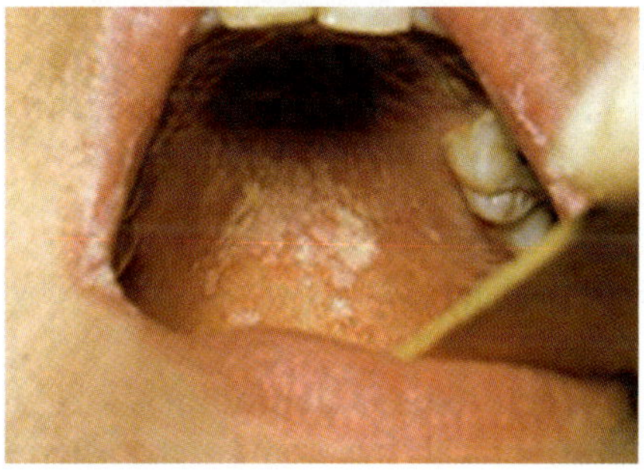

Fig. 2.53: Oral thrush

CANDIDIASIS OF SKIN AND GENITAL MUCOUS MEMBRANES

Clinical Types

- Candidal intertrigo/flexural candidiasis.
- Vulvovaginitis.
- Balanoposthitis (Fig. 2.54).
- Perianal and scrotal candidiasis.
- Napkin candidiasis.
- Nodular or granulomatous candidiasis of napkin area (Granuloma gluteale infection).
  Candidal paronychia.

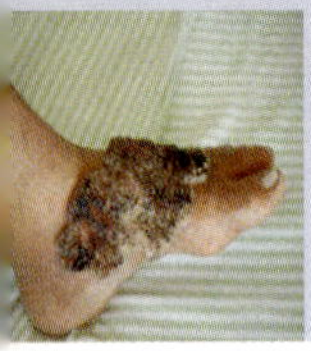

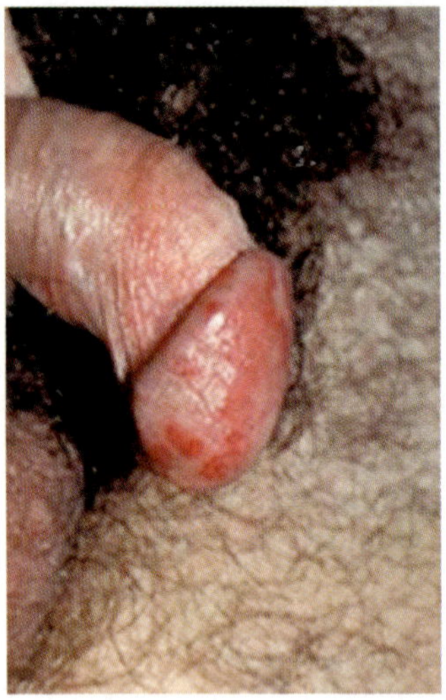

Fig. 2.54: Whitish debris on the glans

- Candidal onychomycosis (Fig. 2.55).
- Congenital candidiasis.

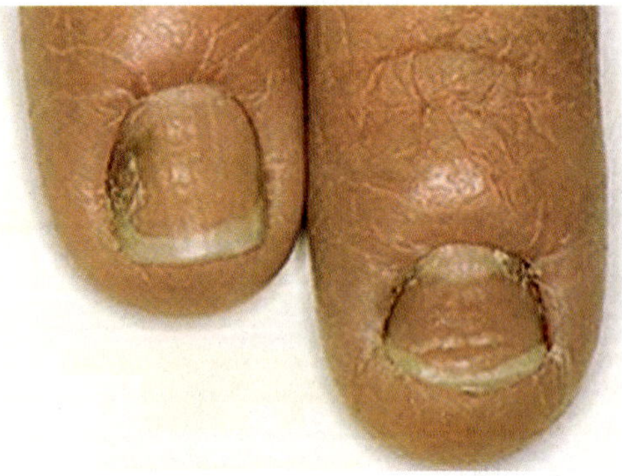

Fig. 2.55: Periungual swelling with nail dystrophy

Chronic mucocutaneous candidiasis—A heterogeneous group of clinical syndromes characterized by chronic, treatment resistant, superficial candidal infections of skin, nails and oropharynx.

—No propensity for disseminated visceral candidiasis .

—Defects in C.M.I.

TREATMENT OF CANDIDIASIS

Oral Candidiasis

Topical agents are 1st line of treatment for uncomplicated cases:

- Nystatin suspension (4-6 lac U q.i.d.) held in mouth and then swallowed.
- Clotrimazole troches (10 mg 5 times a day).
- Chlorhexidine rinses.

Oral Therapy

For unresponsive and chronic cases.

- Ketoconazole 200 mg/day for 1-2 weeks.
- Fluconazole 50-100 mg/day × 1 week.
- Itraconazole 100 mg/day × 2 weeks.

Vulvovaginits: Topical preparation (pessary) of Clotrimazole, Econazole, Miconazole.

Single dose oral therapy—Fluconazole 150 mg or Itraconazole 600 mg.

Flexural candidiasis: Topical therapy as azole or polyene creams usually for 2 weeks is effective.

Napkin candidiasis: Topical antifungals + frequent changes of napkins.

Paronychia and onychomycosis: Minimize wet work. Prolonged topical therapy with lotion form of polyenes. Imidazoles or non-specific remedies such as 4% thymol in chloroform.

Chronic mucocutaneous candidiasis: A combination of anti-fungal drugs and immune deficiency correction will produce best results.

SUBCUTANEOUS AND DEEP MYCOSIS

Table 2.5

Diseases	*Main endemic areas*
Sporotrichosis	Most countries—rare in Europe
Mycetoma	Dry tropics: Latin America, Africa, Middle East, Indian subcontinent
Chromoblastomycosis	Humid tropices—Latin America, Africa, Far East
Subcutaneous phaeohyphomycosis	Can occur anywhere
Rare infections	
• Subcutaneous zygomycosis due to conidiobolus or basidiobolus	Africa, Latin America, Far East
• Lobomycosis due to Loboa loboi	Restricted to South America

Sporotrichosis

Linear eruption of nodules along the lymphatics following trauma on the distal extremity (Fig. 2.56).

Types:

- Fixed.
- Linear lymphatic.
- Systemic.
- Atypical forms.

Characterized by **Asteroid bodies.**

Treatment by KI (Potassium Iodide), Terbinafine, Itraconazole.

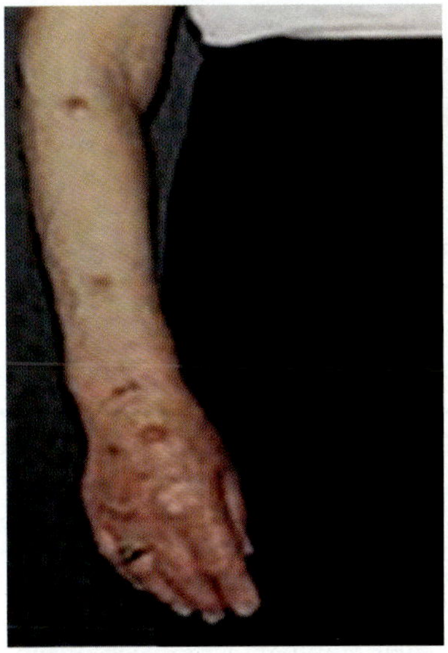

Fig. 2.56: Linear nodules on a limb

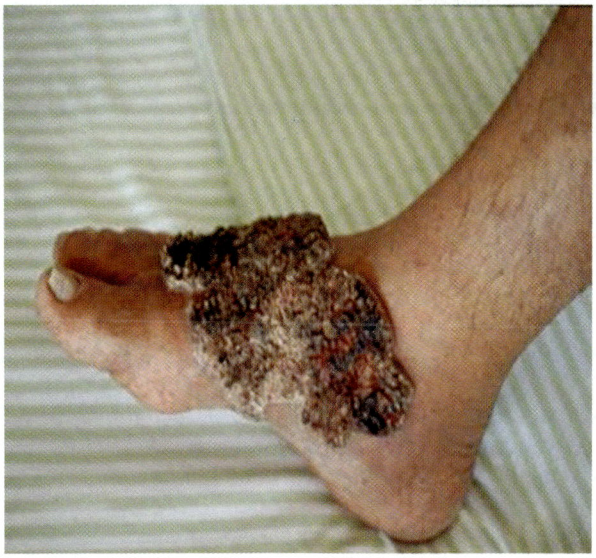

Fig. 2.58: Verrucous plaque on the lower limb

Mycetoma (Fig. 2.57)

- **Eumycetoma**—Caused by fungi like *Madurella mycetomatis*.

  Actinomycetoma—Nocardia and actinomycetes.

  Characterized by swelling, tumefaction, nodules, sinus with discharge of colonies of organism in the form of grains.

Treatment

A combination of aminoglycoside, sulfonamide and penicillin in case of actinomycetoma.

Systemic antifungal with debulking and surgery in case of eumycetoma.

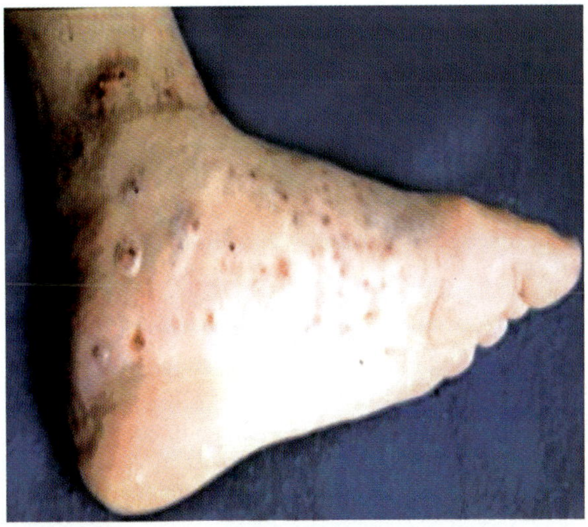

Fig. 2.57: Swelling, sinus with nodules

Chromoblastomycosis (Fig. 2.58)

An infection caused by *Fonsecaea pedrosi* and *Cladosporium carrionii* characterized by warty papillomatous plaques.

They show *medlar bodies* or *copper pennies* on microscopy.

Treatment

Itraconazole,Terbinafine, Amphotericin B.

Cryptococcosis (Fig. 2.59)

Molluscoid papule and nodules on the face with characteristic **double walled yeast cells** on India ink mount. Responsive to Azoles, Amphotercin B and Flucytosine.

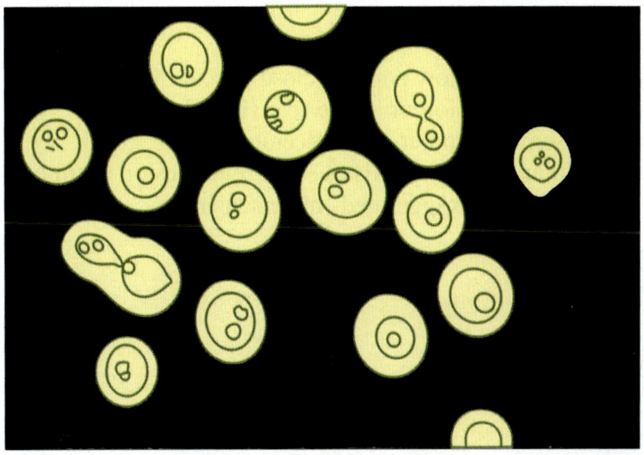

Fig. 2.59: Double walled yeast cells

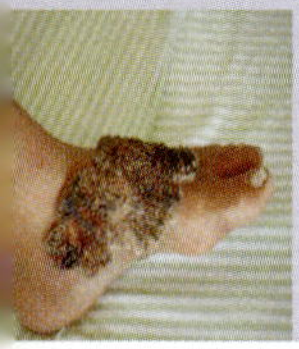

Leishmaniasis

CLASSIFICATION

Cutaneous Leishmaniasis

Old world	*L. major, L. tropica, L. acthiopica, L. infantum*
New world	*L. mexicana complex, L. braziliensis complex*
Mucocutaneous Leishmaniasis	- Old world – *L. aethiopica* - New world – *L. braziliensis*
Visceral Leishmaniasis	*L. donovani, L. infantum*
Other forms	Leishmania recidivans PKDL (post kala-azar dermal leishmaniasis)

Modes of Transmission

- Bite of **sand fly**.
- Congenital infection.
- Blood transfusion.
- Possibly by coitus.

I. OLD WORLD LEISHMANIASIS ACUTE ORIENTAL SORE/ DELHI-BOIL

- *L.major*–I.P. (2 months).
  Nodule → central crusting → Ulcer→Scar (2-6 months).
- *L.tropica*—nodule → crusting → ulcer and lasts for (1 year).
- *L. aethiopica*—mostly central on face and single.
- *L. infantum*—in infants (severe systemic-visceral involvement); in adults (simple self-healing cutaneous disease).

Leishmania Recidivans (Lupoid Leishmaniasis)

Brown red or yellow papules-close to scar of old cutaneous leishmaniasis lesion or in the scar (Fig. 2.60).

- Worsen in summer, may ulcerate.
- Cellular immunity fails to sterilize the lesion despite the presence of exaggerated hypersensitivity.

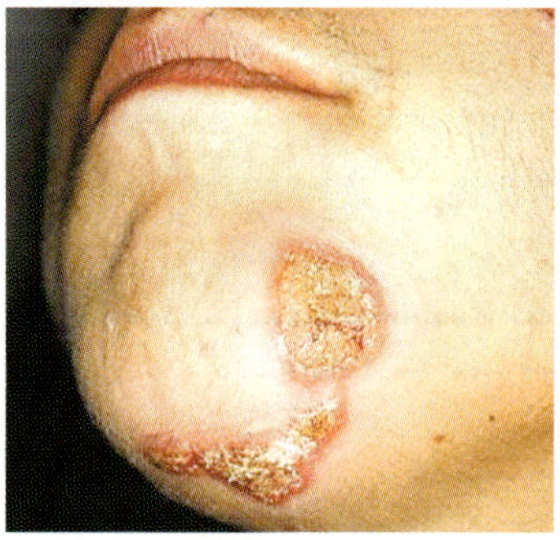

Fig. 2.60: Red plaque over the chin (Lupoid leishmaniasis)

- Common in the Middle East. May closely mimic **Lupus vulgaris**.

Diffuse Cutaneous Leishmaniasis

- *L. aethiopica.*
- Multiple nodules (don't ulcerate).
- Parasites in abundance in the lesions.
- Internal organs are not involved.
- Leishmanin test is negative.
- Chronic disease and relapses common.

II. NEW WORLD CUTANEOUS LEISHMANIASIS

- *L. Mexicana complex*—lesions similar to *L. tropica* most of them on face or behind ears.
- Severe destructive lesions—**Espundia** (invasion of oronasal mucosa).
- *L. brasiliensis* complex–large deep ulcers.

III. MUCOCUTANEOUS LEISHMANIASIS

L. brasiliensis (40% cases).
L. panamensis, L. guyanensis (uncommon).

- 50% of mucosal lesions appear within 2 years of skin lesions.
- 15% have no history of any skin lesions.
- Nasal mucosa is almost always affected.
- Pharynx, palate or upper lip, can also be involved.

IV. VISCERAL LEISHMANIASIS (KALA AZAR)

- *L. donovani, L. infantum.*
- Parasite multiplies in the reticuloendothelial cells.
- Splenomegaly, anaemia, leukopenia and thrombocytopenia, fever, cough, epistaxis, pedal edema.

POST-KALA AZAR DERMAL LEISHMANIASIS

P.K.D.L.

African PKDL	*Indian PKDL*
• Seen in 5% of pts of K.A. • Begins during convalescence	• Seen in 20% • Appears 1-2 years after recovery
• Present on cheek, chin, ears and extensor aspects of forearms and buttocks (Discrete papules)	• Hypopigmented macules similar in appearance to LL.
H/P – Tuberculoid features with scanty parasites	Poorly diff. infiltration of inflammatory cells with variable no. of parasites
Leishmanin test is positive	Usually negative but becomes positive after successful treatment
Heal spontaneously over a few months.	Progressive over many years, seldom heal spontaneously.

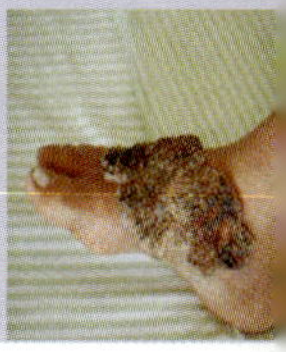

Variants of P.K.D.L.

- Hypopigmented macules (Fig. 2.61) (upper trunk, arms, thighs abdomen).
- Papules and nodules (Fig. 2.61).
- Annular type.
- Hypertrophic forms (like warty or papillomatous).
- Fibroid type.
- Xanthomatous transformation.
- P. Rosea like.
- Mucous membrance involvements.
- Scleral nodules and keratitis.

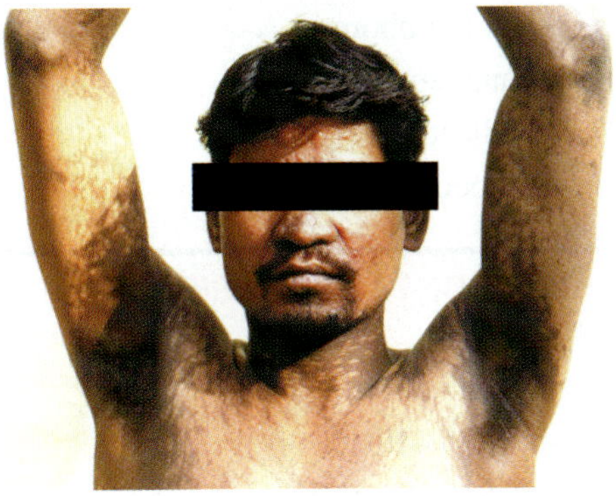

Fig. 2.61: Macules, papules and nodules on face perioral area and chest

Important

- Previous history of K.A. is not necessarily obtained in every case of PKDL.
- Youngest case reported is 4 years.
- Interval between KA and PKDL can vary from 6-60 months (average 26 months).

Serious Complications

- Blindness due to corneal involvement.
- Laryngeal lesions lead to dysphonia, may even cause laryngeal obstruction.

Differential Diagnosis

Most important is **Leprosy:**

- Vitiligo.
- Secondary syphilis.
- Lupus vulgaris.
- Sarcoidosis.

LAB DIAGNOSIS

1. **Slit skin smear:** From the edge of the lesion stained with Giemsa.
   OR
   Leishmanin stain: Amastigotes are seen as pale, blue, oval bodies with dark blue nucleus in the cytoplasm of macrophages.
2. **Culture:**
   NNN Media: Novy Mc, Neal Media
   – a liquid media.
   In these promastigotes can be grown in 4 weeks.
3. **Histopathology:**
   Macular—Mixed inflammatory cells in upper dermis.
   Nodular—Infiltrate is seen in entire dermis.
4. **Splenic/Bone marrow/Liver Aspirate:**
   In case of visceral leishmaniasis parasites can be obtained from the aspirates.
5. **Leishmanin test (Montenegro):**
   To measure CMI (type IV hypersensitivity).
6. **Serological tests:**
   a. Recombinant *L. donovani* gene B protein (r GBP).
   b. ELISA–from urine sample by Anti *L. donovani* IgG-95% (Sensitivity and specificity).
7. **PCR**–Sensitivity–92%
   Specificity–100%
8. **K-39 Antigen**–Sensitivity–91%
   –Specificity–100%

Treatment

1. **SAG (Sodium-Antimony Gluconate)**
   Test dose followed by 20 mg/kg/day–max 850 mg
   - 3 months–4 months–PKDL.
   - 28 days–Visceral, MCL.
   - 20 days–Cutaneous leishmaniasis.

   S/E—GIT, fever, myalgia, phlebitis, hepatitis, hemolytic anemia, cardiac.
   Monitoring—1st 3 weeks (once weekly blood counts, ECG).
   Discontinue if—AST/ALP increases (3-4 times) or ECG (concave ST) or QT interval > 0.5 sec.
   in case of Relapse—Same dose given for twice duration.
2. **Amphotericin B**—Toxic drug, used in resistant cases only (liposomal formulation).
   3 mg/kg/day.
   S/E—Hypertension, dyspnea, fever, renal failure.
   99% cure rates.
3. **Pentamidine Isothiocyanate**
   2-4 mg/kg I/M or IV daily or alternate days
   - 15 days–VL (Visceral).
   - 4 days–CL (Cutaneous).

   S/E—Histamine release,↓ BP (sudden) Palpitation, Arrhythmia.

4. **Paromomycin**—Cut lesions (topical application) 15% parmomycin + 12% methyl *benzethonium* dichloride – BD × 15 days.
5. **Allopurinol—**4-12 mg/kg TDS (3-4 wccks). Good results when used in combination.
6. **Ketoconazole**—600 mg/day – 4 weeks.
7. **Fluconazole**—200 mg OD – 6 weeks.
8. **Imiquimod**—An immunomodulator which activates macrophage killing. When used in combination in case of resistant cases → 90% cure rates.
9. **Miltefosine**—Used in case of cutaneous leishmaniasis 2.25 mg/kg/day–3-4 weeks.
10. **SSG infiltrate**—In case of oriental sore 2 ml (100 mg/ml) around the sore.

REFERENCES

- Thieme's Pocket Dermatology 2006 by Wolfram Sterry, Walter Burgdorf, Ralf Paus.
- Andrews' Diseases of the Skin: Clinical Dermatology by William D. James, Timothy Berger, Dirk Elston 2005.
- Fitzpatrick's Dermatology in General Medicine, 6th edn 2003.
- Rook's Textbook of Dermatology D. A. Burns , S. M. Breathnach, Neil Cox, Christopher E. Griffiths 7th edn 2004.
- Fitzpatrick's Dermatology in General Medicine, 6th edn 2003.

Tuberculosis

INFECTION WITH *M TUBERCULOSIS* CAN OCCUR FROM

- Contact with contaminated body fluids, secretions or discharges, or through direct contact with diseased skin.

MODES OF TRANSMISSION FOR INFECTION INCLUDE

- Respiratory, Gastrointestinal (from unpasteurized milk from infected animals), Genitourinary (through sexual intercourse), and Inoculation through skin or mucous membranes (e.g., the conjunctiva).

SOURCES OF INFECTION INCLUDE

- Humans, cattle, swine, dogs and cats, monkeys, and laboratory bacteriological cultures. Exogenous iatrogenic inoculation has occurred in laboratory workers.

IMPORTANT FACTORS IN THE INCIDENCE AND PREVALENCE OF TUBERCULOSIS

1. Old age.
2. Poverty.
3. Overcrowding.
4. Inadequate hygiene and nutrition.
5. Immunosuppression.
6. Pregnancy.
7. Diabetes.
8. Sarcoidosis.
9. Leukemia, and lymphoma.
10. HLA-BW15 antigen.
11. Cytotoxic medications.
12. Systemic glucocorticosteroids.

THE FREQUENCY OF THE DIFFERENT FORMS OF TUBERCULOSIS

- Lupus vulgaris (57.5%).
- Scrofuloderma (35.4%).
- Verrucous tuberculosis (4.5%).
- Ulcerative tuberculosis (2.6%).

Epidemiology

The male-to-female ratio is **1:2.05**.

Women are more likely to have lupus vulgaris or scrofuloderma. Men more frequently have verrucous or ulcerative tuberculosis.

The young more frequently have scrofuloderma. The elderly more frequently have lupus vulgaris. A classification of the causative organism and that of TB is given in **Tables 2.6 and 2.7.**

INVESTIGATIONS

Diagnostic Criteria

Absolute

- Recovery of bacilli from the lesion.
- Successful guinea pig inoculation.
- Positive culture.

Relative

- Clinical signs and symptoms.
- Presence of active proved TB elsewhere.
- Histopathology (Tuberculoid).
- Positive tuberculin test.
- Therapeutic response to ATT in 6-8 weeks time.

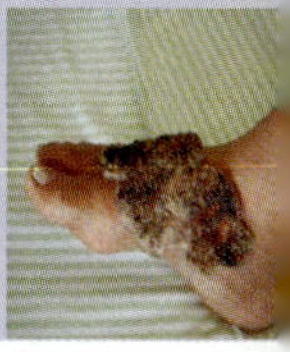

Table 2.6: Classification of mycobacteria

Mycobacterial species	*Skin, subcutis invol.*	*L.N. lung, other invol.*
M. tuberculosis-bovis complex (slow grower, non chromogen) obligate h.p. (human pathogen)	+	+
M. marinum (slow grower, photochromogen facultative h.p.)	+	–
M. kansasii (slow grower, photochromogen facultative h.p.)	+	+
M. avium-intracellulare complex (slow grower, non chromogen facultative h.p.)	+	+
M. haemophilum (slow grower, non chromogen, facultative h.p.)	+	–
M. ulcerans (slow grower, non chromogen, facultative h.p.)	+	–
M. gordonae (slow grower, scotochromogen, facultative h.p.)	+	–
Rapid Grower (*M fortuitiun, chelonae, abscessus, facultative h.p.*)	+	–

Classification of Cutaneous Tuberculosis

Table 2.7: Classification of TB skin

State	*Source*	*Mode*	*Histology*	*Course*	*Disease*	*Immunity*	*Bacilli*
Primary	Exogenous	Inoculation	Non-specific	Localised	**Chancre**	Developing	+++
			TB specific	Localised	**Primary TB complex**	Good	+?
			TB specific	Localised	Lupus vulgaris	Moderate	++
			TB specific	Progressive	TB fungosa serpiginosa	Poor	+++
			TB specific	Generalised	Miliary TB	Poor	+++
Secondary	Exogenous	Reinoculation	TB specific	Localised	**TB verrucosa cutis**	Good	+/–
			TB specific	Progressive	**TB cutis orificialis**	Poor	+++
	Endogenous	Contiguous	TB specific	Localised	**Lupus vulgaris**	Moderate	++
			TB specific	Localised	**Scrofuloderma**	Poor	+++
		Autoinoculation	TB specific	Localised	**TB verrucosa cutis**	Good	+/–
			TB specific	Progressive	**TB cutis orificialis**	Poor	+++
		Hematogenous	TB specific	Localised	**Lupus vulgaris**	Moderate	+++
			TB specific	Localised	**Gumma** (subcutaneous abscess)	Moderate	++
			TB specific	Localised	Ulcerative TB	Moderate	++
			TB specific	Progressive	TB fungosa serpiginosa	Poor	+++
			TB specific	Progressive	**TB cutis orificialis**	Poor	+++
			TB specific	Generalized	Miliary TB	Poor	+++
Tuberculid	Endogenous	Hematogenous	Variable	Localised	Erythema induratum	Moderate-to-good	–/+
			Variable	Scattered crops	Papulonecrotic tuberculid	Moderate-to-good	–/+
			Variable	Generalised	Lichen scrofulosorum	Moderate-to-good	–/+

PRIMARY INOCULATION TUBERCULOSIS

Tuberculous chancre.

Epidemiology

Result of inoculation of M tuberculosis into the skin or mucosa of a **nonimmune host.** An initial negative reaction to PPD reflects the host's **absent immunity.**

Inoculation tuberculosis accounts for only 5% of total primary tuberculosis.

The majority of patients have: Respiratory exposure, Gastrointestinal exposure.

M tuberculosis cannot penetrate intact human skin. Some sort of **injury** must be present for an infection to be established. Portals of entry include minor injuries as abrasions, puncture wounds, hangnails, and pyodermas. **Children** are most frequently affected.

Face and exposed extremities most **common** affected sites.

Clinical Features

After an incubation period of **3 to 4 weeks** following inoculation.

↓

Small inflammatory **papule** develops.

↓

Quickly breaks down into an indolent, firm, nontender, sharply delimited **ulcer** with no tendency for spontaneous healing for several weeks (Fig. 2.62).

↓

After 3 to 8 weeks, tubercle bacilli reach the regional nodes.

↓

Producing a **painless lymphadenitis**.

This **ulceroglandular complex** is the prototype of primary inoculation tuberculosis.The skin analog to the primary pulmonary **Ghon complex.** The PPD usually **becomes positive** after development of lymphadenopathy.

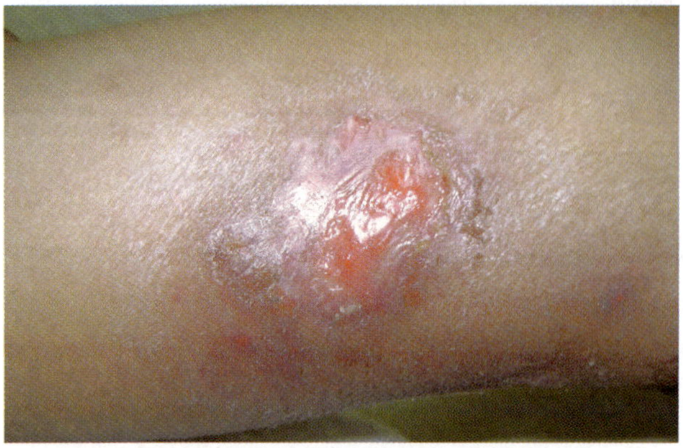

Fig. 2.62: Nontender, *sharply delimited ulcer*

Course and Prognosis

After 1 to 3 months, the primary lesion usually heals with **scarring.** In patients with poor immunity and large bacterial load, **acute miliary tuberculosis** can develop. **Lupus vulgaris** or even **tuberculosis verrucosa cutis** may develop as late sequelae. Regional lymph nodes liquefy producing **scrofuloderma**. In 10% of patients, **erythema nodosum** may develop.

Histopathological Findings

- Epithelioid tubercles, some marked by caseous necrosis in their center, surrounded by dense infiltrates of lymphocytes.
- Fibrocytes, in variable number, present around lymphocytes.
- Uneven psoriasiform acanthosis.
- Sometimes ulceration.

Differential Diagnosis

Primary syphilis, Tularemia, Cat-scratch disease, Sporotrichosis.

TUBERCULOSIS VERRUCOSA CUTIS

Definition: It's a verrucous **(wart like)** form of reinfection tuberculosis.

Syn *warty tuberculosis, prosector's wart, verruca-necrogenica, tuberculosis cutis verruca, postprimary inoculation tuberculosis, and verrucous tuberculosis.*

It occurs when the skin of a previously infected or BCG-immunized host, possessing a **moderate or high degree of immunity**, is subjected to **exogenous reinfection**. Reinoculation occurs at sites of **minor abrasions** or wounds.

It commonly occuss in physicians, pathologists, medical students, laboratory attendants, Veterinarians, farmers, and butchers (tuberculous cattle). Autoinoculation from tuberculous sputum (rare).

Clinical Features

Hands and fingers, lower extremities are affected most frequently.

Initial lesion is a painless, dusky red, firm **papule or papulopustule**.

↓

Expands peripherally and surrounded by **inflammatory halo.**

↓

It quickly develops into a polycyclic, serpiginous, or **annular plaque** with a warty, advancing border and central area of atrophy (Fig. 2.63).

↓

Pus and keratinous material may be expressed from the fissures in the warty areas.

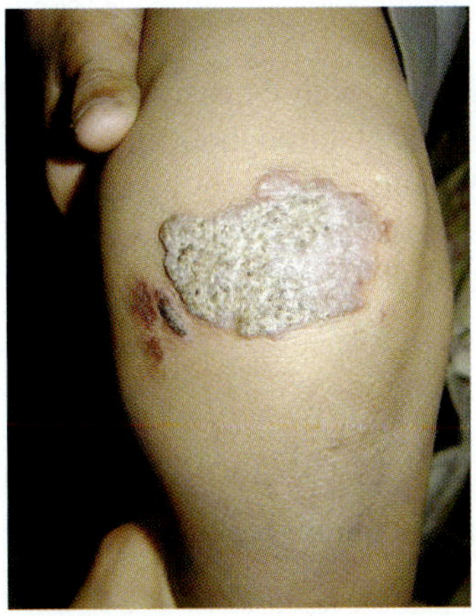

Fig 2.63: Verrucous plaque with an erythematous halo(TBVC)

- Lymphadenopathy is characteristically **absent.**
- Lymph node enlargement, when present, may be the result of secondary infection.
- The lesions rarely ulcerate, and spontaneous invo-lution may occur over months to years.
- Lesions may evolve and last for years or even decades.
- Prognosis is **good.**

Histopathological Findings

- Granulomas with a lichenoid infiltrate of lymphocytes and plasma cells.
- Beneath the zone of lichenoid lymphoplasmacytic infiltration, discrete granulomas surrounded by numerous lymphocytes and plasma cells.
- Multinucleate histiocytes present in granulomas.
- Fibroplasia in the upper part of the dermis in foci.
- Pseudocarcinomatous proliferation of keratinocytes in which collections of neutrophils often are present.
- Papillated epidermal acanthosis in addition to pseudo-carcinomatous proliferation.

Differential Diagnosis

- Iododerma and bromoderma.
- Chronic vegetative pyoderma.
- Squamous cell carcinoma.
- Verrucous carcinoma.
- North American blastomycosis.
- Chromoblastomycosis.
- Verrucous atypical mycobacterial infection.
- Verrucous lupus vulgaris.
- Tertiary syphilis.

SCROFULODERMA

Synonymous

Tuberculosis colliquativa cutis and tuberculous gumma.

Definition

Subacute form of tuberculosis that occurs in patients who have already **have primary tuberculous complex**.

Aetiopathogenesis

The tuberculous foci are commonly in the **lymph nodes, bones and joints, and epididymis** originates as a tuberculous process of the subcutaneous tissues leading to the formation of cold abscesses and then secondary breakdown of the overlying skin. Scrofuloderma is common in **children.**

80% following an oral or tonsillar primary inoculation of bovine tuberculosis from infected milk.The elderly are also susceptible, when their immune defenses are compromised. True tuberculous lymphadenitis is becoming less common in children.

Clinical Features

Initial lesion present with a firm, subcutaneous or deep cutaneous **swelling or nodule**.

↓

Freely movable initially but soon firmly attaches to the skin and later **ulcerates** (Fig. 2.64).

↓

The ulcers tend to have bluish, undermined edges (Fig. 2.65) and soft, granulating floors.

↓

Watery, **purulent, or caseous discharge** may exude from the **sinuses** (Fig. 2.66).

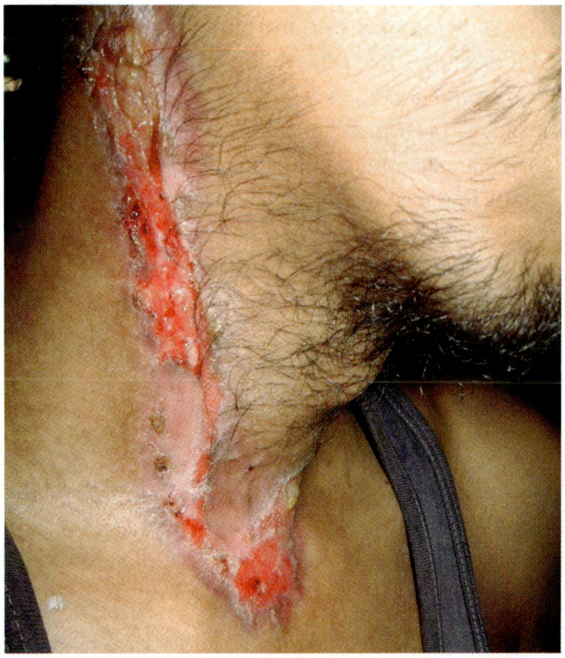

Fig. 2.64: Neck showing ulcers with underlying lymph node (Scrofuloderma)

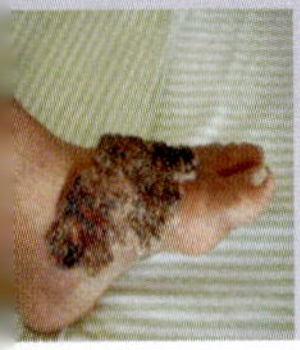

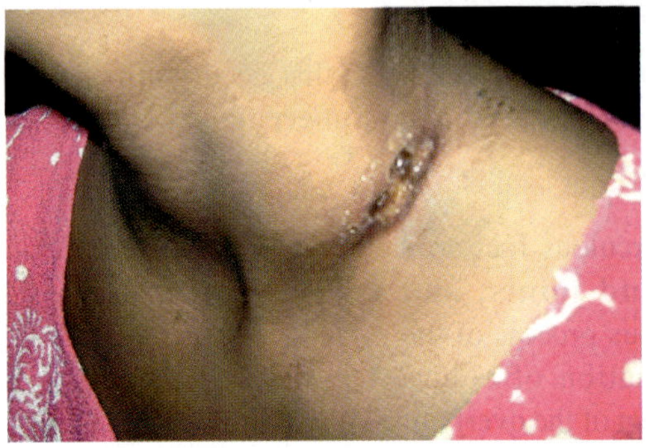

Fig. 2.65: Ulcerated area overlying the neck

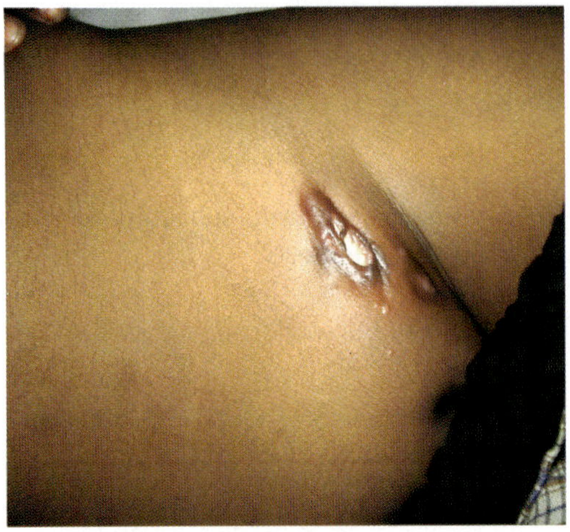

Fig. 2.66: Inguinal area with an ulcer overlying LN

Ulcer showing indurated margins, with black discoloration. Floor shows necrotic yellowish red cheesy material. *Cervical lymph nodes are infected most commonly affected.* In the neck, the tonsillar, submandibular, preauri-cular, postauricular, occipital, and supraclavicular lymph nodes are usually implicated. The parasternal, axillary, inguinal and epitrochlear nodes are potential sites. Over weeks to months the nodes enlarge, turn livid red, suppurate, then perforate with resultant ulceration and fistula formation. Cordlike scarring bridges the ulcerations. Spontaneous healing does occur.

Course and Prognosis

- Scrofuloderma is usually associated with manifest tuberculosis (lungs and abdomen).
- **Lupus vulgaris** may occur in the scar of scrofuloderma.

Complications

Epithelioma
Systemic amyloidosis (rare).

Histopathological Findings

- Tuberculoid granulomas, many with extensive caseous necrosis in their center, present throughout the entire dermis and far into the subcutis.
- Abscesses in some granulomas.
- Fibroplasia in the upper part of the dermis.
- Ulceration common.

Differential Diagnosis

- Tertiary syphilis.
- Deep fungi (sporotrichosis, actinomycosis).
- Severe acne conglobata.
- Hidradenitis suppurativa.
- Chronic granulomatous disease.

TUBERCULOSIS CUTIS ORIFICIALIS

Orificial tuberculosis and tuberculosis ulcerosa cutis et mucosae.

It is the tuberculosis of the **mucous membranes** and the skin of the orifices. It is due to auto inoculation of the tubercle bacilli in patients with advanced visceral tuberculosis. Its occurrence by lymphatic or hematogenous extension is rare.

Affects men > women. Most prevalent in **middle aged or older** individuals. Common in advanced pulmonary, intestinal, or genitourinary tuberculosis.

Clinical Features

Ulcerative lesions commonly occur in the oral cavity and the perineal or perirectal areas.

The tongue particularly its tip and lateral margins. Other sites in the mouth are the soft and hard palate, lips, and in a tooth socket after extraction. Area on and around the anus (intestinal tuberculosis). Vulva, glans, penis and urinary meatus (genitourinary tuberculosis).

A small, yellowish or reddish **nodule** that rapidly breaks down.

↓

Form an exquisitely painful, shallow **ulcer** with bluish, undermined edges.

↓

The surrounding **mucosa is swollen**.

↓

The ulcer is **covered by pseudomembranous** material.

- Ulcers do not heal spontaneously and are signs of a poor prognosis.
- Cutaneous hypersensitivity to tuberculin in these patients is controversial.

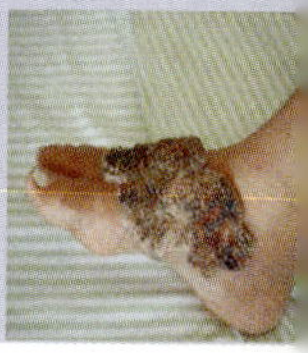

- Ulceration, swelling and crusting of nasal mucosa and upper lip because of pulmonary T.B.

LUPUS VULGARIS

Tuberculosis cutis luposa.

Definition

It is a **reinfection tuberculosis** of the skin. Occurring in previously sensitized individuals. **High degree of tuberculin sensitivity**. Protean and **dramatic** clinical presentations.

Hypersensitivity to tuberculin is high. Immunity is low to moderate.

Epidemiology

- **Most frequent type** of cutaneous tuberculosis.
- Greatest potential for **disfigurement**. Women (2) > men. Tuberculin positive.
- Two thirds of patients with lupus have visceral foci of tuberculosis.
- 40% have tuberculous adenitis or involvement of the mucous membranes.
- 10% to 20% have pulmonary, bone, or joint tuberculosis.

Etiopathogenesis

It is a cutaneous form of **postprimary tuberculosis**.

It may develop in the:

- Site of primary inoculation tuberculosis.
- In the scar of scrofuloderma.
- After BCG immunization.

  Triggered into activity by later trauma or injury.

  The disease can arise from:
- The perforation of tuberculous abscesses into the skin.
- From endogenous dermal inoculation of tubercle bacilli (via lymphatic or hematogenous metastasis).

Clinical Features

Most common on the **face, especially the nose and cheeks.** Followed by the ears, the extensor surfaces of the extremities, the buttocks, and the breasts. **Lower extremities**, especially the buttocks, are the primary site of involvement **(India).**

Mucous membrane involvement (rare).

Earliest lesion appears as small, brownish red **papules** of soft gelatinous consistency.

↓

On diascopy, the characteristic translucent, **apple jelly–colored lupoid infiltrates**.

↓

From these small **granulomas**, the various forms of lupus vulgaris develop over the course of years.

↓

As the lesions enlarge, **caseation necrosis** proceeds, resulting in softening of the lesions.

↓

Accompanied by **central atrophy or scarring**.

Lupus vulgaris shows brown-yellowish nodules which may coalesce into plaques. Typically lupus vulgaris lesions are accompanied with ulceration and scarring.

Clinical Variants are:

Lupus Vulgaris Exfoliativus:

- Characterized by plaques with a psoriatic scale.
- Over time, serpiginous or polycyclic configurations may develop with central clearing and atrophy. Plaque type lesions with scaling and hyperkeratotic margins with central clearing.

Lupus Vulgaris Verrucosus:

Results from a wartlike pseudoepitheliomatous hyperplasia of the epidermis (Fig. 2.67).

Lupus Vulgaris Ulcerosus:

Forms when massive necrosis occurs within the tuberculous granulomas.This ulcerative variant may be accompanied by deep destruction of underlying tissues and cartilage (Fig. 2.68).

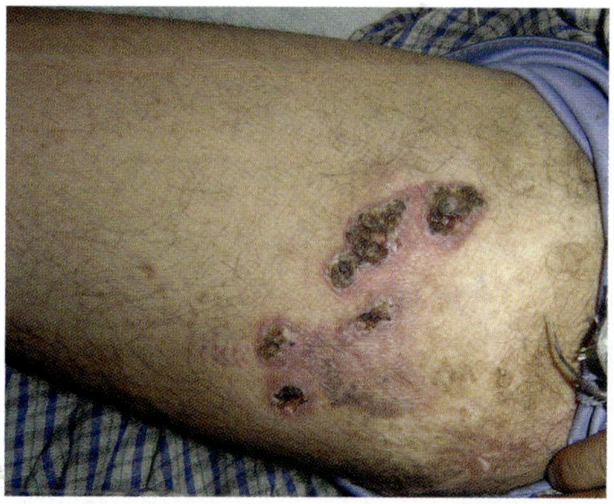

Fig. 2.67: Plaque with serpiginous border showing central healing and scarring

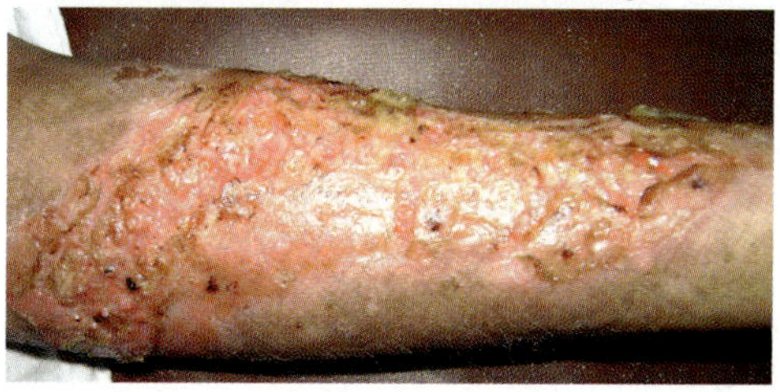

Fig. 2.68: Ulcerative form of lupus vulgaris

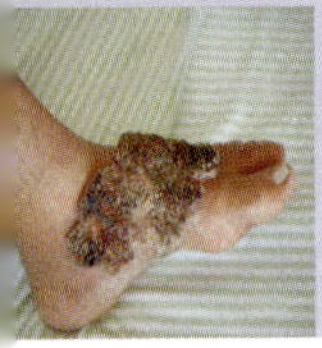

Lupus Vegetans (Lupus Papillomatosus):

It is a vegetative form, occurs in regions of erosive or ulcerative disease.

Lupus Vulgaris Postexanthematicus:

It is a disseminated papular or nodular form. Usually arises during a period of anergy or waning immunity (following measles). Multiple plaque like lesions with scaling and hyperkeratotic margins in lupus vulgaris post exanthematicus.

Lupus Vulgaris of the Mucous Membranes:

It is a rare and special form of lupus vulgaris. Arising by direct extension of skin lupus to the buccal, nasal, or conjunctival mucosa.This form can be highly destructive and disfiguring (Figs. 2.69 and 2.70).

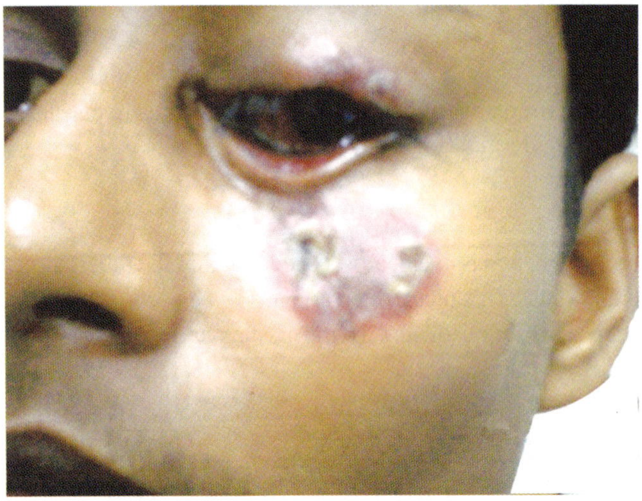

Fig. 2.69: Conjunctival mucosal involvement

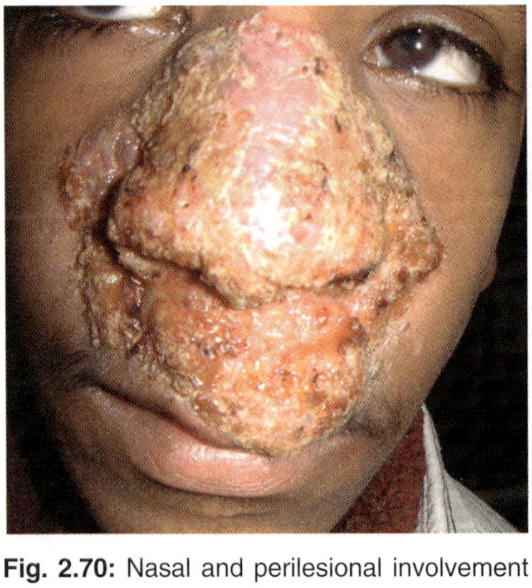

Fig. 2.70: Nasal and perilesional involvement

Histopathology

- Collections of epitheloid histiocytes in the upper half of the dermis, some impinging on the epidermis, which is thinned.
- Dense infiltrates of lymphocytes surrounding granulomas with fibrosis and telangiectases.

Course and Prognosis

- Very protean, destructive disease. Slow progression. Noncontagious. Severe scarring and disfigurement of cosmetic areas.
- Ectropion, distortion of the mouth, or destruction of the nose.
- Lower extremity, distal elephantiasis.
- Squamous cell carcinoma.
- Tuberculids (lichen scrofulosorum and papulonecrotic tuberculid).

Differential Diagnosis

- Presence of apple jelly nodules (lupoid infiltrates) is Characteristic of lupus vulgaris.
- It is not pathognomonic. Identification can be done with a blunt probe, which easily breaks through the overlying epidermis into the nodule, due to the caseous necrosis.

MILIARY TUBERCULOSIS OF THE SKIN

Rare form of acute or subacute cutaneous tuberculosis.

Synonymous

Tuberculosis cutis miliaris disseminata, tuberculosis cutis - miliaris acuta generalisata, and disseminated miliary tuberculosis of the skin.

Infants or children (most common).

Etiopathogenesis

Caused by hematogenous dissemination of *M tuberculosis* from an internal focus of disease, usually pulmonary or meningeal. Following infections that reduce the host immune response (AIDS, measles). Tuberculin sensitivity is usually absent. Bacterial load very high.

Clinical Features

Disseminated lesions occur on all parts of the body. Predilection for trunk, thighs, buttocks and genitalia. The mucous membranes of the mouth can also be affected. Miliary tuberculosis presenting with multifocal oral lesions, extensive proliferative lesion of palate and gingivae.

The primary lesions erupt as discrete, pinhead-sized, bluish red-to-brownish red **macules or papules**.

↓

Often with a **hint of purpura**.

↓

They may be capped with **minute vesicles**, which soon burst and desiccate to **form crusts**.

↓

The lesions are often densely packed.

- Macules, large pustules, ulcerations, subcutaneous nodules, and purpuric lesions may occur.
- Lesions are bacteria rich.

Histopathological Findings

- Sparse infiltrate of neutrophils.
- Necrosis variable, often prominent.
- Epidermis spared.
- Stain for acid fast organisms reveals countless bacilli of *M. tuberculosis*.

Course and Prognosis

Prognosis is poor. Death due to overwhelming infection. In patients whose internal manifestations do not prove fatal, spontaneous healing occurs with significant scarring.

Differential Diagnosis

- Letterer-Siwe syndrome.
- Pityriasis lichenoides acute et varioliformis.
- Secondary syphilis.
- Drug reactions.

Rare Forms of Cutaneous Tuberculosis

- Tuberculous Gumma.
- Tuberculosis Fungosa Serpiginosa.
- Iatrogenic Immunization Tuberculosis.
- Tuberculous Mastitis.

Tuberculous Gumma

- Metastatic tuberculous abscess.
- Results from hematogenous spread during periods of bacillemia and lowered resistance.
- Malnourished children and immunosuppressed patients.

Clinical Features

The lesions are single or multiple, cold, **subcutaneous nodules.** Liquefy into nontender abscesses and perforate the skin, forming **ulcers and sinus tracts** (Fig. 2.71) Tuberculin sensitivity is modest.

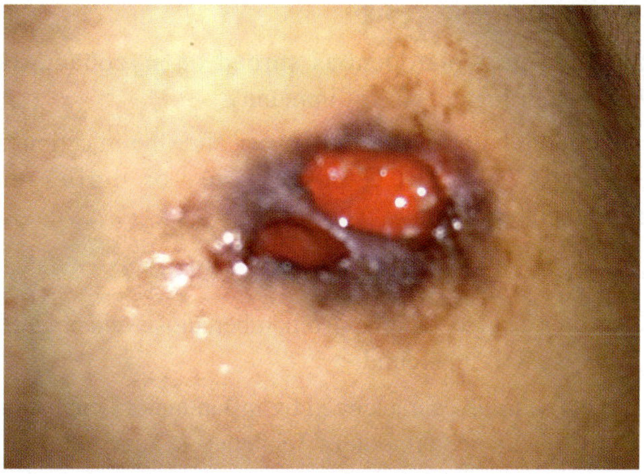

Fig. 2.71: Nontender abscesses perforate the skin, forming ulcers

IATROGENIC IMMUNIZATION TUBERCULOSIS

- Primary inoculation complex, scrofuloderma, lupus vulgaris, exfoliative dermatitis or acute miliary tuberculosis.
- Exfoliative dermatitis after B.C.G. vaccination (in immunodeficient patients).

TUBERCULOUS MASTITIS

- Rare form of tuberculosis involving the breast.
- Present with a nontender, cold abscess.

TUBERCULIDS

- Symmetrical, generalized **exanthem** in the skin of a tuberculous patient.
- Due to an **allergic or hypersensitivity reaction** to the tubercle bacillus or one of its constituent parts.

Tuberculids are:

- Lichen scrofulosrum.
- Papulonecrotic tuberculid.
- Erythema induratum.

Criterion

- Positive tuberculin skin test.
- Tuberculous involvement of lymph nodes or internal viscera or both.
- Absence of tubercle bacilli from skin biopsy and culture.
- Skin lesions that heal on remission of the tuberculous infection.

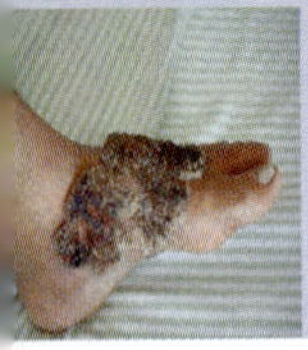

Etiopathogenesis

Result from hematogenous spread of mycobacteria. Moderate or high degree of immunity.

Tuberculids occur rarely. Appear after the injection of tuberculin, after BCG prophylaxis, or during the chemotherapy of active tuberculosis.

Erythema Induratum

- Bazin's disease, tuberculosum, tuberculosis cutis indurativa, nodose tuberculid.

  The disease is characterized by inflammatory cutaneous and subcutaneous nodules.Tendency to ulceration and scarring.
- Occur in **middle-aged women**, with plump extremities and minor peripheral circulatory disturbances. Such as cold feet, erythrocyanosis, or cutis marmorata.

Clinical Features

The eruption is usually symmetric, and typically affects the **calves of pubertal or adult women**.

↓

After some months, these lesions **regress**, especially in the **summer.**

Prognosis

Wax and wane for many years. Worsening in the colder months. New nodules may form, older nodules and ulcerations may show only a slight tendency to heal. A good prognosis can be expected if no general disease is found.

Differential Diagnosis

Erythema nodosum, Subcutaneous lipogranulomatosis, Gummas of tertiary syphilis, Nodular pernio.

Papulonecrotic Tuberculid

- Tuberculosis cutis papulonecrotica.
- The lesions tend to heal with varioliform scarring.
- Occur in patients with active or past tuberculosis.
- It is a reaction pattern reflecting a normal protective immune response in a host with tuberculosis.

Clinical Findings

Girls and young women (more susceptible).Typically, symmetrical, loosely disseminated, grouped eruptions of **papulonecrotic lesions arise in crops**. **Extensor surfaces of the arms and legs**, elbows, knees, backs of the hands, dorsal surfaces of the feet and the lower trunk and buttock region.

The genital region is usually spared.

Symmetric eruption of necrotizing skin papules that appear in crops.

↓

The lesions begin as **pinhead-sized papules** or small nodules.

↓

Over the course of approximately **2 weeks**, may become pustular, vesicular, pemphigoid-like, hemorrhagic, and necrotic.

↓

After another **3 to 6 weeks**, the lesions heal with **varioliform scars**.

Itching and burning sensations in the lesions may occasionally be present.

Differential Diagnosis

Leukocytoclastic vasculitis, Pityriasis lichenoides et varioliformis acuta, Lymphomatoid papulosis, Acne necrotica, Secondary syphilis, Prurigo simplex.

Lichen Scrofulosorum

Synonyms

- Tuberculosis cutis lichenoides.
- Occurs predominantly in **children and adolescents.**
- Sites of predilection are the **sides of the trunk.**
- Lesions arrange **parallel to the skin relaxation lines**.

Clinical Features

Eruption is asymptomatic.The exanthem consists of **symmetrically** arranged groups of **tiny papules**. The primary lesion is a white, pale yellow-brown, pale-red, or skin-colored follicular or perifollicular soft papule. Carry a **fine scale** on its summit.

Prognosis

After a few months eruptions resolve spontaneously without scarring. Recurrences are possible. Transformation to papulonecrotic tuberculid can occur. In patients with normal immunity and chemotherapy, the prognosis is good.

ATYPICAL MYCOBACTERIA

In contrast to *M. tuberculosis*, atypical mycobacteria,

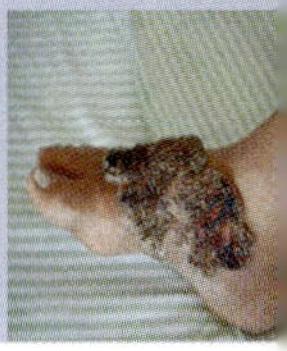

acquired from **environmental sources** (water, soil).They are usually **commensals or saprophytes** than *pathogen*. An **immunosuppressed** state of the host or **damage** to particular organ facilitates these infections. Infection with atypical mycobacteria run a more **benign** and **limited course** than *M. tuberculosis*. They are less responsive to antituberculous **drugs**, but may be senstive to other chemotherapeutic drugs.

I. M. MARINUM (M. BALNEI)

- Slow grower, Photochromogenic, Facultative human pathogen.
- Natural habitat is fresh and salt water (swimming pools, fish tanks).
- Risk factors are: History of trauma and water or fish/ seafood related hobbies.

Clinical Features

- Begin as a **violaceous papule/nodule/psoriasiform or verrucous plaque.**
- I.P is 2 to 3 weeks after inoculation.
- The common sites are **hands, feet, elbow or knee**. Usually lesions are **solitary**, multiple lesions seen in immunocompromised hosts.
- *M. marinum:* Multiple verrucous plaque seen in *immunocompromised hosts*. Sporotrichoid spread of lesions may be seen.
- As a rule regional LN are not involved.
- Lesion may ulcerate and heal spontaneously within 1 to 2 years by residual scarring.

Differential Diagnosis

- Blastomycosis, Coccidioidomycosis, Histoplasmosis.
- Sporotrichosis, Nocardiosis, Tertiary, Syphilis, Yaws.

II. M. ULCERANS

- Slow grower nonchromogenic, Facultative human pathogen.
- Natural habitat is still not known.
- Infection occurs in **wet, marshy or swampy** areas.
- Most commonly occurs in **children and young adults** (female).

Clinical Features

I.P. is about 3 months.

Painless **subcutaneous swelling** develop.

↓

Nodule gradually enlarged and ulcerate.

↓

The **ulcer** is deeply undermined, and necrotic fat is exposed.

↓

The nodule and ulcer are painless.

Buruli ulcer *(M. ulcerans)***:** The ulcer is deeply undermined, and necrotic fat is exposed. It may destroy nerves and blood vessels. Little morbidity occurs with the disease, unless ulcers extend to muscle or bone. Metastatic bone lesions may develop.

The lesion may occur anywhere on the body but **commonly occur on extremities**.

The ulcer **heal spontaneously** in months and years. Healing followed by **scarring and lymphedema**.

Differential Diagnosis

- Foreign body granuloma.
- Phycomycosis.
- Nodular fasciitis.
- Nodular vasculitis.

III. M. KANSASII

- Slow grower.
- Photochromogen.
- Facultative human pathogen.
- Natural habitat is tap water, wild and domestic animals.
- Organism usually acquired from the environment.

Clinical Features

Usually occur in adults with or without Hodgkin's disease, AIDS, immunosuppression.

The route of entry is through **minor trauma** such as puncture wound. Initially there are **papules in sporotrichoid distribution**. Sometimes subcutaneous nodule extend to deeper structures and may result in carpal tunnel syndrome. An ulcerated plaque may also develop in metastatic lesions. In immunocompromised patient it present as cellulitis and abscess formation than granulomatous lesions. Cervical lymphadenopathy may also occur. It also present in nasopharyngeal secretion and can lead to periorificial cutaneous infections.

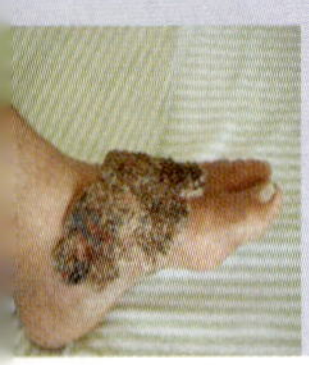

IV. M. SCROFULACEUM

- Slow grower, Scotochromogen, Facultative human pathogen.
- Natural habitat is tap water, soil, other environmental sources.
- Most commonly affects children.
- Route of infection by accidental infestation or inhalation.

Clinical Features

It presents as lymphadenitis in young children of 1 to 3 years. Submandibular and submaxillary nodes are typically involved (TB-tonsilar and anterior cervical). Unilateral lymphadenitis. There is no constitutional symptom except mild pain in neck. Involved L.N enlarged slowly in several weeks and eventually **ulcerate and fistulate**. Disease is **benign and self-limited**.

Differential Diagnosis

All case of cervical lymphadenopathy infectious and neoplastic.

V. M. AVIUM-INTRACELLULARE

- Slow grower.
- Nonchromogen.
- Facultative human pathogen.
- Natural habitat is tap water, soil, other environmental sources.
- This organism often grouped with *M. scrofulaceum* in the **MAIS (M. avium-intercellulare-scrofulaceum).**

Clinical Features

Primary lesion presenting as single or multiple painless, scaling, yellowish **plaques or subcutaneous nodules.** Lesions have tendency to ulcerate and a slowly progressive course.

In immunocompromised host generalized cutaneous ulceration, multiple cutaneous granulomas, pusular lesions or soft tissue swelling may occur.

VII. RAPID GROWER (*M. FORTUITUM, CHELONAE, ABSCESSUS*)

- Facultative human pathogens.
- Also called as *M. fortuitum complex*.
- Commonly found in soil and in water supplies.
- Route of infection by contamination of various materials, including **surgical supplies**.

Clinical Features

Primary cutaneous inoculation occur through skin injuries (**puncture wound or surgical procedure),** in all age group, without immunosuppression. Lesions present as **dark red infiltrated nodule**, often with abscess formation and clear fluid drainage. In immunocompromised host lesions consist of multiple recurrent episodes of abscesses on extremities or generalized macular or papular eruption.

Leprosy

DEFINITION

It is a chronic granulomatous infection of the skin and peripheral nerves with the intracellular bacterium *Mycobacterium leprae*. It affects all organs **except the CNS, *ovary* and heart**. The involvement of **nerves is 100%.** M. leprae was discovered by **Gerhard Armauer Hansen** in 1873 at Norway. It was the first bacillus to be associated with human disease.

M. leprae was cultured in foot pad of mice by *Shephard* in 1960.

Main mode of exit is **nasal mucosa** of untreated cases. Although mode of transmission is still uncertain it seems most likely that *M. leprae are* transmitted via nasorespiratory route. Characteristic virulence factor of *M. leprae* is **phenolic glycolipid I,** a prominent surface lipid, specific of this bacillus. Target organ of *M. leprae* is **Schwann cells** of peripheral nerves.

Generation time is 12 days; Incubation period is 2-7 years (average 3-5 years).

Epidemiology

In India the prevalence is less than 1:10000 and the **most common type is the PB type (indeterminate hansens)**. Risk of transmission of leprosy from a marriage partner is only 5% (Conjugal leprosy).Risk of children acquiring infection from infected adults in the family is 60%.The relative risk for leprosy disease in household contacts is 8-10 for lepromatous disease and 2-4 for tuberculoid forms.

Biology of M. Leprae

M. leprae is an acid-fast gram-positive bacillus and an obligate intracellular parasite with tropism for macrophages and **Schwann cells**. The bacilli show preference for growth

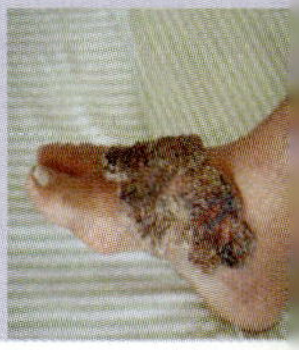

in **cooler regions** of the body. The organism can replicate in the **mouse footpad and the nine-banded armadillo.**

The mycobacterial cell wall contains important targets of the host immune response. These include the species-specific phenolic glycolipid I **(PGL-I),** which stimulates a potent IgM antibody response that is in proportion to the bacterial load in patients and falls with therapy. Other components include lipoarabinomannan, which modulates macrophage bactericidal activities, and proteins involved in cell-wall synthesis.

Host Response

Host genetic factors have a partial effect on both the development of leprosy and the pattern of disease. Whole-genome screening has identified susceptibility loci on chromosome 10p13, close to the gene for the mannose receptor C type 1, a phagocytic receptor on macrophages, and on chromosome 6 within the MHC. Within this region linkage has been shown to HLA class II genes in Indian patients with leprosy and to the gene for tumour necrosis factor (TNF) in Brazilian patients. Polymorphisms in the promoters for genes for both TNF and interleukin 10 are associated with the development of leprosy, and particularly with multibacillary leprosy in the case of the TNF promoter polymorphisms.

The HLA locus also affects the pattern of disease: **HLA DR2 and DR3 alleles are associated with tuberculoid disease, and HLA DQ1 is linked to lepromatous leprosy.** A mutation in the toll-like receptor 2 (TLR2) gene is more common in patients with lepromatous leprosy. Polymorphisms in the *NRAMP1* gene are associated with multibacillary leprosy in African patients.

The varying clinical forms of leprosy are determined by the underlying immunological response to *M. leprae* (Fig. 2.72).

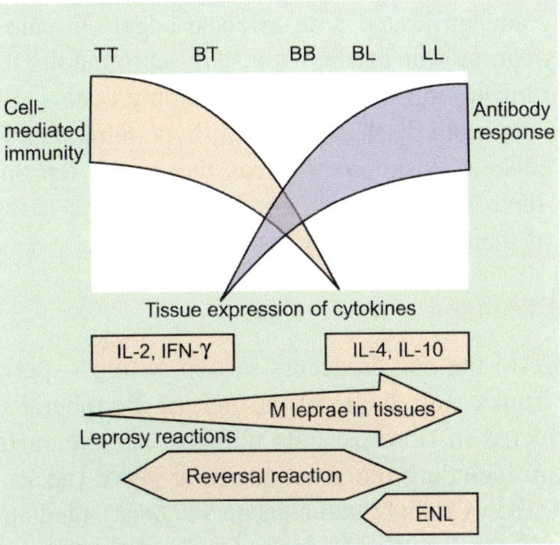

Fig. 2.72: Immunological basis in leprosy

At one pole, patients with tuberculoid leprosy (**TT**) have a **high cellular immune** response to the mycobacterium, which limits the disease to a few well-defined skin patches or nerve trunks. Immune deviation is evident since skin and nerve lesions in tuberculoid leprosy are infiltrated by **Th1-like T cells, which produce abundant interferonα, TNFα, and interleukins 2 and 15.** This leads to well-demarcated granulomas, containing epithelioid and multinucleate giant cells, around dermal nerves. Few, if any, acid-fast mycobacteria can be found in the lesions.

At the other pole, **lepromatous leprosy (LL)** is characterised by the absence of specific cellular immunity but intact immunity to the related *M. tuberculosis*. There is therefore uncontrolled proliferation of leprosy bacilli with many lesions and extensive infiltration of the skin and nerves. The dermis contains foamy macrophages filled with many bacteria, but few CD_4-positive and CD_8-positive T lymphocytes and no organised granulomas. The lepromatous disease contain mRNA for the Th2-like cytokines interleukins 4 and 10. However, the T-cell responses are not completely deviated to the Th2 pattern, since a mixed Th0-like phenotype with concomitant expression of interleukins 4 and 10 and interferon α can be detected in T cells from patients with lepromatous leprosy after stimulation with *M. leprae*. There are **high titres of antibodies to PGL-I** and protein antigens specific for *M. leprae*.

Most patients have the intermediate forms of borderline tuberculoid (BT), mid-borderline (BB), and borderline lepromatous (BL) leprosy. The **borderline forms** are clinically **unstable**, and patients either show slow change towards the lepromatous pole or experience sudden type I or reversal reactions.

Type 1 leprosy reactions or reversal reactions, which occur in a third of patients with borderline forms of disease, are caused by spontaneous increases in T-cell reactivity to mycobacterial antigens. Reversal reactions are associated with the infiltration of **interferon γ** CD_4-positive lymphocytes in skin lesions and nerves, resulting in oedema and painful inflammation.

Type 2 reaction or erythema nodosum leprosum (ENL) is a systemic inflammatory response to the deposition of extravascular immune complexes leading to neutrophil infiltration and activation of complement in many organs. This reaction is accompanied by high circulating concentrations of **TNFα** and striking systemic toxicity. ENL occurs only in **borderline lepromatous and lepromatous leprosy** (Fig. 2.73).

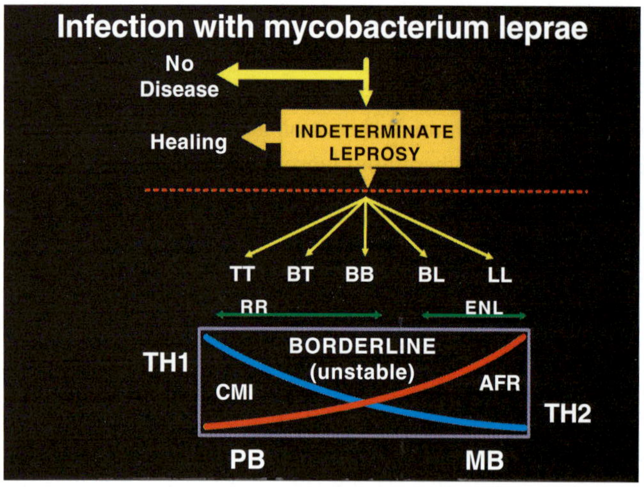

Fig. 2.73: Immunological course

THE IMMUNOPATHOLOGICAL SPECTRUM OF LEPROSY (Fig. 2.73)

Most persons exposed to *Mycobacterium leprae* will not develop leprosy. In susceptible individuals an indeterminate lesion may form. *Indeterminate leprosy often spontaneously heals,* but it may progress into the leprosy spectrum.

The **Ridley-Jopling** classification combines clinical, bacteriological, histopathological, and immunological criteria to identify five forms of leprosy: tuberculoid (TT), borderline tuberculoid (BT), mid-borderline (BB), borderline lepromatous (BL), and lepromatous (LL) leprosy.

Toward the PB end of the spectrum, leprosy lesions have features of a well developed cell mediated immunity (CMI) and contain few acid fast bacilli (AFB), characteristics of a TH1-type immune response. Toward the MB end of the spectrum, the immune response displays a TH2-type profile with a poorly developed CMI and numerous AFB. The borderline area of the spectrum is highly unstable and represents poorly understood immunoregulatory responses; BT and BB (and TT) patients are prone to disfiguring reversal reactions (RR) while BL (and LL) patients are subject to painful ENL (erythema nodosum leprosum) reactions.

CARDINAL SIGNS OF LEPROSY

Diagnostic Signs of Leprosy

Leprosy is diagnosed by finding at **least one** of the following cardinal signs:

1. Definite loss of sensation in a pale (hypopigmented) or reddish skin patch.
2. A thickened or enlarged peripheral nerve, with loss of sensation and/or weakness of the muscles supplied by that nerve (Fig. 2.74).
3. The presence of acid-fast bacilli in a slit skin smear.

   BI–Bacteriological Index: live + dead bacilli (falls by 1 log/year).

   MI—Morphological Index: live bacilli (becomes zero in 6 weeks of therapy—monitor therapy).

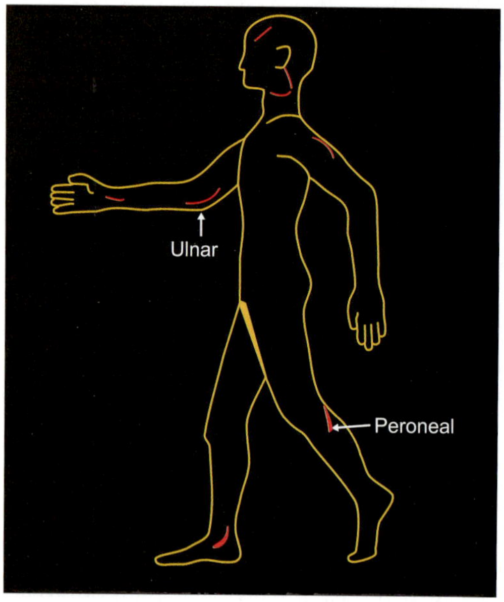

Fig. 2.74: All these nerves can be enlarged in leprosy, the two most commonly affected are the ulnar and the peroneal nerves

Clinical Features of Disease

Skin Involvement

The most common skin lesions are macules or plaques; more rarely papules and nodules are seen. Lesions are hypopigmented in borderline tuberculoid and tuberculoid leprosy and infiltrated with a raised edge. On pale skins, lesions can appear erythematous. In lepromatous leprosy, diffuse infiltration of the skin commonly occurs. Patients with tuberculoid disease have few, hypopigmented lesions with reduced sensation, whereas those with lepromatous forms have many lesions, confluent in some cases, and many of them are not hypoaesthetic.

Nerve Damage

Damage to the nerves occurs in two settings—peripheral nerve trunks and small dermal nerves. Peripheral nerves are affected in fibro-osseous tunnels near the surface of the skin, including the great auricular nerve (neck), ulnar nerve (elbow), radial-cutaneous nerve (wrist), median nerve (wrist), lateral popliteal nerve (neck of the fibula), and

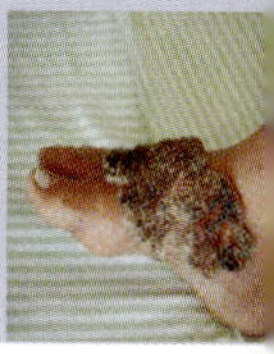

posterior tibial nerve (medial malleolus). The **ulnar nerve is the most commonly affected,** followed by the median, lateral popliteal and facial nerves.

The earliest sensation to be lost is the **cold followed by warm** sensation, touch and pain Small dermal sensory and autonomic nerves are affected producing hypoaesthesia and anhidrosis within borderline-tuberculoid and tuberculoid lesions and glove and stocking sensory loss in lepromatous disease.

Pure neuritic leprosy presents with asymmetrical involvement of peripheral nerve trunks and no visible skin lesions. Histology of a cutaneous nerve biopsy sample might reveal any type of leprosy. This form is seen most frequently, but not exclusively, in India and Nepal, where it accounts for 5-10% of patients.

Systemic Features

These features are seen mainly in lepromatous patients and are due to bacillary infiltration affecting nasal mucosa, bones, and testes. Testicular atrophy results from diffuse infiltration and the acute orchiitis that occurs with ENL reactions. The consequent loss of testosterone leads to azoospermia and gynaecomastia. Renal involvement and amyloidosis are now rarely seen with effective MDT.

Eye Involvement

Resulting from leprosy is devastating for a patient with anaesthetic hands and feet. Eye damage results from both nerve damage and direct bacillary invasion. Lagophthalmos results from paresis of the orbicularis oculi caused by involvement of the zygomatic and temporal branches of the facial (VIIth) nerve.

Other Sites

Leprosy does not involve the CNS and CVS. But traces of AFB have been found at these sites. Also the involvement of the female genital tract is rare, though uncommonly it may involve the uterus and ovary with the ovary being rarer.

Classification

1. **Ridley Jopling:** Clinical, Bacteriological, Immunological and Histological Findings (TT, BT, BB, BL, LL) **Table 2.8.**
2. **Indian—Indeterminate and Neuritic (+RJ types).**
3. **Madrid—Clinical, Bacteriological and Histological Findings.**
4. **WHO.**
5. **Administrative–MB, PB.**

NLEP

Classification of Leprosy

- PB—1-5 skin lesions.
- MB—> 5 lesions.
- Polyneuritic > 1–MB.
- SSL—Single skin lesions—a lesion with sensory loss but no nerve enlargement or infiltration.

WHO

Leprosy is a very variable disease, affecting different people in different ways, according to their immune response. Those at one end of the spectrum, with a high level of immunity harbour a low number of bacilli and are termed Paucibacillary. Those with many bacilli in the body are referred to as multibacillary or MB cases.

1. **The number of individual skin lesions is counted** PB cases have upto 5 skin lesions in total. MB cases have 6 or more skin lesions.
2. **If a skin smear is done and is positive, the patient must be classified as MB** whatever the number of skin lesions. If the smear is negative, the classification is decided by the number of skin lesions.

SUMMARY TO DECIDE MB/PB

Clinical

- >5 lesions—MB.
- ≤ 5 lesions—PB.

Nerve (for neuritic Hansens)

- >1 nerve—MB.
- 1 nerve—PB.

Smear

- BI ≥ 1—MB.

Serology and PCR for Diagnosis

A simple diagnostic test to support the diagnosis of paucibacillary leprosy would be useful. Neither serology nor PCR has a role for this at present. Antibodies to the *M. leprae* specific PGL-I are present in 90% of patients with untreated lepromatous disease, but only 40-50% of patients with paucibacillary disease, and 1-5% of healthy controls. PCR for detection of *M. leprae* DNA encoding specific genes or repeat sequences is potentially highly sensitive and specific, since it detects *M. leprae* DNA in 95% of multibacillary and 55% of paucibacillary patients. Currently PCR is not used in clinical practice.

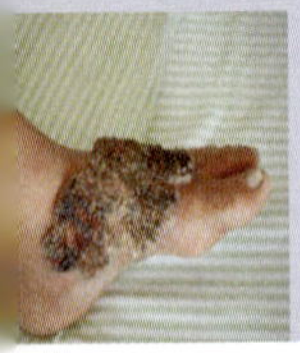

Table 2.8: Clinical findings under Ridley Jopling types

Classification according to Ridley Jopling scheme

	TT	*BT*	*BB*	*BL*	*LL*
Cutaneous lesion	Hypopig/erythematous macules/ plaques **well defined**, **regular-border** dry scaly **saucer right way up** Complete loss of hair/sweat **Anaesthetic.** **Number usually < 3** Nerve to patch Nerve Abscess	Hypopig/erythematous macules/ plaques **well-ill** defined, **irregular** margins, **satellite lesions.** Impaired/complete loss of sweating/hair **Hypoaesthesia** **. <10** Numerous Nerves Assymetrical Nerve Abscess	Morphology of tuberculoid as well as lepromatous **Swiss cheese** **Punched out** **Geographic** Parial loss of sweat hair Hypo-normoaesthesia Numerous B/L sym Countable Numerous Nerves asymmetrical	Variable morphology with papules Shiny to dry **Inverted Saucer** margin well defined Partial to no loss hair and sweat Hypo-normoaesthesia Numerous B/L sym Uncountable Symmetrical	Infiltration, madarosis leonine facies, hypopig/erythematous macules, plaque papules nodules. Margins ill defined No loss of sweat/hair Normoaesthesia Numerous B/L sym - Uncountable Symmetrical
Immunology (lepromin)	Strongly positive (+++)	Weakly positive (+ or ++)	**Negative** (–)	Negative (–)	Negative (–)
Histopath	**Compact granuloma** (tuberculoid) hugging or eroding epidermis. **Cutaneous nerves → destroyed** Langhan Giant Cell	Tuberculoid granuloma less compact than TT. Subepid, **grenz-zone appears.** Nerves → cellular infiltrate	Diffuse epitheloid cell granuloma Grenz zone + nerves → infiltrated epitheloid cell Langhans (-)	Granuloma composed of macrophages + lymphocytes. Grenz zone + Nerves **onion peeling nerve**	Thinned epider. Diffuse lepromatous foamy macrophages few. Lymphocytes + plasma cells. Grenz zone cut nerves are preserved **Virchow cell**
Epilhelioid cells	1+	1 +	1+		
Lymphocytes	3+	2+	1+	3+	0-1+
Langhans' cells	3+	2+	—	—	—
Touton giant cells	—	—	—	—	1+
Globi					1+
Foam cells				1+	2+
CD_4+/CD_8+	1.35 1	—	—	—	0.48 0.50
M. leprae PGL-1 antibodies	1+ (60%+)	2+	2+ 3+	3+	4+ (95%+)
AFB(BI)	0-1+	2-3+	4-5 +	4-6+	globi/normal skin

SALIENT CLINICAL FEATURES OF RIDLEY JOPLING TYPES

1. Tuberculoid (TT)

Single or few, asymmetrical, well-defined, hypopigmented, erythematous or copper-coloured patches.

Clinical

1. The **entire patch (Fig. 2.75) only its edge is raised (Fig. 2.76)** above the surrounding skin.
2. **Hypopigmented patches** not raised above the level of the surrounding skin.
3. Psoriasiform rarely.

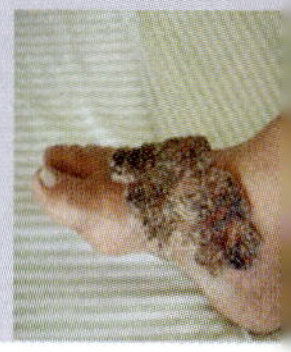

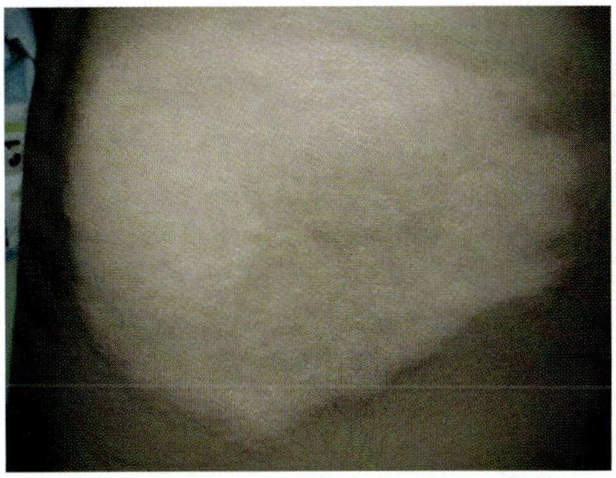

Fig. 2.75: TT– A plaque with uniform infiltration

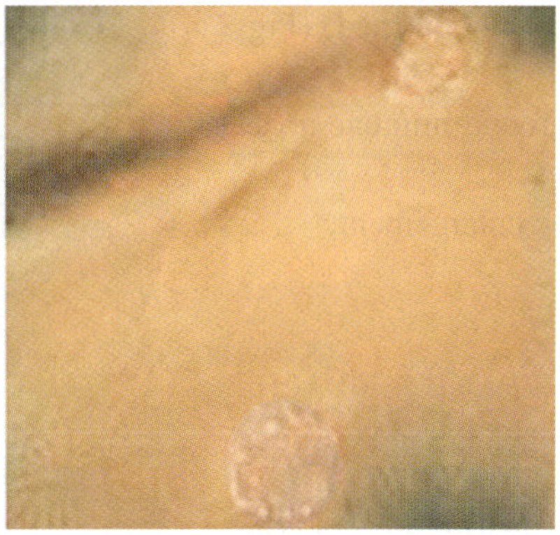

Fig. 2.76

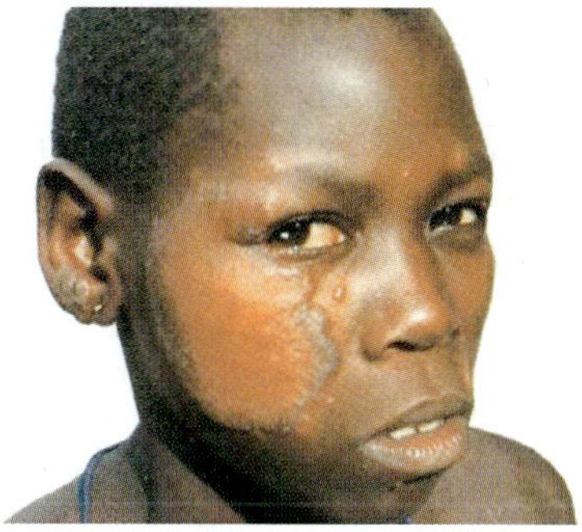

Fig. 2.77: BT–Annular plaque the **outer border** being markedly more **prominent** than the inner border

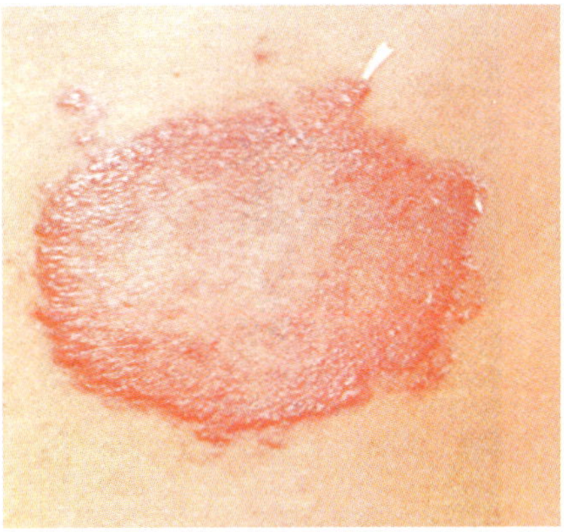

Fig. 2.78: BT–Peripheral border shows pseudopodia with **satellite lesions**

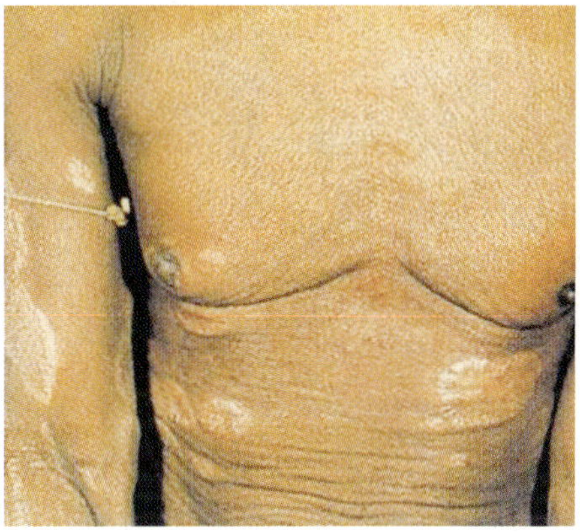

Fig. 2.79: BT–Multiple lesion are seen in BT

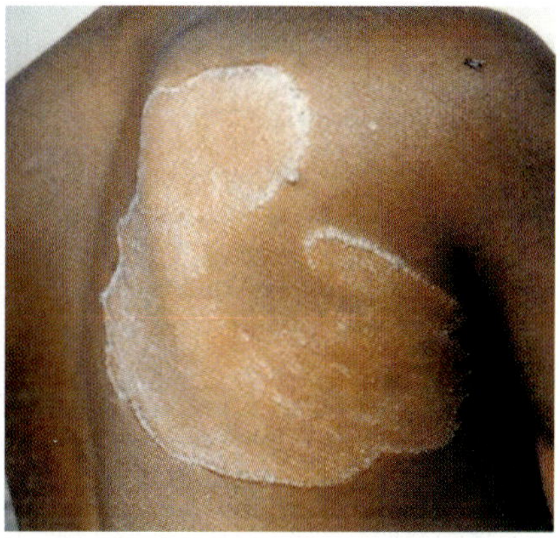

Fig. 2.80: BT–Large lesions with a peripheral infiltration with border ranging from well defined to ill defined

Initially a single peripheral nerve trunk related to the lesion is enlarged; **nerve abscess** may be formed. Foci of lymphocytes, epitheloid cells and Langhans giant cells are seen in the dermis. Nerves are densely infiltrated and often destroyed by the granuloma.

2. Boderline Tuberculoid

Asymmetrical Lesions

1. Usually well-demarcated, somewhat dry.
2. May be annular with *clearly-defined, outer* border (Fig. 2.77).
3. Satellite lesions (Fig. 2.78).

Usually numerous lesions (Fig. 2.79) **and large lesion are seen** (Fig. 2.80).

Widespread and asymmetrical nerve enlargement.

3. Borderline-Borderline (BB)

Asymmetrical less well-demarcated, somewhat shiny lesions.

1. Mixture of lesions of TT and LL type.
2. Often annular lesions with characteristic**, punched-out or swiss cheese** (Fig. 2.81) appearance (**the outer**

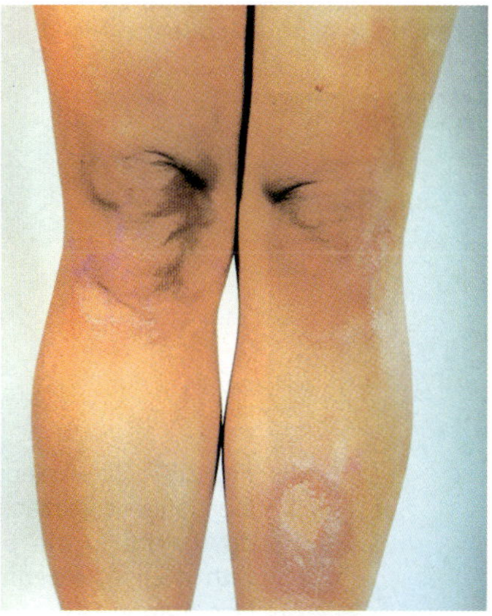

Fig. 2.81: BB–**Classic punched out** lesions

border is vague, *Inner border is clearly* defined) (Fig. 2.82).

3. **Geographic lesions**—Infiltration around immune areas (Fig. 2.83).

   Widespread and asymmetrical nerve enlargement.

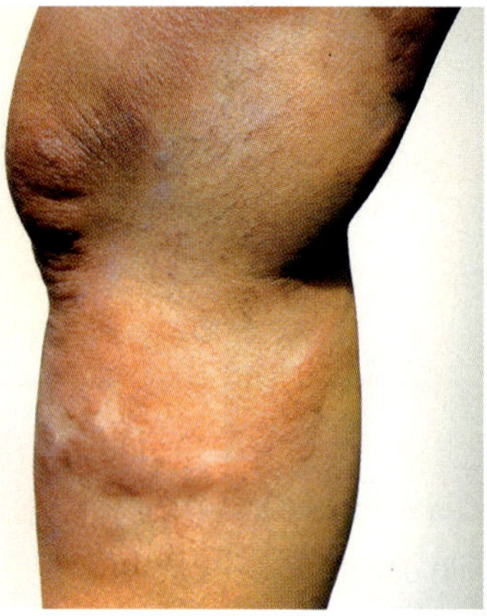

Fig. 2.82:BB–**Inner** border of the annular plaque is more **defined** than the outer and is punched out

4. Borderline-Lepromatous (BL)

Many roughly symmetrical lesions

1. Shiny macules, papules, nodules (Fig. 2.84) and **plaques with sloping edges** (Fig. 2.85).
2. Lesions are **raised in the center and *sloping towards the periphery* "inverted saucer"** (Figs. 2.86 and 2.87).

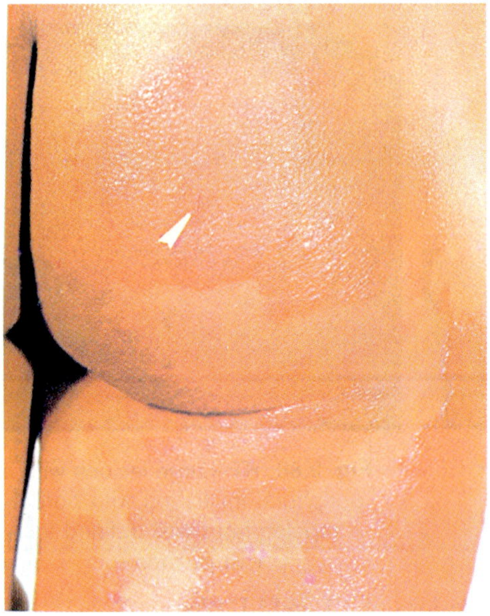

Fig. 2.83: BB–Peripheral infiltrating around an irregular area of central clearing which is the hyperimmune area of previously healed BT–thus representing a geographic lesion

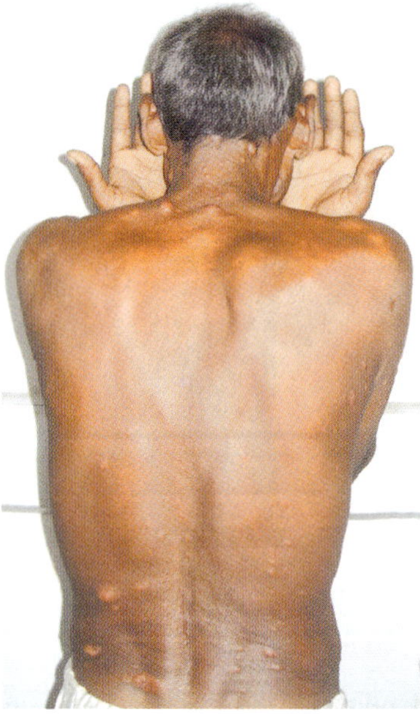

Fig. 2.84: BL–Multiple macules, papules and plaque on the back

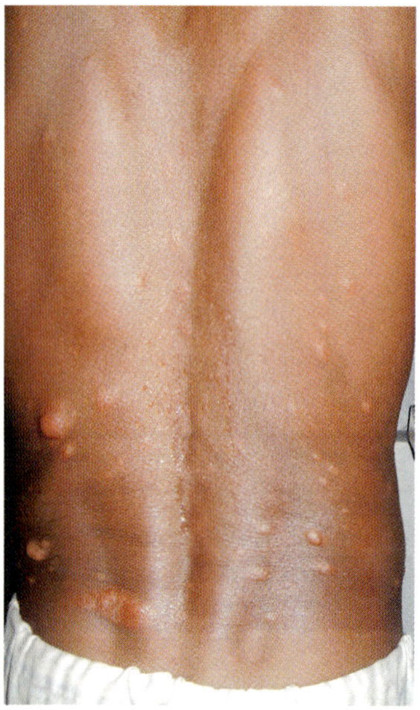

Fig. 2.85: BL–A close up reveals that the **centre is elevated sloping downward** to the periphery representing an **inverted saucer**

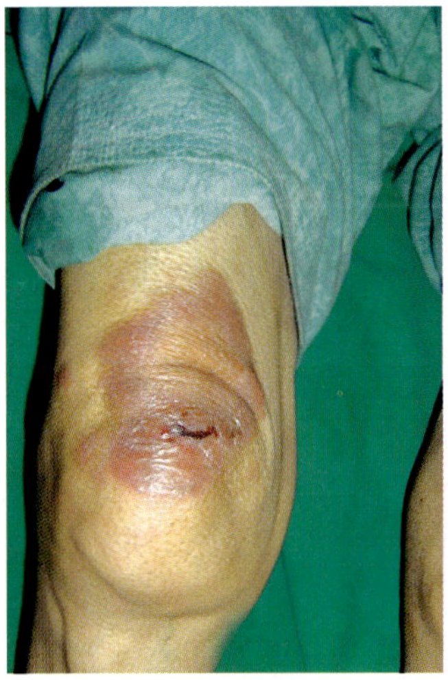

Fig. 2.86: BL– A plaque where the centre is elevated sloping downward to the periphery with a slight clearing (much less than in BB) representing a inverted saucer

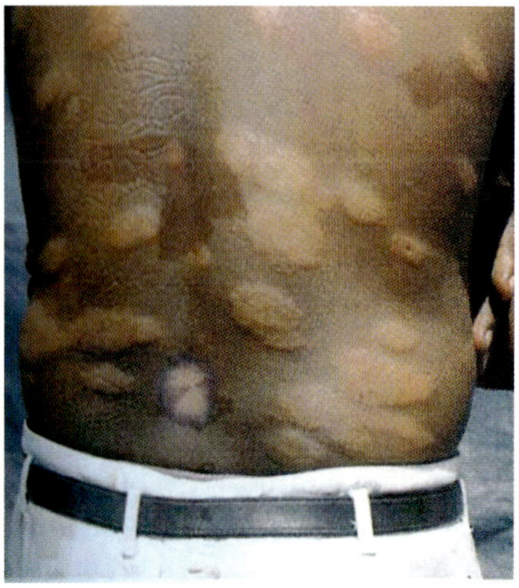

Fig. 2.87: LL–Multiple plaque with inverted saucer appearance

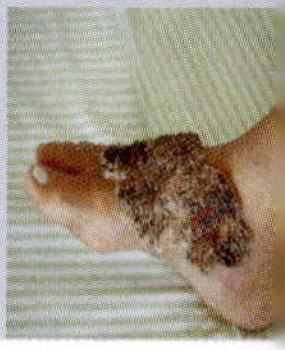

5. Lepromatous

Very numerous symmetrically distributed erythematous or copper-coloured, **shiny**, macules, papules and nodules (Fig. 2.88); the papules lie over infiltrated skin (Fig. 2.89); **macules are ill-defined**; patient may have **leonine face**, loss of eyebrows and eyelashes (Fig. 2.90), with infiltration of the ear lobes (Fig. 2.91).

SALIENT CLINICAL FEATURES OF OTHER TYPES (INDIAN CLASSIFICATION)

Indeterminate Leprosy (Fig. 2.92)

Most common type in India.

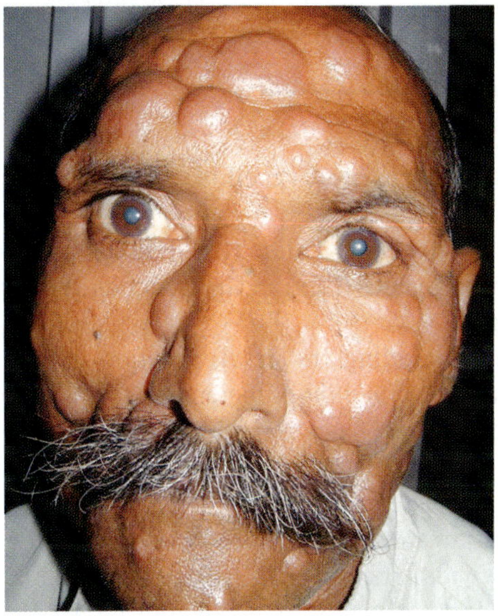

Fig. 2.88: LL–Multiple nodules on the face with loss of hair on the face

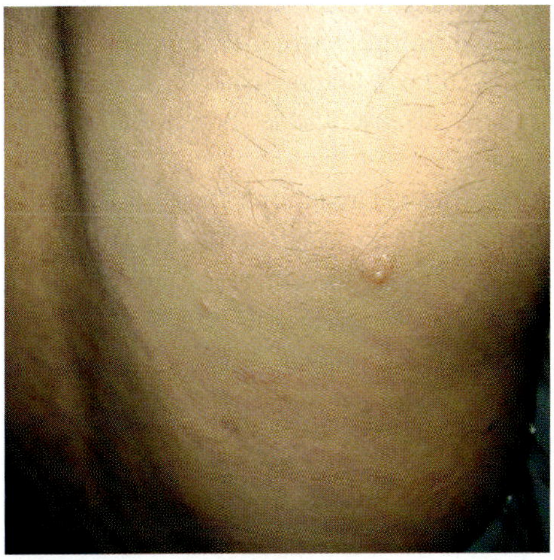

Fig. 2.89: LL–Single papule on an infiltrated plaque

Clinical Features

- Patient is usually a child.
- One or more hypopigmented faintly erythematous **macules**.
- Normoaethesia, no nerve enlarged.
  Lepromin Test: (+/-).
  Slit smear for AFB → (-).
  Biopsy: Mild periappendegeal and perivascular infiltrate.
- **Usually heals spontaneously; about 30% progress to determinate.**

Neural Leprosy

Indian Classification

- Form of leprosy with one or more enlarged nerves but no skin lesions.

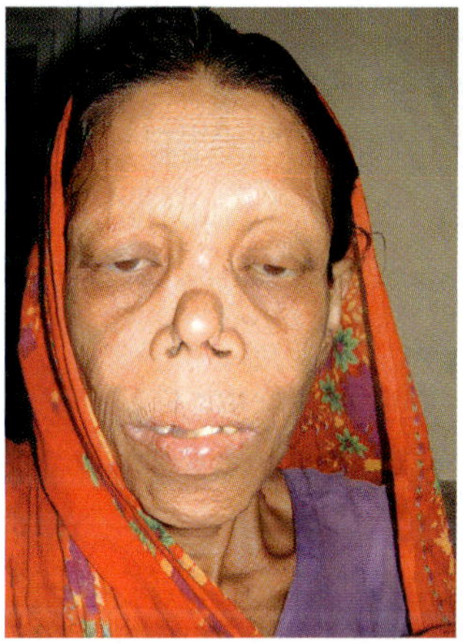

Fig. 2.90: LL: Depressed nose, madarosis, infiltration of the face

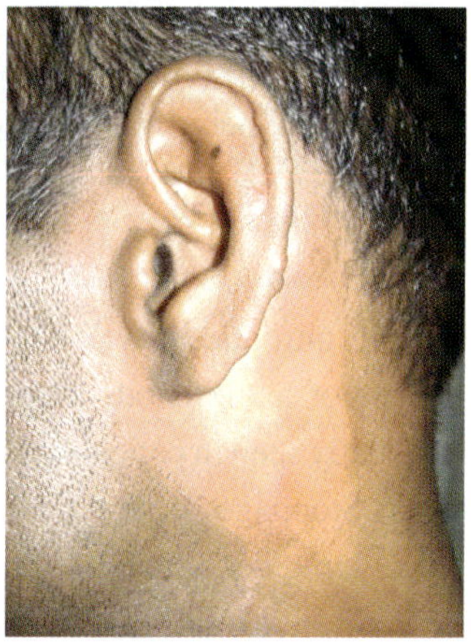

Fig. 2.91: LL: Multiple papules on the ear

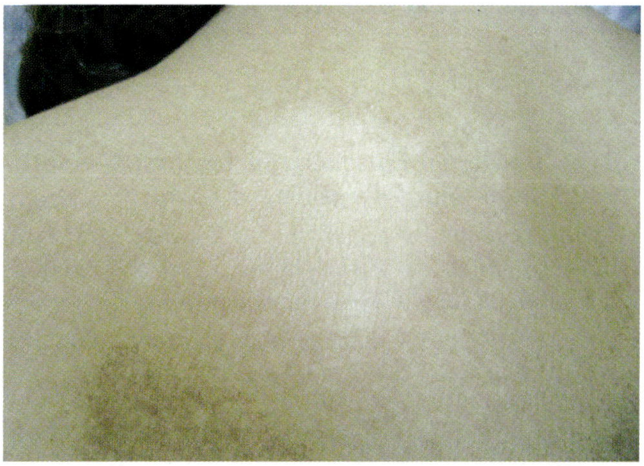

Fig. 2.92: IL: Faint, hypopigmented, non-infiltrated lesion

- MB>1 nerve.
- **Lepromin test** of great value in classification.
  - Strongly + in TT.
  - Weakly + in BT.
  - Negative in BB, BL, LL.

Slit smear for AFB → (-).

SPECIAL VARIANTS

Lucio Leprosy

- Described in Mexico.

Clinical Features

- Diffuse non-nodular.
- Shiny thickened skin, loss of body and facial hair, puffy hands, chronic oedema and ulceration of legs. Widespread sensory loss. Eyes have a shiny, thickened upper eyelids with a sleepy look.
- Ulceration of nasal mucosa presents with epistaxis.
- Laryngeal involvement presents as a hoarse voice. Develop peculiar form of lepra reaction→LUCIO PHENOMENON.

Histoid Leprosy—Variant of LL

- Term introduced by Wade.
- Type of lepromatous leprosy but with better C.M.I.
- Usually seen in patients whose disease is relapsing due to:
  i. Stoppage of treatment.
  ii. Drug resistance.
- Skin lesions—Firm, erythematous, round to oval, shiny, succulent **nodules.**
- **AFB seen of slit smear—longer**, lying singly or in parallel bundles.

PREGNANCY AND LEPROSY

- Worsening of disease especially in 3rd trimester since ↓ CMI.
- **Type 1 reaction especially during first 6 months postpartum→due to regaining of C.M.I.**
- **Type 2 reaction**→especially in 3rd trimester and first 6 months of lactation→since physical stress and return to normal of plasma ACTH + cortisol levels.
- Almost **50% suffer deterioration of nerve function.**
- Babies born to mothers with leprosy weigh less and grew more slowly.
- Rifampicin, Dapsone and Clofazimine, all 3 drugs are considered safe in pregnancy.

REACTION IN LEPROSY

Reactions are acute episodes of hypersensitivity reactions due to fluctuations in the immune status of a leprosy patient. There are three types of reactions: type 1 reaction, type 2 reaction and lucio phenomenon.

How to diagnose a leprosy reaction

Signs of a reaction	
In the skin	– Inflamed skin patches
In the nerves	– Pain or tenderness in a nerve
	– New loss of sensation
	– New muscle weakness
In the eye	– Pain and redness in the eye
	– New loss of vision
	– New weakness in eye closure

TYPE 1 LEPRA REACTION

- **Upgrading (reversal reaction).**
- **Downgrading.**

TYPES: Mostly borderline (BB, BT. BL); may occur in subpolar lepromatous (LLs) and in tuberculoid leprosy **under treatment.**

TIME: Upgrading (reversal) reaction usually occurs during the *first six months* of therapy in BT and BB patients, but longer intervals have been observed in BL patients.

Downgrading reaction occurs spontaneously in untreated patients or in patients whose treatment has been interrupted. On starting treatment, **they may show reversal reaction.**

People with paucibacillary (PB) leprosy and those with multibacillary (MB) leprosy can both get Type 1 reactions. About **25%** of all people with leprosy are likely to get a Type 1 reaction.The most common time is **within six months** of starting treatment. Some people experience a Type 1 reaction before starting treatment – that is, before leprosy has even been diagnosed. The reaction is often the first sign of the disease and is the reason why the person looks for help.

A few patients get reactions later on in the course of their treatment, or even after the treatment has been successfully completed. On rare occasions, a Type 1 reaction can occur upto five years after treatment. Reactions occurring after treatment are sometimes mistaken for a leprosy relapse: that is, a return of the disease itself.

Clinical Features

Upgrading reaction: Some or all the existing leprosy lesions show signs of acute inflammation (pain, tenderness,

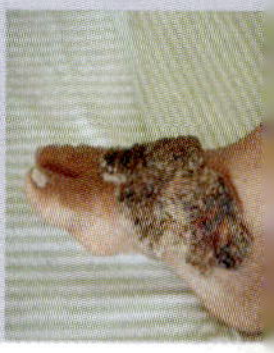

erythema and oedema) (Fig. 2.93). Necrosis and ulceration occur in severe cases. Lesions desquamate as they subside. *New lesions* might appear occasionally in upgrading reactions. As the edema is profound the existing lesion (swiss cheese appearance) becomes more profound (Fig. 2.94).

Downgrading reaction: Lesions worsen and progress towards the lepromatous pole and new skin lesions may appear, each typically **lepromatous in appearance.**

Rapid swelling of one or *more nerves with pain* and tenderness at the site of nerve swelling; oedema of hands, feet or face may be present; *nerve abscesses* may form.

Spl: Very severe reaction with necrosis and ulceration is also called **"Lazarine Leprosy".**

Aetio-Pathogenesis

Cause

Associated with alteration in cellmediated immunity (CMI); upgrading or reversal reactions are due to sudden increase in CMI; *downgrading reactions are due to decrease in CMI.*

It is type 4 hypersensitivity reaction (Coombs and Gell type).

Most type 1 reactions settle down within six months, but without treatment, any effects on the nerves would lead to permanent loss of function.

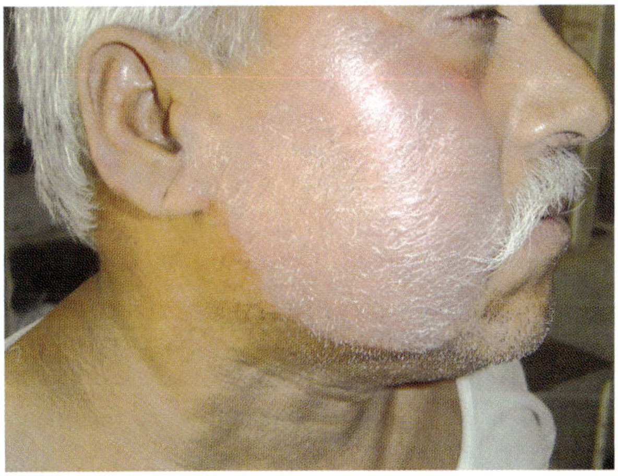

Fig. 2.93: Type 1–A case of BT with edema, erythema and swelling of face showing desquamation due to subsidence of reaction

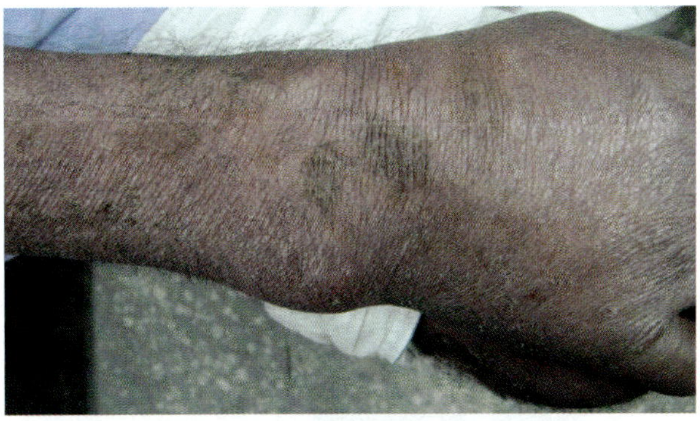

Fig. 2.94: Type 1–A case of BT with edema, erythema and swelling of plaque with a punched out appearance

TYPE 2 LEPRA REACTION

Occurs in **BL, LL after 6 months** of therapy or rarely de novo.

It is also called erythema nodosum leprosum (ENL) reactions. They occur when large numbers of leprosy bacilli are killed and gradually decompose. Proteins from the dead bacilli provoke an allergic reaction. Since these proteins are present in the bloodstream, a type 2 reaction will involve the whole body, causing generalised symptoms.

Type 2 reactions are *less common* than type 1 reactions, although the incidence varies from country to country: in Africa,only about 5 per cent of people with MB leprosy get ENL,whereas in South America upto 50 per cent may get it.

Because it takes the body a long time to clear the dead bacilli, people may still have episodes of type 2 reaction years after stopping treatment.

Clinical Features

Type 2 reactions exhibit the typical signs of erythema nodosum.These are lumps under the skin. There is also inflammation, so that the lumps are painful and red (Fig. 2.95). These lumps may be few or many in number, and

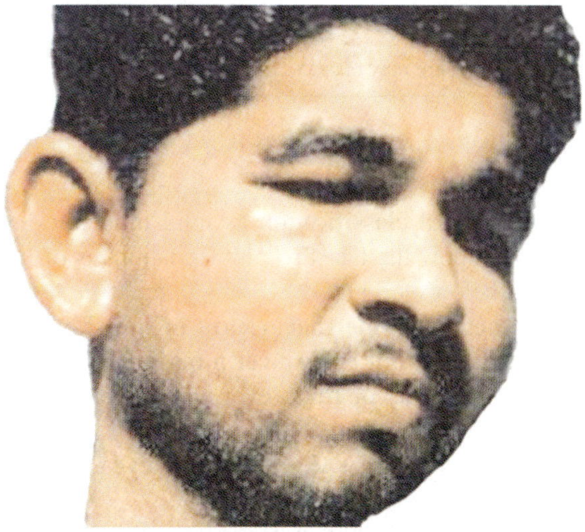

Fig. 2.95: ENL: Red subcutaneous nodules, with edema and swelling of the face

can occur on the legs and arms, and less frequently on the trunk. They are not associated with the leprosy skin lesions. Tenderness of the lumps is an important clinical sign of ENL.

- It is a *type 3 or immune complex* mediated lepra reaction.
- Occurs in *lepromatous spectrum* (Most commonly in LL, occasionally in BL).
- Triggered by *infection, vaccination, drugs and stress.*
- Characterized by tender, erythematous, evanescent nodules called as erythema nodosum leprosum (ENL).
- May have systemic involvement in the form of conjunctivits, keratitis, iritis, iridocyclitis, orchitis, hepatomegaly and lymphadenopathy.

Systemic

- Most common cause of death in lepromatous leprosy is renal failure.
- Type of anaemia seen in leprosy is dimorphic anaemia.
- Cause of blindness in lepromatous variety is due to iridiocyclitis.

Difference between type 1 and type 2

Sign	*Type 1 reaction*	*Type 2 reaction*
Inflammation	The leprosy patches are inflammed, but the rest of the skin is normal	New, tender, red lumps, not associated with the leprosy patches
General condition of the patient	Good, with little or no fever	Poor, with fever and general malaise
Timing of presentation and type of patient	Usually early on in the course of MDT; people with both PB and MB	Usually later in the treatment; only people with MB
Eye involvement	Weakness of eyelid closure may occur	Internal eye disease (iritis) is possible

Grading of Reaction

There was an initial classification as mild moderate and severe ENL but now the latest recommendations is of two type as given below:

- **A mild reaction is one that occurs in the skin only (as long as it does not occur over a major nerve or in the face); there may be mild fever and slight swelling (oedema) of the limbs.**
- **Severe reactions affect the nerves or eyes.**

Signs of Severe Reactions Include

- Pain or tenderness in the nerves.
- New loss of sensation.
- New muscle weakness.
- Reaction in a skin lesion lying over a major nerve.
- Reaction in a skin lesion on the face.
- Signs of inflammation in the eye.
- Severe oedema (swelling) of the limbs (Fig. 2.96).
- Involvement of other organs, such as testes, lymph nodes or joints.
- Ulceration of skin lesions.

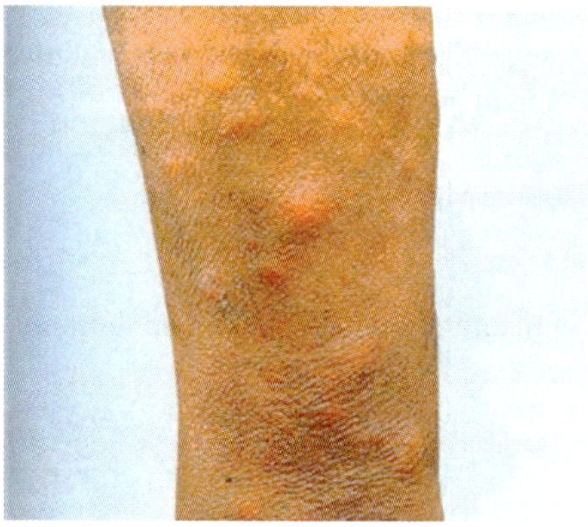

Fig. 2.96

Treatment (Medical)

There are various groups of people who need MDT, recorded as either:

New cases: People with signs of leprosy who have never received treatment before.

Relapse cases receive exactly the same treatment as new cases (either PB or MB).

People who return from default receive exactly the same treatment as new cases (either PB or MB).

PB leprosy treatment: For those over 15 years of age. The course of treatment is given for 6 months.

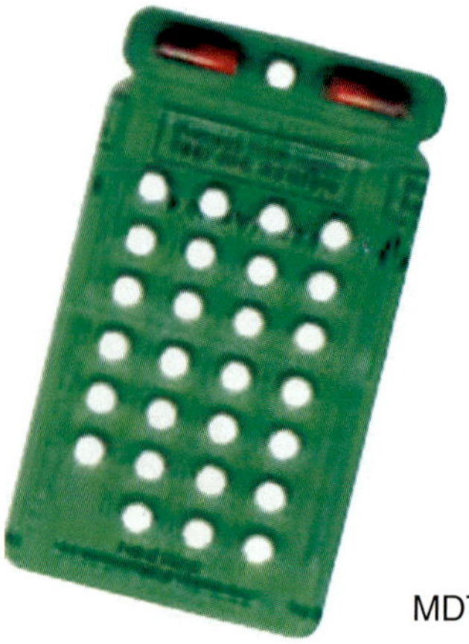

MDT Pack (PB)

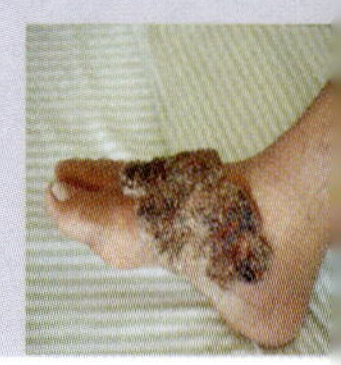

MDT for PB leprosy		
Monthly dose	Rifampicin	600 mg
	Dapsone 100 mg	
Daily dose	Dapsone 100 mg	

MB leprosy treatment for those over 15 years of age. The course of treatment is given for 12 months.

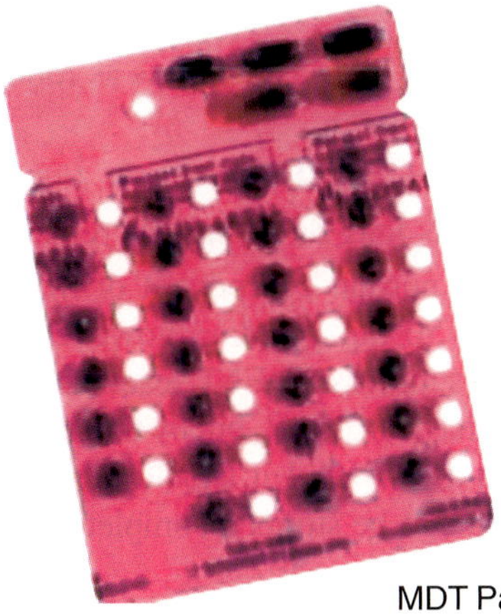

MDT Pack (MB)

MDT for MB leprosy		
Monthly dose	Rifampicin	600 mg
	Clofazimine	300 mg
	Dapsone	100 mg
Daily dose	Dapsone	100 mg
	Clofazimine	50 mg

Leprosy Treatment for Children

The dosage for children varies according to their age, but they must take the same drugs for the same length of time as an adult. That means 6 months for PB and 12 months for MB. As the table below shows, clofazimine is only given for MB leprosy.

MDT for children		Below 10 years	10-14 years
Monthly dose	Rifampicin	300 mg	450 mg
	Dapsone	25 mg	50 mg
MB only	Clofazimine	100 mg	150 mg
Daily dose	Dapsone	25 mg	50 mg
MB only	Clofazimine	50 mg twice a week	50 mg every other day

The appropriate dose for children under 10 years of age can be decided on the basis of body weight [Rifampicin: 10 mg per kilogram body weight, clofazimine: 1 mg per kilogram per body weight daily and 6 mg per kilogram monthly, dapsone: 2 mg per kilogram body weight daily]. The standard child blister pack may be broken up so that the appropriate dose is given to children under 10 years of age. Clofazimine can be spaced out as required.

Newer Forms of MDT

Accompanied-MDT(A-MDT)—Give the full course on the first visit.

Uniform MDT (U–MDT)—6 months to all patients.

Important: As per latest guidelines the therapy is called FDT i.e. Fixed Drug Therapy and at the end of duration irrespective of the activity of disease the medicine is stopped.

NEWER DRUGS IN LEPROSY

1. Quinolones—Perfloxacin, ofloxacin, ciprofloxacin, sparfloxacin.
2. Tetracyclines—Minocycline.
3. Macrolides—Clarithromycin, Roxithromycin.
4. Dapsone analogs.
5. Clofazimine derivatives.
6. Ansamycins—Rifamycin, Rifapentine, Rifabutine.
7. Aminoglycosides—Streptomycin.
8. Cephalosporins—Cefoxitin, Cephaloridin.
9. Beta lactams.
10. Dihydro folate reductase inhibitors—Brodimoprim.
11. Tyrosine inhibitors—Deoxyfructoserotonin.
12. Pyrazinamide.
13. MRRI mycobacterium ribonucleotide reductase inhibitors.
14. Amoxycillin + Clavulanic acid.
15. Fucidic acid.

Vaccines for Leprosy: To be used for:

a. Immunoprophylaxis.
b. Immunotherapy.

FIRST GENERATION VACCINES

- BCG vaccine.
- Killed *M leprae* (armadillo).
- Killed *M leprae*+live BCG (CONVIT).
  a. *M welchii* (Talwars).
  b. ICRC bacillus vaccine (DEO's).
  c. *M vaccae* (Stanfords).
  d. *M leprae*-DCC (Mahadevans).
  e. Vaccine from *M habana* (Singhs).

TREATMENT OF REACTIONS

Type 1 Reactions

The drug of choice remains **Prednisolone**. Other drugs like aspirin, chloroquine are at best adjuvants.

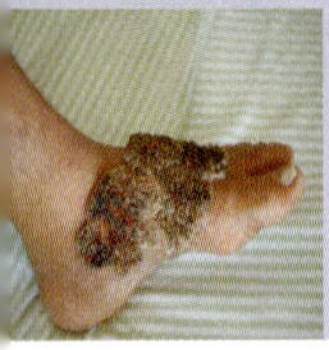

Prednisolone is given by mouth in a decreasing dosage over several months. People with paucibacillary (PB) leprosy receive different duration of steroids from those with the multibacillary (MB) form. People still on anti-leprosy treatment (MDT) must continue their treatment while on steroids; however, those who have completed their course of MDT do not need anti-leprosy treatment while on steroids.

For PB patients the standard treatment is as follows:

Weeks of course	*Daily dose of prednisolone*
1-2	40 mg
3-4	30 mg
5-6	20 mg
7-8	15 mg
9-10	10 mg
11-12	5 mg

The total duration of this course is twelve weeks.

For MB patients the standard treatment is as follows:

Weeks of course	*Daily dose of prednisolone*
1-4	40 mg
5-8	30 mg
9-12	20 mg
13-16	15 mg
17-20	10 mg
21-24	5 mg

This course lasts 24 weeks, exactly double the PB course.

Splinting of the limb in case of neuritis is advisable and drainage of nerve abscess is *not advisable* as this would cause permanent disability as the nerve involved are motor nerves, the systemic steroid is the treatment of choice for abscess.

Newer Drugs: Azathioprine, Cyclosporine.

Type 2 Reactions

Mild—Aspirin, Chloroquine, Clofazamine.
Severe—Thalidomide, Steroids Prednisolone.
Prescribe in the following doses over a short course of 12 weeks:

Weeks of course	*Daily dose of prednisolone*
1	40 mg
2	30 mg
3	20 mg
4	15 mg
5	10 mg
6	5 mg

Prescribing Treatment for Severe Type 2 Reactions

Type 2 reactions can often last for months or even years, and so there is a risk of people becoming dependent on steroids. This makes the reactions very hard to manage, with the result that it can become difficult to reduce and eventually terminate the treatment.

Clofazimine

Clofazimine is given in decreasing doses as follows:

- 300 mg daily for 1 month.
- 200 mg daily for 3-6 months.
- 100 mg daily for as long as symptoms remain.

Clofazimine is a normal component of MDT, and the usual adult dose is 50 mg per day; however, the higher doses are needed to suppress the ENL reaction. Clofazimine takes some time to have an effect, but by the time the steroid dose is reduced to a low level it should be working well, allowing the steroids to be stopped completely.

Thalidomide

Thalidomide is an effective drug for treating type 2 reactions, but because of its side effects one must monitor it very carefully.

It should only be considered for patients whose type 2 reaction cannot be controlled by the first two drugs mentioned above.

The usual dosage is 200-400 mg daily, in divided doses.

REFERENCES

- Ridley Jopling: Hand Book of Leprosy, 2004.
- Hastings: Textbook of Leprosy, 1998.
- Walker SL, Lockwood DN: Leprosy, Clin Dermatol, 2007 Mar-Apr 25(2):165-72.
- WJ Britton, Diana NJ Lockwood: Leprosy, The Lancet 2004; 363:1209-1219.
- Leprosy: SJ Yawalkar, 1992.
- *A New Atlas of Leprosy* by AC McDougall and Yo Yuasa (2000).
- An atlas of Leprosy Guinto RS, Abalos AM, Celona AV, Fajardo TT, Sasakawa Memorial Health Foudation, 1983.
- How to Diagnose and Treat Leprosy ILEP.
- How to Recognize and Manage Leprosy Reactions ILEP.
- Report of the Eighth Meeting of the WHO Technical Advisory Group on Leprosy Control Aberdeen, Scotland 21st April 2006, WHO.

CHAPTER **3**

INSECT BITES AND INFESTATIONS

Insect Bites

Arthropods, the most highly evolved of all invertebrates, are the largest phyla of the animal world. They produce more harm to human beings than any other animal.

Mechanism of Injury to Skin due to Insect Bites

a. Physical trauma.
b. Chemical injuries: This may be due to primary irritation from pharmacologically active substances or sensitization reactions due to antibodies produced against antigenic substances in the venom or saliva of the insect.
c. Secondary pyodermas.
d. Direct invasion of tissues e.g. scabies mite burrows into the superficial layers of the epidermis.
e. Primary irritant contact dermatitis.
f. Chronic inflammatory reactions may be provoked by retained remnants of organisms in the tissues, as in case of scabies, or due to retained mouth parts, as in tick bites.
g. Disease transmission: Infectious diseases are transmitted through mosquitoes, sandflies and ticks.

Diagnosis of Insect Bites

- Possibility should be considered in all cases of pruritic dermatoses.
- Presence of wheals or papules, linear or irregular grouping, asymmetrical distribution, **localisation** to areas accessible to insects.
- Seasonal incidence related to the activities of the insect.

Papular Urticaria (Syn Lichen Urticatus)

- Defined as a chronic recurrent eruption of irritable urticated papules, occurring in patients with an acquired sensitivity to insect bites.
- Lesions tend to have a characteristic distribution and configuration.
- Seasonal incidence.
- Rare in first year of life. Its incidence increases from 2 years onwards and tends to decline after 7 years as repeated bites tend to produce hyposensitisation.
- May be seen in older age groups, although essentially a disease of children.
- Mosquitoes, bed bugs and fleas are the important causes of papular urticaria throughout the world. A number of dipterous flies and mites also produce it.

Clinical Features

Primary lesions are **wheals**, papules or wheals often with a central haemorrhagic **punctum** (Fig. 3.1). Lesions are markedly pruritic. The distribution of lesions depends on the biting habits of the insect and clothing habits of the host, commonly on **exposed** parts of the body. Secondary infections are common.

Differential Diagnosis

Scabies, Atopic dermatitis.

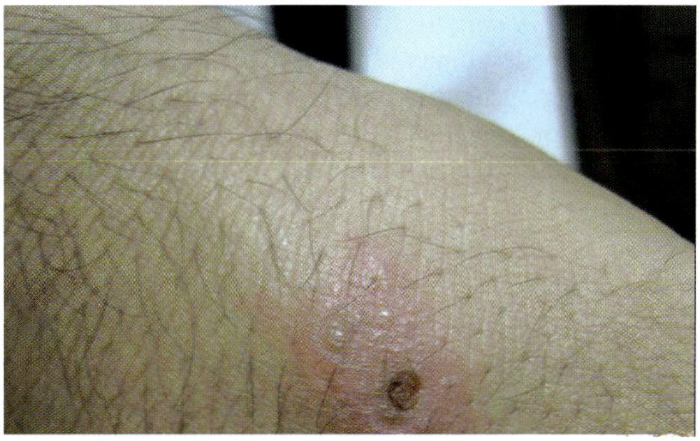

Fig. 3.1: Red lesion with central punctum (Insect bite/Papular urticaria)

Treatment

Insect repellents, antihistaminics, calamine lotion, corticosteroid and antibiotic creams.

Myiasis

- Invasion of mammalian tissues by **dipterous (fly) larvae** is known as myiasis. Myiasis involves different parts of the body, including the skin.
- **Cutaneous myiasis** is classified into 3 forms:
  - i. Creeping **eruption** or creeping myiasis—larvae burrows just under the surface layers of skin.
  - ii. Furuncular myiasis—boil like lesions.
  - iii. Traumatic or wound myiasis—when wound becomes infested with larvae.

Clinical Features

Wound myiasis is seen in neglected ulcers or wounds in most parts of the world. The characteristic larvae, the maggots, are seen in large numbers in the suppurating tissues. May be superficially visible or sometimes hidden, their movements produce pain and distress.

Treatment

No antibiotics are required.

Mechanical removal with forceps.

- If larvae are deep, they can be made to come out by application of open dressings of gauze soaked in turpentine oil.
- In furuncular myiasis—Under local anaesthesia, the lesions can be incised and the larva picked out.
- In creeping eruption larva can be extracted with a needle. Cryotherapy can also be used.

Beetle Dermatitis (Paedrous Dermatitis)

Blister beetle dermatitis: Occurs after contact with 3 major groups of beetles. Injury is produced to the skin by release of vesicating agent **cantharidin or pedrin**. None of the beetles bite or sting; rather they exude their blistering fluid if they are brushed against, pressed, or crushed on the skin (Fig. 3.2).

Clinical Features

Lesions start as **wheals,** blister in about 12 hours. The lesion have a linear distribution. Erythema and swelling are present around the blisters. Kissing lesions are characteristic.

Treatment

Wet compresses. Local corticosteroids application.

INFESTATIONS

Infestations should be distinguished from infections. To be infested is to harbour parasites on the surface. Infestations fall into two main categories:

1. Those due to arthropods.
2. Those due to worms.

PEDICULOSIS (LOUSE INFESTATION)

Two species of blood sucking lice of the order Anoplura have evolved to be obligate ectoparasites of humans. Pediculus humanus and pthirius pubis. The two variants of Pediculus, the head louse and the body louse, are similar morphologically but distinct in the ecologic niches on the body and the clinical manifestations of infestation. Lice are flattened dorsoventrally, and have **3 pairs of leg (Fig. 3.3).**

Pediculosis Capitis

Etiology: The subspecies Pediculus humanus capitis (size 1-2 mm) lays nits within 1-2 mm of scalp. Nits are ova within chitinous case. One female can lay 50 to 150 ova during a 16-day life time. Head louse is not a vector of infectious disease.

Sex, Age of Onset: Girls > boys, 3-11 years, but all ages.

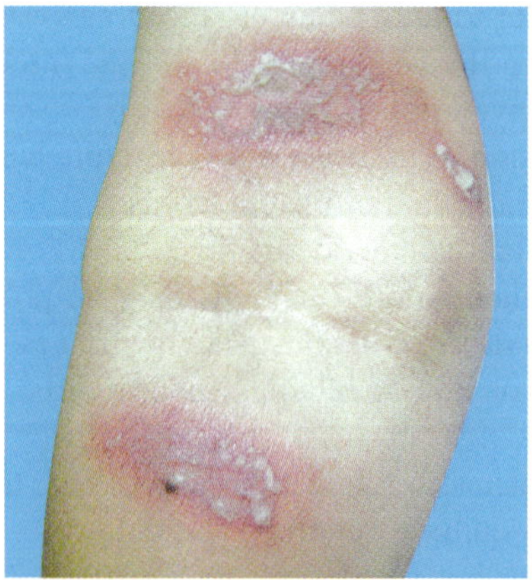

Fig. 3.2: Eczematous plaque with a mirror image (Pedrous dermatitis)

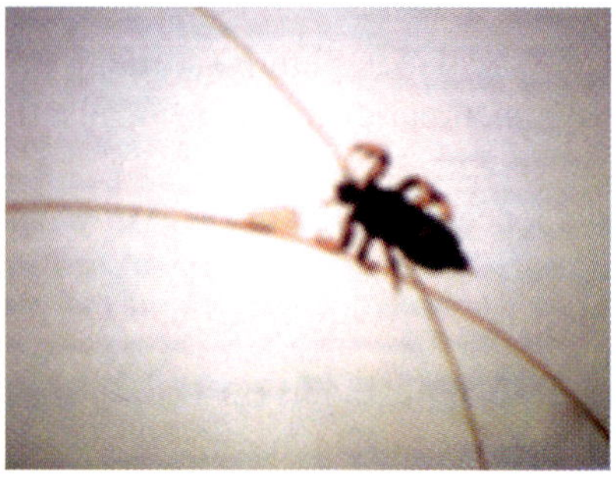

Fig. 3.3: Nits on hair

Transmission: Shared caps, hats, combs, brushes; head to head contact. Epidemics in schools, classrooms are the main source of infestations.

Clinical Features

- Pruritus of the back and sides of scalp. Scratching and secondary infection associated with occipital and/or cervical lymphadenopathy.
- Head lice are identified by eye or with hand lens but are difficult to find. Most patients have a population **of < 10 head** lice, mostly confined to **occipital and post auricular areas**. **Nits** are the oval grayish-white egg capsules (1 mm long) firmly cemented to the hairs; vary in number from only a few to thousands. Nits are deposited by head lice on the hair shaft as it emerges from the follicle.

Complications

- Eczema, excoriation and **lichen simplex chronicus** on occipital scalp and neck.
- Secondary impetignization with S. aureus.
- Confluent, purulent mass of matted hair, lice, nits, crust and purulent exudation '**Plica polonica**'.
- Pediculid is a hypersensitivity rash.

Differential Diagnosis

Dandruff, white piedra, impetigo.

Treatment

Topical therapy

- Permethrin 1%—apply over scalp for 10 min., should be-reapplied in 7 to 14 days.
- Malathion 0.5% applied for 8-12 hours.
- Lindane 1% (GHBC).

Systemic therapy

- Oral Ivermectin 200 μg/kg; repeat on day 10 to kill emerging nymphs.

Secondary infection

Cotrimoxazole, drug of choice which kills bacteria in the gut of lice, which produce nutrients on which the louse survives.

General measures

Fine toothed comb helps to remove empty cased nits.

Pediculosis Corporis

- In body louse infestations, lice remain in clothing except when feeding.

Epidemiology and Etiology

- Pediculus humanus—larger than head louse; 2-4 mm. Life span 18 days. Female lays 270 to 300 ova. Live in seams of clothing, can survive without blood meal for upto 3 days. Grab body hair to feed.
- Risk factors: Poor socio-economic conditions.
- Body lice as vectors of disease: Trench fever, epidemic typhus, relapsing fever.

Clinical Features

- Lice and nits are found in clothing seams.
- Severe widespread itching, especially on the trunk.
- Eczema, excoriation, lichen simplex, secondary impetignization, post-inflammatory hyperpigmentation (**Vagabond's disease**).
- Clothing may be stained with louse feeds, blood/serum.

Differential Diagnosis

Atopic dermatitis, contact dermatitis, scabies.

Management

- Bedding and clothing must be systematically decontaminated.

Hygiene measures: Basic sanitation measures and hygiene measures to assure changes of **clean clothing**, body washing, and sometimes shaving.

Delousing: 1% GBHC or permethrin cream/lotion may be used on patient's skin.

Pediculosis Pubis

Synonymous

Crab lice, pubic lice.

Pediculosis pubis is an infestation of hair-bearing regions, most commonly the pubic area but at times the hairy parts of the chest and axillae and the upper eye lashes.

Epidemiology

Pthirius pubis size 0.8 to 1.2 mm 1st pair of legs vestigial, other 2 clawed. Life span 14 days female lays 25 ova. Adult lice can crawl 10 cm/day.

Most common in young adults, more extensive in males. Transmission is by close physical contact: Sexual exposure (frequent coexistence with other sexually transmitted infection); sharing bed; possibly exchange of towels.

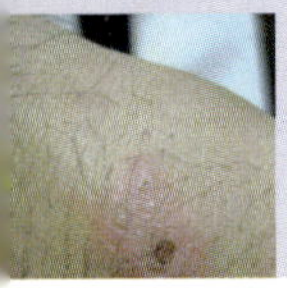

Clinical Features

- Lice 1-2 mm appear as brownish-grey specks.
- Papular urticaria (small erythematous papules) at sites of feeding. Severe itching in pubic areas followed by feeding. Secondary changes of lichenification, excoriation.
- Secondary infections.
- **Maculae cerulae (taches bleues)** are slate grey or bluish grey macules 0.5 to 1 cm in diameter, irregular in shape, non-blanching. Pigment thought to be breakdown product of heme affected by louse saliva. Common on lower abdominal wall, buttocks, upper thighs.
- **Eyelash infestation:** Serous crust may be present along with lice and nits; occasionally, edema of eyelids with severe infestations.

Distribution

Most common in pubic and axillary areas, also in perineum, thighs, lower legs, trunk especially periumbilical.

In hairy males: Nipple areas, upper arms, rarely wrists; rarely, beard and moustache area. Eyelashes and eyebrows may be infested.

Differential Diagnosis

Trichomycosis pubis, white piedra, scabies, mycosis.

Management

30% of persons with pubic lice have another concurrent STI, screen for them.

- 1% permethrin.
- GBHC 1% lotion.
- Malathion 0.5%.

Repeat treatment after 10 days.

For eyelash/eyebrow involvement—Petroleum jelly or anticholinesterase eye ointment for 2 weeks.

SCABIES

Scabies is an infestation by the mite sarcoptes scabiei.

Synonym "7 years itch".

Epidemiology and Etiology

- Scabies is essentially a disease of children. Among children the prevalence is highest in the age group below 5 years.
- Caused by *Sarcoptes scabiei* var hominis. The female mite is about 0.4 × 0.3 mm. They have **four pairs of legs**. The male is much smaller (0.2 × 0.15 mm).
- The female mite burrows though the stratum corneum and granular layer, at the rate of 2-3 mm daily. Usually burrow at night and lay eggs during the day. Female lives 4 to 6 weeks, laying 40 to 50 eggs (Fig. 3.4). The male mite dies after copulation. Usually in classic scabies there are about a **dozen females per patient (10-11 mites)** are present. In hyperkeratotic or crusted scabies, > **1 million mites** may be present.
- Incidence at 300 million cases/year worldwide. In the past, epidemics occurred in cycles every 15 years.
- **Transmission:** Skin to skin contact, can also be sexually transmitted. Mites can remain alive for > 2 days on clothing or bedding; hence, scabies can be acquired without skin-to-skin contact.

Clinical Features

- Incubation period—often varies with immunity to the mite: First infestation, about 3 weeks, reinfestation, immediate i.e. 1-3 days.
- Itching characteristically described as 'worse at night', is the predominant symptom. Similar symptoms may be seen in several family members.

Two types of primary lesions are seen:

1. **Burrows: Pathognomonic** lesion of scabies. Gray or skin (Fig. 3.5) colored ridge 0.5-1 cm in length, either linear or wavy (serpiginous), with minute vesicle or papule at the end of tunnel. They are found in areas with few or no hair follicles, usually where stratum corneum is thin and soft, i.e. interdigital webs of hands > wrists> shaft of penis> elbows> feet> genitals> buttocks> axillae > elsewhere.
2. **Papules and Papulovesicles:** Due to hypersensitivity to the mite and appear as small erythematous papules or papulovesicles, which may be excoriated.

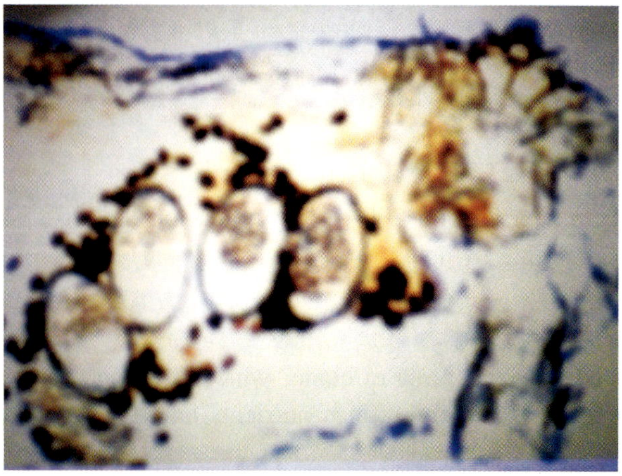

Fig. 3.4: Eggs, with scybala, with nymph (Scabies)

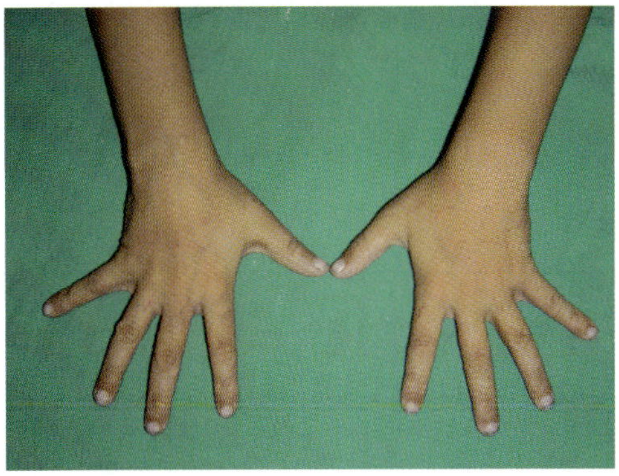

Fig. 3.5: Involvement of web spaces

Secondary lesions seen are:

- **Pustules.**
- Eczematised lesions in infant and children.
- **Nodular** lesions—scrotal skin, penis anterior axillary folds, buttocks and groins.
- Hyperkeratosis/crusting psoriasiform.

Sites of lesions: Papulovesicles or papules appear with crusting over the web spaces, medial aspect of wrist, ulnar border of forearm's, points of the elbow, anterior axillary fold, areola of breasts in female, periumbilical region, groin and thighs, knees, ankles and sole, and gluteal folds (**circle of Hebra**).

Variants of Scabies are:

1. **Infantile***:* Eczematisation with vesicopustules occurs on palms and soles in infants. **Scalp and face** may also be involved. **Vesicles and bullae** are rarely seen.
2. **Nodular scabies** (Fig. 3.6)**:** Develop in 7-10% patients with scabies. They are itchy and due to hypersensitivity reaction **(clean-man scabies)**.
3. **Norwegian scabies:** In immunosuppressed individuals and those with HIV, or lepromatous leprosy, or Down's syndrome and those with neurological disorders, millions of mites are present. In others, clinical appearance is of chronic eczema, psoriasiform dermatitis, seborrheic dermatitis, or erythroderma. Lesions are markedly hyperkeratotic and/or crusted and are generalized.
4. **Scabies incognito***:* Steroid modified scabies.

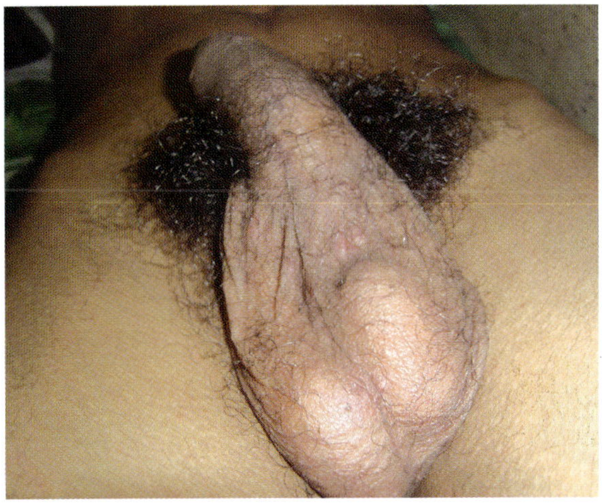

Fig. 3.6: Nodular lesions on the scrotum

Complications

1. Secondary pyodermas.
2. Eczematisation is a frequent manifestation in infants.
3. Acute glomerulonephritis.

Differential Diagnosis

1. Infantile or atopic eczema.
2. Adverse cutaneous drug reaction.
3. Animal scabies.
4. Papular urticaria.
5. Pediculosis corporis.

Diagnosis
- Clinical symptoms
- Demonstration of the mite under microscope is the surest test for diagnosis

Treatment

General Measures

- Treat all members of the family, whether affected or not.
- Ordinary laundering is adequate for bed linen.
- Pruritus can persist for **upto 1-2 weeks** after the end of effective therapy. Try symptomatic treatment with calamine lotion and antihistamines.
- Use an effective **scabicidal**—Apply scabicide **afterbath** on all areas of the body below the jawline in adults. It should be re-applied on hands if they are washed.

Sabicidal drugs used:

Agent	*Strength*	*No. of applications*
1. Benzyl benzoate emulsion	25%	2-3 at 12 hourly interval
2. Gamma Benzene hexachloride Lotion/cream [Contraindication- lactating, pregnant mother and children < 2 years]	1%	Single overnight
3. Permethrin cream (Safe in children, safe in pregnancy)	5%	Single

Contd.

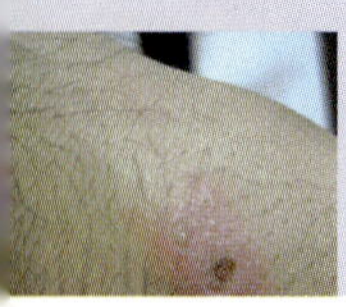

Contd.

4. Crotamiton cream	10%	2 applications on 2 consecutive nights wash off 24 hours after second application
5. Sulfur ointment	6% in petrolatum	Applied to skin for 2-3 days. **Safest in infant and pregnant**

- 5% benzoyl peroxide lotion to which 5% precipitated sulphur is added.

Systemic Ivermectin

200 µg/kg PO single dose to be repeated after 7-10 days. Should be taken empty stomach. Not recommended in children < 5 years, pregnant and lactating women. Useful in epidemic or endemic scabies in institutions such as nursing homes, hospitals, and refugee camps. Also useful in secondarily infected scabies.

Mechanism of Action: It blocks glutamate gated chloride ion channels with effects on nerve and muscle resulting in paralysis of mite.

Treatment of Crusted Scabies

- Multiple scabicide applications.
- Oral ivermectin with topical therapy most effective.

Scabetic Nodules

Intra lesional triamcinolone 5-10 mg/ml into each lesion.

DEMODICOSIS

Caused by Demodex mites, usually found in adults over 30 years of age. There are 2 species:

i. Demodex folliculorum—inhabits pilosebaceous follicles.
ii. Demodex brevis—Lives in sebaceous glands.

The pathogenicity of demodex in man is still disputed. This is because demodices may be readily found in adults without any evidence of disease.

Clinical Features

Burning and itching sensation associated with diffuse erythema of the face.

- Rosacea like lesions.
- Papulonodular eruption in AIDS patients have been reported.

Treatment

- Cleaning with soap water.
- Benzyl benzoate emulsion twice daily.
- Permethrin cream.

Parasitic Worms

1. **Filariasis** (Lymphatic Elephantiasis)
   - Endemic in tropics.
   - Caused by infestation with filarial worms of *Wuchereria bancrofti, Brugia malayi, or B. timori.*
   - Transmitted person to person by the bites of a variety of mosquitoes of the culex, aedes, and anopheles species.
   - The adult worms live in the lymphatic system, where they produce microfilariae. These either remain in the lymphatic vessels or enter the peripheral blood stream in the night.
   - Characterized by lymphoedema, with resulting hypertrophy of the skin and subcutaneous tissues, and by enlargement and deformity of the affected parts, usually the legs, scrotum or labia majora (Fig. 3.7).
   - The onset of elephantiasis is characterized by recurrent attacks of acute lymphangitis in the affected part, associated with chills and fever, that last for several days to several weeks. These episodes recur.
   - After each attack the swelling subsides only partially, and as recrudescences supervene, thickening and hypertrophy become increasingly pronounced.

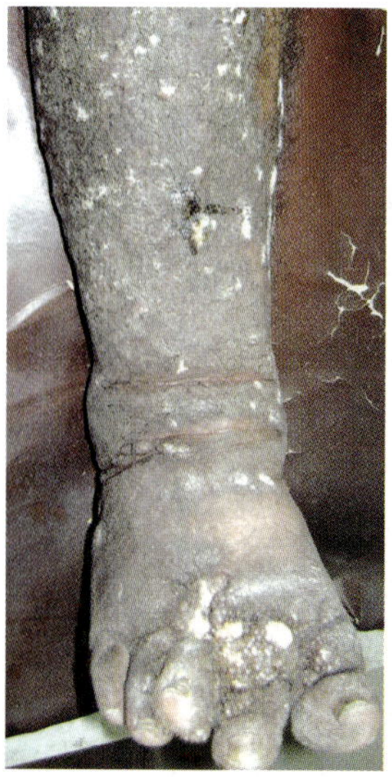

Fig. 3.7: Elephantiasis nostras

Treatment

- DEC Diethyl (*Diethyl*) carbamazine citrate is the drug of choice—Dose.
- Ivermectin 100-440 µg/kg single dose.
- Surgery in late stages.

2. **Cutaneous larva migrans (creeping eruption)**
   - Larva of dog or cat hookworms (mainly *Ancylostoma braziliensis*) may penetrate skin of humans, especially of children walking barefoot on soil contaminated with faeces of these animals.
   - *Clinical features:* Pruritic serpiginous burrows are produced in the sole, buttocks, back and thighs which move at the rate of a few millimeters everyday.
   - The eruption is self limiting, as larva eventually dies. Cryotherapy, 10% thiabendazole suspension topically and oral ivermectin have been used to treat it.
3. **Larva Currens**
   - Intestinal infections with strongyloides stercoralis may be associated with a perianal larva migrans syndrome, called larva currens, because of the rapidity of larval migration (currens means "running" or "racing").
   - Larva currens is an autoinfection caused by penetration of the perianal skin by infectious larvae as they are excreted in the faeces.
   - *Treatment:* Ivermectin 200 µg/kg/day for 2 days.

     or

     Albendazole 400 mg/day × 3 days.
4. **Pinworm infection** (*Enterobius vermicularis*)
   - Most frequent in children, chief symptom is nocturnal pruritus ani. There is intense itching accompanied by excoriations of the anus, perineum and pubic area. The vagina may become infested with the gravid pinworms.
   - *Treatment:* Albendazole 400 mg single dose.
5. **Cysticercosis Cutis**
   - Natural intermediate host of the pork tapeworm, *Taenia solium*, is the pig, but under some circumstances humans act in this role.
   - Larval stage of *T. solium* is cysticercus cellulosae. Infection takes place by the ingestion of food contaminated with the eggs, or by reverse peristalsis of eggs or proglottides from the intestine to the stomach. Eggs hatch here; freeing the oncospheres.
   - These enter the general circulation and form cysts in various parts of the body, as in striated muscle, brain, eye, heart and lung.
   - In subcutaneous tissues the lesions are usually painless nodules that contain cysticerci. They are more or less stationary, usually numerous, and often calcified. Pain and ulceration may accompany the lesion.

Additional Investigations

MRI Brain

Treatment: Praziquantel 10 mg/kg b.w. for 15 days. Calcified parasites need to be surgically removed.

REFERENCE

- Fitzpatrick's Dermatology in General Medicine, 6th edn. 2003.

CHAPTER 4

SEXUALLY TRANSMITTED DISEASES

Chancroid

Haemophilus ducreyi, is the microbial agent of chancroid **Incubation period for chancroid is 3-7 days**.

Clinical Features (Fig. 4.1)

The ulcer is classically described as:
- **Multiple.**
- Not indurated **("soft sore").**
- With a necrotic base and purulent exudate.
- Bordered by **ragged undermined edges.**
- **Bleeding easily on contact.**

There are no prodromal symptoms.

TYPES

- Classical.
- Dwarf.
- Transient.
- Mixed.
- Giant.
- Serpiginous/Herpatiform.
- Pseudogranuloma inguinale.
- Follicular.

REGIONAL LYMPH NODES (Fig. 4.2)

Painful inguinal adenitis is also a characteristic feature of chancroid and may be present in 50% of cases. The **adenitis is unilateral/unilocular** in most patients. Buboes form and can become fluctuant and rupture, releasing thick pus, resulting sometimes in extensive ulceration.

COMPLICATIONS

Mostly seen in men, these may include phimosis and partial loss of tissue, particularly on the glans penis (so-called "phagedenic" ulcers). There can be mild constitutional symptoms but H. ducreyi has not been shown to cause systemic infection or to spread to distant sites.

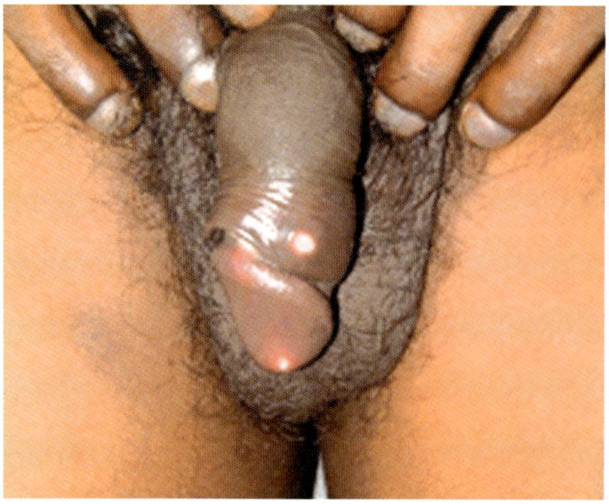

Fig. 4.1: Multiple red ulcers showing necrosis (chancroid)

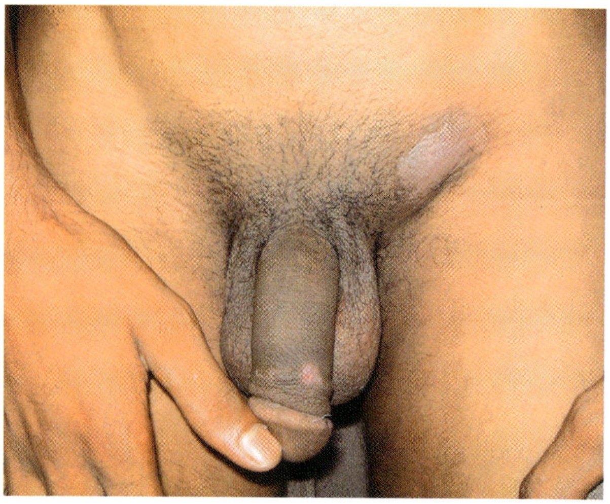

Fig. 4.2: Unilocular unilateral bubo (chancroid)

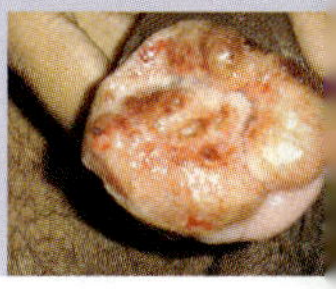

Diagnosis

The main methods of diagnosis revolve around the identification of H ducreyi:

i. **Culture** of scrapings from the ulcer base or of pus aspirate from the bubo; culture media include Mueller-Hinton agar or gonococcal agar base enriched with 1-2% bovine haemoglobin, 5% fetal calf serum, 1% isovitalex and 3 mg/L vancomycin. Since H ducreyi is a fastidious organism, patients' specimens should be plated directly at the clinic or sent rapidly (within 4 hours) to the laboratory; calcium alginate or plastic swabs should be used for sample collection.

ii. **Microscopy of a Gram stained smear** (or other stains) of scrapings from the ulcer base or of pus aspirate from the bubo: demonstration of characteristic **gram-negative coccobacilli** (**school of fish**), with occasional characteristic chaining (Fig. 4.3).

iii. Biopsy 3 zones
   - Superficial→ Necrotic RBC debris
   - Mid→ Thrombosis vascular proliferation
   - Desp→ Fibroblastic, lymphocytes

iv. Detection of nucleic acid (DNA) by amplification techniques such as polymerase chain reaction (PCR), using nested techniques.

Expert opinion has estimated that, in endemic areas, a **positive H ducreyi culture is achievable in 60-80%** of patients considered to have chancroid on clinical grounds.

Microscopy is only 50% sensitive compared to culture, and prone to multiple errors, given the polymicrobial flora of many ulcers. **PCR is the most sensitive** technique, and has been demonstrated to be 95% sensitive compared to culture; conversely culture may be only 75% sensitive relative to PCR.

Other Diagnostic Methods

Antigen-detection techniques involving immunofluorescence or radioisotopic probes. Serologic diagnosis of chancroid has been useful in a number of epidemiological studies, using enzyme-linked immunoassays (EIAs).

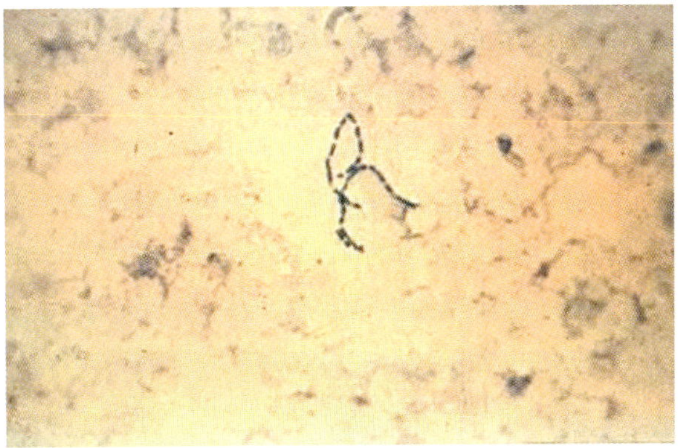

Fig. 4.3: Linear arrangement of cocco-bacilli (School of fish)

Treatment

NACO

Erythromycin stearate/erythromycin base, 500 mg orally 4 times a day for 7 days. Other options:

i. Erythromycin ethyl succinate, 800 mg orally 4 times a day for 7 days.
   N.B In case of concomitant syphilis, treatment can be given for 15 days.
ii. Ciprofloxacin, 500 mg orally twice a day for 3-5 days or till the clearance of lesions, or
iii. Ceftriaxone, 250 mg IM as a single dose, or
iv. Azithromycin, 1 g orally as a single dose, or
v. Doxycycline, 100 mg orally twice daily for 7 days, or
vi. Trimethoprim (80 mg) + sulphamethoxazole (400 mg), 2 tabs orally twice a day for 2 weeks.

CDC

Recommended Regimens

Azithromycin 1 g orally in a single dose.

or

Ceftriaxone 250 mg intramuscularly (IM) in a single dose.

or

Ciprofloxacin 500 mg orally twice a day for 3 days.

or

Erythromycin base 500 mg orally three times a day for 7 days.

If treatment is successful, ulcers usually improve symptomatically within 3 days and objectively within 7 days after therapy.

Sexual Partner(s) Management

Persons who have had sexual contact with a patient who has chancroid within 10 days before onset of the patient's symptoms should be examined, and treated even in the absence of symptoms, as asymptomatic carriage of H ducreyi has been proven to occur.

Management of Lesions

Fluctuant bubo should be aspirated through the surrounding healthy skin. Aspiration should not be done from the dependent side. Incision and drainage or excision of bubo delays healing and is contraindicated.

Chancroid and HIV Infection

In patients with concomitant HIV infection, these regimens are often found to be inadequate. Increased dose and a more prolonged duration of therapy might be necessary.

Some specialists prefer the erythromycin 7-day regimen for treating HIV-infected persons.

Treatment for Pregnant or Lactating Mothers and Children

The erythromycin or ceftriaxone regimens should be applied. No adverse effects of chancroid on pregnancy outcome or on the fetus have been reported.

Genital HSV Infections

Genital herpes has traditionally been **associated with *herpes simplex virus* type 2 (HSV-2)**.

Incubation period for HSV is 7 to 10 days, with a range of 2 to 21 days.

Aetiology

- Roughly speaking, HSV-2 causes 90% and HSV-1 causes 10% of all genital herpes.

Genital herpes is transmitted by sexual intercourse. Direct inoculation of virus occurs through contact with infected secretions or mucosal surfaces. Orogenital contact with a partner with type 1 herpes labialis can also result in genital herpes. **Asymptomatic shedding of HSV is the most common mode of transmission of genital herpes infection.** It is estimated that more than half of the HSV-2 genital infections are asymptomatic.

Types

Asymptomatic

Most common.

Symptomatic

I. **Initial episode:** First episode with either HSV-1 or HSV-2. Dependent on whether the individual has had prior exposure to the other type, this is further subdivided into:

   Primary infection: First infection with either HSV-1 or HSV-2 in an individual with no pre-existing antibodies to either type.

   Non-primary infection: First infection with either HSV-1 or HSV-2 in an individual with pre-existing antibodies to either type.

II. **Recurrent episode:** Recurrence of clinical symptoms due to reactivation of pre-existent HSV-1 or HSV-2 infection after a period of latency.

Primary Genital Herpes

Upto 50% of first-episode cases of genital herpes are caused by HSV-1, but recurrences and subclinical shedding are much less frequent for genital HSV-1 infection than genital HSV-2 infection.

The disease present as multiple painful genital or peri-genital erosions. The polycyclic erosions are preceded by erythematous vesicles (Fig. 4.4). Subsequently, crusts are formed and eventually, they heal spontaneously with no scarring. In women, lesions usually occur on the labia minora (Fig. 4.5), clitoris, perineum, perianal area and the cervix. In men, the penis, perianal area and anus are commonly involved sites.

Cutaneous lesions and viral shedding last about **2 weeks**. It takes **another 1 week** for the lesions to heal. Bilateral

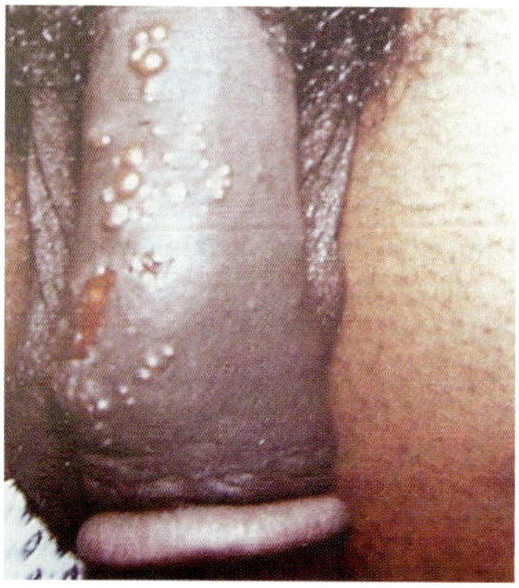

Fig. 4.4: Multiple vesicles on shaft of penis

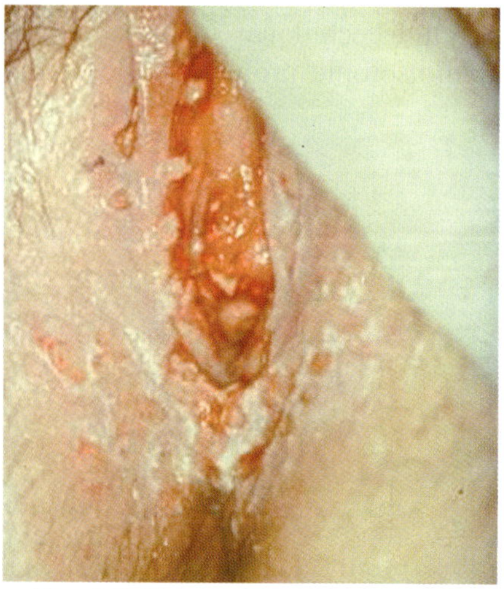

Fig. 4.5: Polycyclic erosions on labia minora and labia majora

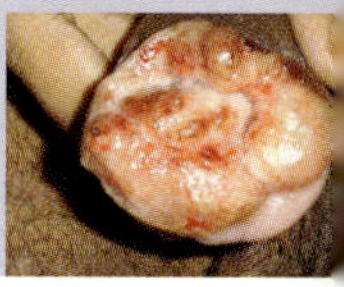

tender inguinal lymphadenopathy is a common associated feature of primary but not recurrent attacks. Primary genital herpes tends to produce more systemic symptoms (i.e. fever, malaise, arthralgia, headache) than recurrent attacks.

Recurrent Infections (Fig. 4.6)

After penetrating the host mucocutaneous surface, HSV is taken up by the peripheral sensory nerves and is carried centripetally to the sensory or autonomic ganglion, where they establish prolonged, latent infection. Reactivation of latent infection gives rise to recurrent skin lesions. Recurrent infection tends to be more localized, of shorter duration and produces less systemic symptoms than the primary attack.

The exact mechanism of reactivation of the virus is unknown but is associated with the following factors:

1. Local trauma (e.g. abrasion resulting from sexual intercourse).
2. Menstruation.
3. Stress.
4. Exposure to sunlight.
5. HSV type: HSV-2 has a higher risk of recurrence than HSV-1.

Prodromal symptoms of local tingling, burning or paraesthesia occur in 50% of recurrent infections. They may precede the localized painful erythematous vesicles or erosions by 24-48 hours. The lesions heal more quickly than the primary attack.

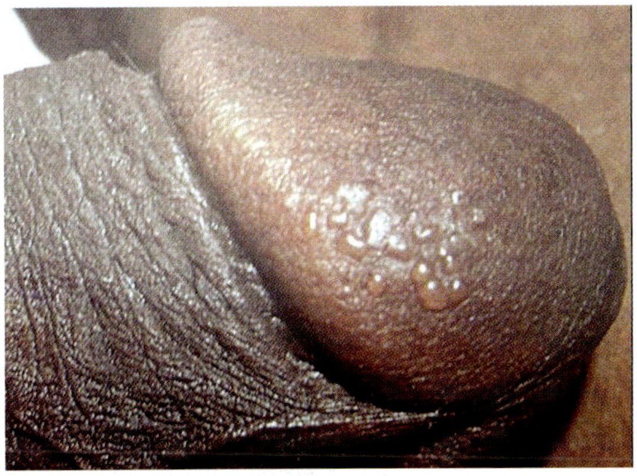

Fig. 4.6: Tense vesicles on glans

DIAGNOSIS

Laboratory Methods

A. Non-culture diagnostic methods
   1. Direct microscopy
      - Giemsa/H and E/Pap stain (Fig. 4.7).

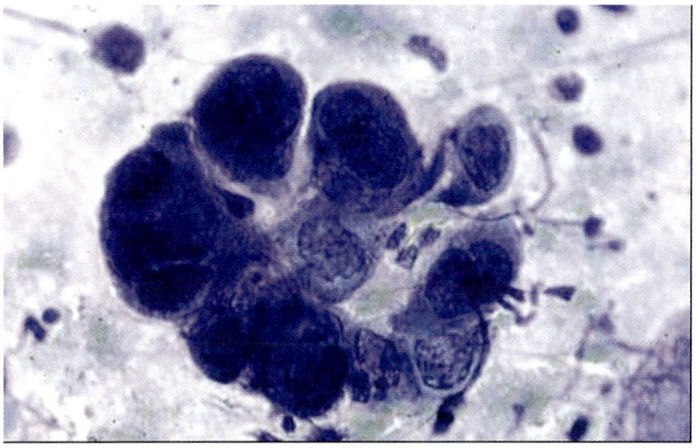

Fig. 4.7: Multinucleate giant cells (Jigsaw puzzle appearance)

   2. Antigen detection
      - IF technique.
   3. Detection of HSV-DNA
      - PCR (Multiplex PCR).

B. Culture.

C. Serology (FDA cleared).

Serology

The detection of HSV-1 IgG or HSV-2 IgG or both, in a single serum sample represents infection with HSV at some time. It is difficult to say whether the infection is recent as IgM detection is unreliable and avidity studies are not commonly available. Collection of serum samples a few weeks apart can be used to show seroconversion and, hence, recent primary infection. HSV-2 antibodies are indicative of genital herpes. HSV-1 antibodies do not differentiate between genital and oropharyngeal infection. Western blot is the diagnostic gold-standard, but it is not commercially available.

Accurate type-specific HSV serologic assays are based on the HSV-specific **glycoprotein G2 (HSV-2) and glycoprotein G1 (HSV-1).** Such assays first became commercially available in 1999, but older assays that do not accurately distinguish HSV-1 from HSV-2 antibody (despite claims to the contrary) remain on the market. Therefore, the serologic type-specific glycoprotein G (gG)-based assays should be specifically requested when serology is performed.

Serology (FDA Cleared)

- Type-specific glycoprotein G (gG)
  e.g.: HSV-specific glycoprotein G2.
- HSV-specific glycoprotein G1
  (sensitivity = 80-96%, specificity >96%).
  Usually takes ~21 days to develop antibodies.
  IgM—new infection (1/2 life ~ 6 weeks), IgG—chronic infection.

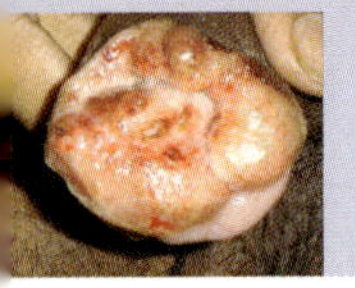

Virus culture is slow, labour-intensive and expensive. Specificity is virtually 100%, but levels of virus shedding, quality of specimens, and sample storage and transport conditions influence sensitivity.

TREATMENT

First Clinical Episode of Genital Herpes

Many persons with first-episode herpes have mild clinical manifestations but later develop severe or prolonged symptoms. Therefore, patients with initial genital herpes should receive antiviral therapy.

Recommended Regimens

Acyclovir 400 mg orally three times a day for 7-10 days.
or
Acyclovir 200 mg orally five times a day for 7-10 days.
or
Famciclovir 250 mg orally three times a day for 7-10 days.
or
Valacyclovir 1 g orally twice a day for 7-10 days.

Suppressive Therapy for Recurrent Genital Herpes

Suppressive therapy reduces the frequency of genital herpes recurrences by 70%–80% in patients who have frequent recurrences (i.e., >6 recurrences per year).

Recommended Regimens

Acyclovir 400 mg orally twice a day.
or
Famciclovir 250 mg orally twice a day.
or
Valacyclovir 500 mg orally once a day.
or
Valacyclovir 1.0 g orally once a day.

Episodic Therapy for Recurrent Genital Herpes

Recommended Regimens

Acyclovir 400 mg orally three times a day for 5 days.
or
Acyclovir 800 mg orally twice a day for 5 days.
or
Acyclovir 800 mg orally three times a day for 2 days.
or
Famciclovir 125 mg orally twice daily for 5 days.
or
Famciclovir 1000 mg orally twice daily for 1 day.

Sexual transmission of HSV can occur during asymptomatic periods. Asymptomatic viral shedding is more frequent in genital HSV-2 infection than genital HSV-1 infection and is most frequent during the first 12 months after acquiring HSV-2.

HIV Infection

Recommended regimens for daily suppressive therapy in persons infected with HIV.
Acyclovir 400-800 mg orally twice to three times a day.
or
Famciclovir 500 mg orally twice a day.
or
Valacyclovir 500 mg orally twice a day.

Recommended regimens for episodic infection in persons infected with HIV.
Acyclovir 400 mg orally three times a day for 5-10 days.
or
Famciclovir 500 mg orally twice a day for 5-10 days.
or
Valacyclovir 1.0 grams orally twice a day for 5-10 days.

All **acyclovir-resistant** strains are resistant to valacyclovir, and the majority are resistant to famciclovir. **Foscarnet,** 40 mg/kg body weight IV every 8 hours until clinical resolution is attained, is frequently effective for treatment of acyclovir-resistant genital herpes. **Topical cidofovir gel 1%** applied to the lesions once daily for 5 consecutive days also might be effective.

Pregnant

Women who are not infected with HSV-1, HSV-2 should be advised to avoid intercourse during the third trimester with men who have genital herpes.

The risk for transmission to the neonate from an infected mother is high (30%-50%) among women who acquire genital herpes near the time of delivery and is low (<1%) among women with histories of recurrent herpes at term or who acquire genital HSV during the first half of pregnancy. However, because recurrent genital herpes is much more common than initial HSV infection during pregnancy, the proportion of neonatal HSV infections acquired from mothers with recurrent herpes is substantial.

Available data does not indicate an increased risk for major birth defects compared with the general population in women treated with acyclovir during the first trimester. Acyclovir treatment late in pregnancy reduces the frequency of cesarean sections among women who have recurrent genital herpes by diminishing the frequency of recurrences at term, and many specialists recommend such treatment. No data support the use of antiviral therapy among HSV seropositive women without a history of genital herpes.

Granuloma-Inguinale (Donovanosis)

Donovanosis is a sexually transmitted infection that usually manifests itself as genital ulceration. It is seen chiefly in small endemic foci in tropical countries. The causative organism, *calymmatobacterium granulomatis* has recently been officially redesignated ***Klebsiella granulomatis***.

Clinical Features (Fig. 4.8)

Type

1. Ulcero granulomatous type.
2. Necrotic type.
3. Verrucous type.
3. Sclerotic/cicatricial type.

- **At site of primary inoculation:** one or more papules/nodules developing into **friable ulcers or hypertrophic lesions** which gradually increase in size. Lesions tend **not** to be **painful.**
- **Regional lymph nodes:** Inguinal nodes are spared and there is spread of infection into overlying tissues, resulting in either abscess formation **(pseudobubo)** or ulceration of the overlying skin.

Untreated infections may either resolve spontaneously or persist and slowly spread. Primary lesions of mouth and cervix occur and the latter have often been mistaken for malignant lesions.

Complications

Haemorrhage, genital lymphoedema, genital mutilation and cicatrisation, development of squamous carcinoma and, on rare occasions, haematogenous dissemination to bone and viscera (particularly during pregnancy).

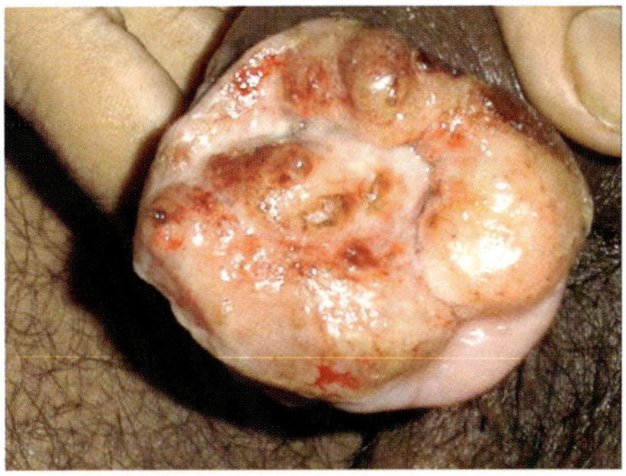

Fig. 4.8: Friable, bleeding, ulcer on penis (Donovaniosis)

Diagnosis

The main method of diagnosis is the demonstration of **Donovan bodies** in either:

i. Cellular material taken by scraping/impression smear/swab/crushing of pinched off tissue fragment on to glass slide; or
ii. Tissue sample collected by biopsy.

Smears can be stained with Giemsa, Wright's stain, or Leishman stain. Biopsies are best stained with silver stains (for example, Warthin-Stary) or Giemsa.

Donovan bodies are characterised by (Fig. 4.9) (i) location within large (20-90 μm) histiocytes, (ii) pleomorphic appearance 1-2 × 0.5-0.7 μm, (iii) bipolar densities and a capsule often visible, (iv) stain gram negative.

In endemic areas identification of Donovan bodies is achievable in 60-80% of patients considered to have donovanosis on clinical grounds.

Culture

Human peripheral blood monocytes and in HEp-2 cells.

Others

(PCR) methods and serological tests for donovanosis have been described but are not yet routinely available.

Treatment (CDC)

Azithromycin 1 g orally once per week for at least 3 weeks or until all lesions have completely healed.

or

Ciprofloxacin 750 mg orally twice a day for at least 3 weeks or until all lesions have completely healed.

or

Erythromycin base 500 mg orally four times a day for at least 3 weeks or until all lesions have completely healed.

or

Trimethroprim-sulfamethoxazole one double-strength (160 mg/800 mg) tablet orally twice a day for at least 3 weeks or until all lesions have completely healed.

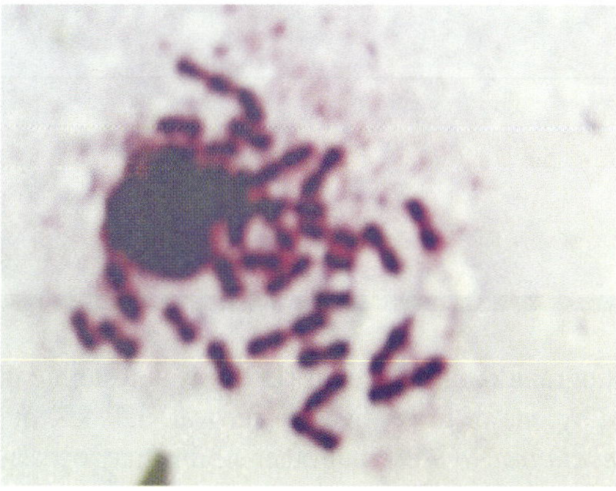

Fig. 4.9: Donovan bodies

Recommended Regimen NACO

i. Doxycycline, 100 mg orally twice a day for 14 days.
   or
ii. Tetracycline HCL, 500 mg orally 4 times a day for 14 days.
   or
iii. Erythromycin stearate or base, 500 mg orally 4 times a day for 14 days.
   or
iv. Trimethoprim (80 mg) + sulphamethoxazole (400 mg), 2 tabs twice a day orally for 14 days or until lesions have completely healed.
v. Lesions should be kept clean.

N.B.: Some patients might require longer treatment than the 14 days as recommended above.

Special Considerations

Pregnancy

Pregnancy is a relative contraindication to the use of sulfonamides. Pregnant and lactating women should be treated with the erythromycin regimen, and consideration should be given to the addition of a parenteral aminoglycoside (e.g., gentamicin). Azithromycin might prove useful for treating granuloma inguinale during pregnancy, but published data are lacking. Doxycycline and ciprofloxacin are contraindicated in pregnant women.

HIV Infection

Persons with both granuloma inguinale and HIV infection should receive the same regimens as those who are HIV negative. Consideration should be given to the addition of a parenteral aminoglycoside (e.g., gentamicin).

Lymphogranuloma Venereum

Lymphogranuloma venereum (LGV) is a systemic disease caused by one of three invasive serovars L1, L2, or L3 of *Chlamydia trachomatis*, but other strains may occasionally be involved.

Clinical Features

The clinical course of LGV is classically divided into three stages.

Primary Stage

The **incubation period is extremely variable (range 3-30 days)** from time of sexual contact with an infected individual; primary lesion is **transient** and often imperceptible, in the form of a painless papule or pustule or shallow erosion; it is found on the coronal sulcus of males and on the posterior vaginal wall, fourchette or on the vulva, and occasionally on the cervix of females.

Extra-genital lesions have been reported such as in the oral cavity (tonsil) and extra-genital lymph nodes.

Secondary Stage, Inguinal Syndrome (Fig. 4.10)

The essential pathological process is thrombolymphangitis and perilymphangitis. Thus, regional dissemination will be characterised by inflammation and swelling of lymph nodes and surrounding tissue.

Lymphadenopathy commonly follows the primary lesion by a period of a few days to weeks (10-30 days, rarely months).

The most common clinical manifestation of LGV (mostly found in heterosexual men) is tender inguinal and/or femoral lymphadenopathy that is typically **unilateral (two thirds of cases)** with considerable periadenitis and bubo formation, which may ulcerate and discharge pus from **multiple points**, creating chronic fistulae.

When both inguinal and femoral lymph nodes are involved, they may be separated by the so-called "**groove sign**", which consists of the separation of these two lymph nodes systems by the inguinal ligament; though considered pathognomonic of LGV, the "groove sign" only occurs in 15-20% of cases.

Tertiary Stage or The Genito-Ano-Rectal Syndrome

The vast majority of patients recover after the secondary stage without sequelae, but in a few patients the persistence

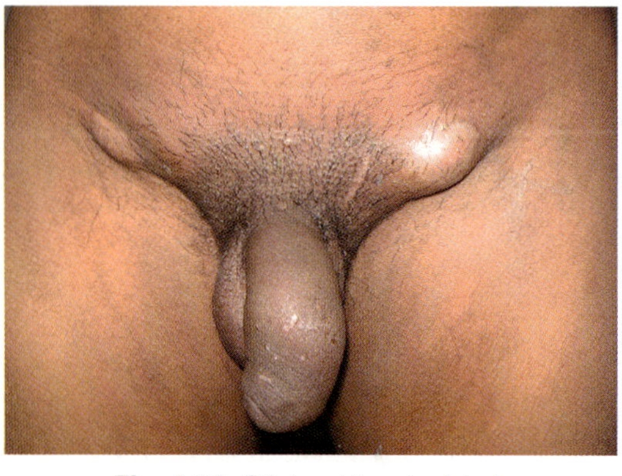

Fig. 4.10: Bilateral inguinal bubo

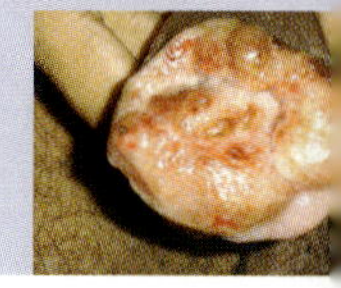

or progressive spread of chlamydia trachomatis in anogenital tissues will incite a chronic inflammatory response, and destruction of tissue in the involved areas, including: proctitis, acute proctocolitis mimicking Crohn's disease, fistulae, strictures and chronic granulomatous disfiguring condition of the vulva (**"esthiomene"**, Greek word meaning "eating away"). These conditions occur most frequently among **women**, reflecting the involvement of retroperitoneal lymphatics (rather than inguinal), and the proximity of the rectal and vaginal tissue, or among homosexual men.

Long-term Complications

- Elephantiasis
- Rectal cancer.

Diagnosis

Diagnosis of LGV is based on both clinical and laboratory investigations which may include the following:

- Mild leukocytosis with an increase in monocytes and eosinophils.
- Elevated gamma-globulin concentration due to an increase of IgA, IgG and IgM.
- Complement fixation test with titres of 1:64 or greater, however the test may cross react with other chlamydial antibodies.
- Microimmunofluorescent test which is diagnostic when the titre is greater or equal to 1:512.
- Isolation of the organism from bubo pus.
- Histological identification of chlamydia in infected tissue.

Definitive diagnosis of LGV is made with cultural (cell cultural lines) isolation of the organism. This method, however, has a recovery rate of less than 30%. Therefore diagnosis is based on serology associated with appropriate clinical findings. A complement fixation titer **(LGV-CF) of greater than 1:16 is strongly suggestive of this diagnosis**. Serology is normally positive within 2 weeks of onset. **Antibody titers do not necessarily correspond with disease activity and may not decline after treatment, as in syphilis.**

TREATMENT

Recommended Regimen (CDC)

Doxycycline 100 mg orally twice a day for 21 days.
Alternative regimen
Erythromycin base 500 mg orally four times a day for 21 days.

Some STD specialists believe that azithromycin 1.0 g orally once weekly for 3 weeks is probably effective, although clinical data are lacking.

NACO

i. Doxycycline, 100 mg orally twice a day for 21days.
   or
ii. Tetracycline, 500 mg orally 4 times a day for 21 days.
   or
iii. Trimethoprim (80 mg) + sulphamethoxazole (400 mg) 2 tabs twice daily for 21 days.
   or
iv. Erythromycin stearate or base, 500 mg orally 4 times a day for 2 weeks.
v. In pregnant and lactating females, erythomycin base/stearate, 500 mg orally 4 times a day for 21 days.

Syphilis

Syphilis is caused by infection with the spirochete bacterium ***Treponema pallidum*** **subsp pallidum (Fig. 4.11)**. This is transmitted from one person to another either by direct contact with an infectious lesion (usually occurring during sexual contact), during pregnancy from mother to child or via infected blood products.

Classification

Syphilis is classified as **acquired or congenital.**

1. **Acquired syphilis**
   Early (primary, secondary, early relapsing syphilis, early latent < 2 years of infection); and
   Late (late relapsing syphilis, late latent > 2 years of infection, tertiary including gummatous, cardiovascular and neurological syphilis).
2. **Congenital syphilis**
   Early (diagnosed in the first two years of life) and late (presenting after two years).

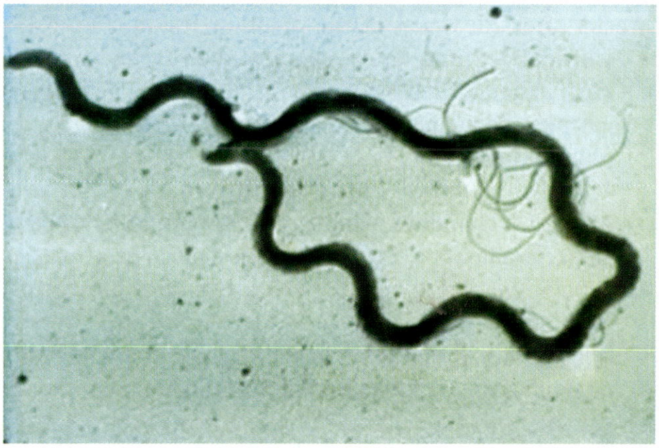

Fig. 4.11: Spirochaete causing syphilis

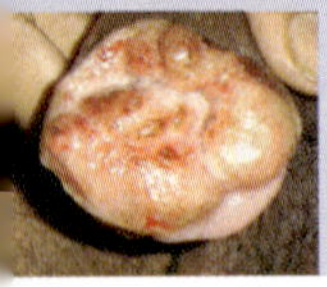

Clinical Features

Primary Syphilis

- **IP—9-90 days**
- *Clinical features:* Characterized by an ulcer (the **hard chancre**) (Fig. 4.12) and regional lymphadenopathy. **Single, painless and indurated** with a clean base discharging clear serum.
- However, chancres may be multiple, painful, purulent, destructive, extragenital (most frequently Lip) and may cause the syphilitic balanitis of Follman.
- **The majority of primary chancres heal within 6 weeks of presentation**. 50% of untreated syphilis infections progress to the second stage, whereas the other 50% enter latency.

  Occasionally the chancre recurs back during relapsing syphilis when it is called **chancre redux.**

  Invg: Dark ground microscopy followed by VDRL. **FTAbs-IgM is + after 2 weeks of initial infection.**

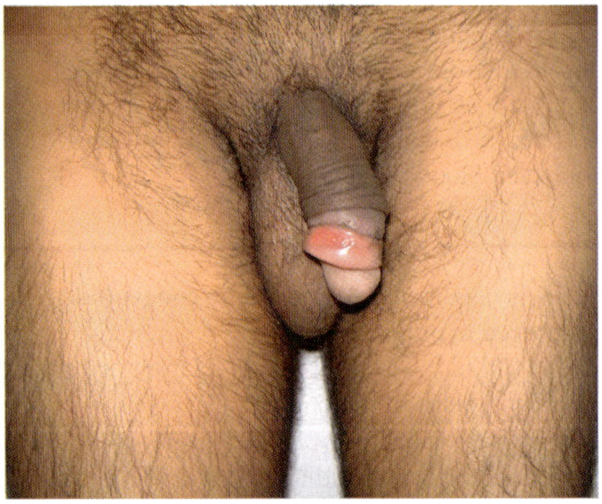

Fig. 4.12: Single, painless, non-bleeding ulcer (Primary chancre)

Secondary Syphilis

The secondary stage of syphilis typically begins 6 to 8 weeks after the onset of the primary lesion (Fig. 4.13).

- **Clinical features:** It is characterised by multisystem involvement. There is often a rash (typically generalised macular, papular or macular-papular often affecting the **palms and soles**) (Fig. 4.14), **condylomata lata** (Fig. 4.15) mucocutaneous lesions (mucous patches), generalized lymphadenopathy and less commonly: patchy alopecia, anterior uveitis, meningitis, cranial nerve palsies, hepatitis, splenomegaly, periosteitis and glomerulonephritis.

  The rash is classically **non-itchy** but may be itchy, particularly in dark-skinned patients and in the follicular variant.
- **Invg:** Dark Ground microscopy followed by VDRL (100% +).

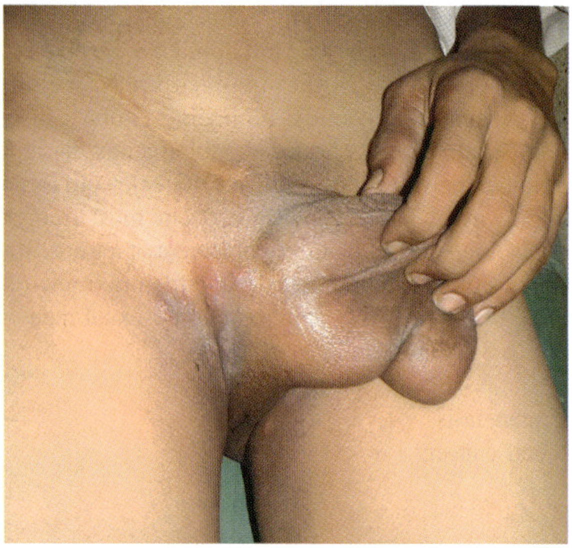

Fig. 4.13: Rash on trunk and the inguinal region (Condylomata lata)

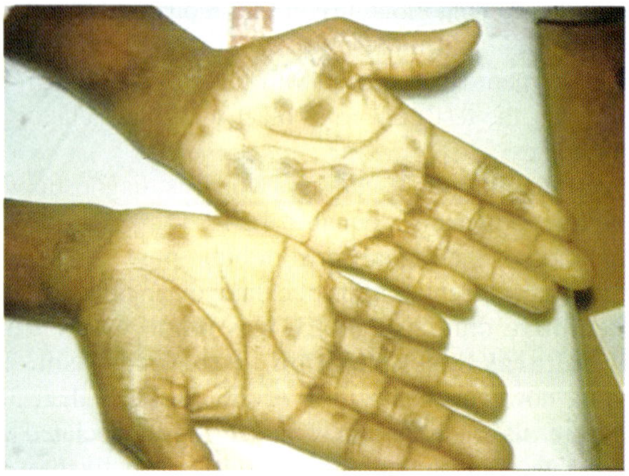

Fig. 4.14: Pigmented macules on palm and sole

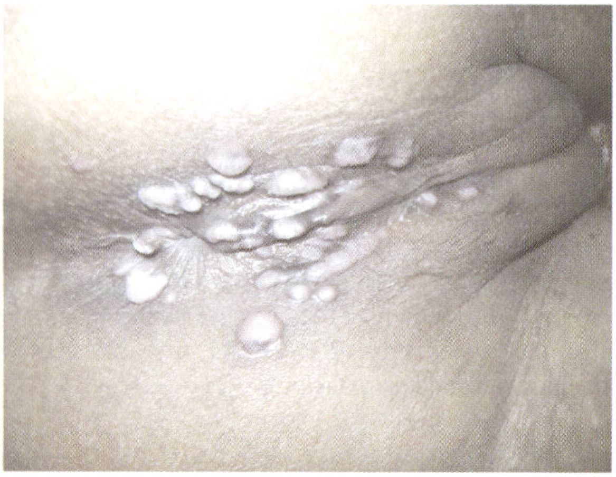

Fig. 4.15: Classic lesions of condylomata lata

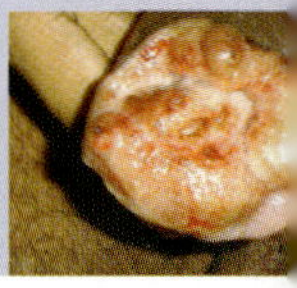

Latent Syphilis

This is when *T. pallidum* infection is diagnosed on serological testing without any symptoms or signs. **Only one third of untreated cases progress to tertiary syphilis. The latent stage is divided into early and late periods. Infection of less than 2 years as early latent disease.**

Invg: VDRL, TPHA +vity.

Tertiary

1. **Cardiovascular syphilis**
   - Heart
   - Great Vessels

   It usually occurs after a latent period of **10-20** or more years.
   a. Angina pectoris due to coronal ostial stenosis.
   b. Aortic incompetence.
   c. Aortic aneurysm (ascending aorta is the most common site).
2. **Neurosyphilis**
   a. *Asymptomatic neurosyphilis:* There is no clinical abnormality but abnormal CSF.
   b. *Meningovascular neurosyphilis:* It usually occurs 3-7 years after infection, affecting cerebral and/or spinal meninges.
   c. *General paralysis of insane (GPI):* This usually occurs 10-20 years or more after infection. The clinical features include dementia with recent memory loss, loss of insight, euphoria with delusion of grandeur, tremor, spastic paraparesis, convulsions, incontinence with patient finally becoming bedridden.
   d. *Tabes dorsalis (TD):* Similarly this occurs 10-20 years or more after infection. The clinical features include lightning pain in legs, paraesthesia, sensory ataxia (positive romberg sign and ataxic gait), sensory loss in proprioception and vibration, deep pain in Achilles tendon, absent reflexes, overflow incontinence, **Argyll Robertson pupils, optic atrophy, Charcot's joints** and visceral crises.
   e. *Ocular syphilis:* The typical features are optic atrophy, optic neuritis, chorioretinitis with salt and pepper fundus.

   Invg: Colloidal gold curve, CSF:
   - Cell
   - Protein
   - Ig Index
   - CSF, VDRL

   (**Quarternary** syphilis includes GPI and TD).
3. **Skin:** Two different types of **cutaneous** lesions may arise:
   - **Nodular or noduloulcerative lesions** are small, firm, nonpruritic, and painless predominantly affecting the back, face and arms. These lesions have the potential for ulceration, with resultant scarring.
   - **Gummas** are painless, deep granulomatous lesions, normally originating from subcutaneous tissue. Predominant locations include the face, scalp, calf, sternum, and sternoclavicular area. Typically heal with retractile scarring. If Gumma occurs on the site of chancre it is called **pseudochancre redux.**

CONGENITAL SYPHILIS

Early (< 2 years)

Includes a rash, condylomata lata, vesiculobullous lesions, snuffles (**earliest sign**), haemorrhagic rhinitis, **osteochondritis, periostitis,** pseudoparalysis, mucous patches, perioral fissures, hepatosplenomegaly, generalised lymphadenopathy, non-immune hydrops, glomerulonephritis, neurological or ocular involvement, haemolysis and thrombocytopenia.

Present at birth: LBW, blisters on palms and soles (**pemphigus syphylitica**).

Develops in the 1st month: Snuffles, periorifacial rhagades, osteochondritis (**Parrot's pseudoparalysis**).

Late (> 2 years)

Hutchinson's triad: Interstitial keratitis, **Clutton's joints**, **Hutchinson's incisors**, mulberry molars, high palatal arch, rhagades, deafness, frontal bossing, short maxilla, protuberance of mandible, saddlenose deformity, sternoclavicular thickening, paroxysmal cold haemoglobinuria, neurological or gummatous involvement.

Stigmata: Saddle nose, Frontal bossing (**Hot Cross Bun), Higoumenaki Sign** (thickening of medial end of clavicle), Saber shin, **Clutton joints**, **Parrots lines** (periorifacial scars), **Dental**–Hutchinson Teeth, mulberry molars.

DIAGNOSIS

Demonstration of Treponema pallidum from lesions by:

- **Dark ground microscopy**
  – If the initial test is negative repeat daily for three days.
  – Less reliable in examining rectal and non-penile genital lesions and not suitable for examining oral lesions due to commensal treponemes.
- **PCR**
  – May be used on oral or other lesions where contamination with commensal treponemes is likely.
- **Serological Tests** (Table 4.1).
  – Treponemal tests
  – Non treponemal tests.

Table 4.1: Serological test for syphilis

Screening tests:	VDRL, RPR, IgG-ELISA
Confirmatory test:	FTA-ABS Test, TPHA
Need for therapy:	IgM-FTA-ABS, IgM-ELISA,VDRL
Follow up:	VDRL, IgM-FTA-ABS, IgM-ELISA

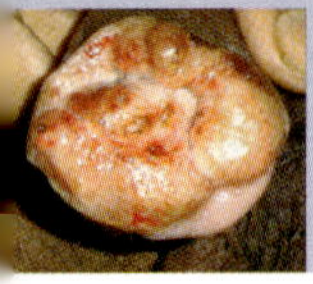

• Specific (Treponemal) Tests

- Treponemal enzyme immunoassay (EIA) to detect IgG, IgG and IgM or IgM.
- *Treponema pallidum* haemagglutination assay (TPHA),
- *Treponema pallidum* particle agglutination assay (TPPA).
- Fluorescent treponemal antibody absorption test (FTA-ABS)
- *Request **EIA for anti-treponemal IgM*** if primary syphilis is suspected **IgM** is detectable towards the end of the **second week** of infection while **IgG** is detectable usually in the **fourth or fifth week**.

The majority of patients who have reactive treponemal tests will have reactive tests for the remainder of their lives, regard-less of treatment or disease activity. However, 15%-25% of patients treated during the primary stage revert to being serologically nonreactive after 2-3 years.

• Cardiolipin (Non-treponemal) Tests

Venereal Diseases Research Laboratory (VDRL), Carbon antigen test/rapid plasma reagin test (RPR). A titer of > 1:8 is positive and it is the best test for **monitoring therapy**. A titre <1:8 is called False Positive VDRL.

Interpretation

A *four fold* change in titer, equivalent to a change of two dilutions (e.g., from 1:4-1:16 or from 1:8-1:32), is considered necessary to demonstrate a clinically significant difference between two nontreponemal test results that were obtained using the same serologic test.

- A **VDRL/RPR titre of >1:16** and/or a positive IgM test indicate **active** disease and the need for treatment, although serology must be interpreted in the light of the treatment history and clinical findings.
- For purposes of partner notification and presumptive treatment of exposed sex partners, patients with syphilis of unknown duration who **have high nontreponemal serologic test titers (i.e.,>1:32)** can be **assumed** to have early syphilis. However, serologic titers should not be used to differentiate early from late latent syphilis for the purpose of determining treatment.

Recommended for Screening

Treponemal EIA (preferably IgG and IgM) or TPPA or VDRL/RPR and TPHA.

EVALUATION OF SEROLOGICAL TESTS

Confirmation of Infection: 2 Positive Tests with Specific Test.

Assessing Degree of Activity: IgM FTA-ABS and VDRL >1:64.

Second Infection: VDRL titre increase by two dilution and new appearance of IgM antibodies.

DIAGNOSIS OF NEUROSYPHILIS

Microscopy: lymphocytes > 5/mm^3.
Biochemistry: protein > 0.4 gm/l.
Serology: VDRL (negative in > *1/4* neurosyphilis).
FTA or TPHA (negative test virtually excludes neurosyphilis).

Neurosyphilis is unlikely when the CSF TPHA *titre is < 1:320 or the TPPA titre <1:640.*

The TPHA index (CSF TPHA/albumin quotient [CSF albumin × 103/serum albumin]) allows for impaired barrier function and is more sensitive than the CSF VDRL whilst maintaining high specificity.

A TPHA index >70 and a CSF TPHA titre >320 are the most reliable in supporting a diagnosis of neurosyphilis but unfortunately determination of the TPHA index is not widely available.

DIAGNOSIS OF CONGENITAL SYPHILIS

- *Direct demonstration* of *T. pallidum* by dark ground microscopy and/or PCR of exudates from suspicious lesions, or body fluids, e.g. nasal discharge.
- *Serological tests* should be performed on **infant's blood** not cord blood and if the infant's serum is positive on screening, perform treponemal IgM EIA, quantitative VDRL/RPR and quantitative TPPA tests on the infant and mother in **parallel.**
- **Serological tests detecting IgG** may be positive due **to passive transfer** of maternal antibodies whether or not the infant is infected.
  - If the IgM test is negative, and the other tests are reactive with titres less than four-fold higher than those of the mother and there are no signs of congenital syphilis, then repeat reactive tests at 3, 6 and 12 months of age or until all tests become negative (usually by 6 months). Also repeat the IgM at 3 months in case the infant's response is delayed or suppressed.
  - If the infant's serum is negative on screening, and there are no signs of congenital infection, no further testing is necessary.
- A positive **IgM EIA test** and/or a sustained **four fold or greater difference of VDRL/RPR titre or TPPA titre above that of the mother** (confirmed on testing a second specimen from the infant) indicates a diagnosis of congenital infection.

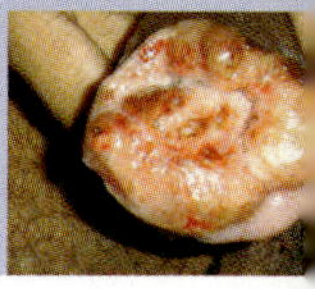

Further investigations required:

– Blood: full blood count, liver function, electrolytes.
– CSF: cells, protein, serological tests.
– X-rays of long bones.
– Ophthalmic assessment as indicated.

DIAGNOSIS IN HIV POSITIVE PERSONS

- HIV infected patients with early syphilis are more likely to have multiple, large and deep genital ulcers and the risk of neurological complications may be higher in HIV-positive patients with early syphilis. However, the clinical features in HIV positive and negative individuals with early syphilis are often similar.
- In a minority of cases, serology may be unreliable: there is a tendency for the RPR/VDRL titre to be lower in primary and statistically significantly higher in secondary syphilis, although lower or false-negative titres have been reported. When clinical findings are suggestive of syphilis but serologic tests are non-reactive, alternative tests (e.g., biopsy of a lesion, dark-ground microscopy) may be useful for diagnosis.

MANAGEMENT: GENERAL CONSIDERATIONS

- A treponemicidal level of antimicrobial should be achieved in serum, and in the case of neurosyphilis in the CSF. A penicillin level of **>0.018 mg/l** is considered treponemicidal, but a higher concentration might be preferable for more rapid elimination of treponemes. The maximal elimination effect is attained at a level of **0.36 mg/l.** Duration of treponemicidal levels of antimicrobial should be at least 7 days to cover a number of division times (30-33 hours) of treponemes in early syphilis with a subtreponemicidal interval of not more than 24-30 hours.

Management in Pregnancy: General Considerations

- Re-treatment in those with a previous diagnosis of syphilis should be considered when there is uncertainty of efficacious past treatment, a 4 fold drop in RPR/VDRL titre has not been achieved, or if the RPR/VDRL titre is serofast at greater than 1:8.
- Non-penicillin alternatives include **ceftriaxone,** for which there is limited data, and **erythromycin or azithromycin.** There are no studies evaluating azithromycin in pregnancy and treatment failure has been reported, with erythromycin the placental penetration is uncertain; for these reasons treatment of the baby at birth with penicillin is recommended following maternal treatment with macrolides.

RECOMMENDED REGIMES

Early Syphilis

Recommended Regimen for Adults

Benzathine penicillin G 2.4 million units IM in a single dose.

Late Syphilis

3 dose of Benzathine Penicillin G.IM, each at 1 week Interval.

Latent Syphils

Recommended Regimens for Adults
Early Latent Syphilis
Benzathine penicillin G 2.4 million units IM in a single dose.

Late Latent Syphilis or Latent Syphilis of Unknown Duration
Benzathine penicillin G 7.2 million units total, administered as 3 doses of 2.4 million units IM each at 1 week intervals.

Some specialists recommend performing a CSF examination on all patients who have latent syphilis and a nontreponemal serologic test of >1:32 or if the patient is HIV-infected with a serum CD_4 count <350.

Neurosyphilis

Recommended Regimen
Aqueous crystalline penicillin G 18-24 million unit per day, administered as 3-4 million units IV every 4 hours or as continuous infusion, for 10-14 days.

Some specialists administer benzathine penicillin, 2.4 million units IM once per week for upto 3 weeks after completion of these neurosyphilis treatment regimens to provide a comparable total duration of therapy.

Follow-up CSF examinations also can be used to evaluate changes in the VDRL-CSF or CSF protein after therapy; however, changes in these two parameters occur more slowly than cell counts, and persistent abnormalities might be less important. If the cell count has ***not decreased after 6 months or if the CSF is not normal after 2 years,*** re-treatment should be considered. Recent data on HIV-infected persons with neurosyphilis suggest that CSF abnormalities might persist for extended periods in these persons, and close clinical follow-up is warranted.

COMPLICATIONS OF THERAPY

- **Jarisch-Herxheimer reaction:** An acute febrile illness with headache, myalgia, chills and rigors, resolving within 24 hours. This is common in **early syphilis** but is usually not important unless there is neurological or ophthalmic involvement or in pregnancy when it may cause foetal distress and premature labour. It is uncommon in late syphilis but can potentially be life threatening if there is involvement of strategic sites (e.g. coronary ostia, larynx, nervous system). Prednisolone can reduce the febrile episode but is not proven to ameliorate local inflammation. Steroids are recommended when there is neurological or cardiovascular involvement and during treatment in pregnancy when additional foetal monitoring is required. Prednisolone 40-60 mg daily for 3 days, starting antitreponemal treatment 24 hours after commencing prednisolone.

- **Procaine reaction (procaine psychosis, procaine mania, Hoignes syndrome):** This is due to inadvertent intravenous injection of procaine penicillin. It is characterised by fear of impending death and may cause hallucinations or fits immediately after injection and lasting less than 20 minutes.

Follow-Up

- For early syphilis, minimum clinical and serological (VDRL or RPR) follow-up should be at months 1, 3, 6 and 12, then 6 monthly until VDRL/RPR negative or serofast.
- For late syphilis minimum serological follow-up is 3 monthly until serofast.
- A sustained two dilution (four-fold) or greater increase in the VDRL or RPR titre suggests **re-infection or treatment failure**.
- **Treatment failure** is characterized by:
  - Four-fold increase in non-treponemal test titre.
  - Recurrence of signs or symptoms.
  - Re-infection excluded.

  Failure of non-treponemal test titers to decline fourfold within 6 months after therapy for primary or secondary syphilis might be indicative of probable treatment failure CSF examination and re-treatment is indicated. The majority of specialists would re-treat patients with benzathine penicillin G administered as 3 doses of 2.4 million units IM each at weekly intervals, if CSF examinations are normal.

CONGENITAL SYPHILIS

The diagnosis of congenital syphilis is complicated by the transplacental transfer of maternal nontreponemal and treponemal IgG antibodies to the fetus.

Diagnosis of Congenital Syphilis

1. Identification of syphilis in the mother.
2. Adequacy of maternal treatment.
3. Presence of clinical, laboratory, or radiographic evidence of syphilis in the infant; and
4. Comparison of maternal (at delivery) and infant nontreponemal serologic titers by using the same test and preferably the same laboratory.

All infants born to mothers who have reactive nontreponemal and treponemal test results should be evaluated with a quantitative nontreponemal serologic test (RPR or VDRL) performed on infant serum because umbilical cord blood can become contaminated with maternal blood and could yield a false-positive result.

All infants born to women who have reactive serologic tests for syphilis should be examined thoroughly for evidence of congenital syphilis (e.g., nonimmune hydrops, jaundice, hepatosplenomegaly, rhinitis, skin rash, and/or pseudoparalysis of an extremity). Pathologic examination of the placenta or umbilical cord by using specific fluorescent antitreponemal antibody staining is suggested. Darkfield microscopic examination or DFA staining of suspicious lesions or body fluids (e.g., nasal discharge) also should be performed.

Diagnosis of Congenital Syphilis

- An abnormal physical examination that is consistent with congenital syphilis.
- A serum quantitative nontreponemal serologic titer that is four-fold higher than the mother's titer, or:
  1. Mother was not treated, inadequately treated, or has no documentation of having received treatment;
  2. Mother was treated with erythromycin or other nonpenicillin regimen; or
  3. Mother received treatment <4 weeks before delivery.
- A positive darkfield or fluorescent antibody test of body fluid(s).

Treatment

Recommended Regimens

Aqueous crystalline penicillin G 100,000-150,000 units/kg/day, administered as 50,000 units/kg/dose IV every 12 hours during the first 7 days of life and every 8 hours thereafter for a total of 10 days.

or

Procaine penicillin G 50,000 units/kg/dose IM in a single daily dose for 10 days.

Follow-Up of Congenital Syphilis

Nontreponemal antibody titers should **decline by age 3 months** and should be **nonreactive by age 6 months** if the infant was not infected (i.e., if the reactive test result

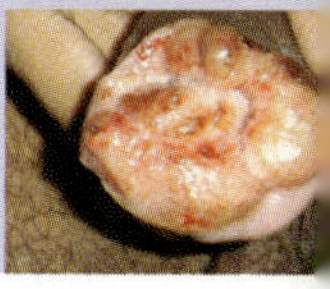

was caused by passive transfer of maternal IgG antibody) or was infected but adequately treated.

Treponemal tests should not be used to evaluate treatment response because the results for an infected child can remain positive despite effective therapy. Passively transferred maternal treponemal antibodies can be present in an infant until age 15 months. A reactive treponemal test after age 18 months is diagnostic of congenital syphilis. If the nontreponemal test is nonreactive at this time, no further evaluation or treatment is necessary. If the nontreponemal test is reactive at age 18 months, the infant should be fully (re)evaluated and treated for congenital syphilis.

Genital Warts

GENITAL WARTS (Fig. 4.16)

As in herpes, only a **minority of human papilloma virus (HPV) infections appear to result in noticeable lesions**. Anogenital warts, also known as **condylomata acuminata**, are benign growths that are most commonly associated with HPV types 6 or 11. These warts typically present as soft, flesh-colored papules that may progress to a cauliflowerlike mass. Multiple clustered lesions are typically present, yet a solitary wart may occasionally occur. **The most common locations in men are the glans, edge of the corona, prepuce, shaft, frenulum, and scrotum. Sites of predilection in women include the labia, perineum, clitoris, and fourchette.** The majority of patients who present with genital warts also have subclinical HPV infection, often including many other HPV types. Therefore **all affected women should be screened for cervical intraepithelial neoplasia.**

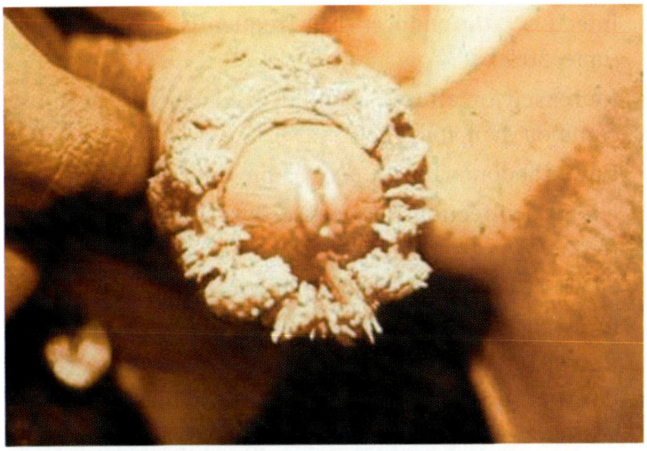

Fig. 4.16: Verrucous growth of C acuminata

Table 4.2: Epithelial anchorage for various HPV types

HPV types	Detected in lesions	
Epithelial anchorage	Immunocompetent	Immunocompromised
Skin	1-4, 7, 10, 28, 41	5, 8, 12, 14-25, 36, 46, 47
Mucous membrane	6, 11, 16, 18, 30, 31, 33-35, 39, 40, 42-45, 51-58	

Table 4.3: Oncogenic potential of mucosotropic HPV types

Oncogenic Potential	HPV Types
Low	6, 11, 34, 40, 42-45, 53-55, 57, 58
High	16, 18, 30, 31, 33, 35, 39, 45, 51, 52, 56

INCUBATION PERIOD

The incubation period of genital warts is long and variable. It is estimated to be around 3 months with a range from 3 weeks to 8 months. Perinatally acquired HPV infection may not manifest for upto two years.

Clinical Variants

1. **Buschke-Lowenstein Tumor**
   This lesion enlarges from a pre-existing benign anogenital wart. This is an extremely rare semi-malignant tumor and can occasionally transform into a squamous cell carcinoma. There is penetration of underlying tissue by compression that sometimes mimics microinvasion and may create difficulties in differentiating it from a true carcinoma.
2. **Bowenoid Papulosis**
   This is a rather common entity in patients of both sexes. **HPV type 16** has been demonstrated in about 80% of cases. It presents clinically as smooth papules that are either erythematous, reddish-violaceous or brownish in colour. Some cases have regressed spontaneously within 1-2 years of observation; in others, the lesions have persisted for more than 10 years. **Progression to carcinoma or true Bowen's disease is very rare**.
3. **Cervical Intra-epithelial Neoplasia (CIN) and Invasive Carcinoma**
   Epidemiological studies have shown that this condition is associated with HPV infection in particular **type 16 and 18**. Patients with history of anogenital warts or history of sexual contact with patient with genital warts should be regularly screened by cervical cytology (Pap Smear).
4. **Laryngeal Papillomas**
   Laryngeal papillomatosis in children is probably acquired from mother with genital warts during delivery. They are usually **caused by type 6 and type 11 HPV**.

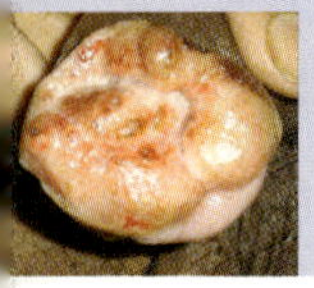

Treatment of genital warts

Therapy of anogenital warts		
Topical	Podophyllin	(10-25%)
	Podophyllotoxin	(0.5%)
	Trichloroacetic acid	(50-90%)
	5-FU	(5%)
	IFN- intralesional, Imiquimod	
Surgery	Curettage and cautery	
	Cryosurgery	
	CO_2 laser	
Systemic	IFNα (subcutaneous, low doses, cyclic therapy)	

i. ***Cervical Warts***

Electrocautery, Cryosurgery

ii. ***Recommended Regimens for Vaginal Warts***

Cryotherapy with liquid nitrogen.**TCA 80%-90%** applied to warts.

iii. ***Recommended Regimens for Urethral Meatus Warts***

Cryotherapy with liquid nitrogen, **Podophyllin 10%-25%** in compound tincture of benzoin.

iv. ***Recommended Regimens for Anal Warts***

Cryotherapy with liquid nitrogen, **TCA 80%-90%** applied to warts.

v. ***Recommended Regimens for Oral Warts***

Cryotherapy with liquid nitrogen.

Surgical removal.

Special Considerations

Pregnancy

Imiquimod, podophyllin and podophyllotoxin should ***not*** be used during pregnancy.

Urethritis

1. **Gonococcal and PGU(Post Gonococcal Urethritis)**
   a. Acute
   b. Chronic
   c. Complicated
2. **NGU** (Non Gonococcal Urethritis) — Chlamydia trachomatis 30-50%
3. **NCNGU** (Non Chlamydial NGU) — Ureaplasma urealyticum, M genitalum Trichomonas vaginalis Candidasis Herpes simplex.
4. NSU (Non-specific urethritis).
5. **Recurrent–T vaginalis,** M genitalum.
6. Persistent–H simplex.
7. Chronic Urethritis.

GONORRHOEA

Symptoms

Men

- Urethral infection commonly causes **urethral discharge (>80%)** and/or dysuria (>50%) (Fig. 4.17).
- Urethral infection can be asymptomatic (<10%).
- Rectal infection in homosexual men is usually asymptomatic but may cause anal discharge (12%) or perianal/anal pain or discomfort (7%).
- Pharyngeal infection is usually asymptomatic (>90%).
  - Itch
  - Ulcer

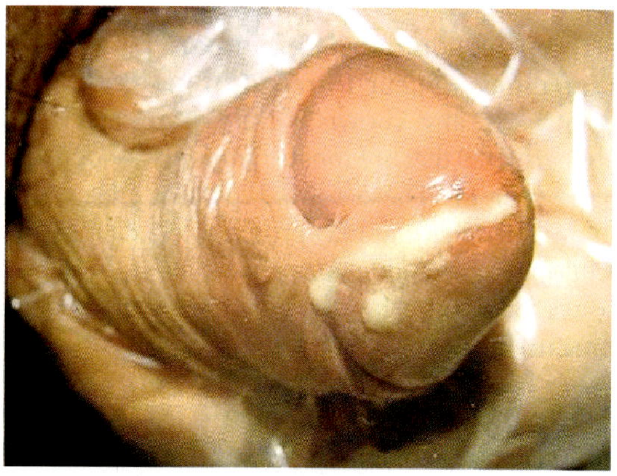

Fig. 4.17: Urethral discharge with purulent yellow discharge (Gonorrhoea)

Women

- Infection at **the endocervix is frequently asymptomatic** (upto 50%).
- Increased or altered vaginal discharge is the most common symptom (upto 50%).
- Lower abdominal pain may be present (upto 25%).
- Urethral infection may cause dysuria (12%) but not frequency.
- Gonorrhoea is a rare cause of intermenstrual bleeding or menorrhagia.
- Rectal infection more frequently develops by trans-mucosal spread of infected genital secretions than from anal intercourse and is usually asymptomatic.
- Pharyngeal infection is usually asymptomatic (>90%).

- Itch
- Ulcer

Complications

Transluminal spread of *N. gonorrhoeae* may occur from the urethra or endocervix to involve the epididymis and prostate in men (1% or less) and the endometrium and pelvic organs in women (probably <10%). Haematogenous dissemination may also occur from infected mucous membranes, resulting in skin lesions, arthralgia, arthritis and tenosynovitis.

Disseminated gonococcal infection is uncommon (<1%).

NGU (NON GONOCOCCAL URETHRITIS)

Symptoms

- Urethral discharge.
- Dysuria.
- Penile irritation.
- Asymptomatic.

Signs

- Urethral discharge. This may only be present on urethral massage. It is **mucoid**. It can also be found in a significant proportion of patients with asymptomatic urethritis.
- Normal examination.

Complications

- Epididymo-orchitis.
- Sexually acquired reactive arthritis/Reiter's syndrome. These are infrequent, occurring in fewer than 1% of cases though incomplete forms may be more common.

MANAGEMENT OF URETHRITIS

Investigations

- **Bedside**–Smear, 2/3 glass test.

1. Smear

Specimen Collection

Men: Routinely from the urethra or by massage, rectal and/or oropharyngeal tests when symptomatic at these sites and as indicated by sexual activity.

Women: Routinely from endocervix if speculum examination performed and from the urethra; rectal and oropharyngeal tests when symptomatic at these sites, when a sexual partner has gonorrhoea and when indicated by the sexual history.

In men, microscopy of **urethral smears** is more sensitive in **symptomatic (90-95%)** than in asymptomatic **(50-75%)** patients. In women, microscopy of gram stained **endocervical smears** is more sensitive than urethral smears (37-50% vs 20%).

Microscopy is not appropriate for pharyngeal specimens.

- **STAIN**= Grams, Geimsa, KOH and saline mount.

i. A Gram stained **urethral smear containing >=5 PMN per oil immersion** (× **1000)** microscopic field (averaged over five fields with greatest concentration of PMNs) (Fig. 4.18).
 and/or
ii. A Gram stained preparation from a **first passed urine (FPU) specimen, containing >=10 PMN per oil immersion (x1000) microscopic field** (averaged over five fields with greatest concentration of PMNs).

Either test can be used: Both tests will identify cases missed by the other test.

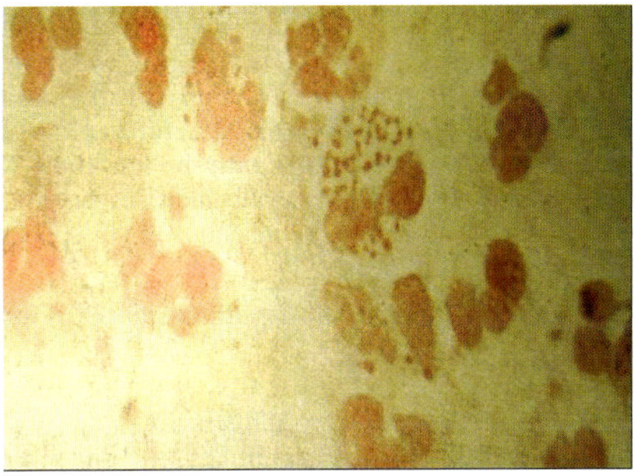

Fig. 4.18: Intracellular diplococci seen

2. Positive Leucocyte Esterase

Positive leucocyte esterase activity on FPU specimen correlate with NGU and is considered diagnostic by some authorities.

Symptomatic patients in whom no urethritis is detected initially, should be retested having held their urine overnight (Four hours is conventional).

3. Specific

Diagnosis

- Direct plating of genital samples and use of transport media with prompt laboratory plating both give acceptable results.
- The use of endocervical samples alone will identify 90-95% of women with gonococcal infection.

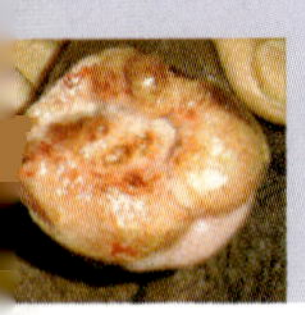

i. **Culture** offers a readily available, specific, sensitive and cheap diagnostic test that readily allows confirmatory identification and antimicrobial susceptibility testing of *N. gonorrhoea*.

Transport Medium

- Stuarts/Amies

Transgrow

- Chocolate agar: 5 % CO_2, ph 7.5, 36 °c.
- Thayer Martin

} Media used

- Martin lewis
- Modified New York medium

Biochemical tests

- Oxidase test.
- Fermentation test: Glucose +.

ii. **Alternative tests** include nucleic amplification tests (NAATs) and nucleic acid hybridization tests. **NAATs are more sensitive than culture** and can also be used as diagnostic/screening tests on non-invasively collected specimens (urine and self-taken vaginal swabs).

Comparisons between NAATs and culture suggest the sensitivity of NAATs exceeds 90% for genital sites, whilst the sensitivity of culture may be less than 75% for endocervical swabs. This probably indicates that NAATs are less affected than culture by inadequacies in collection and transport of specimens.

They are more sensitive in women than the PCR assay.

Management

1. **Uncomplicated gonococcal infection**
   Definition: This includes anterior urethritis and proctitis in males; cervicitis, urethritis and proctitis in females and pharyngitis in both.
   CDC
   Uncomplicated Gonococcal Infections of the Cervix, Urethra and Rectum.
   Ceftriaxone 125 mg IM in a single dose.
   or
   Cefixime 400 mg orally in a single dose.
   or
   Ciprofloxacin 500 mg orally in a single dose.
   NACO
   i. Azithromycin, 2 g orally as a single dose.*
   or
   ii. Cefixime, 400 mg orally as a single dose.
   or
   iii. Ceftriaxone, 250 mg intramuscular (IM) as a single injection.
   * Will treat both gonococcal and chlamydial infections.
2. **Recommended Regimens for MSM or Heterosexuals with a History of Recent Travel**
   Ceftriaxone 125 mg IM in a single dose.
   or
   Cefixime 400 mg orally in a single dose.
   Plus
   Treatment for chlamydia if chlamydial infection is not ruled out.
3. **Uncomplicated Gonococcal Infections of the Pharynx**
   Recommended Regimens
   Ceftriaxone 125 mg IM in a single dose.
   or
   Ciprofloxacin 500 mg orally in a single dose.
   Plus
   Treatment for chlamydia if chlamydial Infection is not ruled out.

Special Considerations

Allergy, Intolerance and Adverse Reactions

Persons who cannot tolerate cephalosporins or quinolones should be treated with spectinomycin. Because spectinomycin is unreliable (52% effective) against pharyngeal infections, patients who have suspected or known pharyngeal infection should have a pharyngeal culture 3-5 days after treatment to verify eradication of infection.

Pegnancy and Breastfeeding

- Ceftriaxone 250 mg IM as a single dose.
- Cefixime 400 mg oral as a single dose.

Co-infection with *Chlamydia trachomatis* Genital infection with *C. trachomatis* commonly accompanies genital gonococcal infection (upto 20% of men and 40% of women with gonorrhoea). Screening for *C. trachomatis* should routinely be performed on adults with gonorrhoea or treatment given to eradicate possible co-infection.

Complicated Infection

Definition

This includes posterior urethritis, prostatitis, epididymo-orchitis, tysonitis, cowperitis and bartholinitis. The patient should, if necessary, be admitted to a hospital.

i. **Ceftriaxone:** 1g IM or IV once daily for 7 days. (An alternative third generation cephalosporin may be required if ceftriaxone is not available, but more frequent daily dosage will be needed).
ii. **Cefixime** 400 mg twice daily orally for 7 days.

Disseminated Gonococcal Infection (DGI)

Recommended Regimen

Ceftriaxone 1 g IM or IV every 24 hours.

All of the preceding regimens should be continued for 24-48 hours after improvement begins, at which time therapy may be switched to one of the following regimens to complete at least 1 week of antimicrobial therapy.

Cefixime 400 mg orally twice daily.

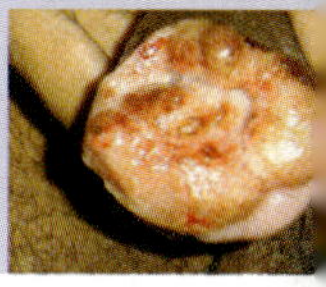

or
Ciprofloxacin 500 mg orally twice daily.
or
Ofloxacin 400 mg orally twice daily.
or
Levofloxacin 500 mg orally once daily.

Gonococcal Meningitis and Endocarditis

Recommended Regimen

Ceftriaxone 1-2 g IV every 12 hours.
Therapy for meningitis should be continued for 10-14 days; therapy for endocarditis should be continued for at least 4 weeks. Treatment of complicated DGI should be undertaken in consultation with a specialist.

Resistance

Two Types

Plasmid (PPNG)
Chromosomal

- High dose azithromycin (2.0 gms as a single dose) has shown acceptable efficacy in clinical trials, but is associated with a high gastrointestinal intolerance. The emergence of azithromycin resistant *N. gonorrhoeae* has been reported and clinical efficacy does not always correlate with *in-vitro* sensitivity testing.

Partner Notification

Male patients with *symptomatic* urethral infection should notify all partners with whom they had sexual contact within the preceding **2 weeks** or their last partner if longer ago. Patients with infection at other sites or *asymptomatic infection* should notify all partners within the preceding **3 months.**

Patients should be assessed after treatment:

- To confirm compliance with treatment.
- To ensure resolution of symptoms.
- To enquire about adverse reactions.
- To re-take the sexual history to explore the possibility of re-infection.
- To pursue partner notification and health promotion.

A microbiological test of cure is *not routinely necessary* when the infection has been treated with a recommended directly observed therapy, the infection is fully sensitive to the antimicrobial administered, symptoms have resolved and there is no risk of re-infection.

If a patient is symptomatic after treatment, has received a suboptimal treatment, a resistant strain is identified or there is a possibility of reinfection, test of cure with culture is recommended. If a test of cure is performed, culture tests should be performed at least 72 hours after completion of antimicrobial therapy and NAATs tests two weeks after therapy.

Infection identified after treatment more commonly indicates *reinfection* rather than treatment failure.

NGU (NON GONOCOCCAL URETHRITIS)

CDC

Recommended Regimens

Azithromycin 1 g orally in a single dose.
or
Doxycycline 100 mg orally twice a day for 7 days.

NACO

Recommended Regimen

(Effective against both *chlamydia trachomatis* and *ureaplasma urealyticum*).

i. Azithromycin, 2 g orally in a single dose.*
 or
ii. Doxycycline, 100 mg orally twice daily for 7 days.
 or
iii. Erythromycin base/erythromycin stearate, 500 mg orally for 7 days.

* Will treat both gonococcal and chlamydial infections.

Regimens in Pregnancy

i. Erythromycin base/stearate, 500 mg orally 4 times a day for 7 days; erythromycin should not be taken on empty stomach.
 or
ii. Amoxycillin, 500 mg orally three times a day for 7 days on empty stomach.
 or
iii. Azithromycin*, 2 g orally as a single dose on empty stomach.

* Azithromycin has not been adequately evaluated during pregnancy.

Follow-up for Patients with NGU

This is an important part of the management of NGU and should take place 2 weeks after initiating therapy. However, some patients may not choose to return, emphasising the importance of the initial consultation. Follow-up has a number of objectives including:

- Following up partner notification.
- Reinforcing health education.
- Providing reassurance.
- Assessment of treatment compliance and efficacy.
- Repeat urethral smear and FPU specimen to look for persistent urethritis only if patient is symptomatic or has a urethral discharge on examination (test of cure).

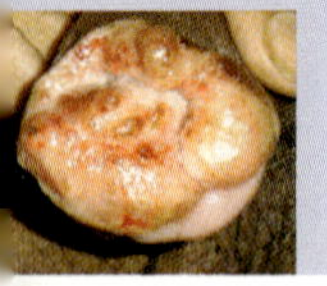

PERSISTENT/RECURRENT NGU

There is no consensus of opinion in either diagnosis or management of this condition. Its aetiology is probably multifactorial. It occurs in 20-60% of men treated for acute NGU.

CHRONIC NGU

Persistent or recurrent urethritis occurring **30-92 days** following treatment of acute NGU. There is evidence that ureaplasmas and *M. genitalium* may be important in the aetiology of chronic NGU with either symptoms or signs.

MANAGEMENT OF PERSISTENT/RECURRENT NGU

Ensure patient has completed initial course of therapy. If not consider re-prescribing initial treatment. Ensure sexual partner(s) have been treated and re-infection is not a possible cause. If patient has no signs or symptoms consider re-assurance.

Recommended Regimens

Metronidazole 2 g orally in a single dose.
or
Tinidazole 2 g orally in a single dose.
Plus
Azithromycin 1 g orally in a single dose (if not used for initial episode).

CONTINUING SYMPTOMS

There is only limited evidence on how best to manage patients who either remain symptomatic following a second course of treatment or who have frequent recurrences after treatment.

Erythromycin 500 mg four times daily for 3 weeks may help.

- Urological investigation is usually normal unless the patient has urinary flow problems.
- Chronic abacterial prostatitis (see guideline on prostatitis).
- Psychosexual causes should be considered in the differential diagnosis.
- There is no evidence to suggest that patient with microscopic urethritis but who have no signs or symptoms after two courses of treatment are persistently infected. They should be reassured.
- Retreatment of the sexual partner may be helpful in recurrent urethritis as it may be due to re-infection. This has not been evaluated in clinical studies.
- For men with persistent urethritis, there is no evidence that retreatment of an appropriately treated sexual partner is beneficial.

Cervicitis

ETIOLOGY

When an etiologic organism is isolated in the setting of cervicitis, it is typically *C. trachomatis* or *N. gonorrhoeae.* Cervicitis also can accompany trichomoniasis and genital herpes (especially primary HSV-2 infection). However, in the majority of cases of cervicitis, no organism is isolated, especially in women at relatively low risk for recent acquisition of these STDs (for example, women aged >30 years). Limited data indicate that infection with *M. genitalium* and BV as well as frequent douching might cause cervicitis. For reasons that are unclear, cervicitis can persist despite repeated courses of antimicrobial therapy. Because the majority of persistent cases of cervicitis are not caused by relapse or reinfection with *C. trachomatis* or *N. gonorrhoeae*, other determinants (e.g., persistent abnormality of vaginal flora, douching or exposure to chemical irritants, or idiopathic inflammation in the zone of ectopy) might be involved.

Recommended Regimens for Presumptive Treatment

Azithromycin 1 g orally in a single dose.

or

Doxycycline 100 mg orally twice a day for 7 days.

VAGINAL DISCHARGE

1. Bacterial Vaginosis

Diagnostic Considerations

BV can be diagnosed by the use of clinical criteria or Gram stain. Clinical criteria require three of the following symptoms or signs: i.e. Amsler's criteria:

- Homogeneous, thin, white discharge that smoothly coats the vaginal walls.
- Presence of clue cells on microscopic examination.
- pH of vaginal fluid >4.5; and
- A fishy odor of vaginal discharge before or after addition of 10% KOH (i.e., the whiff test).

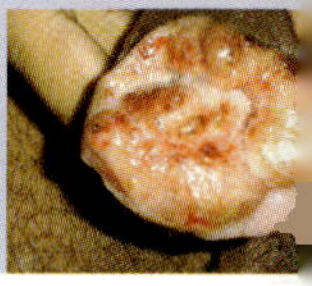

Recommended Regimens

Metronidazole 400 mg orally thrice a day for 7 days. This formulation is not available in India.

or

Metronidazole gel, 0.75%, one full applicator (5g) intravaginally, once a day for 5 days.

or

Clindamycin cream, 2%, one full applicator (5g) intravaginally at bedtime for 7 days.

2. Trichomoniasis

Recommended Regimens

Metronidazole 2 g orally in a single dose.

or

Tinidazole 2 g orally in a single dose.

Alternative Regimen

Metronidazole 500 mg orally twice a day for 7 days.

3. Vulvovaginal Candidiasis

T Fluconazole 150 mg 1 stat or clotrimazole, pessary 100 mg × 7 days..

EPIDIDYMITIS

Ceftriaxone 250 mg IM in a single dose.

PLUS

Doxycycline 100 mg orally twice a day for 10 days.

For acute epididymitis most likely caused by enteric organisms or for patients allergic to cephalosporins and/ or tetracyclines:

Ofloxacin 300 mg orally twice a day for 10 days.

or

Levofloxacin 500 mg orally once daily for 10 days.

SYNDROMIC APPROACH (NACO 2007)

4.1: URETHRAL DISCHARGE

Causative organisms

1. *Neisseria gonorrhoeae*
2. *Chlamydia trachomatis*
3. *Trichomonas vaginalis*

History

- Urethral discharge
- Pain or burning while passing urine, increased frequency of urination
- Sexual exposure of either partner to high risk practices including oro-genital sex

→

Examination

Look for

- The **urethral meatus** for redness and swelling
- If urethral discharge is not seen, then gently **massage** the urethra from the ventral part of the penis towards the meatus and look for thick, **creamy greenish-yellow or mucoid** discharge

→

Gram stain examination of the urethral smear will show gram-negative intracellular diplococci in case of gonorrhoea

In **non-gonococcal urethritis** more than **5 neutrophils per oil immersion field (1000X)** in the urethral smear or more than **10 neutrophils** per high power field in the sediment of the **first void urine** are observed

←

Treatment

- As dual infection is common, the treatment for urethral discharge should adequately cover therapy for both, **gonorrhoea and chlamydial infections**.

Recommended regimen for uncomplicated gonorrhoea + chlamydia:

- Uncomplicated infections indicate that the disease is limited to the anogenital region (anterior urethritis and proctitis).
  i. Tab. **Cefixime 400** mg orally, single dose.
  Plus
  ii. Tab **Azithromycin 1 gram** orally single dose under supervision.
- Advise the client to return after 7 days of start of therapy.

- When symptoms **persist or recur** after adequate treatment for gonorrhea and chlamydia in the index client and partner(s), they should be treated for ***Trichomonas vaginalis***
- If discharge or only dysuria persists after 7 days:
  i. Tab. **Secnidazole 2 gm** orally, single dose (to treat for *T. vaginalis*)
- If the symptoms still persists.

  ↓

  Refer to higher centre as early as possible.
- If individuals are allergic to Azithromycin, give Erythromycin 500 mg four times a day for 7 days.

⇩

Syndrome specific guidelines for partner management:

- Treat all recent partners.
- Treat female partners (for gonorrhoea and chlamydia) on same lines after ruling out pregnancy and history of allergies
- Advise sexual abstinence during the course of treatment.
- Provide condoms, educate about correct and consistent use.
- Refer for voluntary counselling and testing for HIV, Syphilis and Hepatitis B.
- Schedule return visit after 7 days.

  Follow-up

  After seven days
- To see reports of tests done for HIV, Syphilis and Hepatitis B.
- If symptoms persist to assess whether it is due to treatment.

PREGNANCY

- Cephalosporins to cover gonococcal infection are safe and effective in pregnancy.
- Tab. Cefixime 400 mg orally, single dose;

  Or

  Ceftriaxone 125 mg by intramuscular injection

  +

  Tab. Erythromycin 500 mg orally four times a day for seven days;

  Or

  Cap. Amoxicillin 500 mg orally, three times a day for seven days to cover chlamydial infection.

  (Quinolones (like ofloxacin, ciprofloxacin), doxycycline are contraindicated in pregnant women.)

4.2: SCROTAL SWELLING

Causative Organisms

- *Neisseria gonorrhoeae*
- *Chlamydia trachomatis*

Investigations

- Gram stain examination of the urethral smear will show gram-negative intracellular diplococci in case of complicated gonococcal infection
- In non-gonococcal urethritis more than 5 neutrophils per oil immersion field in the urethral smear or more than 10 neutrophils per high power field in the sediment of the first void urine are observed.

Differential Diagnosis (non RTIs/STIs) Infections causing scrotal swelling:

i. Tuberculosis, filariasis, coliforms, pseudomonas, mumps virus infection.

ii. **Non infectious** causes:

Trauma, Hernia, Hydrocele, Testicular torsion and Testicular tumors.

Treatment

⇩

- Treat for both gonococcal and chlamydial infections:

  Tab **Cefixime 400 mg** orally BD for 7 days.
- Plus Cap. **Doxycycline 100 mg orally, twice daily for 14 days** and refer to higher centre as early as possible since complicated gonococcal infection needs parenteral longer duration of treatment.
- Supportive therapy to reduce pain (bed rest, scrotal elevation with T-bandage and analgesics).

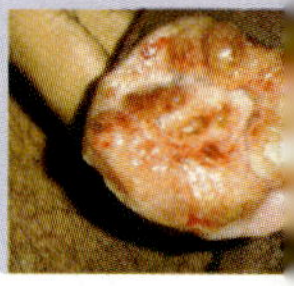

Note:
If quick and effective therapy is not given, damage and scarring of testicular tissues may result causing sub-fertility.

Pregnancy

- Depending on the clinical findings in the pregnant partner (whether vaginal discharge or endocervical discharge or PID is present) the drug regimens should be used.
- Doxycycline is contraindicated in pregnancy.
- Erythromycin/Amoxicillin can be used in pregnancy.
  (Erythromycin estolate is contraindicated in pregnancy due to hepatotoxicity. Erythromycin base or erythromycin ethyl succinate should be given).

4.3: INGUINAL BUBO

Causative Organisms

- *Chlamydia trachomatis* serovars *Ll, L2, L3,* causative agent of lympho granuloma venerum (LGV).
- *Haemophilus ducreyi* causative agent of chancroid.

History

- Swelling in inguinal region which may be painful
- Preceding history of genital ulcer or discharge
- Sexual exposure of either partner to high risk practices including orogenital sex
- Systemic symptoms like malaise, fever.

⇨

Examination

Look for
Localized enlargement of lymph nodes in groin which may be tender and fluctuant
- Inflammation of skin over the swelling
- *Presence of multiple sinuses*
- Edema of genitals and lower limbs
- Presence of genital ulcer or urethral discharge and if present refer to respective flowchart

⇨

Laboratory Investigations

Diagnosis is on clinical grounds

Differential Diagnosis

- *Mycobacterium tuberculosis*, filariasis.
- Any acute infection of skin of pubic area, genitals, buttocks, anus and lower limbs can also cause inguinal swelling. If malignancy or tuberculosis is suspected refer to higher centre for biopsy.

Treatment

- Start Cap. **Doxycycline 100 mg** orally twice daily for 21 days **(to cover LGV).**

  Plus
- Tab **Azithromycin** 1gm orally single dose.

  OR
- Tab. **Ciprofloxacin 500 mg** orally, twice a day for three days **(to cover chancroid).**
- Refer to higher centre as early as possible.

Note:
- *A bubo should never be incised and drained at the primary health centre, even if it is fluctuant, as there is a high risk of a fistula formation and chronicity. If bubo becomes fluctuant always refer for aspiration to higher centre.*
- *In severe cases with vulval edema in females, surgical intervention may be required for which they should be referred to higher centre.*

Syndrome Specific Guidelines for Partner Management:

- Treat all partners who are in contact with client in last 3 months.
- Partners should be treated for chancroid and LGV.
- Tab Azithromycin 1gm orally single dose (chancroid).

  \+

  Cap Doxycycline 100 mg orally, twice daily for 21 days to cover LGV.

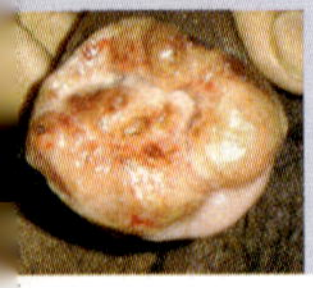

Management of Pregnant Partner:

- Quinolones (like ofloxacin, ciprofloxacin), doxycycline, sulfonamides are contraindicated in pregnant women.
- Pregnant and lactating women should be treated with the **erythromycin regimen**, and consideration should be given to the addition of a **parenteral amino glycoside (e.g., gentamicin).**
  Tab. Erythromycin base, 500 mg orally, 4 times daily for 21 days and refer to higher centre.
  (Erythromycin estolate is contraindicated in pregnancy due to hepatotoxicity. Erythromycin base or erythromycin ethyl succinate should be given).

4.4: GENITAL ULCERS

Causative Organisms

- *Treponema pallidum* (syphilis)
- *Haemophilus ducreyi* (chancroid)
- *Klebsiella granulomatis* (granuloma inguinale)
- *Chlamydia trachomatis* (lymphogranuloma venerum)
- *Herpes simplex* (genital herpes)

History

- Genital ulcer/vesicles
- Burning sensation in the genital region
- Sexual exposure of either partner to high risk practices including orogenital sex

Examination

- Presence of vesicles
- Presence of genital ulcer–single or multiple
- Associated inguinal lymph node swelling if present refer to respective flowchart

Ulcer Characteristics:

- Painful vesicles/ulcers, single or multiple **—Herpes simplex**
- Painless ulcer with shotty lymph node **—Syphilis**
- Painless ulcer with inguinal lymph nodes**–G inguinale and LGV**
- Painful ulcers
  Chancroid associated with painful bubo

Laboratory Investigations

RPR test for syphilis
For further investigations refer to higher centre

Treatment

- If vesicles or multiple painful ulcers are present treat for **herpes** with **Tab. Acyclovir 400 mg orally, three times a day for 7 days.**
- If vesicles are not seen and only ulcer is seen, treat for **syphilis and chancroid** and counsel on herpes genitalis.

To cover syphilis
(Inj **Benzathine penicillin 2.4 million** I.U. 1M after test dose in two divided doses (with emergency tray ready). (In individuals allergic or intolerant to penicillin, Doxycycline 100 mg orally, twice daily for 14 days).

To cover chancroid.

Tab Azithromycin 1 gm orally single dose

or

Ciprofloxacin 500 mg orally, twice a day for three days.

Treatment should be extended beyond 7 days if ulcers have not epithelialized i.e. formed a new layer of skin over the sore.
Refer to higher centre:

- If not responding to treatment.
- Genital ulcers co-existent with HIV.
- Recurrent lesion.

Syndrome Specific Guidelines for Partner Management:

- Treat all partners who are in contact with client in last 3 months.
- Partners should be treated for syphilis and chancroid.
- Advise sexual abstinence during the course of treatment.
- Provide condoms, educate about correct and consistent use.
- Refer for voluntary counseling and testing for HIV, Syphilis and Hepatitis B.
- Schedule return visit after 7 days.

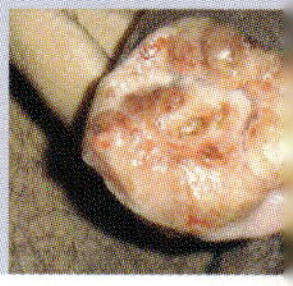

Management of Pregnant Women:

- Quinolones (like ofloxacin, ciprofloxacin), doxycycline, sulfonamides are contraindicated in pregnant women.
- **Pregnant women who test positive for RPR** should be considered infected unless adequate treatment is documented in the medical records and sequential serologic antibody titers have declined.
  (i) Inj Benzathine penicillin 2.4 million i.u. 1M after test dose (with emergency tray ready).
  (ii) A **second dose** of benzathine penicillin 2.4 million units 1M should be administered 1 week after the initial dose for women who have **primary, secondary, or early latent syphilis**.
- **Pregnant women who are allergic to penicillin** should be treated with erythromycin and the neonate should be treated for syphilis after delivery.
  Tab. Erythromycin 500 mg orally four times a day for 15 days.
  (Note: Erythromycin estolate is contraindicated in pregnancy because of drug related hepatotoxicity.
  Only Erythromycin base or erythromycin ethyl succinate should be used in pregnancy).
- All pregnant women should be asked history of genital herpes and examined carefully for herpetic lesions.
- Women without symptoms or signs of genital herpes or its prodrome can deliver vaginally.
- Women with genital herpetic lesions at the onset of labour should be delivered by caesarean section to prevent neonatal herpes.
- Acyclovir may be administered orally to pregnant women with first episode genital herpes or severe recurrent herpes.

4.5: VAGINAL DISCHARGE IN FEMALES

SYNDROME: VAGINAL DISCHARGE

Causative Organisms for Vaginitis

- *Trichomonas vaginalis* (TV)
- *Candida albicans*
- *Gardnerella vaginalis, Mycoplasma* causing bacterial vaginosis (BV)

Causative Organisms for *Cervicitis*

- *Neisseria Gonorrhaeae*
- *Chlamydia trachomatis*
- *Trichomonas vaginalis*
- *Herpes simplex virus*

History

- Menstrual history to rule out pregnancy
- Nature and type of discharge (amount, smell, color, consistency)
- Genital itching
- Burning while passing urine, increased frequency
- Presence of any ulcer, swelling on the vulval or inguinal region
- Genital complaints in sexual partners
- Low backache

⇒

Examination

Per speculum examination to differentiate between vaginitis and cervicitis

a. **Vaginitis:**
Trichomoniasis—greenish frothy discharge
Candidiasis - curdy white discharge
Bacterial vaginosis - adherent discharge
Mixed infections may present with atypical discharge

⇒

Laboratory Investigations

(If available)

- **Wet mount** microscopy of the discharge for Trichomonas vaginalis and clue cells
- **10% KOH** preparation for Candida albicans
- **Gram stain** of vaginal smear for **clue cells** seen in bacterial vaginosis
- **Gram stain** of endocervical smear to detect gonococci

Treatment

Vaginitis (TV+BV+Candida)

- Tab. **Secnidazole** 2 gm orally, single dose.
  Or
  Tab. **Tinidazole** 500 mg orally, twice daily for 5 days.
  } TV+BV
  (Tab. Metoclopropramide taken 30 minutes before Tab. Secnidazole to prevent gastric intolerance).
- **Tab Fluconazole** 150 mg orally single dose or local **Clotrimazole 500 mg** vaginal pessaries once.} Candida

Treatment for Cervical Infection (Chlamydia and Gonorrhoea):

- Tab. cefixime 400 mg orally, single dose.
  Plus
  Azithromycin 1 gram, 1 hour before lunch. If vomiting within 1 hour, give anti-emetic and repeat.
- If vaginitis and cervicitis are present treat for both.
- Instruct client to avoid douching.
- Pregnancy, diabetes, HIV may also be influencing factors and should be considered in recurrent infections.
- Follow-up after one week.

Management in Pregnant Women:

Per speculum examination should be done to rule out pregnancy complications like abortion, premature rupture of membranes.
Treatment for vaginitis (TV + BV +Candida):

i. **In first trimester of pregnancy**
   - Local treatment with **Clotrimazole vaginal pessary/cream only** for candidiasis.
     (Oral Flucanozole is contraindicated in pregnancy).
   - **Metronidazole pessaries or cream intravaginally** if ***trichomoniasis or BV*** is suspected.

ii. **In second and third trimester**
   - Oral metronidazole can be given.
   - Tab. Secnidazole 2 gm orally, single dose.
   - Tab. Tinidazole 500 mg orally, twice daily for 5 days.
     (Tab. Metoclopropramide taken 30 minutes before Tab. Metronidazole to prevent gastric intolerance).

4.6: MANAGEMENT OF LOWER ABDOMINAL PAIN IN FEMALES

SYNDROME: LOWER ABDOMINAL PAIN

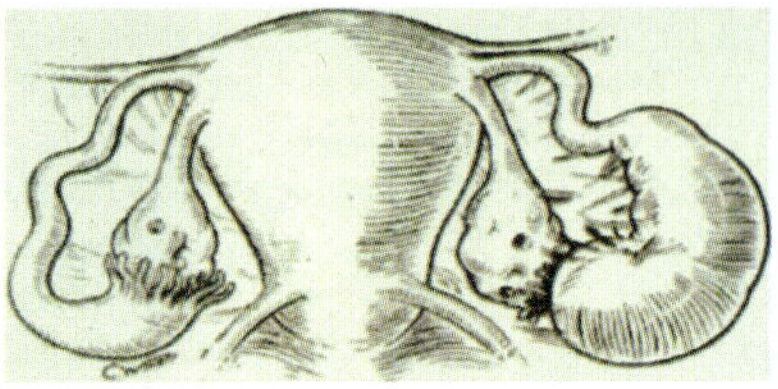

Pelvic inflammatory disease

Treatment

In mild or moderate PID (in the absence of tubo ovarian abscess), outClient treatment can be given. Therapy is required to cover ***Neisseria gonorrhoeae, Chlamydia trachomatis*** **and anaerobes.**

- Tab. **Cefixime 400 mg orally BD for 7 days**
  +
  Tab. Metronidazole 400 mg orally, twice daily for 14 days.
  +
  Doxycycline, 100 mg orally, twice a day for 2 weeks.
- Tab. Ibuprofen 400 mg orally, three times a day for 3-5 days.
- Tab. Ranitidine 150 mg orally, twice daily to prevent gastritis.
- Remove intrauterine device, if present, under antibiotic cover of 24-48 hours.
- Advise abstinence during the course of treatment and educate on correct and consistent use of condoms.
- Observe for 3 days. If no improvement (i.e. absence of fever, reduction in abdominal tenderness, reduction in cervical movement, adnexal and uterine tenderness) or if symptoms worsen, refer for inclient treatment.

Caution: PID can be a serious condition. Refer the client to the hospital if she does not respond to treatment within 3 days and even earlier if her condition worsens.

Management of Pregnant Women:

Though PID is rare in pregnancy

- Any pregnant woman suspected to have PID should be referred to district hospital for hospitalization and treated with a parenteral regimen which would be safe in pregnancy.
- Doxycycline is contraindicated in pregnancy.

Note: Metronidazole is generally not recommended during the first three months of pregnancy. However, it should not be withheld for a severely acute PID, which represents an emergency.

Hospitalization for acute PID should be seriously considered when:

- The diagnosis is uncertain.
- Surgical emergencies e.g. appendicitis or ectopic pregnancy cannot be excluded.
- A pelvic abscess is suspected.
- Severe illness precludes management on an out Client basis.
- The woman is pregnant.
- The client is unable to follow or tolerate an out Client regimen.
- The client has failed to respond to out Client therapy.

Note: *All Clients requiring hospitalization should be referred to the district hospital.*

REFERENCES

- Thieme's Pocket Dermatology 2006 by Wolfram Sterry, Walter Burgdorf, Ralf Paus.
- Sexually Transmitted Diseases, Holmes May 2007, McGraw-Hill.
- King A, Nicol C, Rodin P.: Venereal Diseases, 4th edn., ELBS 1980; 251.
- Sexually Transmitted Diseases Treatment Guidelines, 2006 CDC.
- Flow Charts on the Syndromic Management of Sexually Transmitted Infections NACO, Aug 2007.

CHAPTER 5

HIV

Biology, Diagnosis Investigations Treatment, PEP

THE BIOLOGY OF HIV INFECTION

A brief overview of the HIV virus is elucidated below:

The HIV Virus Structure (Fig. 5.1)

- Spherical enveloped virus, 90-120 nm in size.
- Nucleocapsid – outer icosahedral shell.
- – inner cone shaped core.
- Viral RNA – Diploid, 2 identical copies of single stranded positive sense RNA.
- Reverse transcriptase enzyme (RNA dependent DNA polymerase).

VIRAL GENES AND ANTIGENS (Fig. 5.1)

HIV genome – Structural genes.
– Non-structural and regulatory genes.

A. Genes Coding for Structural Proteins:

1. **gag**–core and shell of virus
   Expressed as precursor protein, p55
   P55 cleaved into p15, p18 and p24.

p24 is the major core antigen which can be detected during early stages of inflammation before antibodies appear. Late in course, anti-p24 declines and p24 Ag reappears in circulation indicating exacerbation. Within the envelope of a mature HIV particle is a bullet-shaped core or capsid, made of 2,000 copies of another viral protein, p24. The capsid surrounds two single strands of HIV RNA, each of which has a copy of the virus' nine genes. Three of these genes, *gag, pol* and *env*, contain information needed to make structural proteins for new virus particles.

The core of HIV also includes a protein called p7, the HIV nucleocapsid protein. Three enzymes carry out later steps in the virus' life cycle: reverse transcriptase, integrase, and protease. Another HIV protein called p17, or the HIV matrix protein, lies between the viral core and the viral envelope.

2. **env**–Envelope glycoprotein gp 160 – gp 120
   – gp 41

The Viral Envelope

HIV has a diameter of 1/10,000 of a millimeter and is spherical in shape. The outer coat of the virus, known as the viral envelope, is composed of two layers of fatty molecules called lipids, taken from the membrane of a human cell when a newly formed virus particle buds from the cell.

Embedded in the viral envelope are proteins from the host cell, as well as 72 copies (on average) of a complex HIV protein (frequently called "spikes") that protrudes through the surface of the virus particle (virion). This protein, known as Env, consists of a cap made of three molecules called glycoprotein (gp) 120, and a stem consisting of three gp41 molecules that anchor the structure in the viral envelope. Much of the research to develop a vaccine against HIV has focused on these envelope proteins.

3. **Pol**–Reverse transcriptase, protease, endonuclease, integrase (Antigens P31, P51, P66).

B. Non-structural and Regulatory Genes:

1. **tat** (Trans activating gene) increases expression of all viral genes.
2. **nef** (Negative factor gene) down regulating viral replication.

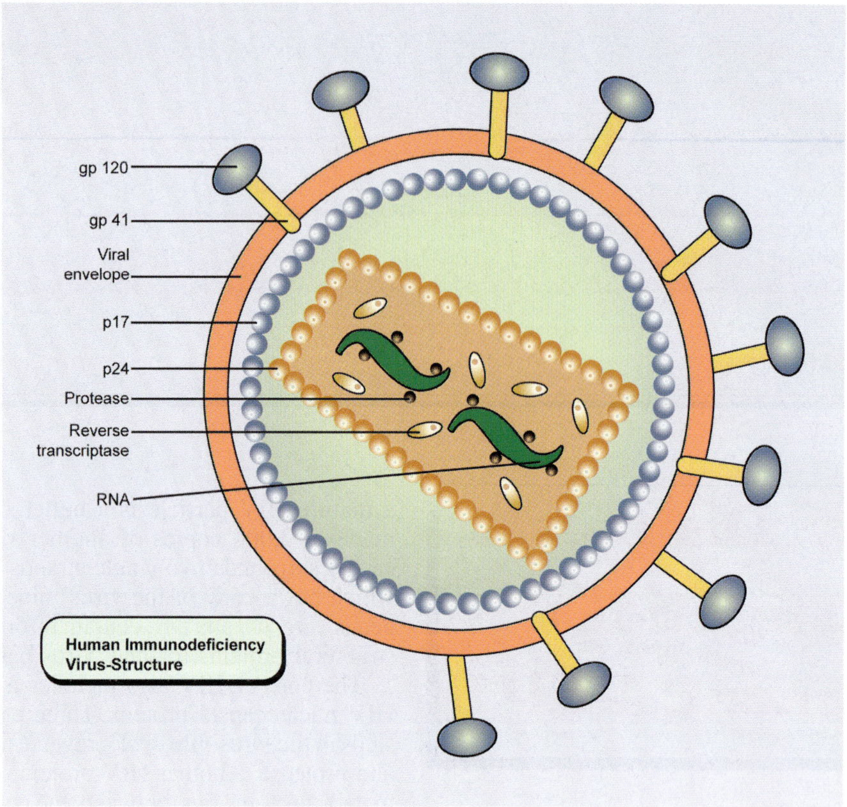

Fig. 5.1: Structure of HIV virus

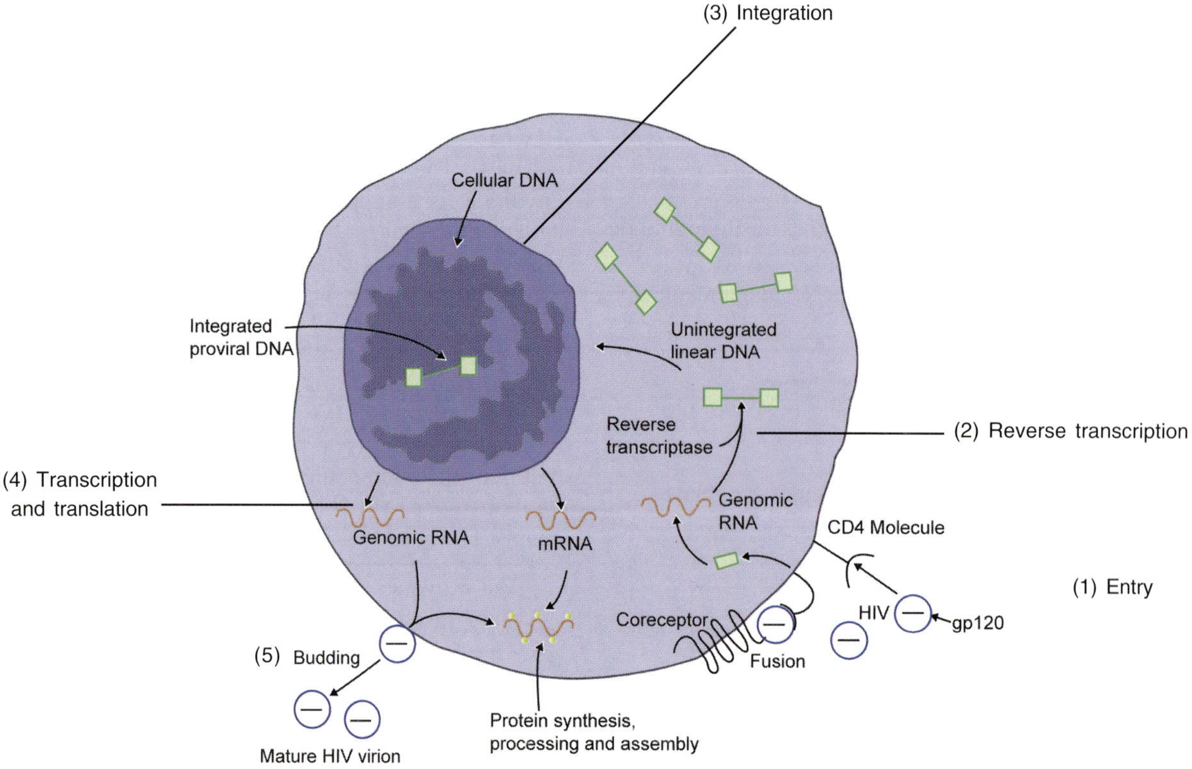

Fig. 5.2: Mode of invasion of host cell by HIV virus

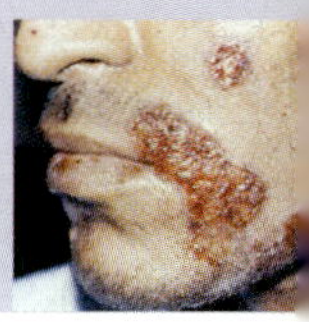

3. **rev** (Regulator of virus gene) increases structural protein expression.
4. **vif** (Viral infectivity factor gene).
5. **vpu** (HIV-1); vpx (HIV-2) increase maturation and release of progeny virus from cells.
6. **vpr–**Stimulates promoter region of virus.

   Six regulatory genes, *tat, rev, nef, vif, vpr,* and *vpu*, contain information necessary to produce proteins that control the ability of HIV to infect a cell, produce new copies of virus, or cause disease. The protein encoded by *nef*, for instance, appears necessary for the virus to replicate efficiently, and the *vpu*-encoded protein influences the release of new virus particles from infected cells.
7. **LTR** (At each end) give promoter, enhancer and integration signals.

The ends of each strand of HIV RNA contain an RNA sequence called the long terminal repeat (LTR). Regions in the LTR act as switches to control production of new viruses and can be triggered by proteins from either HIV or the host cell.

ANTIGENIC VARIATION AND DIVERSITY OF HIV

- Based on molecular and Ag differences 2 types:

  HIV-1 and 2.
- **HIV-1 subtypes**

  [Group M (Major –11 subtypes A-K)]

  [Group O (outlier – 9 subtypes)]

  [Group N (New virus)]

  Subtypes A, C and D predominate in Africa.

  Subtype B and E predominate in Thailand.

  Subtype C predominate in India.

  Subtype B predominate in U.S. and Western Europe.
- **HIV-2**

Table 5.1

Major epidemic pattern	*Geographic region*	*HIV-1 subtype*				
		A	*B*	*C*	*D*	*E*
Heterosexual hosts	Sub-Saharan Africa	+	-	+	+	+
	South East Asia	-	-	-	-	-
	India	+	+	+	-	-
Intravenous drug users and homosexual hosts	North America	-	+	-	-	-
	Western Europe	-	+	-	-	-
	South East Asia	-	+	-	-	-
	India	-	+	+	-	-

REPLICATION CYCLE OF HIV (Fig. 5.2)

Entry of HIV into Cells

Infection typically begins when an HIV particle, which contains two copies of the HIV RNA, encounters a cell with a surface molecule called cluster designation *4* (CD_4). Cells carrying this molecule are known as CD_4+ cells.

One or more of the virus' **gp 120** molecules binds tightly to CD_4 molecule(s) on the cell's surface. The binding of gp120 to CD_4 results in a conformational change in the gp120 molecule allowing it to bind to a second molecule on the cell surface known as a co-receptor. The envelope of the virus and the cell membrane then fuse, leading to entry of the virus into the cell. The **gp 41** of the envelope is critical to the *fusion process.* Drugs that block either the binding or the fusion process are being developed and tested **in clinical trials.**

Studies have identified multiple *coreceptors* for different types of HIV strains. These coreceptors are promising targets for new anti-HIV drugs, some of which are now being tested in preclinical and clinical studies. Agents that block the coreceptors are showing particular promise as potential microbicides that could be used in gels or creams to prevent HIV transmission. In the early stage of HIV disease, most people harbor viruses that use, in addition to CD_4, a receptor *called CCR5* to enter their target cells. With disease progression, the spectrum of co-receptor usage expands in approximately 50 percent of patients to include other receptors, notably a molecule called CXCR4. Virus that uses CCR 5 is called R5 HIV and virus that uses CXCR4 is called X4 HIV.

Although CD_4+ T cells appear to be the main targets of HIV, other immune system cells with and without CD_4 molecules on their surfaces are infected as well. Among these are long-lived cells called **monocytes** and **macrophages**, which apparently can harbor large quantities of the virus without being killed, thus acting as reservoirs of HIV. CD_4+ T cells also serve as important reservoirs of HIV; a small proportion of these cells harbor HIV in a stable, inactive form. Normal immune processes may activate these cells, resulting in the production of new HIV virions.

Cell-to-cell spread of HIV also can occur through the CD_4-mediated fusion of an infected cell with an uninfected cell.

Reverse Transcription

In the **cytoplasm** of the cell, HIV reverse transcriptase converts viral RNA into DNA, the nucleic acid form in which the cell carries its genes.

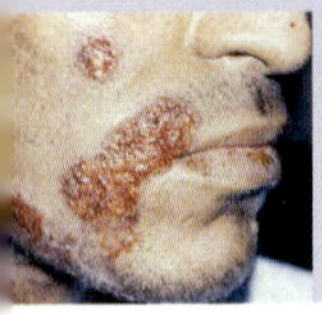

Integration

The newly made HIV DNA moves to the cell's nucleus, where it is spliced into the host's DNA with the help of HIV *integrase.* HIV DNA that enters the DNA of the cell is called a provirus.

Transcription

For a provirus to produce new viruses, RNA copies must be made that can be read by the host cell's protein-making machinery. These copies are called messenger RNA (mRNA), and production of mRNA is called transcription, a process that involves the host cell's own enzymes. Viral genes in concert with the cellular machinery control this process; the tat gene, for example, encodes a protein that accelerates transcription. Genomic RNA is also transcribed for later incorporation in the budding virion.

Cytokines, proteins involved in the normal regulation of the immune response, also may regulate transcription. Molecules such as tumor necrosis factor (TNF)-alpha and interleukin (IL)-6, secreted in elevated levels by the cells of HIV-infected people, may help to activate HIV proviruses. Other infections, by organisms such as *Mycobacterium tuberculosis*, also may enhance transcription by inducing the secretion of cytokines.

Translation

After HIV mRNA is processed in the cell's nucleus, it is transported to the cytoplasm. HIV proteins are critical to this process; for example, a protein encoded by the *rev* gene allows mRNA encoding HIV structural proteins to be transferred from the nucleus to the cytoplasm. Without the *rev* protein, structural proteins are not made. In the cytoplasm, the virus co-opts the cell's protein-making machinery—including structures called ribosomes—to make long chains of viral proteins and enzymes, using HIV mRNA as a template. This process is called translation.

Assembly and Budding

Newly made HIV core proteins, enzymes and genomic RNA gather inside the cell and an immature viral particle forms and buds off from the cell, acquiring an envelope that includes both cellular and HIV proteins from the cell membrane. During this part of the viral life cycle, the core of the virus is immature and the virus is not yet infectious. The long chains of proteins and enzymes that make up the immature viral core are now cut into smaller pieces by a viral enzyme called protease.

This step results in infectious viral particles. Drugs called protease inhibitors interfere with this step of the viral life cycle. FDA has approved eight such drugs—saquinavir, ritonavir, indinavir, amprenavir, nelfinavir, fosamprenavir, atazanavir and lopinavir.

NATURAL HISTORY OF HIV DISEASE

Natural History of HIV/AIDS (Fig. 5.3)

Four stages of HIV infection can be described:

i. **Primary infection:** Infection with HIV results in rapid proliferation of the virus in blood and lymph nodes. The infected person may experience a seroconversion illness, which usually resolves within weeks. The CD_4 cell count declines rapidly before virus is controlled by the immune system, whereupon the count returns to near normal.
ii. **Early immune deficiency (CD_4 cell count > 500/ml):** During this phase the immune system has controlled the virus, which is largely restricted to lymphoid tissue. In this phase, the damage inflicted by the virus is limited to the regenerative capacity of the immune system and people with HIV are usually without symptoms.
iii. **Intermediate immune deficiency (CD_4 cell count 200-500/ml):** Viral replication is very high and CD_4 cell turnover is rapid. Subtle signs and symptoms indicating compromise of immune system begin to appear.
iv. **Advance immune deficiency (CD_4 cell count < 200/ ml):** The virus which proliferates throughout the body overcomes the immune system. Major opportunistic infections and malignancies become increasingly common and require increasing medical intervention (Fig. 5.3). Depicts the natural history of HIV/AIDS.

CLINICAL STAGES OF HIV DISEASE

Infection with HIV leads to a progressive impairment of cellular immune function, characterized by a gradual decline in peripheral blood CD_4+T – lymphocyte levels which results in an increasing susceptibility to wide variety of opportunistic viral, bacterial, protozoal and fungal infections and to certain malignancies also.

Stage I: Acute (Primary) Infection (Sero Conversion)

Initial primary infection with HIV is usually asymptomatic. However, after an incubation period of **2-6** weeks (longest upto **36** weeks), there is a phase of viraemia and upto 50% of individuals experience an acute infection mononucleosis like illness or a viral syndrome. There may be high fever, lymphadenopathy, pharyngitis, arthralgia, a morbillifom rash and myalgia. The illness usually lasts 2 weeks or less and may even go uninvestigated as possibility of HIV infection is frequently not explored at this stage.

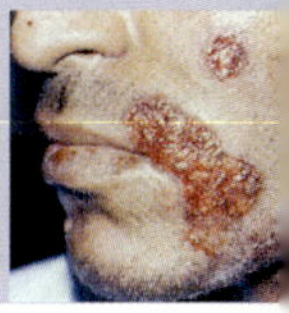

Exposure to HIV Infection	Seroconversion illness	Asymptomatic period	Subtle symptoms and signs of immunodeficiency	Full blown AIDS symptoms and signs of opportunistic infections
Antibody Titre and Infectivity	Not detectable (window period) highly infectious	Detectable antibodies infectious	Detectable antibodies infectious	Antibodies may or may not be detectable highly infectious
Time Period	12 weeks	3-5 years	2-3 years	1-2 years
Stage of HIV Disease	Primary infection (CD_4 cell count near normal)	Early immunodeficiency (CD_4 cell count >500 cell mm^3)	Intermediate immunodeficiency (CD_4 cell count <500 >200 cells mm^3)	Terminal illness (CD_4 cell count <200 cell mm^3)

Fig. 5.3: Natural history of HIV

Around 10-20% patients may present with headache, meningoencephalitis, peripheral neuropathies, myelopathy, Bell's Palsy or G.B. Syndrome. One may occasionally also get oropharyngeal candidiasis.

There is severe CD_4 lymphopaenia and this may drop to levels indicative of advanced HIV disease but typically it rebounds to near normal in 2-3 weeks in most of cases. In some cases CD_4 count may remain suppressed and this may be harbinger of a more accelerated course of disease. HIV antibody tests are often negative in early stages of HIV seroconversion illness:

The **diagnosis** depends on tests to detect viral antigen (e.g. p24 antigen and PCR tests).

Stage II: Early (Asymptomatic) Disease (CD_4 Count>500/mm^3)

This is the *longest period* in course of HIV disease in which patient is asymptomatic and remains apparently healthy for a few years or more. This period may be, on an average, 8-10 years in Western countries but in India it has been found to be 5-7 years. But there are still no large epidemiological studies to confirm this.

Clinical Features

The relatively symptom free period may be punctuated by various ***dermatological conditions*** like seborrheic dermatitis, pruritis, cellulitis, reactivation of latent herpes zoster infection, worsening of psoriasis. Sometimes oral hairy leukoplakia may be identified at this stage of disease.

There may be symptoms and sign suggestive of *polyclonal activation of immune* system manifesting as ITP, G.B. Syndrome, auto-immune demyelination of peripheral nerves, polymyositis and mononeuritis multiplex. The manifestation of HIV infection in this period correlates poorly with risk of disease progression.

Another feature seen frequently is symptomless *Persistent Generalised Lymphadenopathy (PGL)*. This is seen 3-5 years after HIV infection and usually involves one or more extra inguinal lymph nodes (cervical or axillary) with nodes being more than 1 cm in diameter, not matted and persisting for more than three months duration.

Laboratory data shows leukopenia, thrombocytopenia, polyclonal gammopathy and altered serum transaminase levels. Even without ARV therapy chances of patients in this stage progressing to AIDS within 2 years is less than 5%. The CD_4 count continues to decline progressively and though difficult to predict, on an average there is decrease of 40-80 cells/mm^3/year without ARV therapy.

Stage III: Intermediate HIV infection (CD_4 Count 200-500/mm^3)

As CD_4 count falls, the complications of HIV infection begin to occur more frequently or worsen in severity.

The person gets other disorders (earlier referred to as ARC) like recurrent HSV and HZV infection (shingles), mild oropharyngeal or vaginal candidiasis, oral hairy leukoplakia indicates a higher risk of progression to AIDS. *Mycobacterium tuberculosis* is seen commonly with a CD_4 count around 250/mm^3. Atypical and extrapulmonary tuberculosis (affecting lymph nodes or causing tubercular meningitis) are also common.

When left untreated, patients with intermediate HIV disease have 30-50% chance of developing an AIDS defining conditions or dying within next 18-28 months. With ARV therapy, however, the risk is reduced two to three folds.

Stage IV: Late Stage HIV Disease (CD_4 count 50-200/mm^3)

According to revised CDC definition of AIDS, all patients in this group are now defined as *having AIDS*.

The most commonly noted *opportunistic infections* during this stage include cerebral toxoplasmosis, PCP, cryptococcal meningitis, cytomegalovirus retinitis etc.

Stage V: Advanced HIV Disease (CD_4 count <50/ mm^3)

Even with therapy, the patients with advanced HIV disease have a likelihood of dying within a 2-year period due to any of the opportunistic infections.

As the CD_4+ count gets depleted further, the spectrum of infections widens and frequent relapses are seen despite treatment and secondary prophylaxis.

The common infections seen in this stage are those with *M. Avium Complex (MAC),* systemic histoplasmosis, cryptococcal meningitis, progressive multifocal leukoencephalopathy, CMV retinitis, CMV colitis and CMV encephalitis.

Many patients with CD_4 count < 50/mm^3 present with direct neurological effects of HIV known as AIDS Dementia Complex (ADC). It is a subcortical dementing process which causes motor abnormalities, cognitive impairment and behavioural changes. The incidence of ADC is decreasing over years with use of ARV therapy. Many patients in this stage develop significant weight loss, wasting of muscles, various types of malabsorptions, various features of Addison's disease etc. (HIV wasting syndrome).

The latest clinical stages are given below:

Table 5.2: WHO clinical staging of HIV/AIDS for adults and adolescents, 2006

Clinical Stage 1
Asymptomatic
Persistent generalized lymphadenopathy
Clinical Stage 2
Unexplained moderate weight loss (<10% of presumed or measured body weight)[1]
Recurrent respiratory tract infections (sinusitis, tonsillitis, otitis media, pharyngitis)
Herpes zoster
Angular cheilitis
Recurrent oral ulceration
Papular pruritic eruptions
Seborrheic dermatitis
Fungal nail infections
Clinical Stage 3
Unexplained[2] severe weight loss (>10% of presumed or measured body weight)
Unexplained chronic diarrhoea for longer than one month
Unexplained persistent fever (above 37.5°C is intermittent or constant for longer than one month)
Persistent oral candidiasis
Oral hairy leukoplakia
Pulmonary tuberculosis
Severe bacterial infections (e.g. pneumonia, empyema, pyomyositis, bone or joint infection, meningitis, bacteraemia)
Acute necrotizing ulcerative stomatitis, gingivitis or periodontitis
Unexplained anaemia (<8g/dl), neutropenia (<0.5 x 10^9/litre) and or chronic trombocytopenia (<50 x 10^9/litre[3])
Clinical Stage 4[3]
HIV wasting syndrome
Pneumocystis pneumonia
Recurrent severe bacterial pneumonia
Chronic herpes simplex infection (orolabial, genital or anorectal of more than one month's duration or visceral at any site)
Oesophageal candidiasis (or candidiasis of trachea, bronchi or lungs)
Extrapulmonary tuberculosis
Kaposi sarcoma
Cytomegalovirus infection (retinitis or infection of other organs)
Central nervous system toxoplasmosis
HIV encephalopathy
Extrapulmonary cryptococcosis including meningitis
Disseminated non-tuberculous mycobacteria infection
Progressive multifocal leukoencephalopathy
Chronic cryptosporidiosis
Chronic isosporiasis
Disseminated mycosis (extrapulmonary) histoplasmosis, coccidiomycosis)
Recurrent septicaemia (including non-typhoidal salmonella)
Lymphoma (cerebral or B cell non-Hodgkin)
Invasive cervical carcinoma
Atypical disseminated leishmaniasis
Symptomatic HIV-associated nephropathy or symptomatic HIV-associated cardiomyopathy

1. Assessment of body weight in pregnant woman needs to consider expected weight gain of pregnancy.
2. Unexplained refers to where the condition is not explained by other conditions.
3. Some additional specific conditions can also be included in regional classifications (e.g. reactivation of American trypanosomiasis meningoencephalitis and/or myocarditis) in Americas region, Penicilliosis in Asia.

Tests (Table 5.3)

- ***HIV:** At least 2 different antigen or principles based Rapid/ELISA tests in symptomatic HIV patients* (Western blot no longer required as a must in our country).

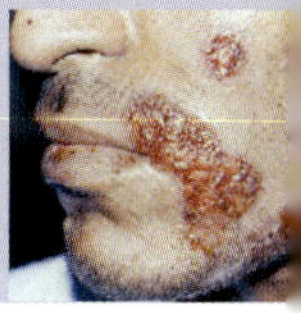

Table 5.3: Investigations

Essential	*Optional*
Confirm HIV infection: HIV status must be documented. Refer to ICTC if in doubt	**Fasting lipid profile:** May be recommended in patients with established coronary disease risk factors, or if stavudine, efavirenz, protease inhibitor (PI) use is contemplated
Specific investigations: To rule out Ols, depending on the clinical need	**Pregnancy test:** EFV is contraindicated in pregnancy during the first trimester of pregnancy
***CD_4 counts:** All patients should have a baseline screening	**Anti-HCV screening:** The prevalence of hepatitis C virus (HCV) is low in HIV-infected patients, except, for example, in the northeastern states of India, where injecting drug use is a risk factor. Such screening is also recommended in HIV-infected haemophiliacs and thalassaemics
CBC: Hb, TLC, DIC, ESR	**Chest X-ray:** To rule out TB or other pulmonary infection based as symptoms
LFTs: Necessary to find evidence of hepatitis, particularly when NVP use is contemplated	**Plasma viral load (PVL):** A baseline PVL is not necessary. With optimum adherence and a potent regimen, undetectable levels should be achieved at 6 months after ART initiation
Urine routine: To evaluate proteinuria and sugar (may necessitate estimation of blood glucose)	
HbsAg: To rule out concomitant hepatitis B infection as this can influence choice of ARV regimen. The abrupt stopping of anti-HBV drugs such as lamivudine and tenofovir is not recommended in patients with chronic hepatitis B co-infection since it may result in hepatitis B flare-up. This screening is mandatory for IDUs and those with transfusion-associated HIV infection	
HCV screening: Mandatory for IDUs and those with transfusion-associated HIV infection	
VDRL/TPHA (syphilis screening): Especially for persons from high-risk behaviour groups, those with history of STIs and/or symptoms suggestive of syphilis	
Pap smear: Helps in earlier diagnosis of cervical intraepithelial neoplasia (CIN). Or Trichloroacetic acid staining at district facilities where Pap smear is not available	

***** CD_4 count**	***Repeat at***
< 350 and not on ART	3 months
> 350 and not on ART	6 months
On ART (any value)	6 months
> 500	Annual screening

- ***Immune functions:*** CD_4+, CD_8+ Cell counts, CD_4/CD_8 ratio.
- Plasma viral loads (wherever possible).
- Full blood counts, liver and renal function tests.
- Mantoux test.
- X-ray chest.
- Co-infections: Tests for syphilis, gonorrhoea, hepatitis A, B and C, Toxoplasma, E-B virus, pap smear for women.

National Guidelines on Testing Adults

- **For symptomatic persons:** The sample should be **reactive with two different kits.**
- **For asymptomatic persons:** The sample should be **reactive with three different kits.**
- The blood sample collected at one time is tested with the first kit. If it is reactive, it is then retested sequentially with the second and third kits.

DRUGS (Fig. 5.4) (Table 5.4)

Antiretroviral agents are drugs which act at various stages of the life-cycle of HIV in the body and work by interrupting the process of viral replication. Theoretically, ARV drugs can act in any of the following ways during different stages of viral replication:

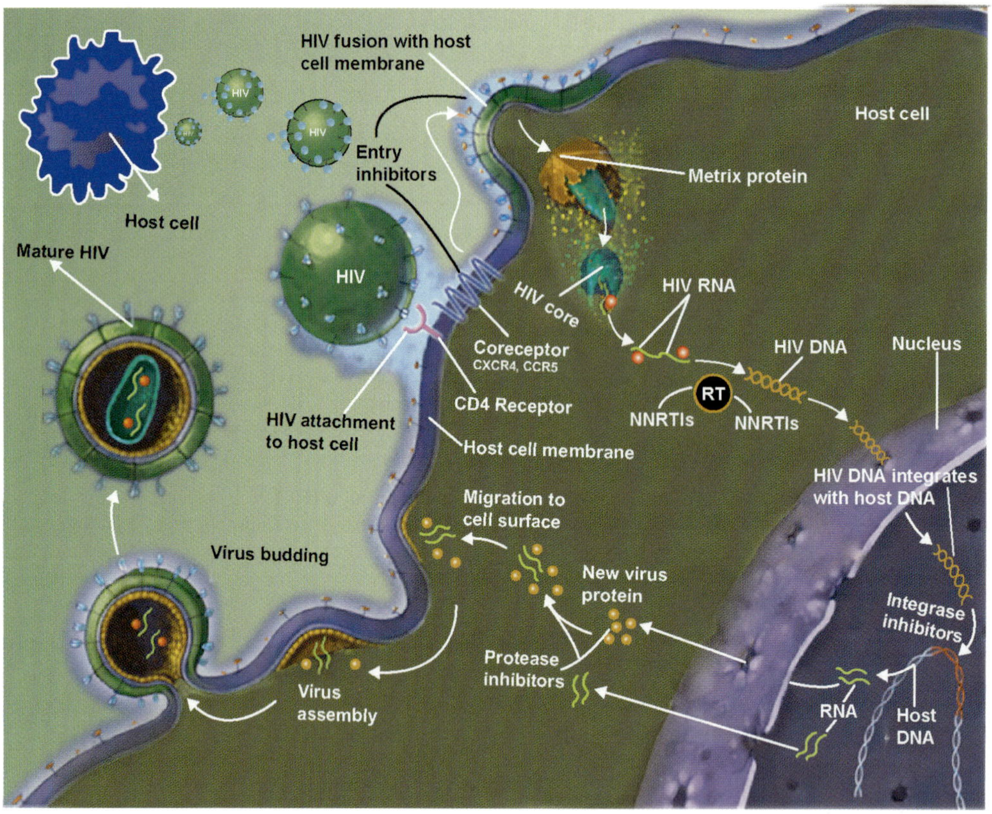

Fig. 5.4: Drugs

i. Block binding of HIV to target cell **(fusion inhibitors).**
ii. Block viral RNA cleavage and one that inhibits reverse transcriptase **(reverse transcriptase inhibitors).**
iii. Block the enzyme, **integrase**, which helps in the incorporation of the proviral DNA into the host cell chromosome (**integrase inhibitors**).
iv. Block the RNA to prevent viral protein production.
v. Block the enzyme protease (**protease inhibitors**).
vi. Inhibit the budding of virus from host cells.

Table 5.4

Nucleoside reverse transcriptase inhibitors (NRTI)	*Non-nucleoside reverse transcriptase inhibitors (NNRTI)*	*Protease inhibitors (PI)*
Zidovudine (AZT/ZDV)*	Nevirapine*(NVP)	Saquinavir*(SQV)
Stavudine (D4T)*	Efavirenz*(EFV)	Ritonavir* (RTV)
Lamivudine (3TC)*	Delavirdine (DLV)	Nelfinavir* (NFV)
Didanosine (ddl)*		Amprenavir (APV)
Zalcitabine (ddC)*	*Fusion inhibitors (FI)*	Indinavir* (INV)
Abacavir (ABC)*	Efuviritide (T-20)	Lopinavir/Ritonavir (LPV)*
Emtricitabline (FTC)		Foseamprenavir (FPV)
(NtRTI)	*Integrase Inhibitors (new)*	Atazanavir (ATV)*
Tenofavir (TDF)*	Tipranavir (TPV)	
	CCR5 Entry Inhibitor (new)	

* Available in India

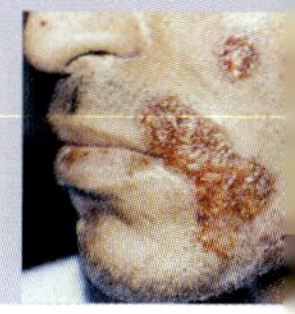

The currently available agents target the virus mainly by inhibiting the enzymes reverse transcriptase (RT inhibitors) and protease (protease inhibitors), and preventing fusion of the virus with CD_4 cells (fusion inhibitors). New classes of drugs are emerging.

Goals of Antiretroviral Therapy

The currently available ARV drugs cannot eradicate the HIV infection from the human body. This is because a pool of latently infected CD_4 cells is established during the earliest stages of acute HIV infection and persists within the organs/ cells and fluids (e.g., liver and lymphoid tissue) even with prolonged suppression of plasma viraemia to <50 copies/ml by antiretroviral therapy. The goals of therapy are as follows:

When to Start ART in Adults and Adolescents (Tables 5.5 and 5.6)

The initiation of ART is based on the clinical stage and the CD^4 count is used to guide treatment and follow-up. The lack of a CD_4 result should not delay the initiation of ART if the patient is clinically eligible according to the WHO clinical staging, but a CD_4 test should be done as soon as possible.

All HIV-positive persons are eligible for CD_4 testing for the purpose of screening for ART eligibility, under the national programme. Priority is given to the following groups:

- All HIV-positive persons in WHO clinical stages 3 and 4.
- All persons tested HIV-positive 6-8 years ago.
- PLHA with a history of pulmonary TB and/or herpes zoster.
- If the CD_4 count assessed by a private laboratory is less than 350 cells/mm^3.
- HIV-infected partners of AIDS patients.
- All pregnant HIV-positive women.
- All HIV-positive children (<15 years of age).

Starting ART by Using CD_4 Guidance

The optimum time to start ART is before the patient becomes unwell or presents with the first OI. The progression of the disease is faster in patients who commence ART when the

Table 5.5

- **Clinical goals:** Polongation of life and improvement in quality of life.
- **Virological goals:** Greatest possible reduction in viral load for as long as possible.
- **Immunological goals:** Immune reconstitution that is both quantitative and qualitative.
- **Therapeutic goals:** Rational sequencing of drugs in a fashion that achieves clinical, virological and immunological goals while maintaining treatment options, limiting drug toxicity and facilitating adherence.
- **Reduction of HIV transmission in individuals:** Reduction of HIV transmission by suppression of viral load.

Table 5.6

Classification of HIV-associated	*WHO clinical stage clinical disease*	*CD_4 test not available (or result pending)*	*CD_4 test available*
Asymptomatic	1	Do not treat	Treat if CD_4 < 200
Mild symptoms	2	Do not treat	
Advanced symptoms	3	Treat	Consider treatment if CD_4 < 350 and initiate ART before CD_4 drops below 200
Severe/Advanced symptoms	4	Treat	Treat irrespective of CD_4 count

Notes:

- Determining the clinical stage is part of the baseline assessment (first visit) on entry into the case and treatment programme. Clinical staging is used to guide decisions on initiating co-trimoxazole prophylaxis and ART CD_4 testing facilities are not immediately available (or the result is pending).
- Offer ART to symptomatic patients if the CD_4 count is 200-350 cells/mm^3.
- Consider ART for asymptomatic patients with CD_4 count between 200-350 cells/mm^3 and monitor closely for new symptoms.
- If the CD_4 counts 200-250 cells/mm^3, physicians can repeat the CD_4 test in 4 weeks in asymptomatic patients. This is to rule out the possibility of a 20% margin of error in laboratory results.
- Patients should start ART before the CD_4 count drop below 200 cells/mm^3.

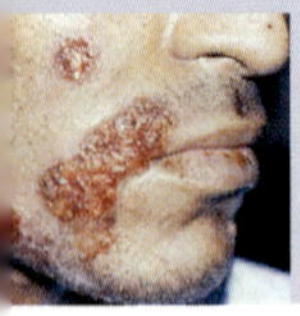

CD_4 count falls below 200 cells/mm^3 than in those who start ART before the count drops to this level. Patients should start ART before the CD_4 count drops below 200 cells/mm^3.The CD_4 count should be assessed after stabilization of any concurrent illness because the absolute CD_4 count can vary with illness. The CD_4 count should be used as a supplement to clinical assessment for determining the stage of the disease in matters of decision-making. All HIVconfirmed persons should be referred to ART centres for registration into care and screening for medical eligibility for ART.

Do not delay ART initiation if the patient is clinically eligible according to the WHO clinical staging criteria, in absence of a CD_4 count.

Manage OIs Before Starting ART Commencing ART in the Presence of Active OIs (Table 5.7)

Do not start ART in the presence of an active OI. In general, OIs should be treated or stabilized before commencing ART. *Mycobacterium Avium Complex (MAC) and Progressive Multifocal Leukoencephalopathy (PML)* are exceptions, in which commencing ART may be the preferred treatment, especially when specific MAC therapy is not available.

Table 5.7

Clinical picture	*Action*
Any undiagnosed active infection with fever	Diagnose and treat first; start ART when stable
TB	**Treat TB first**; start ART as **recommended** in TB sections (5.10 and 5.11)
PCP	Treat PCP first; start ART when PCP treatment is completed
Invasive fungal diseases: oesophageal candidiasis, cryptococcal meningitis, penicilliosis, histoplasmosis	Treat esophageal candidiasis first; start ART as soon as the patient can swallow comfortably Treat cryptococcal meningitis, penicilliosis, histoplasmosis first; start ART when patient is stabilized or OI treatment is completed
Bacterial pneumonia	Treat pneumonia first; start ART when treatment is completed
Malaria	Treat malaria first; start ART when treatment is completed
Drug reaction	Do not start ART during an acute reaction
Acute diarrhoea which may reduce absorption of ART	Diagnose and treat first; start ART when diarrhoea is stabilized or controlled
Non-severe anaemia (Hb < 8 g/litre)	Start ART if no other cause for anaemia are found (HIV is often the cause of anaemia); avoid AZT
Skin condition such as PPE and seborrheic dermatitis, psoriasis, HIV-related exfoliative dermatitis	Start ART (ART may resolve these problems)
Suspected MAC, cryptosporidiosis and microsporidiosis	Start ART (ART may resolve these problems)
Cytomegalovirus infection	Treat if drugs available; if not, start ART
Toxoplasmosis	Treat; start ART after 6 weeks of treatment and when patient is stabilized

Contd.

Contd.

Some conditions which may *regress* following the commencement of ART include candidiasis and cryptosporidiosis.

The following OIs and HIV-related illnesses need treatment or stabilization before commencing ART.

Antiretroviral Therapy Regimens (Tables 5.8 to 5.11)

Currently, the **national programme** provides the following combinations for first-line regimens.

i. **Stavudine (30 mg) + Lamivudine (150 mg).**
ii. Zidovudine (300 mg) + Lamivudine (150 mg).
iii. Stavudine (30 mg) + Lamivudine (150 mg) + Nevirapine (200 mg).
iv. Zidovudine (300 mg) + Lamivudine (150 mg) + Nevirapine (200 mg).
v. Efavirenz (600 mg).
vi. Nevirapine (200 mg).

Fixed-dose combinations (FDCs) are preferred because they are easy to use, have distribution advantages (procurement and stock management), improve adherence to treatment and thus reduce the chances of development of drug resistance. The current national experience shows that bid (twice a day) regimens of FDCs are well tolerated and complied with. At present, second-line drug regimens are not available under the national programme.

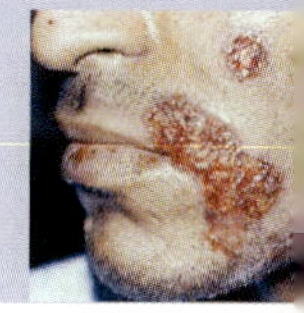

Table 5.8

Principles for selecting the first-line regimen

1. Choose 3TC (lamivudine) in all regimens
2. Choose one NRTI (AZT or d4T) to combine with 3TC
3. Choose one NNRTI (NVP or EFV)

First choice: AZT + 3TC + NVP (for patients with Hb>8g/dl) Second choice: D4T + 3TC + NVP	Substitute NVP with EFV, for patients with TB or toxicity to NVP

Table 5.9

Recommendation	*Regimen*	*Comments*
Preferred first line regimen	AZT + 3TC + NVP	AZT may cause anaemia, which requires Hb monitoring, but is preferred over d4T because of d4T toxicity (lipoatrophy, lactic acidosis, peripheral neuropathy)
		Patients who develop severe anemia while on an AZT-based regimen should not be re-challenged with AZT. In such cases, the patient should receive either d4T or TDF in place of AZT
		For women with CD4 > 250 cells/mm^3, monitor for hepatotoxicity closely if started on the NVP-based regimen
Alternative first line regimens	AZT + 3TC + EFV	EFV is substituted for NVP in cases of intolerance to the latter or if patients are receiving rifampicin-containing anti TB treatment
		EFV should not be used in patients with grade 4 or higher elevations of ALT
	D4T + 3TC + (NVP or EFV)	It the patients have anaemia, a d4T-based regimen should be prescribed
Other options	TDF + 3TF + (NVP or EFV) or AZT + 3TC + TDF	TDF is supplied on a case-to-case basis by SACS after evaluation by the SACS clinical expert panel

Initiation of First-line ART in Relation to Anti-TB Therapy

(Based on 2006 WHO guidelines)

Table 5.10

CD4 cell count (cells/mm^3)	*Timing of ART in relation to initiation of TB treatment*	*ART recommendations*
CD_4 < 200	Start ATT first Start ART as soon as TB treatment is tolerated (between 2 weeks and 2 months)[i]	*Recommended ART*[ii] EFV-containing regimens [iii]
CD_4 between 200-350	Start ATT first Start ART 8 weeks after starting ATT (i.e. after completion of TB-intensive phase)	Recommend ART [vi]
CD_4 > 350	Start ATT first Re-evaluate patient for ART at 8 weeks and at end of TB treatment	Defer ART[v]
CD_4 not available	Start ART 2-8 weeks after ATT initiation	Recommend ART[iv]

i. Timing of ART initiation is based on clinical judgment, in accordance with other signs of immunodeficiency and WHO clinical stages. In the case of extrapulmonary TB, ART should be started as soon as TB treatment is tolerated, irrespective of the CD_4 count.
ii. ART should be started as soon as TB treatment is tolerated, particulary in patients with severe immunosuppression.
iii. EFV-containing regimens include D4T/3TC/EFV and AZT/3TC/EFV (Nevirapine should not be used).
iv. ART should be started if other non-TB stage 3 or 4 events are present.
v. For some types of TB that generally respond well to anti-TB therapy (i.e. lymph node TB, uncomplicated pleural effusion), or some cases where uncomplicated pulmonary TB disease is responding well to TB treatment, consider deferring ART initiation.

Rationale for ART Recommendation During TB Treatment

Table 5.11

- HIV-infected patients with a CDR count of 200-350 cells/mm^3 are at an increased risk of developing active tuberculosis, even in regions with high-baseline TB prevalence.
- HIV-infected patients with a CD_4 count of 200-350 cells/mm^3 and active tuberculosis are at a greater risk of AIDS and death than those without TB and with CD_4 counts in the same range.
- In the absence of ART, TB therapy alone does not significantly increase the CD_4 cell count. Nor does it significantly decrease the HIV viral load. Thus, CD_4 counts measured during active TB are likely to reflect the actual level of immunosuppression.
- The use of HAART in patients with TB can lead to a sustained reduction in the HIV viral load. it can also facilitate immunological reconstitution, and decrease AIDS-defining illness and mortality. This benefit is seen across different ranges of CD_4 counts.

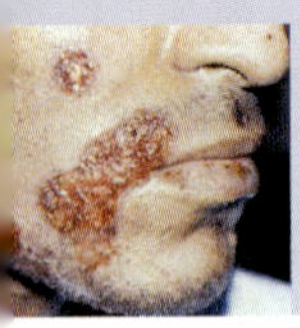

POST EXPOSURE PROPHYLAXIS (Tables 5.12 and 5.13)

The average risk of acquiring HIV infection after different types of occupational exposure is low compared to risk of infection with HBV or HCV. In terms of occupational exposure the important routes are *needle stick exposure* (0.3% risk for HIV, 9–30% for HBV and 1–10% for HCV) and *mucous membrane exposure* (0.09% for HIV).

Table 5.12

Exposure to body fluids considered 'at risk'	*Exposure to body fluids considered not at risk'**
Blood	Tears
Semen	
Vaginal secretions	Sweat
Cerebrospinal fluid	
Synovial, pleural, peritoneal, pericardial fluid	Urine and faeces
Amniotic fluid Other body fluids contaminated with visible blood.	Saliva

* Unless these secretions contain visible blood

Table 5.13

Exposure route	*Risk of HIV*
Blood transfusion	90-95%
Perinatal	20-40%
Sexual intercourse	0.1 to 10%
Vaginal	0.1 to 10%
Anal	0.065-0.5%
Oral	0.0005-0.01%
Injecting drugs use	0.67%
Needle stick exposure	0.3%
Mucous membrane splash to eye, oro-nasal	0.09%

Note: Needle-stick exposure for HBV is 9-30% and HCV is 1-10%.

Step 1: Management of Exposure Site–First Aid

For skin: If the skin is broken after a needle-stick or sharp instrument:

Immediately wash the wound and surrounding skin with water and soap and rinse. Do not scrub.

Do not use antiseptics or skin washes (bleach, chlorine, alcohol, betadine).

After a splash of blood or body fluids:

To unbroken skin:

- Wash the area immediately.
- Do not use antiseptics.

For the eye:

- Irrigate exposed eye immediately with water or normal saline.
- Sit in a chair, tilt head back and ask a colleague to gently pour water or normal saline over the eye.
- If wearing contact lens, leave them in place while irrigating, as they form a barrier over the eye and will help protect it. Once the eye is cleaned, remove the contact lens and clean them in the normal manner. This will make them safe to wear again.
- Do not use soap or disinfectant on the eye.

For mouth:

- Spit fluid out immediately.
- Rinse the mouth thoroughly, using water or saline and spit again. Repeat this process several times.
- Do not use soap or disinfectant in the mouth.

Step 2: Establish Eligibility for PEP

The HIV seroconversion rate of 0.3% after an AEB (for percutaneous exposure) is an average rate. The real risk of transmission depends on the amount of HIV transmitted (= amount of contaminated fluid and the viral load).

A designated person/trained doctor must assess the risk of HIV and HBV transmission following an AEB. This evaluation must be made rapidly, so as to start any treatment as soon as possible after the accident (Ideally **within 2 hours** but certainly **within 72 hours**). This assessment must be made thoroughly (because not every AEB requires prophylactic treatment).

The **first dose** of PEP should be administered within the first 72 hours of exposure and the risk evaluated as soon as possible. If the risk is insignificant, PEP could be discontinued, if already commenced.

Two main factors determine the risk of infection: the nature of exposure and the status of the source patient.

I. *Assessing the Nature of Exposure and Risk of Transmission (Table 5.14)*

Three categories of exposure can be described based on the amount of blood/fluid involved and the entry port. These categories are intended to help in assessing the severity of

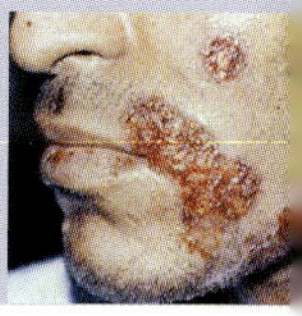

the exposure but may not cover all possibilities. PEP must be initiated as soon as possible, preferably within 2 hours.

TYPE OF EXPOSURE

Table 5.14

Category	*Definition and example*
Mild exposure:	Mucous membrane/non-intact skin with small volumes e.g.: A superficial wound (erosion of the epidermis) with a plain or low calibre needle, or contact with the eyes or mucous membranes, *subcutaneous* injections following small-bore needles
Moderate exposure:	Mucous membrane/non intact skin with large volumes OR Percutaneous superficial exposure with solid needle e.g. a cut or needle stick injury penetrating *glovers*
Severe exposure:	Percutaneous with large volume e.g.: • An accident with a high calibre needle (> 18G) visibly contaminated with blood; • A deep wound (hemorrhagic wound and/or very painful); • Transmission of a significant volume of blood; • An accident with material that has previously been used intravenously or intra-arterially.
The wearing of gloves during any of these accidents constitutes a protective factor.	

Note: In case of an AEB with material such as discarded sharps/needles, contaminated for over 48 hours, the risk of infection becomes negligible for HIV but still remains significant for HBV. HBV survives longer than HIV outside the body.

II. *Assessing the HIV Status of the Source of Exposure (Table 5.15)*

PEP needs to be started as soon as possible after the exposure and within 72 hours. In animal studies, initiating PEP within 12, 24 or 36 hours of exposure was more effective than initiating PEP 48 hours or 72 hours following exposure. PEP is not effective when given more than ***72 hours*** after exposure. A baseline rapid HIV testing should be done before starting PEP.

Table 5.15

Source HIV status	*Definition of risk in source*
HIV negative	Source is not HIV infected but consider HBV and HCV
Low risk	HIV positive and clinically asymptomatic
High risk	HIV positive and clinically symptomatic (see WHO clinical staging)
Unknown	Status of the patient is unknown, and neither the patient nor his/her blood is available for testing (e.g. injury during medical waste management the source patient might be unknown). The risk assessment will be based only upon the exposure (HIV prevalence in the locality can be considered)

Initiation of PEP where indicated should not be delayed while waiting for the results of HIV testing of the source of exposure. Informed consent should be obtained before testing of the source as per national HIV testing guidelines.

HIV infection is not detected during the primary infection period by routine use HIV tests. During the "window period", which lasts for approximately 6 weeks, the antibody level is still too low for detection – but infected persons can still have a high viral load. This implies that a positive HIV test result can help in taking the decision to start PEP, but a negative test result does not exclude HIV infection. In districts or some population groups with a high HIV prevalence, a higher proportion of HIV-infected individuals are found in the window period. In these situations, a negative result has even less value for decision-making on PEP.

III. *Assessment of the Exposed Individual*

The exposed individual should have confidential counselling and assessment by an experience physician. The exposed individual should be assessed for pre-existing HIV infection intended for people who are HIV-negative at the time of their potential exposure to HIV. Exposed individuals who are known or discovered to be HIV-positive should not receive PEP. They should be offered counselling and information on prevention of transmission and referred to clinical and laboratory assessment to determine eligibility for antiretroviral therapy (ART).

Step 3: Prescribe PEP (Table 5.16)

Deciding on PEP regimen.
There are two types of regimens:

- **Basic regimen: 2-drug combination.**
- **Expanded regimen: 3-drug combination.**

The decision to initiate the type of regimen depends on the type of exposure and HIV serostatus of the source person

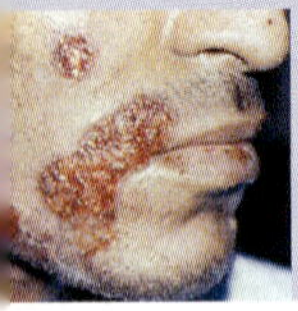

Table 5.16

Exposure	*Status of source*		
	HIV+ and asymptomatic	HIV+ and Clinically symptomatic	HIV status unknown
Mild	Consider 2-drug PEP	Start 2-drug PEP	Usually no PEP or consider 2-drug PEP
Moderate	Start 2-drug PEP	Start 3-drug PEP	Usually no PEP or consider 2-drug PEP
Severe	Start 3-drug PEP	Start 3-drug PEP	Usually no PEP or consider 2-drug PEP

HIV testing of the source patient should not delay the decision about whether or not to start PEP.

Start 2 drugs first if required, then send for consultation or refer.

In the case of a high risk exposure from a source patient who has been exposed to or is taking antiretroviral medications, consult an expert to choose the PEP regimen, as the risk of drug resistance is high.

Initiate HIV Chemoprophylaxis (Table 5.17)

Because post-exposure prophylaxis (PEP) has its greatest effect if begun within 2 hours of exposure, it is essential to act immediately. There is little benefit if >72 hours later. The prophylaxis needs to be continued for **4 weeks.**

Table 5.17

Medication regimen	*2-drug*	*3-drug regimen*
Zidovudine (AZT)	300 mg twice a day	300 mg twice a day
Stavudine (d4T)	30 mg twice a day	30 mg twice a day
Lamivudine (3TC)	150 mg twice a day	150 mg twice a day
Protease inhibitors		**1st choice:**Lopinavir/ritonavir (LPV/r) 400/100 mg twice a day or 800/200 mg once daily with meals **2nd choice:** Nelfinavir (NLF) 1250 mg twice a day or 750 mg three times a day with empty stomach. **3rd choice:** Indinavir (IND) 800 mg every 8 hours and drink 8-10 glasses (> 1.5 litres) of water daily.

Note: If protease inhibitor is not available and the 3rd drug is indicated, one can consider using Efavirenz (EFV 600 mg once daily). Monitoring should be instituted for side effects of this drug e.g. CNS toxicity such as nightmares, insomnia etc.

The Tests to be Done for PEP are given below:

Table 5.18

Timing	*In persons taking PEP (standard regimen)*	*In persons not taking PEP*
Weeks 2 and 4	Transaminases* Complete blood count[ξ]	Clinical monitoring for hepatitis
Weeks 6	HIV-Ab	HIV-Ab
Months 3	HIV-Ab, anti-HCV, HBsAg Transaminases*	HIV-Ab, anti-HCV, HBsAg
Months 6	HIV-Ab, anti-HCV, HBsAg Transaminases*	HIV-Ab, anti-HCV, HBsAg

* Transaminases should be checked at weeks 2 and 4 to detect hepatitis in case the exposed person contracted HBV from the AEB.

ξ For persons started on AZT-containing PEP regimens.

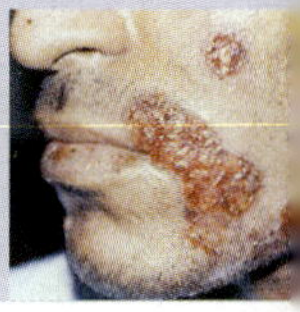

A Brief Outline of the Management Protocol is given below: (Table 5.19)

Table 5.19: Steps for managing occupational exposure

time line: 0 hr 0 min → As soon as possible → Ideally with 2 hours, but certainly within 72 hours → 6 months

Step 1: Manage exposure site	Step 2: Establish eligibility for PEP	Step 3: Counsel for PEP	Step 4: Prescribe PEP	Step 5: Laboratory evaluation	Step 6: Follow-up and monitor adherence
↓ Wash wound and surrounding skin with water and soap OR Irrigate exposed eye immediately with water or normal saline OR Rinse the mouth throroughly, using water or saline and spit again ↓ Refer to physician ↓	↓ Exposure within 72 hours ↓ Assess exposed individual ↓ Assess exposure source ↓ Assess type of exposure ↓ Determine risk of transmission ↓ Determine eligibility for PEP	↓ Provide information on HIV and PEP ↓ Obtain consent for PEP ↓ Offer speical leave from work	↓ Assess source patient's ARV status ↓ Check for pregnancy if exposed female HCP ↓ Explain side effects of ARVs ↓ Explain post exposure measures against HBV and HBC	↓ Provide HIV pretest counselling ↓ Check immunization status for hepatitis B ↓ Offer HIV, HBV, HBC test ↓ Draw blood to include CBC, liver function tests, pregnancy test, if applicable ↓ Provide HIV post-test counselling	↓ Record-keeping ↓ Follow-up visits for clinical assessment at 2 weeks and hepatitis B vaccination if needed ↓ HIV test at 3 and 6 months

REFERENCES

- Rook's Textbook of Dermatology D. A. Burns, S. M. Breathnach, Neil Cox, Christopher E, Griffiths 7th edn 2004.
- Fitzpatrick's Dermatology in General Medicine, 6th edn 2003.
- NACO Guidelines 2007.
- WHO Guidelines 2006.

Cutaneous Manifestations

PURPOSE OF STUDYING CUTANEOUS MANIFESTATIONS OF HIV INFECTION

- To know which dermatoses correlates with immunosuppression.
- To know which dermatoses are specific of HIV.
- IRIS (Immune Reconstitution Inflammatory Syndrome).

SPECIFIC DERMATOSES

- Exanthem of acute retroviral syndrome (ARS).
- PSO (Proximal subungual onychomycoses).
- OHL (oral hairy leucoplakia).
- Chronic herpetic ulcer.
- Eosinophilic folliculitis.
- Papular eruption.
- Kaposi sarcoma (KS).
- Facial molluscum contagiosum in adults.

NON-SPECIFIC DERMATOSES

- **Infections** –Fungal
  –Viral
  –Bacterial.
- Eczema.
- Seborrhoeic dermatitis, Xerosis.
- Psoriasis.
- Lichen planus.
- **Miscellaneous** –Photosensitivity
  –Malignancy
  –PCT
  –Vasculitis.
- Oral–OHL,Thrush, Aphthous Ulcer, Gingivitis, Ulcer.

CLASSIFICATION ON THE BASIS OF CD_4 CT

Early Symptomatic Stage

CD_4 cell count falls below 500 cells/mm^3

- Oral candidiasis.
- Oral hairy leukoplakia.
- HSV infection–recurrent and chronic.
- Herpes zoster–multi-dermatomal, recurrent and disseminated.
- Recurrent oral and genital ulcers.
- Itchy papular dermatoses.

Advanced Symptomatic Stage

CD_4 cell count falls below 200 cells/mm^3

- Opportunistic infections.
- Neoplasms.

CLASSIFICATION ON THE BASIS OF CUTANEOUS ASSOCIATION

Muco-Cutaneous Disorders Indicative of HIV Infection

Highly Indicative of HIV Infection

- Exanthem of ARS, proximal subungual onychomycosis.
- Chronic herpetic ulcers.
- OHL, KS, Eosinophilic folliculitis.

Strongly Associated with HIV Infection

- Any STD, HZ.
- Signs of injective drug abuse.
- Candidiasis–oropharyngeal or recurrent vulvovaginal candidiasis.

May be Associated with HIV Infection

- Generalized lymphadenopathy.
- Seborrhoeic dermatitis.
- Apthous ulcers.

SPECIFIC DERMATOSES

Acute HIV-Seroconversion

Non-specific rash is seen.

Eosinophilic Folliculitis

It is characterized by follicular, red, itchy, persistent, folliculitis, classically occurring above the nipple line (Fig. 5.5).

Treatment: Steroids are usually the only alternative.

INFECTIONS COMMONLY SEEN

1. **Bacterial**
   - Staphylococcal.
   - Mycobacterial.

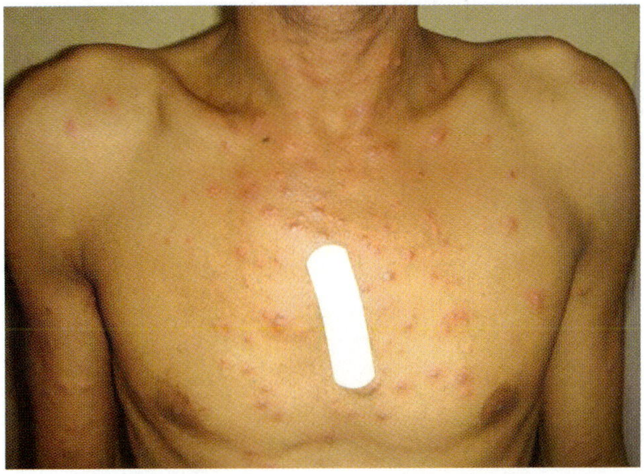

Fig. 5.5: Red pustules, eosinophilic folliculitis

- M. tuberculosis.
- M. leprae.
- Atypical mycobacteria.

2. **Ectoparasitic Infection**
   - Scabies.
3. **Fungal**
   - Dermatophyte.
   - Candida.

Treatment
Candidiasis
Oropharyngeal
Fluconazole 200 mg stat followed by
Fluconazole 100 mg OD –10/14 days.
Esophageal
Fluconazole 200 mg stat followed by
Fluconazole 100 mg OD (max 400 mg)–21 days.
Resistant
Amp B, Capsofungin, Voriconazole.

- **Pityrosporum.**
- **Deep Fungal.**

1. Cryptococcus

Treatment–Cryptococcosis
Induction
Amp B 0.7 mg/kg IVOD and/or 5 FC 25 mg/kg QID –2 weeks.
Consolidation
Fluconazole 400 mg OD 8 weeks.
Maintenance
Fluconazole 200 mg OD

2. Histoplasma and Peniciliosis

Induction
Amp B 0.7 mg/kg IV OD 3-10 days.
Consolidation
Itraconazole 200 mg BD 12 weeks.
Maintenance
Itraconazole 200 mg OD.

4. **Viral**
   a. Molluscum contagiosum—typical, involving the face, or with occasional plaque form (Fig. 5.6).
   b. HIV rash at seroconversion.
   c. Herpes simplex—Atypical, persistent and recurrent (Fig. 5.7).

Treatment HSV
- Famciclovir 500 mg BID.
- Valaciclovir 1 g BID 7-14 days.
- Acyclovir 400 mg TID.

Resistant
Foscarnet/Cidofovir.

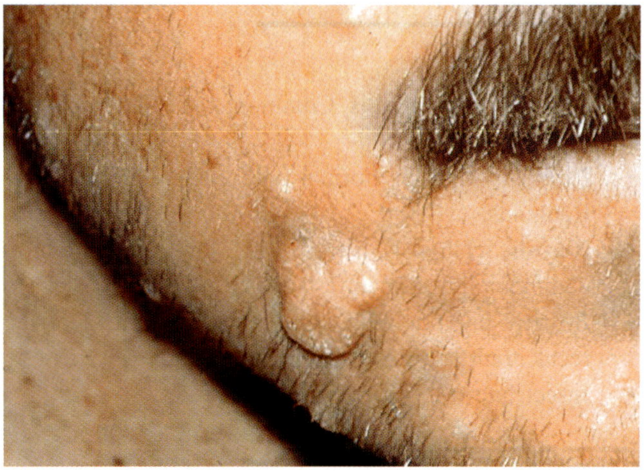

Fig. 5.6: Molluscum contagiosum on the face with a single plaque

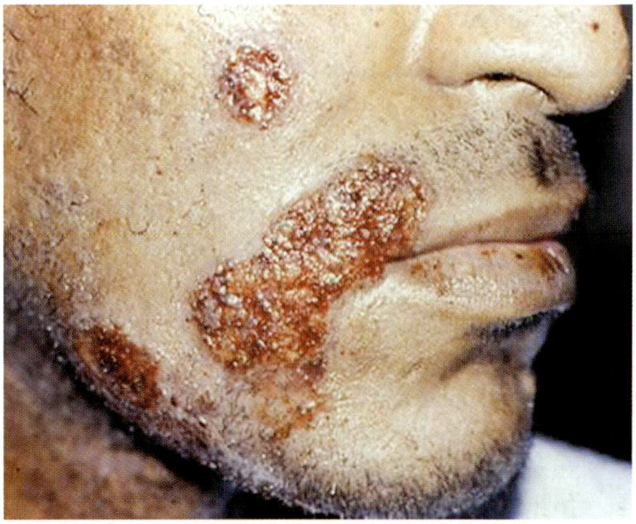

Fig. 5.7: Persistent erosions: Atypical HSV 1

d. **Varicella Zoster** Atypical, multidermatomal and hemorrhagic (Fig. 5.8). Also one of the most common manifestations of IRIS.

Treatment HZ
Famciclovir 500 mg TID.
Valaciclovir 1 g TID 7-10 days.
Treatment Varicella
Acyclovir 800 mg TID.
Famciclovir 500 mg TID.
Valaciclovir 1 g TID 7-10 days.
Resistant
Acyclovir 10 mg/kg IV 8 hourly–then oral.

e. HPV.
f. EB virus.

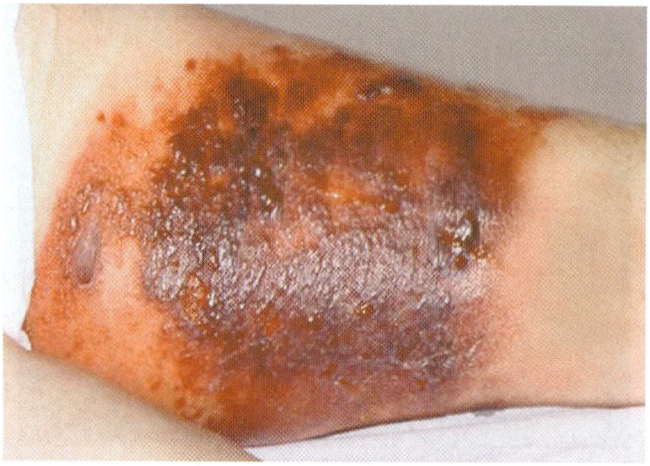

Fig. 5.8: Hemorrhagic zoster

INFLAMMATORY DERMATOSES

- Seborrheic dermatitis–Common, but not typical nor diagnostic.
- Psoriasis–Usually normal course, drug of choice is Retinoids.
- Xerosis, ichthyosis–Non-specific, but one of the most common clinical manifestations.
- Pruritic papular rash–Non-specific, multifactorial, recalcitrant and relapsing rash.
- Insect bite reactions.

ORAL DISORDERS

- **Oral Candidiasis (Fig. 5.9)**
- **Oral Hairy Leukoplakia–**Vertical striations on the side of the tongue–EBV induced (Fig. 5.10).
- **Aphthosis.**

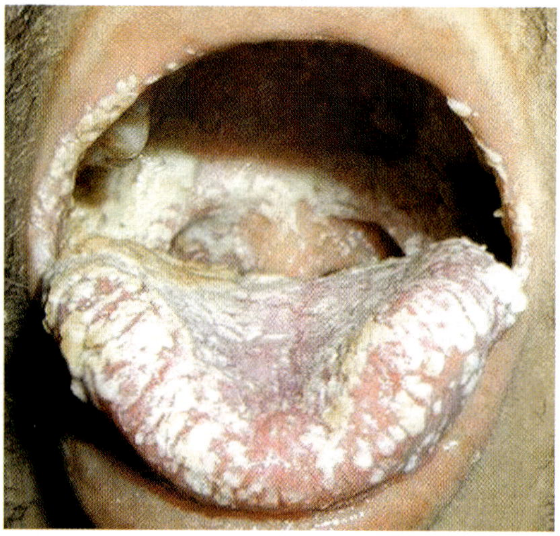

Fig. 5.9: Candidiasis

NEOPLASTIC DISEASES

- Kaposi's sarcoma.
- Lymphoma.
- Other skin malignancies.

DRUG ERUPTIONS

NNRTI—Skin manifestations:

- Maculopapular rash.
- Hypersensitivity syndrome.
- Stevens-Johnson syndrome.
- Toxic epidermal necrolysis.
- Hepatitis.

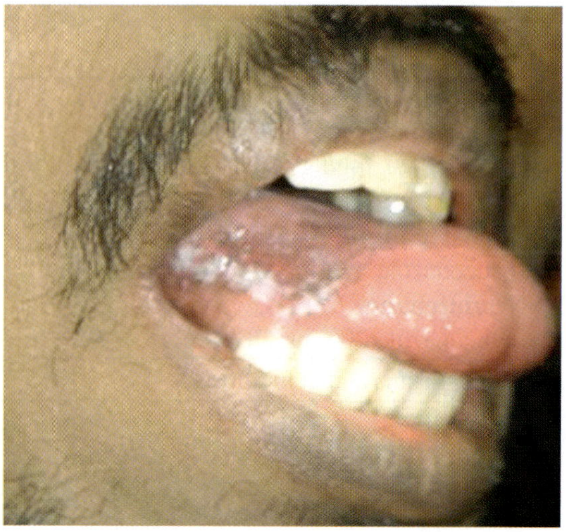

Fig. 5.10: Oral hairy leukoplakia

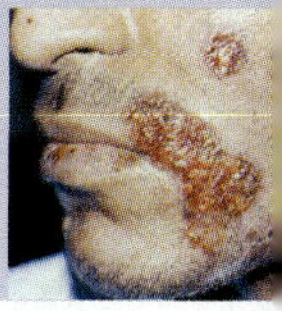

Rash to NNRTI

Females and persons with earlier HIV disease or with a large rise in CD_4+ cell count after starting therapy are at greater risk for NNRTI-related rash.

Strategies to Prevent Rash to NNRTI

- Do not co-administer prednisolone to prevent rash.
- If rash develops within *'lead in'* dose period, do not increase dose.
- Do not continue drug if there is extensive rash, vesicles/ bullae, mucosal involvement, liver enzymes elevated.

Zidovudine–Skin Manifestations

- Nail hyperpigmentation.
- Mucocutaneous hyperpigmentation.
- Hypertrichosis.
- Eyelash hypertrichosis.
- Leukocytoclastic vasculitis.
- Nail-fold pyogenic granuloma.

Lamivudine–Skin Manifestations

- No rash.
- Paronychia.

Protease Inhibitors

- Lipodystrophy.
- Hypersensitivity reaction.

IRIS
(Immune Reconstitution Inflammatory Syndrome)

- First occurrence or recurrence of previously treated opportunistic infections.

Infections Seen

- CMV, PCP, TB, MAIC.
- Herpes zoster and herpes simplex, HPV, fungal infections, eosinophilic folliculitis, leprosy, sarcoidosis.

Which Patient Gets IRIS

- HAART initiated closer to the diagnosis of their underlying opportunistic infection.
- Robust response to HAART.

REFERENCES

- Rook's Textbook of Dermatology, D. A. Burns , S. M. Breathnach, Neil Cox, Christopher E., Griffith's 7th edn 2004.
- Fitzpatrick's Dermatology in General Medicine, 6th edn 2003.
- NACO Guidelines 2007.
- WHO Guidelines 2006.

CHAPTER **6**

ALLERGIC DISORDERS

Urticaria

DEFINITION

Urticaria is characterized by transient, superficial cutaneous swellings (wheals or hives) caused by transudation of plasma from the dermal capillaries.

It is not a single disease but a reaction pattern that represents cutaneous mast cell degranulation.

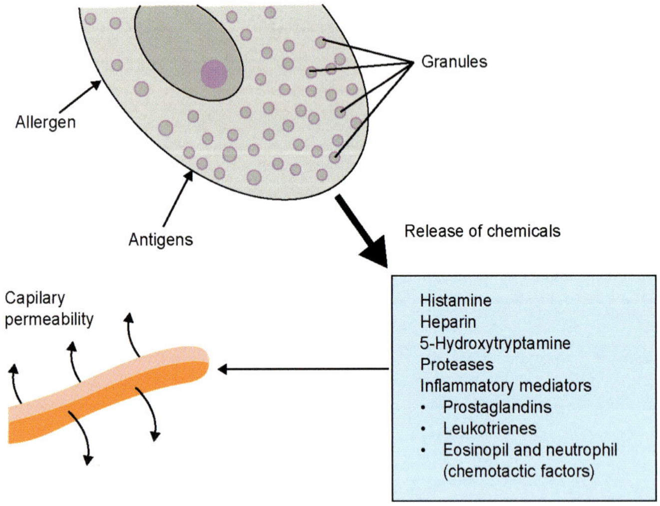

Angioedema is a more generalized swelling, caused by the same process but occurring at deeper levels (i.e. in the dermis and subcutaneous tissue).

Clinical Features

Urticaria is due to localized capillary vasodilatation, followed by extravasation of protein-rich fluid into the surrounding tissues.

It is characterized by the appearance of a transient, migratory pruritic rash with raised, round, oval, or serpiginous patches that blanch on pressure **(wheals)** (Fig. 6.1). Lesions often have a pale centre and are surrounded by an area of erythema.Lesions may vary in diameter from a few millimeters to the size of a hand or more and may be confluent.Persistent erythema after trauma is called Dermographism (Fig. 6.1).

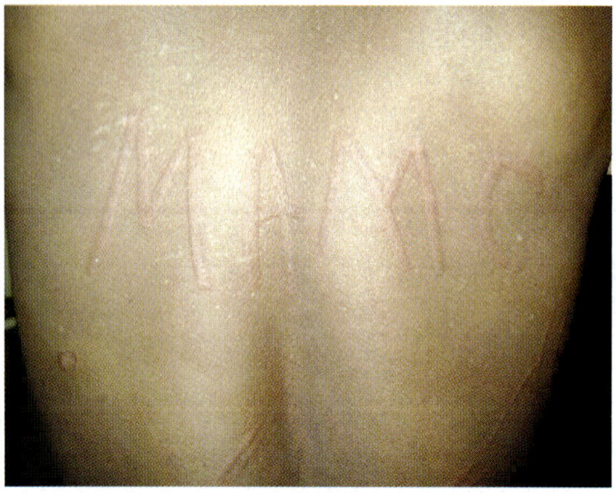

Fig. 6.1: Persistent erythema after trauma: Dermographism

Angioedema (Fig. 6.2) is due to the same process occurring at deeper levels. It presents as a poorly-defined swelling that may be painful rather than pruritic and often occurs on the face, and nasal, laryngeal, GI mucosa.

Demographics

Age

- Acute urticaria is more common in children and young adults.
- Chronic urticaria is more common in adults.

Gender

- Overall, the male: female ratio for chronic urticaria is 1: 2.

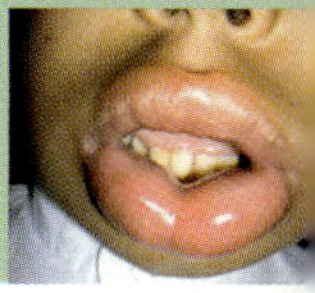

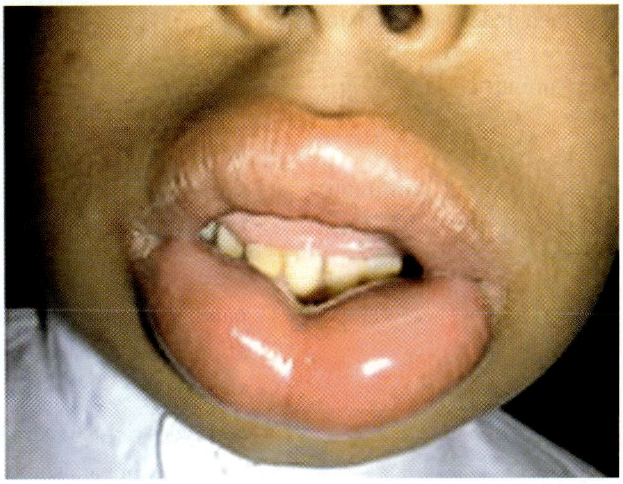

Fig. 6.2: Swelling of mucosa: Angioedema

Classification of urticaria

Type	*Provocative agents/tests*	*Comments*
Acute urticaria	• Foods (nuts, shellfish, eggs, fruits) • Insect stings • Drugs (especially aspirin, NSAIDs. • Contactants—cosmetics, work exposures • Infection-viral (hepatitis, upper respiratory), bacterial, parasitic • Systemic diseases—SLE, endocrinopathy (thyroid), neoplasm • Stress • Idiopathic	• Attack lasts <6 weeks • Each lesion lasts <24 hours • Occurs with or without angioedema
Chronic urticaria	• Most commonly idiopathic • Aggravating and causative factors may be similar to those in acute urticaria	• Attack lasts >6 weeks • Each lesion lasts <24 hours
Cholinergic urticaria	• Increased core body temperature • Hot shower, exercise	• Tiny flesh coloured wheals with surrounding red flare
Contact urticaria	• Latex rubber—patch test, allergy test	
Physical urticarias		
• Aquagenic urticaria	• Exposure to water	
• Adrenergic urticaria	• Stress	
• Cold urticaria	• Ice cube, swimming pool	Can be life threatening
• Dermographism	• Friction, rubbing skin	Immediate and possible delayed types

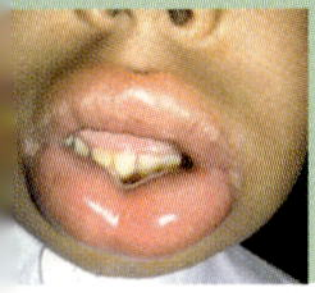

- Women significantly outnumber men in dermographism and cold urticaria.
- More men develop delayed pressure urticaria.

Genetics

- Hereditary angioedema has an autosomal dominant inheritance pattern and occurs in approximately 1:150,000.
- Familial cold urticaria, a rare condition, is inherited as an autosomal dominant trait.

CLASSIFICATION

Duration

Acute or Chronic

Acute urticaria is usually defined as urticaria lasting less than 6 weeks, and the etiology can be inferred in upto 50% of new cases. In general, more than 80% of cases of new-onset urticaria resolve in 2 weeks.

Chronic urticaria is usually defined as urticaria lasting for more than 6 weeks. More than 50% of these cases will resolve spontaneously within 6 months. An etiology is difficult to determine in the majority of cases.

Causes of urticaria and angioedema

Immunologic Causes

Type I IgE-mediated

Foods: Nuts, legumes, crustacea, fish eggs, milk, soy, wheat.
Organic substances: Preservatives, latex, hymenoptera venom.
Medications: Penicillin, cephalosporin, aspirin, NSAIDs.
Aeroallergens: Dust mites, pollens, molds, animal dander.
Type II cytoxic antibody-mediated: Transfusion reaction.
Type III antigen-antibody mediated: Serum sickness reaction.
Type IV delayed hypersensitivity: Medication, food handling, or exposure to animals.
Autoimmune disease: Hashimoto's disease, systemic lupus erythematosus, vasculitis, hepatitis.
Infection: Viral (e.g., cytomegalovirus, Epstein-Barr, hepatitis), parasitic, fungal or bacterial.

Nonimmunologic causes

Physical stimuli: Exposure to sun, water or temperature extremes; delayed pressure (e.g., wearing a heavy backpack); vibration.
Direct mast cell degranulation: Opiates, vancomycin (Vancocin), aspirin, radiocontrast media, dextran, muscle relaxants, bile salts, NSAIDs.
Foods containing high levels of histamines: Strawberries, tomatoes, shrimp, lobster, cheese, spinach, eggplant.

Physical Urticarias

Physical urticarias are characterized by the predominant physical stimulus that elicits them. They may overlap:

i. **Dermatographia:** This is the most common physical urticaria. It may be elicited by firmly stroking the skin.
ii. **Cold urticaria:** More common in children and young adults. Wheals occur in areas exposed to cold.
iii. **Solar urticaria:** Exposure to the sun results in the rapid onset of urticaria; usually short-lasting.
iv. **Cholinergic urticaria:** Wheals (typically small, papular) occur when the individual becomes hot (e.g. after exercise, as a result of heat exposure or emotional stress).
v. **Delayed pressure urticaria/angioedema:** Typically, urticaria appears some 4-6 hours after the area has been subjected to pressure (e.g. on the shoulder after carrying an object or on the feet after walking).
vi. **Vibratory urticaria/angioedema:** Occurs in response to a vibratory stimulus such as working with a jack hammer or sander.
vii. **Water (aquagenic) urticaria.**

Nonimmunologic (Contact) Urticaria

- Plants (e.g. nettles).
- Animals (e.g. jellyfish, caterpillar).
- Therapeutic agents (e.g. cinnamic aldehyde, dimethyl sulfoxide).

AETIOLOGICAL FACTORS

Infections

Certain infections have been implicated in the etiology of urticaria, including dental and sinus infections, HBV, *Helicobacter pylori* infection, and herpes simplex virus infection.

Urticaria has also been reported with chronic parasitic infections such as intestinal strongyloidosis.

Autoimmune Diseases

Urticaria has been associated with a number of autoimmune diseases, including SLE, juvenile rheumatoid arthritis.

Recent studies have shown that 25-60% of these patients have autoantibodies directed against their high-affinity IgE receptors. 5-10% have autoantibodies directed against the IgE molecule.

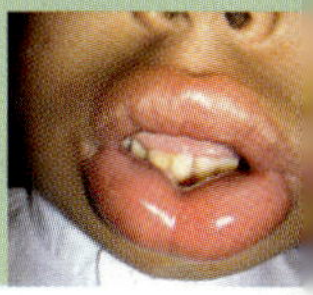

Unknown Causes

In the remaining cases no cause can be found. Some researchers have found a higher frequency of thyroid autoimmunity in this group, but others have been unable to reproduce this finding.

Malignant Disease

Urticaria has been associated with malignant conditions, but the evidence is sparse and should not prompt vigorous investigation unless other factors (e.g. history, clinical examination) warrant it.

Rare Causes

A number of conditions have in rare instances been associated with urticaria (e.g. endocrine tumors, ovarian pathology, **cryoglobulinemias** and serum sickness).

Urticaria may be a feature of rare metabolic disorders such as **Schnitzler** syndrome (pyrexia, arthralgia, and monoclonal gammopathy), **Muckle-Wells** syndrome (amyloidosis and sensorineural deafness), and familial **Mediterranean** fever (urticaria, fever and amyloidosis).

Familial cold urticaria is a rare variant inherited as an autosomal dominant disorder.

Chronic Idiopathic Urticaria (CIU)

Patients in whom no cause is established for their urticaria are said to have CIU. However, recent research suggests that in upto 50% of cases of CIU there is an autoimmune basis.

Clinical clues and associated rationale for diagnosis of urticaria and angioedema

Clinical clue	*Rationale for diagnosis of urticaria or angioedema*
Wheals and swelling develop immediately or upto 60 minutes after food ingestion, recent change in diet, ingestion of processed foods	Allergy to foods, preservatives, or food colouring agents
Medication usage: New medication or supplement started or dosage changed (prescription or over-the-counter, particularly NASAIDs and ACE inhibitors)	Allergy to medication or related molecules, preservatives, or food colouring agents
Exercise (particularly jogging), sun exposure, cold or heat exposure, water exposure, pressure, vibration	Physical or environmental exposure
Occupational exposure latex products, chemical irritants (particularly formaldehyde)	Allergy (can manifest as IgE-mediated reaction, contact dermatitis or irritant dermatitis)
Fatigue, weight gain, family history of thyroid disease	Hypothyroidism or Hashimoto's disease
Weight loss and fatigue in patient with family history of lymphoma	Malignancy or lymphoma
Travel out of country	Parasitic, fungal, bacterial or viral infection

INVESTIGATION

Acute Urticaria

Laboratory testing for acute urticaria is not indicated unless a particular medical condition is suspected. A careful history and clinical examination are all that is required.

Chronic Urticaria

The extent to which laboratory testing should be carried out in chronic urticaria is controversial.

In general, relentless laboratory investigation is not justified unless there is evidence of an underlying condition; it generates anxiety in the patient and is rarely fruitful. Any investigations should be prompted by the history and examination and individualized for each patient.

Common Screening Tests Might Include

- Complete blood count with differential.
- Erythrocyte sedimentation rate.
- Urinalysis followed by urine culture if there are symptoms suggestive of urinary infection.
- Antinuclear antibody (ANA) titers may be indicated if urticarial vasculitis is being considered.
- Skin biopsy may be helpful if urticarial vasculitis or mastocytosis is suspected, although it is not routinely indicated.

Additional tests should be guided by the history and clinical findings. According to the history the following might be added if relevant in the individual case:

- Stool analysis for ova and parasites.
- TSH and thyroid autoantibody levels can be considered because there may be an association between chronic urticaria and autoimmune thyroid disease. The patient may be euthyroid.

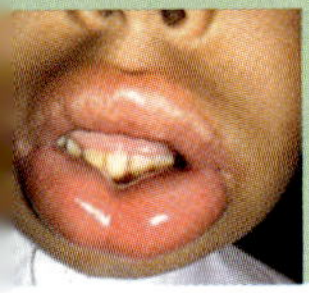

The patient is often advised to keep a diary of events to try to associate dietary and other factors with the onset or worsening of urticaria. This is rarely successful and may be unhelpful by focussing the patient's attention on the condition and generating anxiety.

Skin tests or radioallergosorbent assay test (specific IgE) may be performed but are rarely helpful.

Treatment

Type	*Treatment*
Cold urticaria	Avoid cold Protective clothing Antihistamines
Cholinergic urticaria	Avoid heat Minimize anxiety Avoid excessive exercise Anticholinergics Antihistamines Tranquillizers
Dermographism	Avoid trauma Antihistamines
Hereditary angioedema	Avoid trauma Attenuated androgenic steroids as prophylaxis Tracheostomy may be necessary
Hypersensitivity urticarias	Remove cause Antihistamines (H1+H2) Sympathomimetics Systemic steroids (rarely justified) Avoid aspirin-containing drugs
Solar urticaria	Avoid sun exposure Protective clothing Sunscreens and sun blocks Beta-carotene Antihistamines

Therapeutic Options

Summary of Therapies

- Precipitating factors should be avoided whenever appropriate
- Antihistamine therapy with H_1 antagonists should be the mainstay of therapy and therapy should be individualized according to the patient's response. Sometimes a combination of H_1 and H_2 antagonists is found to be the most effective strategy.
- First-generation H_1 antagonists are usually sedating. Diphenhydramine and chlorphenamine (chlorpheniramine) and hydroxyzine.
- Second-generation H_1 antagonists are less sedating but more expensive. Examples include cetrizine and levocetrizine, fexofenadine, loratadine and desloratadine.
- Second-generation H_1 antagonists may be taken during the day and first-generation H_1 antagonists at night, when sedation may be desirable (e.g. because of pruritus).
- H_2 antagonists (such as famotidine, ranitidine, nizatidine, and cimetidine) may be added when the urticaria does not respond to H_1 antagonists alone.
- If this strategy is ineffective, doxepin may be added (an antidepressant and potent H_1 receptor antagonist).
- Oral corticosteroids (prednisone or prednisolone) may be used in cases of refractory urticaria or angioedema.
- Intravenous gammaglobulin, plasmapheresis and cyclosporine have been shown to be effective in a limited number of studies but are reserved for the most severe and refractory cases.
- Colchicine, hydroxychloroquine, sulfasalazine, methotrexate and dapsone have also been used in treatment, but evidence for their effectiveness is sparse and their efficacy has not been proven in large controlled studies.

Pharmacotherapeutic management of chronic urticaria

↓

Patient diagnosed with chronic urticaria

↓

Second-generation H_1-receptor antagonist:

Cetrizine, 5 to 10 mg per day for several weeks, then 10 to 20 mg per day, depending on symptom control

OR

Fexofenadine, 180 mg per day or 60 mg twice daily

OR

Desloratadine, 5 mg per day

OR

Loratadine, 10 mg per day

↓

Symptoms are not controlled

↓

Add first-generation sedating H_1-receptor antagonist:

Hydroxyzine (Atarax), 10 to 50 mg at night

OR

Diphenhydramine (Benadryl), 25 to 50 mg at night

OR

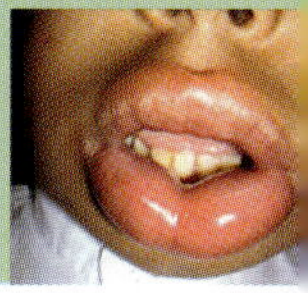

Add H_2-receptor antagonist
Ranitidine, 150 mg twice daily
OR
Add H_1-plus H_2-receptor antagonist.
Doxepin, 10 to 50 mg at night
OR
Cyproheptadine, 4 mg, upto three times daily

OR
Add leukotriene modifier:
Montelukast, 10 mg per day
OR
Zafirlukast, 20 mg twice daily

↓

Symptoms remain severe

↓

Add oral corticosteroid:
Prednisone as short-term therapy of 20 to 40 mg per day or 1 to 10 mg daily as a short term measure

↓

Symptoms are servere and are not controlled by above medications

↓

Consider investigative therapy, such as intravenous immunoglobulin, plasmapheresis, cyclosporine, anti-IgE therapy, azathioprine, cyclophosphamide, autologous serum

Flowchart: Treatment of urticaria

REFERENCES

- Barbara A, Muller, Urticaria and Angioedema: A Practical ApproachAm Fam Physician 2004; 69:1123-28.
- The diagnosis and management of urticaria: A practice parameter. Ann Allergy Asthma Immunol 2000; 85:521-44.
- Grattan C, Powell S, Humphreys F; British Association of Dermatologists, Management and diagnostic guidelines for urticaria and angio-oedema, Br J Dermatol 2001; 144:708-14.
- Bowen T, Cicardi M, Farkas H, et al. Canadian 2003 International Consensus Algorithm for the Diagnosis, Therapy, and Management of Hereditary Angioedema, J Allergy Clin Immunol. 2004 114:629-37.

Drug Reactions

Cutaneous drug reactions (CDRs) are adverse drug reactions that appear on the skin. An adverse drug reaction is any unintended or undesirable response to a medication given *at an appropriate dose.*

The overwhelming majority of CDRs are thought to be immunologic.

The spectrum of CDRs is wide, ranging from transitory exanthematous rash to the potentially fatal toxic epidermal necrolysis (TEN) and Stevens-Johnson Syndrome (SJS).

CARDINAL FEATURES

- Cutaneous drug reactions (CDRs) are unintended, undesirable changes in the structure or function of the skin, its appendages, or mucous membranes, that occur because of oral or parenteral drugs administered *at appropriate dosages.*
- As the most commonly encountered type of adverse drug reactions, CDRs include: exanthems, urticaria and angioedema, cutaneous lupus erythematosus (CLE), contact dermatitis, photodermatitis, acute generalized exanthematous pustulosis (AGEP), vasculitis, fixed drug eruptions, anticoagulant skin necrosis, erythema multiforme, which includes erythema multiforme minor and erythema multiforme major—also known as Stevens-Johnson syndrome (SJS), and toxic epidermal necrolysis (TEN). *Besides SJS (<10% epidermal detachment) and TEN (>30%), there is an SJS/TEN overlap (10-30%).*
- A further complication of CDRs is the development of drug rash with eosinophilia and systemic symptoms (DRESS syndrome). Hepatic inflammation and lymphadenopathy are also features.
- Of the common types of adverse CDRs: Exanthems or morbilliform rash constitute 46%, urticaria 23%, fixed drug eruptions 10%, and erythema multiforme 5.4%.
- Drug-induced SLE rarely has cutaneous findings, usually only systemic. Drug-induced SCLE and CLE do have cutaneous findings.
- The drugs most commonly associated with CDRs are amoxicillin, ampicillin, and trimethoprim-sulfamethoxazole.

CAUSES

- **Urticaria and angioedema:** Antibiotics, radiographic contrast media, anaesthetics, angiotensin-converting enzyme (ACE) inhibitors, nonsteroidal anti-inflammatory drugs (NSAIDs), opiates, curare.

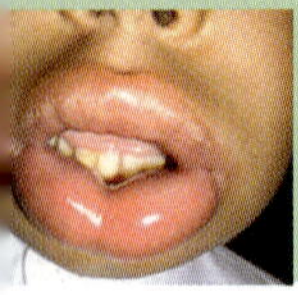

- **Erythema multiforme (Fig. 6.3), SJS, TEN:** Sulfonamides, aromatic anticonvulsants (phenobarbital, phenytoin, carbamazepine), penicillins, quinolone, cephalosporins, NSAIDs, allopurinol, aspirin.
- **DRESS syndrome:** Sulfonamides, aromatic anticonvulsants (phenobarbital, phenytoin, carbamazepine), also other antiepileptics (valproic acid), allopurinol, NSAIDs, antibiotics and dapsone.
- **Systemic lupus erythematosus (SLE):** Hydralazine, procainamide, isoniazid, chlorpromazine, penicillamine, phenytoin, sulfasalazine, minocycline.
- **Contact dermatitis:** Neomycin, benzocaine, paraben, ethylenediamine, formaldehyde, p-aminobenzoic acid (PABA), topical antihistaminics, topical corticosteroids.
- **Photodermatitis:** Coal tar derivatives, psoralen, chlorpromazine, tetracycline, doxycycline, promethazine, PABA, nonsteroidal anti-inflammatory agents (NSAIDs), sulfonamides, griseofulvin.
- **Exanthems:** Beta-lactam antibiotics, sulfonamides, erythromycin, gentamicin, anticonvulsants, gold salts.
- **AGEP (Acute generalized exanthematous pustulosis)** (Fig. 6.4) beta-lactam antibiotics, macrolides, calcium channel blockers, terbinafine.
- **Vasculitis:** Allopurinol, cimetidine, furosemide, penicillins, sulfonamides, hydantoin, thiazide, diuretics.
- **Fixed drug eruption** (Fig. 6.5) penicillins, tetracycline, sulfonamides, barbiturates, phenolphthalein, gold salts, NSAIDs, carbamazepine.
- **Anticoagulant skin necrosis:** Warfarin, heparin.

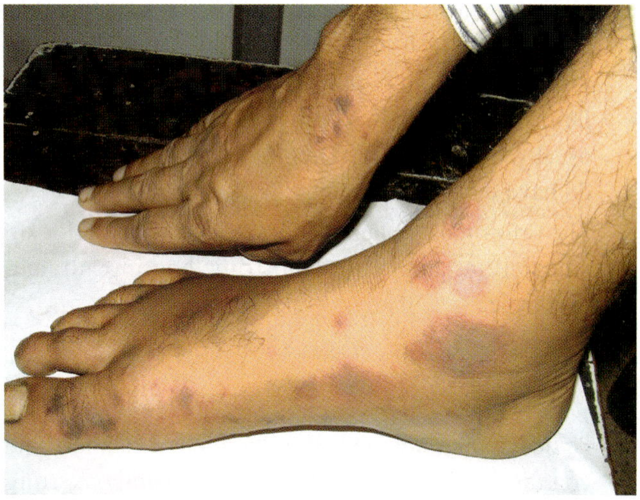

Fig. 6.3: EM lesions with central dusky hue: "iris-like" lesions

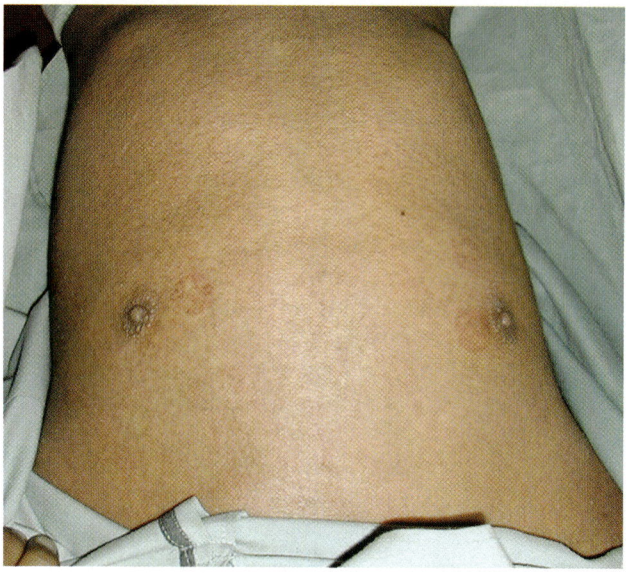

Fig. 6.4: Multiple pustules all over the body Acute Generalised Exanthematous Pustulosis

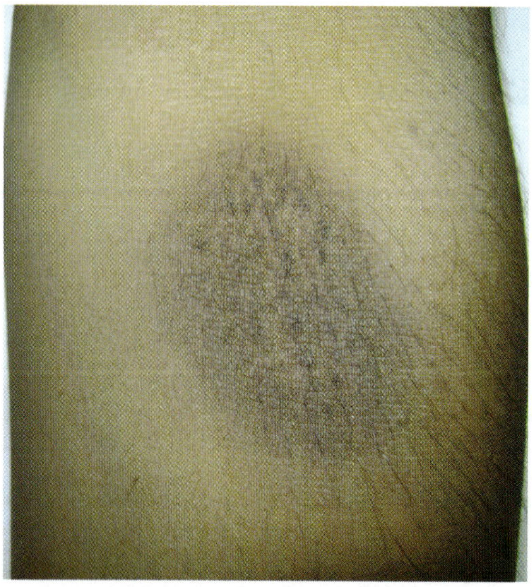

Fig. 6.5: Fixed drug eruption

- **Pigmentary changes:** Oral contraceptives, phenothiazines, heavy metals, antimalarials, clofazimine, tetracycline, minocycline, amiodarone.

Mechanism of drug reactions are either immunologic or nonimmunologic:

Immunologic reactions are independent of dose; they can persist long after the causative drug has been stopped.

Immunologic reactions are classified by the Gell and Coombs classification system, which describes the predominant mechanisms of immunologic reactions that lead to the clinical symptoms of drug hypersensitivity (type IV reactions are the most common):

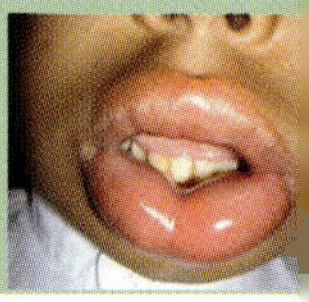

1. **Type I reactions** (immediate hypersensitivity reactions) are mediated by immunoglobulin E (IgE) antibodies, which induce the release of inflammatory mediators from mast cells and basophils (result in urticaria and angioedema; and are associated with insulin and other proteins; frequently caused by antibiotics (especially penicillin), radiographic contrast media and anaesthetics.
2. **Type II reactions** (cytotoxic antibody reactions) are driven by immunoglobulin E (IgE) or immunoglobulin M (IgM) antibodies, which develop several hours after drug intake (result in hemolysis and purpura; caused by: penicillin, cephalosporins, sulfonamides, rifampicin).
3. **Type III reactions** (immune complex reactions) are driven by immunoglobulin E (IgE) or immunoglobulin M (IgM) antibodies, which develop several hours after drug intake (result in vasculitis, serum sickness, urticaria; possible causes: quinine, salicylates, chlorpromazine, sulfonamides).
4. **Type IV reactions** (delayed hypersensitivity reactions) are mediated by drug-specific T lymphocytes (result in allergic contact dermatitis, exanthematous reactions, photoallergic reactions); often encountered in cases of contact hypersensitivity to topical medications, such as neomycin sulfate, benzocaine, paraben, formaldehyde, para-aminobenzoic acid (PABA), and topical antihistaminics.

   Nonimmunologic reactions are dose-dependent; their symptoms resolve shortly after the causative drug has been stopped.

   Nonimmunologic CDRs are associated with toxicity, drug-drug interactions, exacerbation of pre-existing dermatologic diseases, and nonimmunologic activation of effector pathways.

CONTRIBUTORY OR PREDISPOSING FACTORS

Patient Factors

Age: Especially neonates and elderly patients.
Sex: More common in females.

Underlying disease: Infectious mononucleosis increases risk of skin rash to ampicillin or its analogues; human immunodeficiency virus (HIV) increases risk of development of sulfonamide rash; pre-existing disease (e.g. impaired hepatic and renal function) increases risk of development of drug rashes.

Genetics: Individual genetic variations in drug metabolism (e.g. a drug which body has not adequately metabolized may cause direct toxicity to cells or immune-mediated hypersensitivity); TEN has been associated with HLA B_{12}; TEN due to sulfonamides with HLA-A29, B_{12} and DR7; and oxicam-related TEN with HLA-A2 and A-12.

Erythema multiforme has been associated with HLA B 62 (B15), HLA B-35 and HLA A-33, HLA DR-53, HLA DQB1* 0301. Recurrent erythema multiforme has been shown to be strongly associated with HLA DQB.

Drug Factors

Route of administration: Oral route is safest; reactions are more common with topical and intramuscular administration and less so with intravenous administration.

Duration of medication: Reactions are more common with chronic or frequent use than with short-term or intermittent use.

Therapeutic indices: Reactions are more common for drugs with low therapeutic indices, high levels of drug-drug interactions, and a tendency to form reactive intermediates or toxins.

Use of multiple drugs: Associated with higher incidence of drug reactions: as observed in increased frequency in hospitalized patients.

Environmental Factors

Ultraviolet light can alter the immunogenicity of certain medications.

SUMMARY OF TESTS

1. Medical history and physical examination are essential components of the clinical evaluation because they aid in distinguishing drug reactions from viral exanthems or pre-existing skin disease.
2. Obtain a detailed drug history, and a clear history of the onset and duration of the skin eruption.
3. If clinical findings suggest a drug-related cause, the eruption should be classified clinically (and the offending drug discontinued if possible).
4. Patch testing evaluates the possibility of allergic contact dermatitis; photo patch test helps to evaluate photoallergic reactions. Patch tests use small doses of suspected allergens on adhesive bandages that are placed on the skin (usually on the back). The patches are left in place for 2 days and the skin is checked for signs of an allergic reaction.
5. Radioallergosorbent test (RAST) measures IgE level - may be helpful if clinical diagnosis is in doubt. Sensitivity and specificity for diagnostic purposes is between 80-90% depending on the test method and the allergen being tested for.

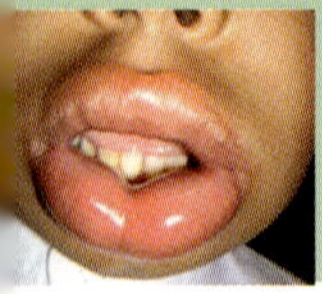

6. Skin biopsies can help to confirm the diagnosis of a CDR; the presence of eosinophils, edema, and inflammation is indicative of hypersensitivity; vasculitis and necrotic changes may suggest erythema multiforme, SJS or TEN. Direct immunofluorescent testing uses the patient's skin as substrate, exposed to fluorescein-conjugated antibodies directed against human immunoreactants (e.g. IgG or C3). *In vivo* deposition of immunoreactants is reflected as specific patterns of immunofluorescence in the basement membrane zone when examined with a fluorescence microscope.
7. Rechallenge test with the offending drug to confirm diagnosis is considered the most sensitive, specific test for drug reactions, but has been associated with anaphylaxis and erythroderma, and therefore is not routinely recommended.
   - Introduce a suspected drug again after initial adverse result, to observe effects.
   - Only restart one medication at a time otherwise picture can get cloudy.
   - Should be only undertaken when the benefits clearly outweigh the risks.
   - Patients should be fully informed of the risks (anaphylaxis or severe eruptions) and monitored closely.
   - Never perform a drug challenge test in patients with suspected SJS.

Treatment

General

- Treatment of most CDRs is, for the most part, supportive. Symptomatic treatment is contingent on the withdrawal of the offending medication.
- For a morbilliform eruption or fixed drug eruption, if no systemic involvement is present it is permissible to continue the medication and 'treat through the rash'.
- In DRESS syndrome, SJS, and TEN in particular, it is imperative that the offending medication is always discontinued immediately.

Specific

1. Mild topical corticosteroids and antihistamines such as hydroxyzine are used to relieve dermatologic symptoms, such as pruritus, that accompany morbilliform drug eruptions (or exanthems). Moisturizing agents may also be helpful.
2. **Urticaria and angioedema** often resolve spontaneously; H_1 antihistamines provide effective symptomatic relief. A combination of H_1 and H_2 antihistamines or systemic corticosteroids helps in resistant urticaria. If anaphylaxis occurs, the universally accepted treatment is epinephrine (Fig. 6.6).
3. **Hypersensitivity vasculitis** is treated primarily by identifying and ceasing the offending medication, after which the disease usually clears spontaneously in most cases. In persistent cases, systemic corticosteroids may be used to control systemic symptoms. Nonsteroidal anti-inflammatory drugs (NSAIDs) and antihistamines may be used for symptomatic relief. Colchicine may be helpful for chronic disease, and dapsone may be used if disease is confined to the skin. Immunosuppressant therapy (e.g. azathioprine, cyclophosphamide, methotrexate, or cyclosporine) is usually reserved for severe or recalcitrant disease, with or without a corticosteroid.
4. No treatment is usually required for the minor form of erythema multiforme. If recurrent, antivirals may prevent further recurrence. Use of corticosteroids is controversial.

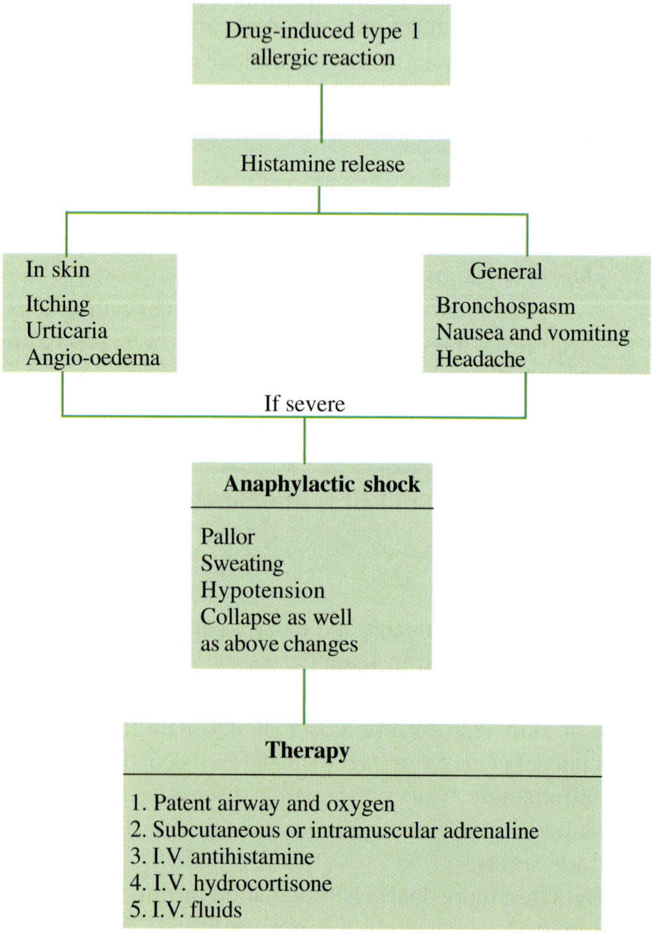

Fig. 6.6: Management of type I allergic reaction

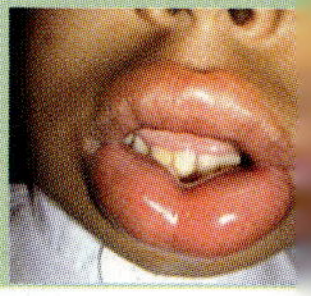

5. Treat erythema multiforme major (SJS and TEN) supportively, with aggressive fluids, analgesia, aseptic handling, nutritional support, and antibiotics (to prevent secondary infection). In addition, SJS and TEN may be treated with systemic corticosteroids, intravenous immune globulin (IVIG), plasmapheresis, thalidomide, and cyclosporine; these treatments are controversial because they are thought by some to adversely affect outcome (e.g. by risking infection, hypertension, fluid retention, and diabetes). They have not been consistently shown to be beneficial in double-blind, placebo-controlled studies. Use of IVIG (although in need of further testing) looks promising.
6. **Drug-induced lupus (can include SLE, SCLE and CCLE):** First-line therapy for cutaneous lupus erythematosus (CLE) is an antimalarial agent. Second-line therapy includes corticosteroids, dapsone, thalidomide, retinoids, and immunosuppressants/cytoxic agents. Third-line therapy includes IVIG and interferon alfa. Hydroxy-chloroquine is commonly used and is the medication of choice. Response to hydroxy-chloroquine and azathioprine (as separate treatments) usually occurs in 4-8 weeks; for thalidomide, 3 months, and for chloroquine and systemic prednisone (as separate treatments) 3-4 weeks.
7. **Fixed drug eruptions:** Withdrawal of the offending drug is often all that is needed; topical steroids after withdrawal tend to speed resolution.
8. **Exanthems (morbilliform rash):** Rechallenge has been successful in determining etiology, especially graded or gradual challenge.
9. **Contact allergic dermatitis:** Since the effects of the offending drug tend to worsen after withdrawal in allergic dermatitis, glucocorticoid therapy (topical or systemic) helps to prevent a prolonged rash.
10. **Photodermatitis:** Phototoxic, photoallergic, and phytophotoallergic reactions respond well to avoidance of the implicated agent. Polymorphous light eruption responds to phototherapy as well as UV avoidance and use of sunscreen.
11. **Anticoagulant skin necrosis:** Vitamin K successfully reverses warfarin-induced necrosis. Treatment with heparin.
12. **Pigmentary changes:** Sunlight protection and laser therapy have been successful treatments. If pigmentary changes do not fade after the offending medication is stopped, sunlight protection is recommended, because many of the same causative medications also cause photosensitivity reactions.

Table 6.1: Morphological classification of drug eruptions

Acanthosis nigricans-like eruption
Corticosteroids, Hydantoin, Nicotinic Acid, OCP Pills, Stilbestrol
Acneiform eruption
Anticonvulsant (phenytoin, phenobarbital, trimethadione), Antituberculous (isoniazid, ethionamide, rifampicin), Azathioprine, Chloral hydrate, Corticosteroids, Corticotropin (ACTH), Cyanocobalamin, Cyclosporin, Halogens (bromides, chlorides, iodides, halothane), Haloperidol, Lithium, Pills, Psoralens, Quinine.
Acral erythema/red palms
Adriamycin (Doxorubicin), Cystosine arabinoside, 5-fluorouracil
Acrodynia
Mercury
Alopecia
Allopurinol, Bromocriptine, Carbimazole, Chlorambucil, Chloramphenicol, Cholesterol lowering agents, Cimetadine, Colchicine, Coumarin, Cytotoxic drugs, Diazoxide, Ethionamide, Fluconazole, Gentamicin, Gold, Heavy metals, Heparin, Hydantoin, Levodopa, Methotrexate, Methyldopa, NSAID (indomethacin, piroxicam), Pills, Propanolol, Sodium valproate, Thiouracil, Vitamin A or Retinoids
Anaphylactic Reaction
Acetylsalicylic acid, ACTH, Meprobamate, Mercurial Diuretics, Para-aminosalicylic Acid, Penicillin, Succinylcholine, Tetracycline, Thiouracil
Angiitis, Necrotizing
Bishydroxycoumarin (Dicumarol)
Angioedema
Meprobamate, Penicillin, Stilbestrol, Sulfonamides
Argyria
Silver Salts
Arteritis
Chlorpromazine, Iodides, Phenylbutazone, Phenytoin, Poison Ivy Extract, Sulfonamides, Thiouracil
Black hairy tongue
Tetracycline, Penicillin
Bowen's disease
Arsenic, Fowler's solution
Candidiasis
Tetracyclines
Chilblains-like erythema
Coumarins, Phenindione, Sulindac
Cyanosis
Acetanilide
Depigmentation
Chloroquine
Eczematous reactions (other than contact eczema)
Aminophylline, Antibiotics, Antihistaminics, B-blockers, Benzocaine, Bleomycin, Carbamazepine, Diphenhydramine, Disulfuram, Fluorouracil, Fucidin, Methaminodiazepoxide, Minoxidil, Neomycin, Nystatin, Phenothiazines, Procainamide, Procaine, Quinidine, Streptomycin (cross-reaction with neomycin), Sulphonamide, Thiazide
Edema
Arsenic, Chlorpromazine, Penicillin, Phenytoin, Promethazine, Chloroquine
Elastosis perforans serpiginosa
Penicillamine
Erythema/exanthem
1. Maculopapular rash Allopurinol, Chloroquine, Meprobamate, Penicillin, Promethazine, Streptomycin, Sulfamethoxypyridazine
2. Morbilliform erythema Acetylsalicylic acid, Ampicillin, Barbiturates, Bromides, Chlorpromazine, Griseofulvin, Insulin, Meprobamate, Penicillin, Promethazine, Salicylates, Streptomycin

Contd.

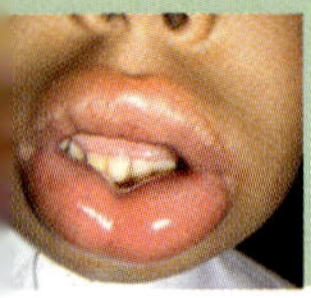

Contd.

3. Scarlatiniform erythema
Barbiturates, Mercury, Morphine, Opium, Penicillin, Phenobarbital, Pituitary Extract, Quinine, Salicylates, Streptomycin, Sulfonamides
4. Toxic erythema.

Drugs most commonly responsible (upto 5% of patients affected): Allopurinol, Carbamazepine, Cephalosporins, Gold, Nalidixic acid, Penicillins, Sulphonamides

Other drugs commonly responsible (1-4% of patients affected): Isoniazid, Para-amino salicylic acid, Phenytoin, NSAIDs, Nitrofurantoin, Streptomycin

Erythema multiforme (including Stevens-Johnson syndrome and toxic epidermal necrolysis)
Acetylsalicylic acid, Allopurinol, Amidopyrine, Antihistaminics, Antipyrines, Barbiturates, Bromides, Carbamazepine, Chloral hydrate, Cimetadine, Corticotropin (ACTH), Furosemide, Griseofulvin, Hydantoins, Iodides, Mercury, NSAIDs (especially piroxicam), Para-aminosalicyclic Acid, Penicillins, Phenytoin, Phenolphthalein, Phenothiazine, Phenyl-butazone, Procaine, Streptomycin, Sulfamethoxy-pyridazine, Sulphonamides, Tetracycline

Erythema Nodosum
Acetylsalicylic Acid, Bromides, Gold, Iodides, Penicillin, Phenacetin, OCP, 13-cis-retinoic acid, Salicylates, Sulfathiazole, Tetracycline

Erythroderma (Exfoliative dermatitis)
Allopurinol, Aminosalicylic Acid, Arsenicals, Barbiturates, Bismuth, Captopril, Carbamazepine, Chlorpromazine, Chloroquine, Cimetadine, Dapsone, Diltiazem, Gold, Griseofulvin, Hydantoin, Iodides, Isoniazid, Lithium, Mercury, Nitrofurantoin, NSAID, Penicillin, Phenothiazines, Phenytoin, Quinidine, Quinacrine, Sodium Thiosulfate, Stilbestrol, Streptomycin, Sulphonamides, Sulphonylurea, Tetracycline, Thiouracil, Retinoid

Erythromelalgia
Bromocriptine, Nifedipine, Pergolide, Verapamil

Fixed drug eruption
Aminopyrine, Amphetamines, Antihistaminics, Antimony Compounds, Antipyrines, Arsenic, Barbiturates, Chlordiazepoxide, Chloral Hydrate, Chloroquine, Codeine, Dapsone, Gold, Digitalis, Ephedrine, Ergot, Hydantoin, Hydralazine, Iodides, Mercury, Metronidazole, Morphine, NSAIDs, Opium, Para-aminosalcylic acid, Paracetamol, Penicillin, Phenacetin, Phenolphthalein, Phenothiazine, Phenylbutazone, Potassium Chlorate, Quinine, Reserpine, Salicylates, Streptomycin, Sulfonamides, Tetracyclines.

Gangrene
Coumarin

Gingival hyperplasia
Cyclosporin, Nifedipine, Hydantoin

Hair color changes
Carbamate, Chloroquine, Chlorpromazine

Henoch-Schonlein purpura-like eruption
Diltiazem, Frusemide

Hirsutism/hypertrichosis
Acetazolamide, Anabolic agents, Bromocryptine, Chlorobenzene, Corticosteroid, Cyclosporin, Cyproterone, Danazol, Diazoxide, Digoxin, Diphenylhydantoin, Dyazide, Metyrapone, Minoxidil, Penicillamine, Phenothiazine, Progestogens, Psoralens, Spironolacton, Streptomycin

Ichthyosis, acquired
Butyrophenone, Nicotinic acid, Triparanol

Jaundice
Aurothioglucose, Para-aminosalicylic Acid, Phenobarbital, Thiouracil

Keratoderma
Gold

Keratoses
Arsenic, Fowler's Solution, Gold

LE-like syndrome
Acebutolol, Allopurinol, Aminoglutethimide, Aminosalicylic acid, Captopril, Carbamazepine, Chlorpromazine, Cimetidine, Ethosuximide, Gold, Griseofulvin, Hydantoin, Hydralazine, Isoniazid, Lithium, Mephobarbital, Methyldopa, Minocycline, Penicillin, Phenylbutazone, Phenytoin, Procainamide, Reserpine, Streptomycin, Sulfamethoxypyridazine, Sulphonamide, Tetracycline HCl (degraded), Thiazide, Thionamide, Thiouracil

Lichenoid eruption
Beta-blocker (Practolol), Bismuth, Captopril, Carbamazepine, Chloroquine, Cholorpropamide, Gold, Hydroxyurea, Meprobamate, Mepacrine, Methyldopa, Para-amino-salicyclic acid, Penicillamine, Phenothiazine, Quinine, Quinidine, Streptomycin, Sulphonylurea, Tetracycline, Thiazides

Linear Ig-A dermatosis
Amiodarone, Captopril, Cefamandole, Diclofenac, Lithium, Vancomycin

Livedo reticularis
Amantadine

Lymphoproliferative disease/Pseudolymphoma
ACE-inhibitor, Carbamazepine, Cyclosporin, Dantrolene, Diltiazem, Hydantoin, Pyrazolone, Pyrimethamine

Mucosal ulcerations, Oral
Foscarnet, DDC, Interferon

Nail changes
Amodiaquin (hyperpigmentation), arsenic (longitudinal white stripes), argyria (dark blue nail bed), Chloroquine (blue-black nail bed), Phenolphthalein (dark blue fixed eruption), tetracycline (yellow nail and yellow fluorescence), demethylchlortetracycline (phototoxic onychomadesis)

Ochronosis-like pigmentation
Phenol, Quinacrine, Resorcin

Onycholysis
Demethylchlortetracycline

Pellagra-like eruption
Isoniazid

Pemphigoid-like eruption
1. Bullous
5-Fluorouracil (topical), Frusemide, Ibuprofen, Penicillamine, Penicillin, Sulphasalazine, PUVA
2. Cicatrical
Anti-glaucoma agent (topical), Clonidine, Indomethacin, D-penicillamine, Practolol, Sulphadoxine

Pemphigus-like eruption
Ampicillin, Captopril, Enalapril, Pencillamine, Penicillin, Phenylbutazone, Pyrazolan derivative, Rifampicin, Sulphydryl groups (pyritinol, thiopronin)

Photosensitivity
Amiodarone, Chlorthiazide, Chlorpromazine, Chlorpropamide, Cytotoxic (Dacarazine, Methotrexate, Fenofibrate, 5-fluorouracil, Furocoumarins, Griseofulvin, Nalidixic acid, NSAID (benoxaprofen, piroxicam, naproxen), Phenothiazine, Promethazine, Psoralen (Methoxsalen, Trimethylpsoralen), Quinidine, Quinine, Quinolones, Reserpine, Retinoids, Sulphonamides, Sulphonylureas, Sunscreen (PABA, oxybenzone), Tetracyclines (demeclote-tracycline, doxycycline, tetracycline), Tolbutamide, Tricyclic antidepressant (Clomipramine, Carbamazepine)

Pigmentation
Amiodarone *(slate grey pigmentation on light-exposed skin)*
Antimalarials *(diffuse generalized grey/brown pigmentation; mepacrine causes generalized yellow/orange discoloration resembling jaundice*
Antipyrines, Bismuth (gums)
Clofazimine
Chlorpromazine *(slate-colored)*
Chloroquine (bleaching of hair)

Contd.

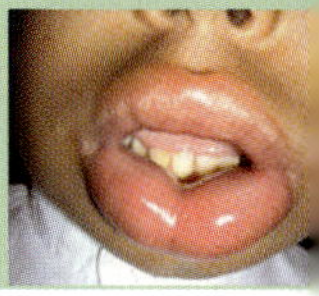

Contd.

Cytotoxic drugs (busulphan, bleomycin, cyclophosphamide, fluorouracil, hydroxyurea, may cause generalized brown pigmentation)
Gold/silver (chrysiasis) *blue/grey pigmentation on light-exposed skin*)
Minocycline hydrochloride (blue/grey pigmentation on light-exposed skin and in scars)
Oral contraceptives (melasma-brownish pigmentation on face)
Phenformin (brown pigmentation on light-exposed skin)
Phenytoin (melasma-like pigmentation on face)
Phenothiazines (bluish pigmentation on light-exposed skin, especially on the face)
Streptomycin, Tetracosactide, Tetracyclines, Thiouracil
Zidovudine (AZT) (melanonychia, diffuse cutaneous/oral mucosal pigmentation, acral hyperpigmented macules)

Pityriasis rosea-like eruption
Arsenicals, Bismuth, Gold, Barbiturates, Clonidine, Captopril, Isotretinoin, Ketotifen, Methoxypromazine, Metronidazole

Porphyria
(Drugs provoke variegate porphyria):
Alcohol, Androgens, Barbiturates, Carbamazepine, Chlordiazepoxide, Chloroquine, Griseofulvin, Hexachlorobenzene, Hydantoin, Meprobamate, Nortriptyline, Pills, Oestrogens, Sodium valproate, Sulphonamides, Sulphonylureas
(Drugs provoke porphyria cutanea tarda):
above + Busulphan, Quinidine, Quinine, Rifampicin

Pseudo-porphyria
Amiodarone, Bumetamide, Ciprofloxacin, Frusemide, Nalidixic aid, NSAID, Ofloxacin, Tetracycline

Pruritus
Alkaloid, Antidepressive, Antimalarial, Atropine, Aurothioglucose, Barbiturates, Belladonna, Bismuth, Cimetadine, CNS stimulant, Cocaine, Codeine, Coumarin, Griseofulvin, Heparin, Insulin, Iodide, Niacinamide, Opiates, Penicillin, Phenobarbital, Procaine, Quinacrine, Streptomycin, Tetracyclines, Thiamine Chloride, Thiouracil

Pruritus ani
Chloroquine, Codeine, Liver Extract, Tetracyclines

Purpura Fulminans
Acetylsalicylic acid, Coumarin, Iodides

Pustuloderma
Bromides, Chloral hydrate, Iodides, Penicillin, Macrolide

Seborrhoeic dermatitis
Methyldopa, Phenothiazines

Scleroderma-like eruption
Epoxy resin monomer, Organic solvent, Perchlorethylene, Trichlorethylene, Vinyl chloride monomer
Bleomycin, Carbidopa, Penicillamine, Pentazocine, Organic solvent, Sodium valproate, Injection of paraffin or silicone

Stomatitis
Aurothioglucose, Bismuth, Chlorpromazine, Dilantin (gingivitis), Fluorides, Methotrexate, Phenobarbital, Streptomycin, Thiouracil

Striae
Corticosteroids, Isoniazid

Urticaria
1. *Immunological mediation*
   Drugs most commonly responsible:
   Enzymes, Penicillins, Pollen vaccines, Polypeptide hormone, Serum, Sulphonamides
   Other drugs responsible, but lower incidence:
   Barbiturate, Carbimazole, Cephalosporins, Cimetidine, Griseoful-vin, Insulin, Metronidazole, Phenytoin, Quinidine, Synthetic adrenocorticotrophin, Tetracycline
2. *Non-immunological mediation*
   Alcohol, Aspirin and other salicylates, Atropine, Chlortetracycline, Codeine, Dextran, Decamethonium, Morphine, NSAID, Oestrogen, Pilocarpine, Polymyxin antibiotics, Quinine, Radiographic contrast media, Scopolamine, Snake venoms, Thiamine, d-Tubocurare, Vancomycin

Vasculitis
Anti-influenza, vaccine, Allopurinol, Arsenic, Captopril, Chlorpromazine, Cimetidine, Clindamycin, Corticosteroids, Ethacrynic acid, Gold, Griseofulvin, Guanethidine, Heparin, Hydantoin, Hydralazine, Indomethacin, Insulin, Iodide, Ketoconazole, Methylthiouracil, Penicillin, Phenothiazine, Phenylbutazone, Phenytoin, Poison ivy extract, Quinidine, Serum, Streptomycin, Streptokinase, Sulphonamides, Tamoxifen, Tetracycline, Thiazide, Thiouracil, Vancomycin

Table 6.2: Syndromes: Clinical features of drug-hypersensitivity syndrome, serum sickness-like reaction, Stevens-Johnson syndrome and toxic epidermal necrolysis

	Drug-hypersensitivity syndrome	*Serum sickness-like reaction*	*Stevens-Johnson syndrome and toxic epidermal necrolysis (215 pg)*
Symptoms	Fever, cutaneous eruption, internal organ involvement	Fever, cutaneous eruption, arthralgias	Fever, cough, malaise, macular exanthem with mucosal involvement
Laboratory abnormalities	Atypical lymphocytosis with prominent eosinophilia; laboratory abnormalities dependent on the organ involved	Mild leukocytosis with eosinophilia	Leucopenia, occasional liver function test abnormalities
Onset of symptoms	2-8 weeks	7-14 days	2-8 weeks
Implicated drugs	Aromatic anticonvulsants (phenytoin, phenobarbital, carbamazepine), lamotrigine, allopurinol, dapsone, sulfonamide	Beta-Iactam antibiotics (especially cefaclor), sulfonamide, minocycline	Aromatic anticonvulsants, lamotrigine, allopurinol, dapsone, piroxicam

DRUG HYPERSENSITIVITY SYNDROME

Skin Involvement

A generalized exanthem (Fig. 6.7) occurs in approximately 85% of patients and usually occurs simultaneously with the appearance of the fever or shortly after. Skin manifestations can range from an exanthematous eruption to more serious eruptions, such as exfoliative dermatitis. Conjunctivitis and angioedema of the face may also be present in some patients with anticonvulsant-induced hypersensitivity syndrome.

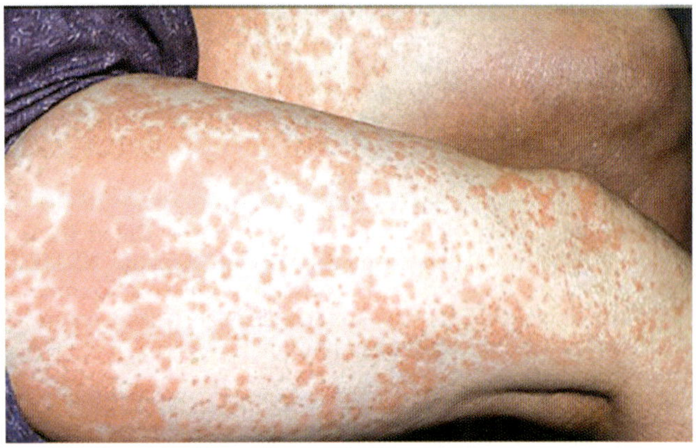

Fig. 6.7: A diffuse maculopapular rash

Lab Abnormalities

Liver abnormalities, presenting as elevated transaminases, alkaline phosphatase, prothrombin time, and bilirubin, are present in approximately 50% of patients. In some patients, development of severe hepatitis with jaundice may occur.

Systemic

Other organs, such as the kidney (interstitial nephritis, vasculitis), central nervous system (encephalitis, aseptic meningitis) or the lungs (interstitial pneumonitis, respiratory distress syndrome, vasculitis) may less commonly be involved. A small subgroup of patients may become hypothyroid as part of an autoimmune thyroiditis within 2 months of initiation of symptoms . This is characterized by a low thyroxine level, an elevated level of thyroid-stimulating hormone and thyroid autoantibodies, including anti-microsomal antibodies. An under-reported toxicity with hypersensitivity syndrome is colitis. This presents with bloody diarrhoea and abdominal pain and has led to fatal surgical intervention. The pathology shows a mixed inflammatory infiltrate analogous to the renal histologic changes.

Management

Although the role of systemic corticosteroid therapy is controversial, most clinicians would elect to start prednisone at a dose of 1 to 2 *mg/kg/d* if symptoms are severe. In contrast to the issue of corticosteroids in Stevens-Johnson syndrome and Toxic Epidermal Necrolysis, there is no significant barrier function alteration (i.e., skin sloughing) leading to the potential for sepsis in the hypersensitivity syndrome. There are cases of patients who have been treated with cyclosporine or intravenous immunoglobulin. Antihistamines or topical corticosteroids can also be used to alleviate symptoms. Because the risk of hypersensitivity syndrome is substantially increased in first-degree relatives of patients who had hypersensitivity syndrome reactions, counselling of family members is a crucial part of the assessment of this syndrome.

SERUM SICKNESS LIKE REACTION (SSLR)

Fever, rash (usually urticarial), and arthralgias occurring 1 to 3 weeks after drug initiation. Other findings, such as lymphadenopathy and eosinophilia may also be present. However, immune complexes, hypocomplementemia, vasculitis, and renal lesions are absent in SSLRs. Epidemiologic studies in children suggest that the risk of SSLRs is greater with cefaclor as compared with other antibiotic therapy, including other cephalosporins. Other drugs that have recently been implicated in the causation of SSLRs include minocycline, bupropion and rituximab.

Management

Discontinuation of the culprit drug and symptomatic treatment with antihistamines and topical corticosteroids are recommended in patients with SSLR. A short course of oral corticosteroids may be required in patients with more severe symptoms. The drug causing the SSLR should be avoided in the future.

STEVENS-JOHNSON SYNDROME AND TOXIC EPIDERMAL NECROLYSIS

The spectrum of severe cutaneous adverse reactions, which may represent variants of the same disease process, includes Stevens-Johnson syndrome and toxic epidermal necrolysis.

Erythema multiforme (EM), EM major, and atypical EM major are cutaneous reactions that are usually seen postinfection rather than postdrug. Severe cases of EM major and atypical EM major can be confused with Stevens-Johnson syndrome. Most investigators believe that Stevens-

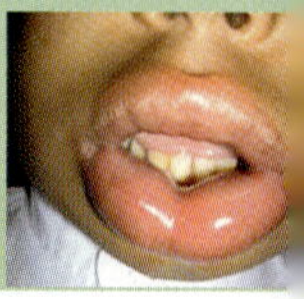

Johnson syndrome and toxic epidermal necrolysis are on a spectrum of severity and are different than the EM diseases.

Clinical Features

A prodromal phase of fever, cough, and malaise is followed by a macular exanthem, which progresses to become Nikolsky positive. In patients with toxic epidermal necrolysis, the gastrointestinal tract can be involved, and up to 30% of cases may have respiratory involvement. In addition, abnormalities in liver function tests have been reported. Significant leucopenia is a common finding as well.

Differentiation among cases of Stevens-Johnson syndrome and toxic epidermal necrolysis depends on the nature of the skin lesions and extent of body surface area involvement. The more severe forms of toxic epidermal necrolysis have a greater *percentage of body surface area of epidermal detachment(Fig. 6.8). Target lesions tend to change from the classic, raised, three-ringed iris lesion (Fig. 6.9). to a more purpuric or erythematous two ringed lesion (Fig 6.10).*

Clinically, each of these reaction patterns is characterized by the presence of the triad of *mucous membrane erosions, target lesions, and epidermal necrosis with skin detachment* (Fig 6.11). Some Stevens-Johnson syndrome cases are not drug related and may develop after a variety of other predisposing factors, including infections (e.g, mycoplasma-induced pneumonia), neoplasia, and autoimmune diseases.

The most frequent drugs cited as causes for Stevens-Johnson syndrome and toxic epidermal necrolysis are the anticonvulsants, sulfonamide nonsteroidal anti-inflammatory drugs (especially piroxicam), and allopurinol.

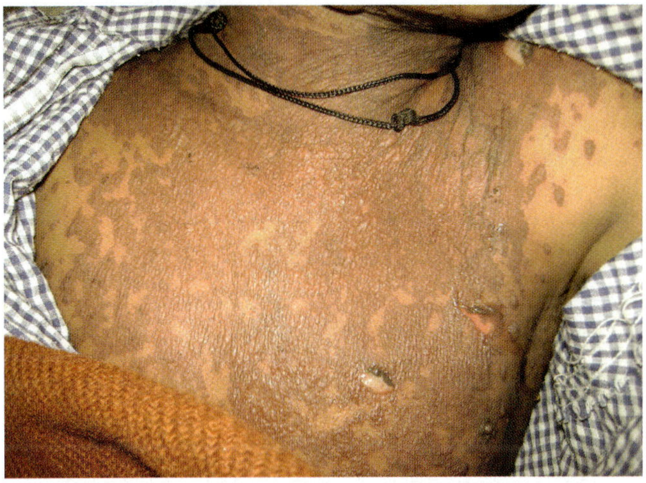

Fig. 6.8: Epidermal detachment, early stage of TEN

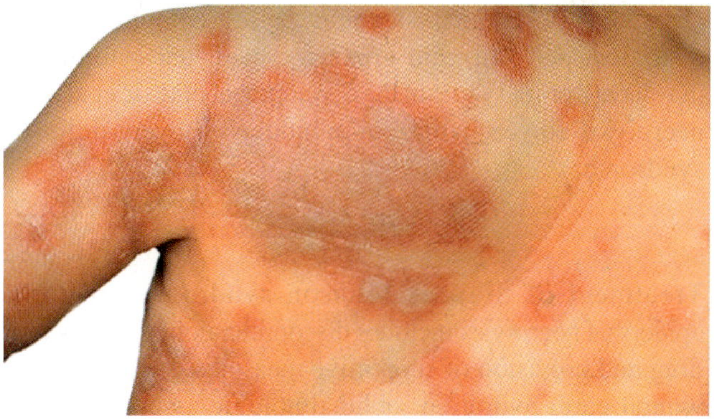

Fig. 6.10: Two rings of EM

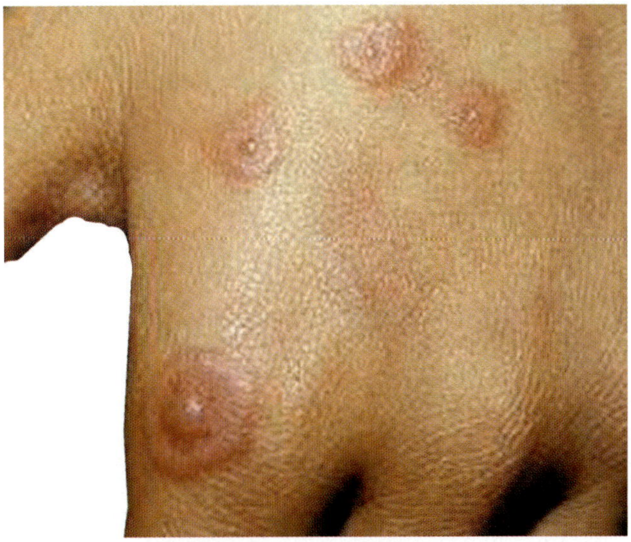

Fig. 6.9: Three ring of EM

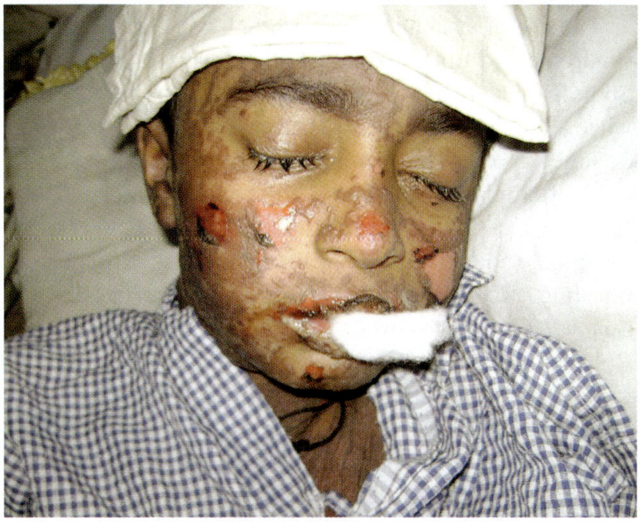

Fig. 6.11: Mucosal involvement, with eye involvement, with skin detachment

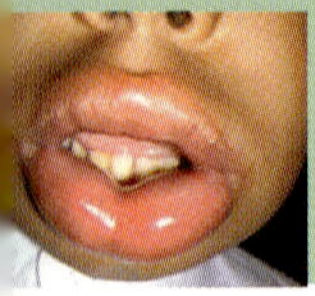

PATHOGENESIS

The pathogenesis of Stevens-Johnson syndrome and toxic epidermal necrolysis is unknown, although a metabolic basis has been hypothesized. Sulfonamides and anticonvulsants, which are the two group of drugs most frequently associated with Stevens-Johnson syndrome and toxic epidermal necrolysis, are metabolized to toxic metabolites that are subsequently detoxified in most individuals. However, in predisposed patients with a genetic defect, the metabolite may bind covalently to proteins. In some of these patients, the metabolite-protein adducts may trigger an immune response that may lead to cutaneous adverse drug reactions. Some evidence supports the role for the "cell death" receptor Fas and its ligand FasL in the pathogenesis of keratinocyte apopotosis during toxic epidermal necrolysis. In addition, activated T cells, macrophages, and neutrophils may be triggers for the development of toxic epidermal necrolysis . Drug specific major histocompatibility complex class I-restricted, perforin- and granzyme-mediated cytotoxicity may have a primary role in the development of toxic epidermal necrolysis for carbamazepine-induced Stevens-Johnson syndrome.

Management

Treatment of Stevens-Johnson syndrome and toxic epidermal necrolysis includes discontinuation of a suspected drug and provision of supportive measures, such as careful wound care, hydration, ophthalmologic assessment, and nutritional support. Ocular complications are not infrequent and have a significant impact on long-term morbidity. In one study, 79% of patients with ocular involvement in the acute phase of toxic epidermal necrolysis had long-term ocular complications.

The use of systemic corticosteroids in Stevens-Johnson syndrome and toxic epidermal necrolysis is controversial. Some clinicians believe corticosteroids may be beneficial when administered early in the disease and at relatively high dosage. However, other investigators suggest that corticosteroids do not shorten the recovery time and may increase the risk of complications, including secondary infections (potentially leading to sepsis) and gastrointestinal bleeding. *Most clinicians avoid systemic corticosteroids, especially in severe cases.*

Uncontrolled studies showed that plasmapheresis and cyclosporine, may be beneficial. Some centers use high-dose human intravenous immunoglobulin.

A **summary of diagnosis and management** of adverse drug reactions is depicted in (Fig. 6.12).

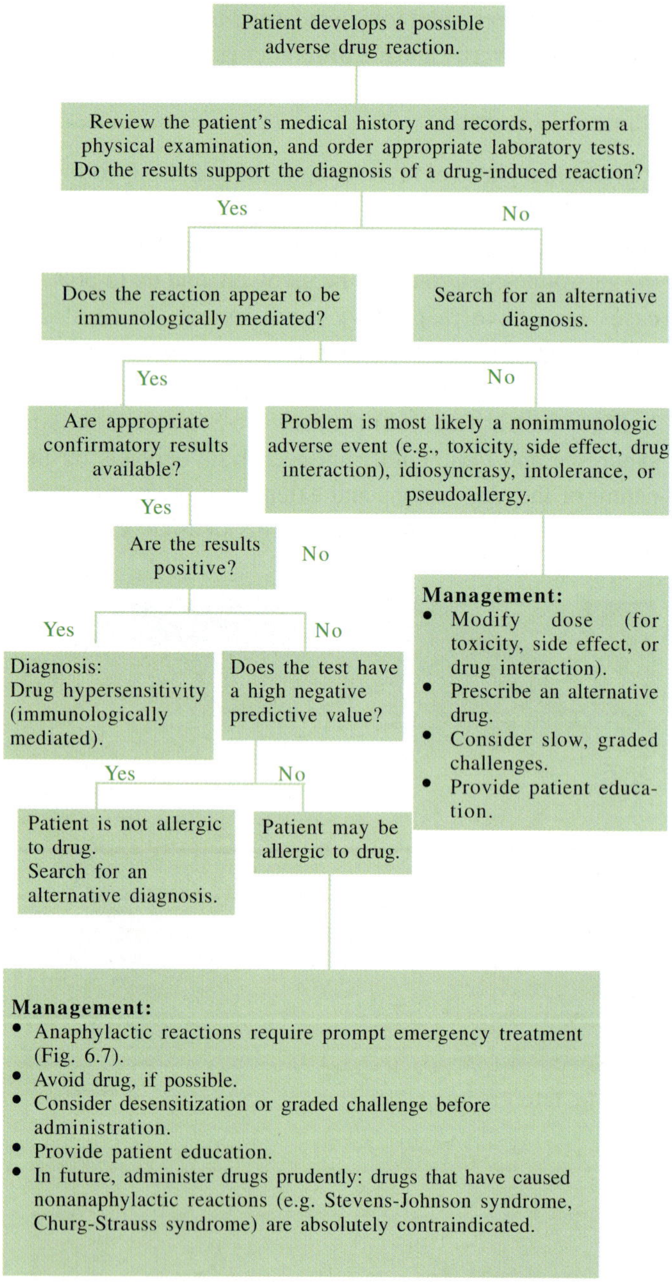

Fig. 6.12: Adverse drug reactions (Management)

REFERENCES

- Drake LA, Dinehart SM, Farmer ER, *et al.*: Guidelines of care for cutaneous adverse drug reactions, American Academy of Dermatology J Am Acad Dermatol 1996; 35: 458-61.
- Adverse Drug Reactions: Types and Treatment Options, Am Fam Physician 2003; 68:1781-90.
- Drug actions, reactions and interactions, Dermatological Clinic, April 2007; 25:2:245-60.

CHAPTER 7

ECZEMA AND DERMATITIS

The word 'eczema' comes from the Greek for 'boiling', a reference to the tiny vesicles (bubbles) that are often seen in the early acute stages of the disorder, but less often in its later chronic stages.

'Dermatitis' means inflammation of the skin and is therefore, strictly speaking, a broader term than eczema which is just one of several possible types of skin inflammation. It may be allergic or irritant.

Eczema can be defined histologically by the presence of a predominantly lymphohistiocytic infiltrate around the upper dermal blood vessels, associated with varying degrees of spongiosis and acanthosis.

CLASSIFICATION OF ECZEMA (Table 7.1)

Eczema may be classified according to the appearance of the lesions, site of involvement or according to the putative causative mechanism. Eczema is a reaction pattern and many different stimuli can make the skin react in the same way, and several of these may be in action at the same time. This complicates classification and only upto 2/3rd of cases can be accurately diagnosed.

Pathogenesis

The pathways leading to an eczematous reaction are likely to be common to all subtypes and to involve similar inflammatory mediators (prostaglandins, leukotrienes and cytokines). Helper T cells, sometimes activated by superantigens from *Staphylococcus aureus*, predominate in the inflammatory infiltrate. One current view is that epidermal cytokines help to produce spongiosis and that their secretion by keratinocytes can be elicited by T lymphocytes, irritants, bacterial products and other stimuli.

Table 7.1: Classification of eczemas

Type	*Variety*
EXOGENOUS	Irritant
	Allergic
	Photodermatitis
	Infective eczematoid dermatitis
ENDOGENOUS	Atopic
	Seborrhoeic
	Discoid (Nummular)
	Venous (stasis, gravitational)
	Pompholyx
	Pityriasis alba
	Hyperkeratotic eczema
UNCLASSIFIED	Asteatotic eczema
	Juvenile plantar dermatosis
	Neurodermatitis

Histology (Fig. 7.1)

The clinical appearance of the different stages of eczema mirrors their histology. In the acute stage, oedema in the epidermis (spongiosis) progresses to the formation of intraepidermal vesicles, which may coalesce into larger blisters or rupture. The chronic stages of eczema show less spongiosis and vesication but more thickening of the prickle cell layer (acanthosis) and horny layers (hyperkeratosis and parakeratosis).

Clinical Appearance (Table 7.2)

The different types of eczema have their own distinguishing marks, and these will be dealt with later; most share certain general features, which it is convenient to consider here. The *absence of a sharp margin* is a particularly important feature that separates eczema from most papulosquamous eruption.

Acute Eczema

Acute eczema is recognized by its:

- Weeping and crusting.
- Blistering—usually with vesicles but, in fierce cases, with large blisters.
- Redness, papules and swelling—usually with an ill-defined border.

Chronic Eczema

Chronic eczema may show all of the above changes but in general is:

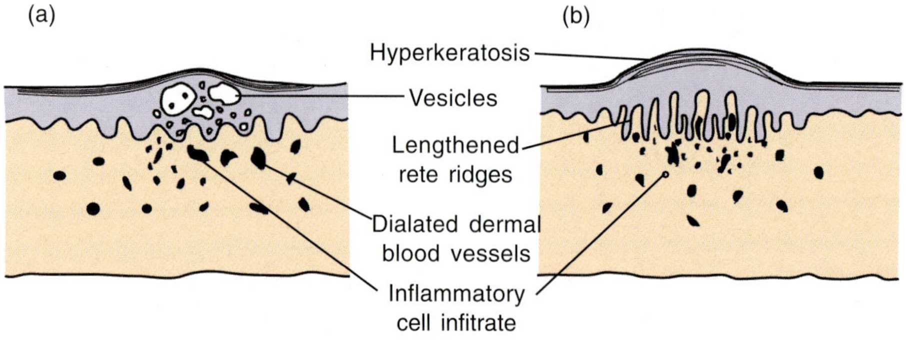

Fig. 7.1: The histology of (a) Acute dermatitis and (b) Chronic dermatits

Table 7.2: Stages of eczematous inflammation

Stage	*Morphology of lesions*	*Symptoms*	*Examples*	*Treatment*
Acute	Vesicles, blisters, intense red	Intense itch, stinging, burning	Acute contact dermatitis, acute nummular eczema, stasis dermatitis, pompholyx,	Cold wet compresses, steroid, antihistamine, antibiotics
Subacute	Red, scale, fissuring, parched appearance, scalded appearance	Slight to moderate itch, stinging, burning	Contact allergy, irritation, atopic dermatitis, stasis dermatitis, nummular eczema, asteatotic eczema	Topical steroid emollients, antihistamine antibiotics
Chronic	Thickened skin, lichenified excoriation, fissuring	Moderate to intense itch	Atopic dermatitis, lichen simplex chronicus, fingertip eczema, hyperkeratotic eczema	Topical steroid anti-histamine antibiotics, emollients

- Less vesicular and exudative.
- More scaly, pigmented and thickened.
- More likely to show lichenification – dry leathery thickened state, with increased skin markings, secondary to repeated scratching or rubbing.
- More likely to fissure.

Common Patterns of Eczema

IRRITANT CONTACT DERMATITIS

This accounts for more than **80%** of all cases of contact dermatitis, and for the vast majority of industrial cases. However, it can also occur in children, e.g. as a reaction to play dough or lip-licking.

Cause

Strong irritants elicit an acute reaction after brief contact. This involves necrosis of epithelial cells and the diagnosis is then usually obvious. Prolonged exposure, sometimes over years, is needed for weak irritants to cause dermatitis, usually of the hands and forearms. This is also known as cumulative contact irritant dermatitis or '*wear and tear* dermatitis'. Detergents, acids and alkalis, solvents, cutting oils, water and abrasive dusts are common culprits. There is a wide range of susceptibility: those with very dry skin especially vulnerable. Past or present atopic dermatitis doubles the risk of irritant hand eczema developing.

Course

The need to continue at work, or with housework, often stops the skin regaining its normal barrier function. Even under ideal circumstances this may take several months. All too often therefore irritant eczema, probably reversible in the early stages, becomes chronic.In housewives detergents are the most common cause.

Clinical Features

Acute Irritant Type: Vesicle, Itch/stinging/Burning sensation, oozing of fluid (Fig. 7.2).

Chronic Type: Cumulative Irritant CD: Can mimic Psoriasis. *It is the most common type* (Fig. 7.3).

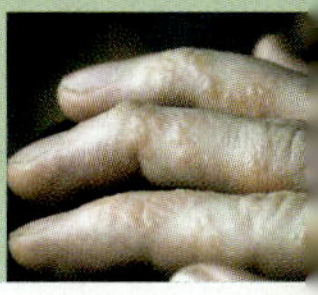

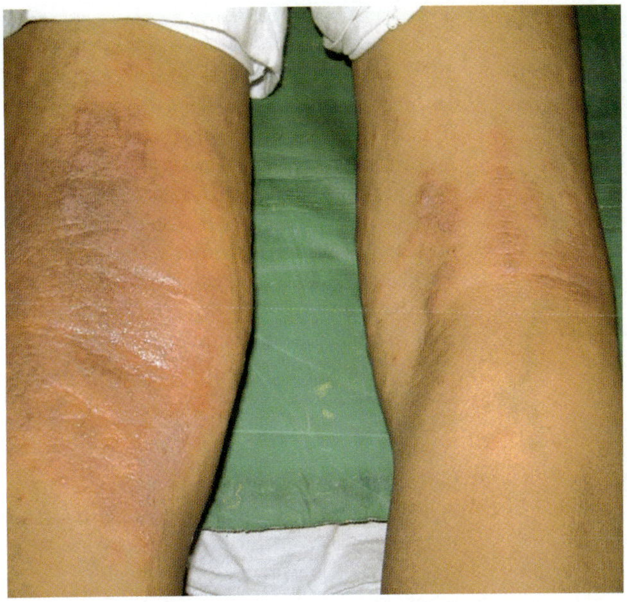

Fig. 7.2: Acute irritant dermatitis

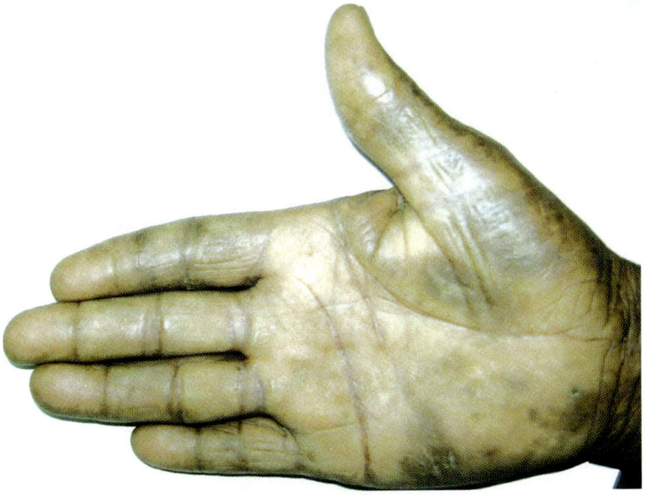

Fig. 7.3: Areas of scaly plaques seen in cumulative irritant dermatitis

Differential Diagnosis

It is often hard to differentiate irritant from allergic contact dermatitis and from atopic eczema of the hands—the more so as atopic patients are especially prone to develop irritant eczema.

Investigations

Patch testing with irritants is not helpful and may be misleading; but patch testing to a battery of common allergens is worthwhile if an allergic element is suspected.

Treatment

Management is based upon avoidance of the irritants responsible for the condition, but often this is not possible and the best that can be achieved is reduced exposure by the use of protective gloves and clothing.

Washing facilities at work should be good. Barrier creams seldom help established cases, and dirty hands should not be cleaned with harsh solvents.

Prevention is better than cure because, once started, irritant eczema can persist long after contact with offending substances has ceased, despite the vigorous use of emollients and topical corticosteroids. Vulnerable people should be advised to avoid jobs that carry an especially heavy exposure to skin irritants. Moderately potent topical corticosteroids and emollients are valuable, but are secondary to the avoidance of irritants and protective measures.

ALLERGIC CONTACT DERMATITIS

Cause

The mechanism is that of delayed (type IV) hypersensitivity. It has the following features:

- Previous contact is needed to induce allergy.
- It is specific to one chemical and its close relatives.
- After allergy has been established, all areas of skin will react to the allergen.
- Sensitization persists indefinitely.
- Desensitization is seldom possible.

Allergens

Most allergens are relatively simple chemicals that have to bind to protein to become 'complete' antigens. These are known as *haptens*. Their ability to sensitize varies from substances that can do so after a single exposure (e.g. poison ivy), to those that need prolonged exposure (e.g. chrome-brick layers take an average of 10 years to become allergic to it).

Presentation and Clinical Course (Tables 7.3 and 7.4)

The original site of the eruption gives a clue to the likely allergen but secondary spread may later obscure this. Easily recognizable patterns exist. Nickel allergy, for example, gives rise to eczema under jewellery, bra clips and jean studs. The lax skin of the eyelids and genitalia is especially likely to become edematous. Possible allergens are numerous and to spot the less common ones in the environment needs specialist knowledge. The **Most common** allergens identified are **Nickel+ Cobalt**.

Allergic contact dermatitis should be suspected if:

1. Certain areas are involved, e.g. the eyelids, external ear, hands or feet, and around gravitational ulcers.
2. There is known contact with allergens mentioned in table below (Table 7.3).
3. Individual's work carries a high risk, e.g. hairdressing, working in a flower shop, or dentistry.

Table 7.3: The sources of common allergens

Allergen	*Source*
Nickel	Jewellery, zips, fasteners, scissors, instruments
Cobalt	Pigment, paint, ink, metal alloys
Chromate	Cement, tanned leather, primer paint, anticorrosives
Rubber chemicals	Tyres, boots, shoes, belts, condoms, gloves
Paraphenylene-diamine (PPD)	**Dye** (clothing, hair), shoes, colour developer
Epoxy resins	Adhesives, plastics, mouldings
Colophony	Glue, adhesives, varnish, polish
Fragrance	Cosmetics, creams, soaps, detergents
Plants	Parthenium sp., primula sp., chrysanthemum, poison ivy, oak, garlic
Preservatives	Cosmetics, creams, oils

Both allergic contact dermatitis and irritant contact dermatitis bear similar clinical signs. In acute cases weeping and crusting will be present, while in chronic cases scaling and fissuring are the dominant findings. Sometimes, allergic contact dermatitis differs from irritant contact dermatitis in that erythema and edema may be more prominent and pruritus more troublesome in the former.

Systemically induced allergic contact dermatitis: Patients who have been sensitized to topical allergens may develop generalized eczematous inflammation if these allergens or chemically related substances are ingested, e.g. Patient with a history of nickel allergy may get a widespread flare when he takes food rich in nickel; patient sensitized to topical ethylenediamine may develop generalized inflammation following treatment with aminophylline.

Airborne allergic contact dermatitis (ABCD) and photodermatitis may look similar. However there is a characteristic sparing of the upper eyelids, submental region, and the Wilkinson's triangle (behind the ear in case of photodermatitis) while ABCD begin in the flexures and typically spares the tip of the nose (Nose-tip sign). The most common cause of ABCD in India in **Parthenium** and it is seen in **farmers** (Fig. 7.5).

The characteristic distribution of the lesions can often give clue to a particular allergen (Table 7.4). Removal of the suspected allergen leads to resolution of the dermatitis. A positive patch test to a suspected offending allergen supports the clinical diagnosis.

Table 7.4: Distribution of allergens

Location	*Material*
Scalp and ears	Shampoo, hair dyes, topical medicaments (Fig. 7.4)
Eyelid	Nail polish, cosmetics, contact lens solution, metal eyelash curlers, topical medicaments
Face	Airborne allergens, cosmetics, sunscreen, acne medications, aftershave lotion
Neck	Necklaces, airborne allergens, perfumes, aftershave lotion
Trunk	Topical medicaments, sunscreens, plants, clothing, undergarments (e.g., elastic waist band, spandex bra), metal belt buckles
Axilla	Deodorant, clothing
Arms	Watch and watchband
Hands	Soaps and detergents, foods, poison ivy, cement, metals, topical medications, rubber gloves
Genitals	Rubber condom, allergens transfers by hands
Anal region	Haemorrhoid preparations, antifungal preparations
Lower legs	Topical medicaments, dye in socks
Feet	Shoes, cement spilling into boots

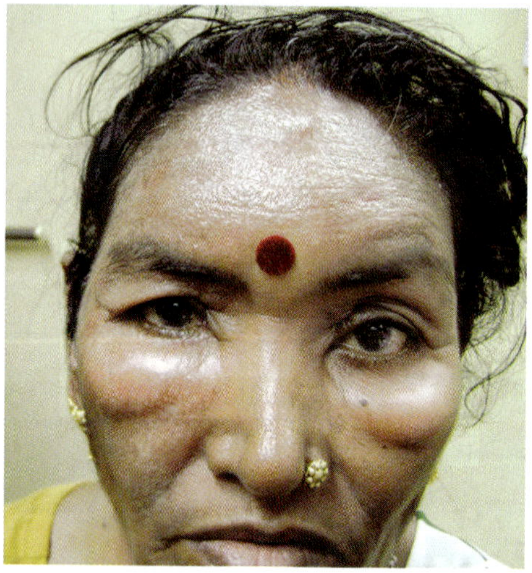

Fig. 7.4: Edema of the eyes and forehead due to a reaction to hair dye

Diagnosis

The gold standard is Patch Testing and it is read at 2,4 days. A summary of Standard Screening Series is given in Table 7.5.

Treatment

Topical corticosteroids give temporary relief, but far more important is avoidance of the relevant allergen. Patch testing can be helpful in identifying the relevant allergen. However it must be kept in mind that all positive reactions are not relevant in an individual case. Reducing exposure is usually not enough: active steps have to be taken to avoid the allergen completely. Job changes are sometimes needed to achieve this. Even then, other factors may come into play; e.g. some believe that reactions to nickel can be kept going by nickel in the diet, released from cans or steel utensils, as changes in diet and cooking utensils have sometimes been helpful.

Table 7.5: Standard screening series and examples of common sources

1.	**Potassium dichromate**	**Cement**
2.	Neomycin sulphate	Topical medicaments
3.	**Thiuram mix**	**Rubber products (shoes, balloons), pesticides**
4.	**Paraphenylenediamine free base**	**Hair dyes**, azo dyes, fur dyes, leather dyes, photodeveloper
5.	Cobalt chloride	In almost all trades and industry, **nickel and cobalt often occur together**
6.	Benzocaine	Topical anaesthetics
7.	**Formaldehyde**	**Glues, paper, clothing, cosmetic e.g. shampoo**
8.	Colophony	Adhesive plasters, paper, plaster, polishes and waxes
9.	Quinoline mix	Antiseptics in topical therapeutics
10.	Balsam of Peru	Cosmetics (perfumes, flavours)
11.	Black rubber mix	Rubber products
12.	Wool alcohols	Lanolin, vehicles
13.	Mercapto mix	Shoes, rubber products
14.	Epoxy resin	Glues, pastes, insulator, building material
15.	Paraben mix	Preservatives and vehicles in medicine and cosmetics
16.	Paratertiarybutyl phenol formaldehyde resin	Leather, adhesive and rubber systems
17.	Fragrance mix	Stabilizer in medical products
18.	Ethylenediamine Dihydrochloride	Medicaments
19.	Quaternium 15	Cosmetics
20.	**Nickel sulphate**	**Earrings, metal tools, clothing accessories, cheap ornaments**
21.	Primin	The allergen in P obconica, which mingle with house dust causing dermatitis.
22.	**Mercaptonbenzo-thiazole**	**ABCD (Fig. 7.5)**
23.	**Sesquiterpene lactone mix**	**ABCD (Parthenium)**

SEBORRHEIC DERMATITIS

Seborrheic dermatitis is a chronic, scaly inflammatory eruption usually affecting the scalp and face.

Cause

Sebum production is normal, but the eruption often occurs in the sebaceous gland areas of the scalp, face and chest. Endogenous and genetic factors, and an overgrowth of the commensal yeast *Pityrosporum ovale,* are involved. The condition is severe in some patients with HIV infection.

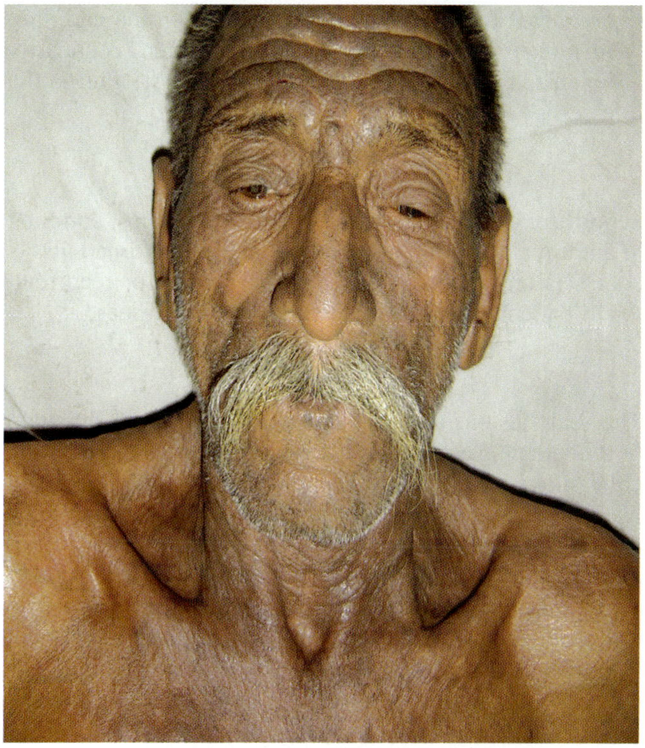

Fig. 7.5: Farmer with lichenified plaques of air borne contact dermatitis

Clinical Presentation (Fig. 7.6)

There are four common patterns:

- *Scalp and facial involvement:* Excessive dandruff, with an itchy *scaly* erythematous eruption affecting the sides of the nose, scalp margin, eyebrows and ears. The scales have a greasy appearance. Blepharitis may occur. Most common in young adult males.
- *Petaloid:* A dry scaly eczema over the presternal area.
- *Pityrosporum folliculitis:* An erythematous follicular eruption with papules or pustules over the back.

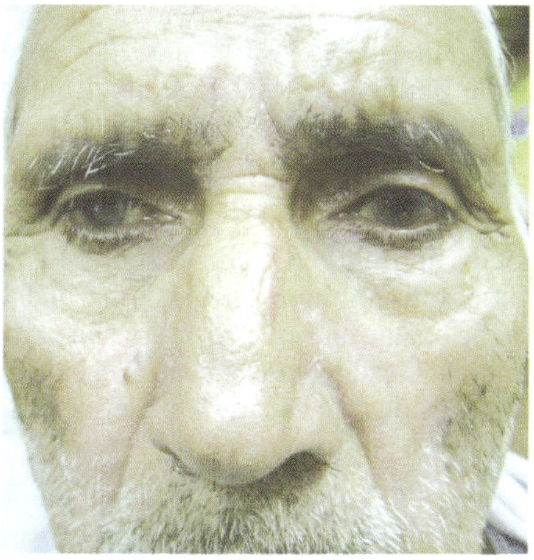

Fig. 7.6: Itchy scaly erythematous eruption affecting the sides of the nose, eyebrows and ears

- *Flexural:* Involvement of the axillae, groins and submammary areas by a moist intertrigo, often secondarily colonized by *Candida albicans.* Seen most often in the elderly.

Course

Seborrheic eczema may affect infants but is most common in adult males. In infants it clears quickly but in adults its course is unpredictable and may be chronic or recurrent. AIDS patients may have particularly severe disease.

Treatment

The scalp lesions require the use of a medicated shampoo (e.g. containing coal tar, selenium sulphide or ketoconazole), either alone or following the application of 2% sulphur and 2% salicylic acid cream left on for several hours. Facial, truncal and flexural involvement respond to an imidazole or antimicrobial, often combined with 1% hydrocortisone, in a cream or ointment base. Lithium succinate cream is also effective. Recurrence is common and repeated treatment often necessary.

DISCOID (NUMMULAR) ECZEMA

Nummular Eczema

Nummular eczema, also termed discoid eczema, is a specific variant of eczema in which the lesions occur in round or oval shapes, resembling a coin.

Types

- Dry discoid.
- Discoid eczema of hands and feet.
- Discoid eczema of other areas.

Cause

Risk factors include excessive bathing (e.g. more than 10 minutes) or other prolonged water exposure (e.g. swimming). Some studies have found it to be common in atopics, while others have not. Lesions usually occur in crops, and adults are more commonly affected than children.

Presentation and Course (Fig. 7.7)

Coin-shaped (nummular), red, eczematous areas are characteristic and common on the arms and legs. The surface may be oozing and crusted or dry and scaly. Pruritus may be significant leading to secondary lichenification. The margins of the lesions are usually well defined. The lesions often recur on stopping treatment.

Treatment

Prolonged water exposure should be avoided. A medium- to high-potency topical steroid ointment should be applied after the bath or shower. Petrolatum or a heavy cream applied to the skin immediately after a bath or shower is helpful. Superinfection with *staph aureus* is common and may have to be treated. Crude coal tar ointment (3-5%) is also useful.

PUVA and narrow band UVB (311nm) are very effective for resistant or widespread cases.

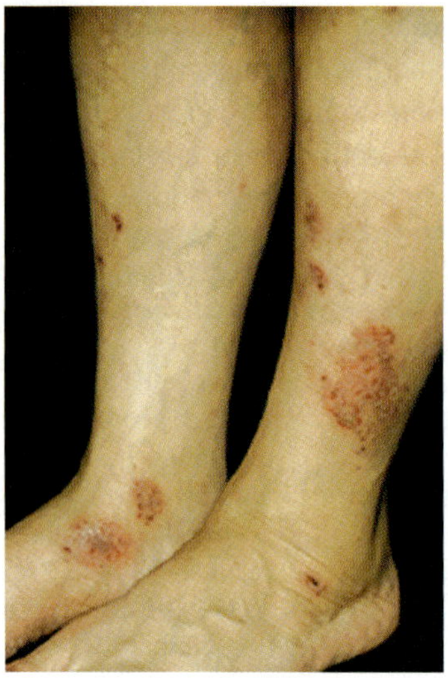

Fig. 7.7: Coin-shaped (nummular), red, eczematous areas

DYSHIDROTIC ECZEMA (*POMPHOLYX*)

Dyshidrotic eczema is a recurrent or chronic relapsing form of vesicular palmoplantar dermatitis of unknown etiology. Dyshidrotic eczema is also termed pompholyx, which derives from *cheiropompholyx*, meaning "hand and bubble" in Greek.

Types

- Acute.
- Subacute.
- Chronic.

Cause

The etiology of dyshidrotic eczema is unresolved and believed to be multifactorial. It is considered a reaction pattern caused by various endogenous conditions and exogenous factors.

Dyshidrotic eczema may be associated with atopy. Of patients with dyshidrosis, 50% have atopic dermatitis.

Exogenous factors (e.g., contact dermatitis to nickel, balsam, cobalt; sensitivity to ingested metals; bacterial and fungal infection) may trigger episodes. These antigens may act as *haptens* with a specific affinity for palmoplantar proteins of the stratum lucidum of the epidermis. The binding of these haptens to tissue receptor sites may initiate pompholyx.

Emotional stress and environmental factors reportedly exacerbate dyshidrosis.

Presentation and Course (Fig. 7.8)

Dyshidrotic eczema occurs in as many as 5-20% of patients with hand eczema and more commonly occurs in warmer climates and during spring and summer months. Symmetric crops of clear vesicles and/or bullae on the palms and lateral aspects of fingers characterize dyshidrotic eczema. Feet, soles and the lateral aspects of toes also may be affected. Vesicles are deep seated with a tapioca-like appearance, without surrounding erythema. Secondary infection and lymphangitis may occur.

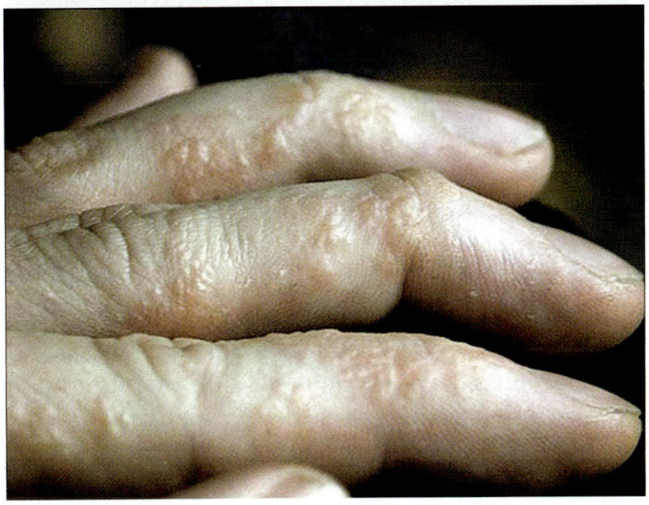

Fig. 7.8: Clear vesicles on the lateral aspects of fingers (Pompholyx)

Hands are involved solely in 80% of patients, feet solely in 10%, and both hands and feet are involved in 10% of patients. The condition is recurrent, with each bout lasting a few weeks.

Treatment

Appropriate antibiotics should be given for bacterial infections. Aluminium acetate or potassium permanganate soaks, followed by applications of a very potent corticosteroid cream, are often helpful.

ASTEATOTIC ECZEMA

Cause

Many who develop asteatotic eczema in old age will always have had a dry skin and a tendency to chap. Other contributory factors include the removal of surface lipids by over-washing, the low humidity of winter and central heating, the use of diuretics, and hypothyroidism.

Presentation and Course (Fig. 7.9)

Often unrecognized, this common and itchy pattern of eczema usually occurs on the legs of elderly patients. Against a background of dry skin, a network of fine red superficial fissures creates a *crazy paving* appearance. Very extensive cases may be part of malabsorption syndromes, zinc deficiency or internal malignancy.

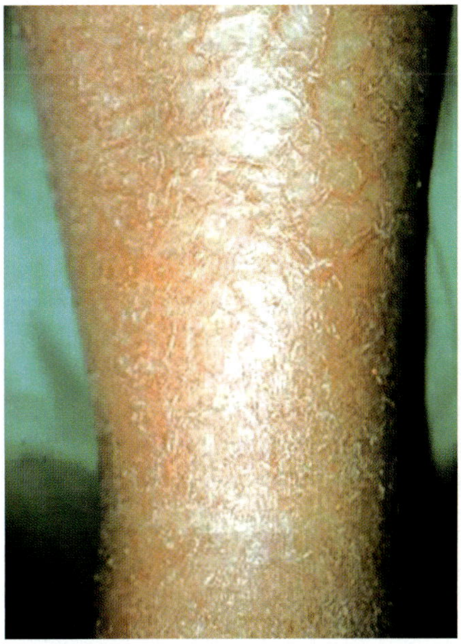

Fig. 7.9: *Crazy paving* appearance (Asteatotic eczema)

Treatment

Topical steroid ointments with 24 to 48-hour occlusion is the treatment of choice for the rapid resolution of asteatotic dermatitis. Many patients heal with mild topical steroids (class III-VI) alone, depending on the severity of the dermatitis, compliance with treatment, and the reduction in the use of soap and hot water over the involved areas. The liberal use of moisturizers, especially petrolatum-based preparations, alone or in combination with topical steroids for mild cases of asteatotic dermatitis is recommended.

The soak-and-smear method of hydrating the skin by bathing or soaking the affected area followed by immediate application of steroid ointment once daily has been shown to clear more that 90% of patients in 4-14 days. This is best performed at night.

VENOUS (STASIS/GRAVITATIONAL) ECZEMA

Cause

Venous eczema affects the lower legs and is associated with underlying venous disease, which may not always be obvious.

Incompetence of the deep perforating veins increases the hydrostatic pressure in the dermal capillaries. *Pericapillary fibrin* deposition leads to the clinical changes.

Presentation and Course

Most patients are middle-aged or elderly women. Varicose veins of venules and haemosiderin pigmentation around the ankles are early signs. Eczema develops later, sometimes with fibrosis of the dermis and subcutaneous tissue (*lipodermatosclerosis*), and ulceration.

Allergy to an applied medicament can complicate the picture, particularly relevant to topical antibiotics.

Treatment

This should include the elimination of oedema by elevation, pressure bandages or diuretics. A moderately potent topical steroid may be helpful, but stronger ones are best avoided. Bland applications, e.g. Lassar's paste or zinc cream daily or medicated bandages (Tar-impregnated), applied once or twice a week, are useful especially when ulceration coexists.

Stasis eczema is liable to persist, despite surgery of the underlying veins.

PITYRIASIS ALBA

Pityriasis alba is a common hypopigmented dermatitis that occurs primarily in preadolescent children. It is often an incidental finding on clinical examination. This is a self-limited disorder that usually resolves by adulthood. Pityriasis alba is relatively common, occurring in upto 5% of children.

Cause

No definitive etiologic agent has been described. Unlike the conventional belief it has *nothing* to do with nutritional deficiency. It may be more common in atopic children. An eczematous process occurs first, followed by loss of pigment.

Presentation and Course

Ill defined hypopigmented, macules or patches are found typically over the face and, at times, the neck and shoulders (Fig. 7.10).

These are preceded by an erythematous stage which is overlooked by most patients.

The lesions of pityriasis alba tend to have less well-defined, *scaly* (Fig. 7.11) borders than lesions seen in vitiligo, and they do not coalesce as seen in tinea versicolor. It is easily distinguished from *Indeterminate Hansen* as the latter is usually *not scaly*.

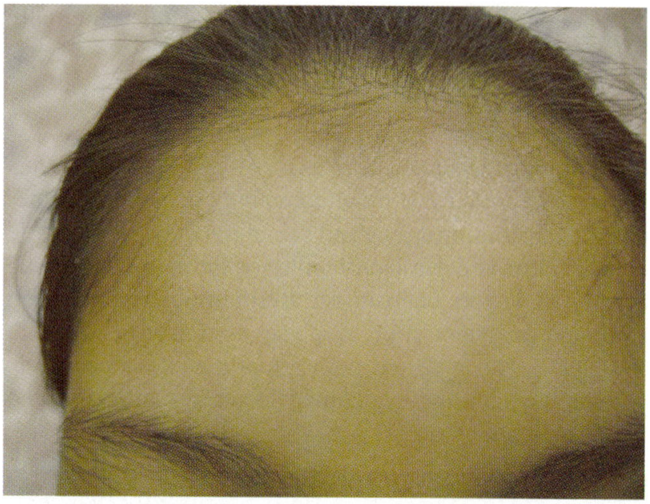

Fig. 7.10: Hypopigmented macules on the face

Lesions are more visible over dark skin, hence some patients may complain of a summer exacerbation due to tanning of surrounding skin.

Treatment

Since the disease usually is self-limited and asymptomatic, medical therapy is often unnecessary. Pityriasis alba has no medical consequences, and the side effects of the medications may outweigh the cosmetic benefit of intervention. The most commonly used remedies (e.g., emollients, topical steroids, PUVA) appear to have limited efficacy.

Emollients are used to reduce the scaling of the lesions, especially on the face.

Topical steroids may help with erythema and pruritus during the initial lesions and may accelerate repigmentation of existing lesions.

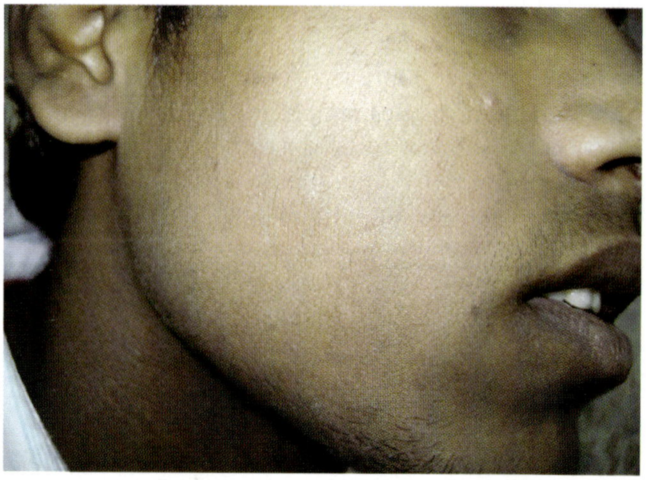

Fig. 7.11: Scaly macules on the face

Psoralen plus ultraviolet light A photochemotherapy (PUVA) may be used to help with repigmentation in extensive cases, although the recurrence rate is high after treatment is stopped.

LICHEN SIMPLEX (CIRCUMSCRIBED NEURODERMATITIS)

Lichenification denotes a cutaneous response to repeated rubbing or scratching. It is characterized clinically by a *thickened appearance of the skin, darkening of skin colour*, and *accentuation of the surface markings* so that the affected skin surface resembles a tree bark. **Lichen simplex** is a circumscribed area of lichenification resulting from repeated rubbing and scratching occurring on some predilected sites. This term is used when there is *no known predisposing skin disorder.*

Type

- Nuchal.
- Pebbly.
- Giant variant.

Presentation and Course (Fig. 7.12)

Women are more commonly affected than men. Pruritus is the predominant symptom and is often out of proportion to the extent of the objective changes. During the early stages the skin is reddened and slightly oedematous, and the normal markings are exaggerated. The **redness and oedema subside with time the central area becomes scaly, thickened** and pigmented. Almost any site is affected, but the most common sites are those that are conveniently reached. The usual sites are the nape and sides of the neck, lower legs and ankles, scalp, upper thighs, vulva, pubis or scrotum and the extensor forearms. The pruritis is typically worse when the patient is not distracted by some other activity, e.g. many patients have no itching while working.

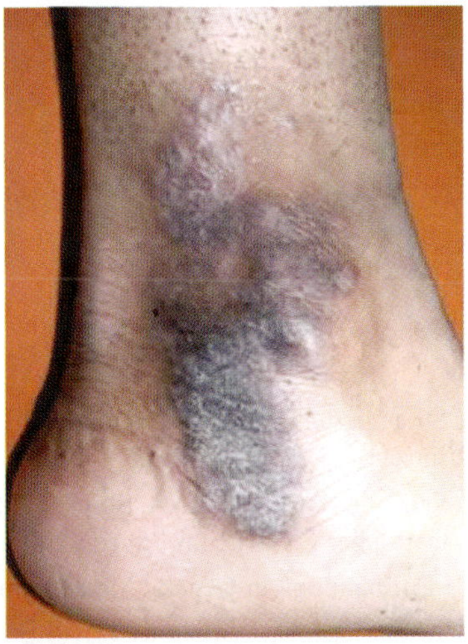

Fig. 7.12: Thickening of skin and increased markings (Lichen simplex chronicus)

Treatment

A search for a causation should be made before the lichenification is considered to be primary, then a careful psychological history should be taken and the patient given some assistance in reducing her tensions. Careful counselling is necessary to explain the importance of breaking the 'itch-scratch cycle'. Topical steroid is the treatment of choice, sometimes with occlusion to enhance absorption and prevent further scratching. Intralesional triamcinolone is useful for circumscribed chronic lesions.

HYPERKERATOTIC ECZEMA

This condition can be a very persistent and bothersome problem to middle-aged men. There may be a significant negative impact on work. The clinical appearance is somewhere between that of eczema and a keratoderma. Patch testing and mycology are important for excluding other causes. In some patients, this condition may be a type of lichen simplex chronicus of the palms. In such cases, any friction (e.g. work-related friction) should be minimized.

Presentation and Course

A diffuse, thickened, fissured hyperkeratosis of the palms occurring in a middle-aged man is characteristic.

Treatment

The disease is usually resistant to treatment. Potent topical steroids, lubrication, and keratolytics may be tried. Hand PUVA may be of some benefit. Acitretin may be used and the effectiveness of Cycosporin A has been reported.

INFECTIOUS ECZEMATOID REACTION

In this variant of eczema, a progressive, moist, eczematous process seems to result from a combination of eczema and superficial bacterial infection with *Staphylococcus aureus*.

Clinical

The skin surrounding an obvious focus of infection like impetigo is erythematous, wet, and oozing. At the edge, small, circular lesions appear and coalesce as the condition spreads. Those lesions are eczematous in nature.

Treatment

Treatment should involve both a potent topical steroid and an oral antibiotic.

SECONDARY ('AUTOSENSITIZATION') ECZEMA

This condition (also termed an **'id' reaction**) is an eczematous reaction pattern to inflammation at other skin sites. It may be widespread or may be clinically identical to pompholyx.

Presentation and Course

A *diffuse, symmetric eczematous* rash may occur after a flare of a localized eczematous eruption. Such reactions have occurred after nummular eczema, stasis dermatitis, lichen simplex chronicus, allergic contact dermatitis, radiation dermatitis, *tinea, or scabies*.

Treatment

The inciting eczematous eruption should be treated. Topical and systemic steroids may be given.

PRURIGO NODULARIS

In 1909, Hyde and Montgomery first described prurigo nodularis (PN) as pruritic nodules on the extensor surfaces of the lower extremities in middle-aged women. Today, PN is still a condition of unknown etiology. PN has been documented to be much more common in immunocompromised and HIV populations. Some associations have been made between PN and internal malignancy as well as severely decreased kidney function.

Presentation and Course (Fig. 7.13)

Chronic mechanical trauma to the skin causes thickening of the skin proportionate to the trauma. Repetitive rubbing, scratching, and touching results in plaque or nodular lichenification and hyperkeratosis. Pigmentary changes often result from such repetitive trauma to the skin. Mature nodules rarely increase or decrease in size; spontaneous resolution is even more rare. PN is usually bilaterally symmetric.

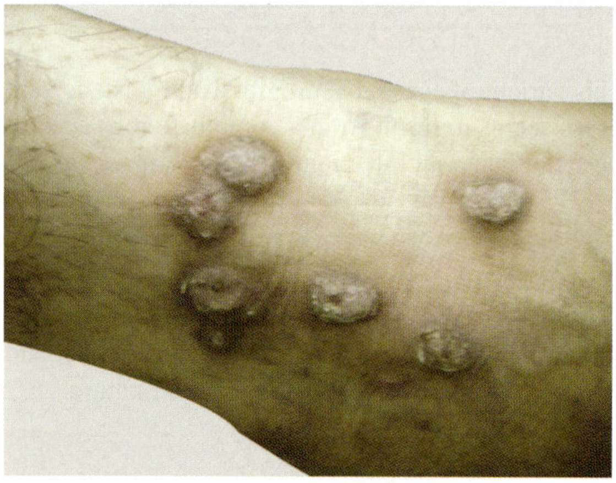

Fig. 7.13: Nodules which resemble localized lichen simplex chronicus (Prurigo nodularis)

Histological Findings

The histologic features of prurigo nodularis include a hyperkeratotic epidermis with acanthosis and parakeratosis. Rete ridges are elongated and irregular with a dense dermal infiltrate consisting of neutrophils, eosinophils, histiocytes, and monocytes. Also notable in the dermis are *thickened nerve fibers* and fibrosis with thickened collagen bundles. Axons and Schwann cells both show hyperproliferation.

Treatment

Currently available treatments for PN have had mild-to-moderate success at best. Often, combinations of several medications or physical modalities may be used in an attempt to control this process.

Topical, oral, and intralesional corticosteroids have all been used in attempts to decrease inflammation and itching, and to soften and smooth out firm nodules. The improvement with corticosteroids is variable, and corticosteroids are sometimes not helpful.

Menthol, phenol, pramoxine, capsaicin cream, vitamin D-3 ointment, and topical anesthetics are some other topical agents used to reduce pruritus. Treatment with occlusive therapies has been suggested to flatten lesions while at the same time preventing patients from directly scratching nodules.

UV light treatment using UV-B or UV-A plus psoralen may be beneficial for severe pruritus.

Antihistamines, anxiolytics, opiate receptor antagonists, and (most recently) thalidomide are oral medications used for PN. Thalidomide has been shown to aid in several severe dermatoses, including PN with or without associated HIV disease.

Cryotherapy and pulsed dye laser have been used for resistant cases.

REFERENCES

- Therapeutic Strategies in Dermatology; Timothy G. Berger, M.D. Bruce U. Wintroub, M.D.
- Rook's Textbook of Dermatology D.A. Burns , S. M. Breathnach, Neil Cox, Christopher E., Griffiths 7th edn 2004.
- Fitzpatrick's Dermatology in General Medicine 6th edn 2003
- Lever's Histopathology of the Skin by David E Elder, Rosalie Elenitsas, Bernett L Johnson, George F Murphy, 9th edition 2004.

Hand Eczema

COMMON PATTERNS

I. ACD (Allergic-Contact-Dermatitis)

15% of all causes:
- Acute.
- Chronic.

Clinical Features

- Initially localised.
- Later involves distant sites.
- Palms are relatively resistant – involved in floral workers.
- Dorsum and fingers usually involved.
- Allergens—Rubber mix, Nickel, Chromium, PPD, Paraben, lanolin, Balsam of Peru, Colophony, Epoxy Resins, Formaldehyde, Fragrances, *Medications*.

II. ICD (Irritant-Contact-Dermatitis)

50%.

Cause

- Alkalis.
- Alcohols.
- Solvents.
- Adhesives.
- Metal salts.
- Plants.
- Chronic and Cumulative damage due to Wear and Tear and Trauma.
- Chemical factors.
- **Soaps, detergents,** cleansers, solvents, cutting oils, raw foods.

Clinical Features

- Localised to web-spaces, sides of fingers and dorsum of hands, palmar surface.
- Volar aspect of wrist is spared.
- Predisposing factors.

III. Atopic Hand Eczema

- Usually >15 years.
- Patchy vesicular and eczematous lesions on the back of hands may turn to chronic lichenfied lesions.
- Associated involvement of feet common.
- Manifestations of atopy present.
- Prone to infections.
- Increased predisposition to allergic nummular and hyperkeratotic lesions.

IV. Wear and Tear Dermatitis

Syn: Asteatotic Hand Eczema/Housewife's Dermatitis/ Dry Palmar Eczema/*Dermatitis Palmaris Sicca (Fig. 7.14)*
- Housewives/Laundry workers/Cleaners/Dishwashers/ Bartenders/Atopics.
- Dry hands with criss-crossed superficial white cracks over an erythematous background.
- Chapping over the palms and dorsum of fingers.
- Irritant dermatitis.
- Associated with ring eczema and fingertip dermatitis.

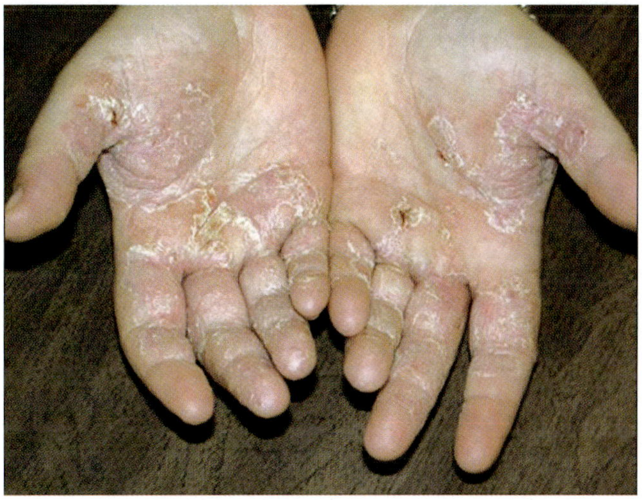

Fig. 7.14: Bilateral symmetrical areas of scaling

V. Pompholyx

1. Recurrent eruptions of minute, non-inflammatory, vesicles on fingers, palms and soles is characteristic. Pruritus is common, sometimes lesions can be painful or it may be asymptomatic. Scratching of vesicles leads to weeping and crusting.
2. *Management:* $KMnO_4$ soaks, oral antihistamines and application of mid to high potency steroids for mild cases. A short course of oral steroid is required for severe cases. Psychological factors are important. Counselling, behavioral modification may be necessary.

VI. Keratolysis Exfoliativa

This is a common chronic asymptomatic non-inflammatory bilateral peeling of the palms and soles. Its cause is unknown. The eruption is most common during the summer months and often associated with sweaty palms and soles. Scaling starts simultaneously from several points on the palms or soles with 2 or 3 mm in diameter round scales. The scales continue to peel and extend peripherally, forming larger roughly circular areas that resemble ringworm, while the central area become slightly red and tender.

VII. Fingertip Eczema (Fig. 7.15)

A very dry chronic condition of the palmar surface of finger tip. Usually of unknown cause, but may be the result of an allergic reaction. One or several fingers may be involved. Initially the skin is moist; gradually becomes dry, cracked and scaly. The process usually stops shortly before the distal interphalangeal joint is reached. Fingertip eczema may last for months or years and is resistant to treatment. Treatment is by avoiding irritants and frequent lubrication. Topical steroid with or without occlusion may give temporary relief. Tar is an alternative treatment. Allergy and psoriasis may have to be excluded.

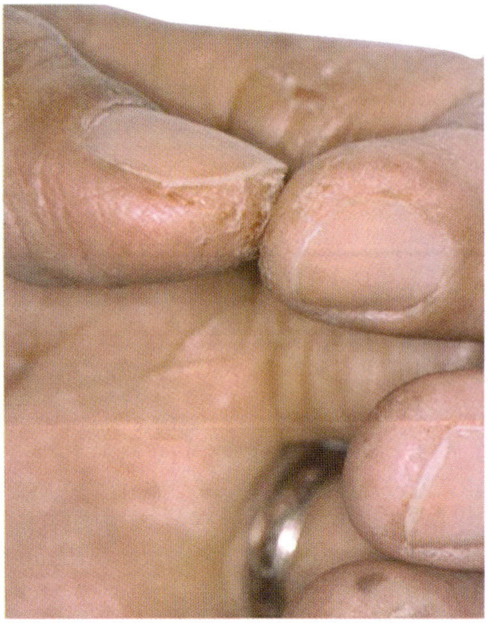

Fig. 7.15: Fingertip eczema

VIII. Ring Eczema

An irritable patch of eczema under a ring and tends to spread to adjacent area. This affects mainly young women soon after marriage or childbirth. If the ring is transferred to the other hand, the eczema will appear at the new site. The cause is due to concentrations of detergent beneath the ring and repeated friction. Removal of the ring often brings remission.

TREATMENT

General and specific.

General

- Emollients.
- Hypo-allergenic tapes.
- Cyanoacrylates and superglues, should be avoided.
- Dietary modifications, may be helpful.
- Barrier creams.
- Other protective measures (tincture benzoin).

Specific

Depending on whether the condition is acute or chronic.

Acute Weeping Eruptions

Wet dressings in saline, aluminum subacetate, silver nitrate
Steroid creams.

Chronic Eruptions

- Emollients.
- Steroid ointments.
- Salicylic acid combination.

Topical Steroids

- Cornerstone of therapy.
- Used in all but the mildest cases.
- Should be used sparingly and in the weakest effective potency.
- May require to be used under occlusion or in combination with antibiotics and salicylic acid.
- For maintenance purposes, intermittent dosing used.
- Recalcitrant cases may require intra-lesional injections.

Other Topical Treatments

Tar Paste

- Messy preparations (5% crude tar).
- Used in combination with steroid and salicylic acid.

Salicylic Acid

- Hyperkeratotic and scaly lesions.
- Increased penetration and decreased steroid doses.
- Used with propylene glycol under occlusion before applying steroids.

Topical Antibiotics

- Used in fissured and acute oozing eczemas.
- Mainly against staphylococcus.
- Used in combination with steroids.
- Neomycin sensitivity known.

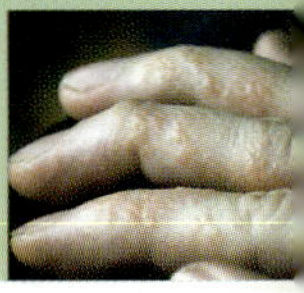

Topical Immuno-Modulators

- Tacrolimus–Macrolactam compound.
- Concentration available—0.03% and 0.1%—to be applied twice daily.
- **Side effects**—Burning and irritation.

Pimecrolimus

- Ascomycin compound.
- 1% concentration—to be applied twice daily.

Topical Puva Soaks and Baths.

SYSTEMIC THERAPY

- Systemic steroids.
- PUVA, UVB Radiation.
- Systemic anti-histaminics.
- Methotrexate, azathioprine.
- Low dose cyclosporine.
- Isotretinoin.
- Etretinate.

NEWER TREATMENTS

- Rotational Therapy.
- Hyposensitization/Desensitization.
- Tolerance Induction.
- Intra Lesional Botulinum Toxoid.
- Bexarotene Gel.

REFERENCES

- Rooks Book of Dermatology (7th Edition).
- Fischer's Book of Contact Dermatitis.
- Fitz Patrick Book of Dermatology.

Atopic Dermatitis

Eczematous disorder with intense itching, relapsing course in infants and children with family history of atopy.

Incidence

- 10-15% (prevalence).
- 65% (before 1st year).
- 90% (before 5 years).

Etiopathogenesis

1. Genetic Factors

- 70-90% have family history of atopy.
- 81% risk if both parents are affected.
- 56% risk if 1 parent affected.
- Chromosome 11q 12-13.

2. Immunological Factors

- 80% have increased IgE, decreased IgA levels.
- Langerhan cells and monocytes have a role to play.
- Increase TH2 response.
- Decreased cAMP (Negative modulator of immune response).
- Basophils—release of histamine and degranulation.

3. Disruption of Epidermal Barrier

- ↓ in ceramide in both lesional and non-lesional skin.
- ↓ in linoleic and linolenic acid metabolism.
- Itch-scratch cycle.

4. Role of Super Antigens

- 90% colonization with *staph aureus*.
- Similarly *pityrosporum ovale* also elicits immune response by super antigens.

Antigen	*Super Antigen*
• Processed by APC	• By pass APC
• Subject to MHC-II restriction	• Not restricted by MHC II
• 0.01% T cells activated	• 30% of T cells activated
• Anti bodies neutralize Ag	• Ab are not protective

E.g.

- Staphylococcal enterotoxin A, B, C, D, E.
- Toxic shock syndrome toxin-I.
- Streptococcal S-Ag.

TRIGGERING FACTORS

Irritants

- Lipid solvents (soaps/detergents).
- Disinfectants/occupational irritants.

Contact and Aeroallergens

Dust mite/furry animals/pollen/dander mould/synthetic-woollen/cigarette smoke.

Microbial agents.

Food allergy.

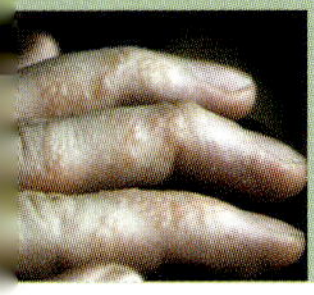

Psychogenic.
Hormonal influence.
Climate.

Clinical Features

Infantile Phase	Childhood Phase	Adult Phase
3 m/1year	2-12 years	>12 years

Seventy-five per cent of cases of atopic eczema begin before the age of *6 months*, and *80-90%* before the age of *5 years*. It affects at least 3% of infants, but the onset may be delayed until childhood or adult life.

Some 60-70% of children with atopic eczema will clear by their early teens, although subsequent relapses are possible. The distribution and character of the lesions vary with age but a general dryness of the skin may persist throughout life.

- In **infancy**, atopic eczema tends to be vesicular and weeping. It often starts on the face with a non-specific distribution elsewhere, commonly sparing the napkin (diaper) area.

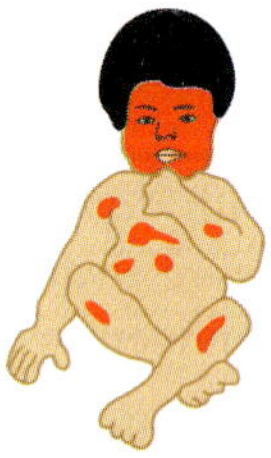

Infant: Distribution of lesions

- **In childhood,** the eczema becomes leathery, dry and excoriated, affecting mainly the **elbow and knee flexures** (Fig. 7.16), wrists and ankles. A stubborn 'reverse' pattern affecting the extensor aspects of the limbs is also recognized.
- In adults, the distribution is as in childhood with a marked tendency towards **lichenification** and a more widespread but low-grade involvement of the trunk, face and hands. **White dermographism** is often striking, but not diagnostic of atopic eczema.

The cardinal feature of atopic eczema ***is itching***; and scratching may account for most of the clinical picture. Luckily, the condition remits spontaneously before the age of *10 years in at least two-thirds* of affected children, although it may come back at times of stress.

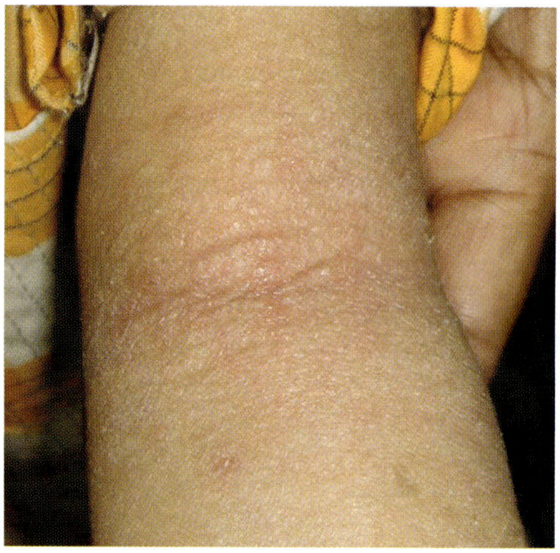

Fig. 7.16

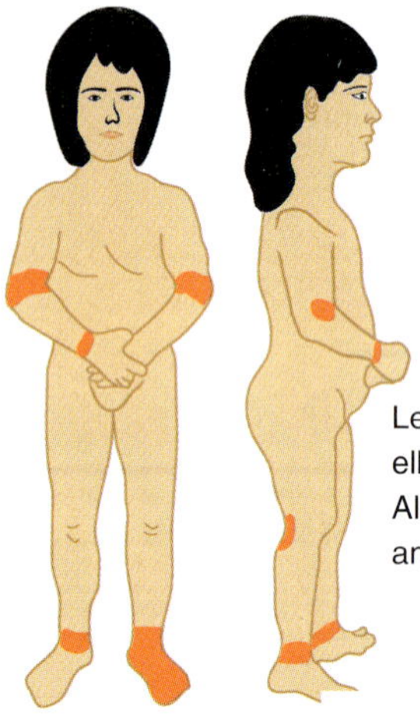

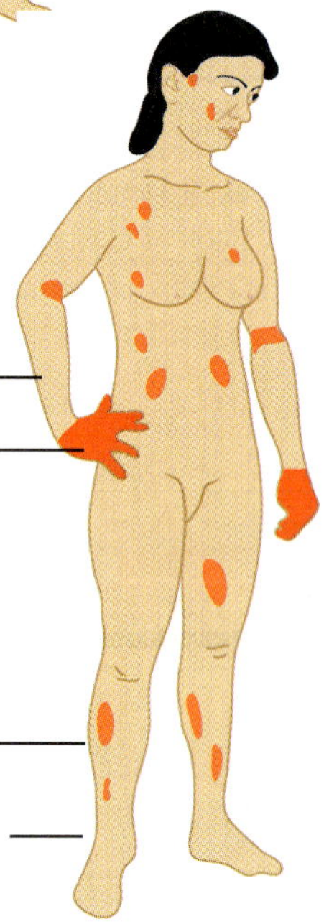

Adult

SECTION - 3

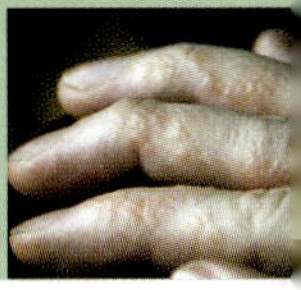

ASSOCIATED DISORDERS

- Allergic Rhinitis/asthma – 30-50%.
- Dry skin, Icthyosis vulgaris.
- Netherton's syndrome.
- Allergic contact dermatitis.
- Alopecia areata.
- Migraine.
- Urticaria.
- Drug sensitivity (Anaphylaxis).

DIAGNOSIS (HANIFIN AND RAJKA'S CRITERIA)

Major (3 should be present)
- Pruritus
- Chronic relapsing course.
- Typical distribution.
- Personal or family history.

Minor (3 should be present).

Eye

Cataract, recurrent kerato conjunctivitis, keratoconus.

Skin

- Facial pallor or erythema, Headlight sign, Dennie-Morgan fold (Fig. 7.17), perifollicular accentuation, Hertoghes sign keratosis pilaris.
- Nipple dermatitis, orbital darkening, Hand dermatitis, Hyperlinear palms (Fig. 7.18), P. alba, white dermographism.
- Icthyosis, xerosis
- Infections.
- Food intolerance.
- ↑ IgE levels/Immediate (type 1 skin reactivity), Wool intolerance.

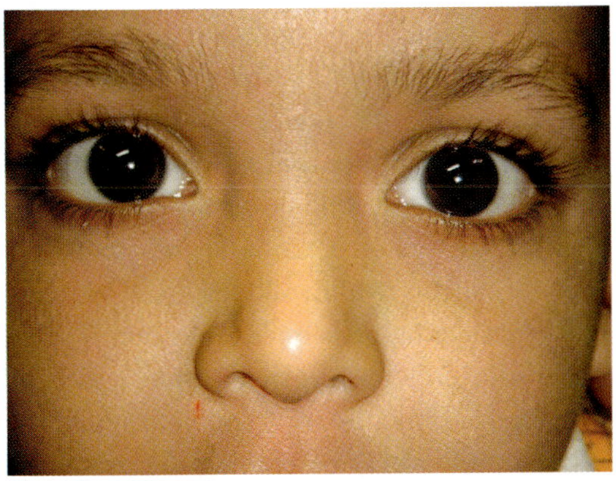

Fig. 7.17: Dennie-Morgan fold

UK WORKING GROUP CRITERIA'S

Major Criterion– Itchy Skin Condition

+ 3 minor
- Onset < 2 years of age.
- General dry skin.

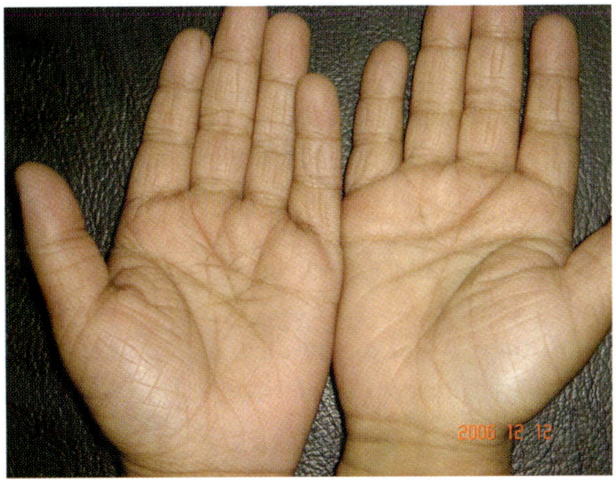

Fig. 7.18: Hyperlinear palms

- History of skin crease involvement and face (< 10 years of age).
- Visible flexural dermatitis (cheeks/forehead < 4 years).
- Personal history of atopy (history of any atopy in 1st degree relative in children < 4 years).

LAB DIAGNOSIS (SUPPORTIVE)

1. Cord blood IgE level > 0.7 KUIL
   Total serum IgE – > than the (N) value of – 50-350 KUIL.
2. **Prick Test**
   For detection of **IgE bound to mast cells in skin**
   To measure IgE Ab in the serum
   ↓ ↓ ↓
   Prausnitz Kustner Test | RAST | ELISA
   - **RAST** (Radio allegro sorbent test)
     Pt's sera + Readymade Ag impregnated disc
     ↓
     IgE Ab in sera get fixed
     ↓
     Radiolabelled antiserum against IgE added

- Sensitive and specific test.
- 420 allergens.
- Costly and should be selective and based on history of exposure.

3. **Mixed Allergen Test**
   - Cost effective.
   - If mixed allergen test is +ve, then specific CAP-RAST test can be done.
4. **Food Allergy**–especially useful in children.
   - Food elimination and provocation tests.
   - DBPCFC (double blind placebo controlled food challenges) are gold standard.
   - (Specific levels IgE to milk/egg/peanut/wheat/fish/soya).
5. **Eosinophilia.**
6. **Gram Stain/KoH/Tzanck smear/pus—C/S.**
7. **Patch Testing.**
8. **Skin Biopsy—not diagnostic.**
   (No investigation is diagnostic for AD)

MANAGEMENT

General Measures and Advice

- Counselling of parents/patients.
- Avoidance of triggers.
- Use of dust mite proof pillows/mattresses.
- Air conditioning.
- Cutting of nails.
- Cotton and loose fitting clothes.
- Use of less alkaline soaps (pH =5.5).

FIRST LINE OF THERAPY

Hydration–most important.
Affected sites–steroids, emollients.
Normal sites–emollients.

Make sure they are applied when the skin is moist Prescribe plenty (at least 500 g/week for the whole skin of an adult and 250 g/week for the whole skin of a child) and ensure they are used at least 3-4 times a day.

For maximal effect, combine the use of creams, ointments, bath oils and emollient soap substitutes.

Skin Care

Atopic dermatitis is associated with a loss of skin lipids such as ceramides. This results in dry skin (xerosis) and enhanced transepidermal water loss. Irritants such as soaps or detergents, contact with chemicals, smoke, alcohol and astringents found in toiletries as well as abrasive clothing can worsen the dry skin. Soaps with minimal defatting activity and a neutral pH should be used in this patient. Xerosis contributes to the development of microfissures and cracks in the skin. This favors the entry of skin pathogens, irritants and allergens that can trigger further skin inflammation. Wet dressings can be used to hydrate and protect severely affected or chronic lesions refractory to skin care. Such dressings may serve as an effective barrier against persistent scratching and enhance absorption of topical medications, thus allowing more rapid healing of excoriated lesions.

Every attempt should be made to allow patients to have normal activity. Certain sports such as swimming are better tolerated than other sports that involve intense perspiration and physical contact. After swimming, chlorine should be rinsed off immediately and the skin lubricated.

Topical Steroids—Mainstay

Choice depends – severity/extent/location/age.
Mild to moderate potency:
E.g. Fluticasone propionate, Mometasone, Prednicarbate, Clobetasone butyrate.

Use the weakest steroid that controls the eczema effectively. Review their use regularly: check for local and systemic side-effects.

ICTHAMMOL and TAR – Over Lichenified Lesions

Antibiotics–Bacterial/Viral/Fungal Infections

Antistaphylococcal antibiotics can be helpful in the treatment of poorly controlled patients with atopic dermatitis that is heavily colonized or infected with *S. aureus*. Topical mupirocin or fusidic acid may be useful in the treatment of localized impetiginized lesions but is expensive in the treatment of patients with extensive skin disease. In the latter situations, patients with sensitive *S. aureus* strains may benefit from a course of systemic antibiotics such as erythromycin and the newer macrolide antibiotics (azithromycin and clarithromycin). However, for macrolide-resistant *S. aureus*, a penicillinase-resistant penicillin (*e.g.*, dicloxacillin) and first-generation cephalosporins may be preferred. In patients with a sudden flare of their atopic dermatitis, consider herpes simplex infection. The presence of punched-out erosions, vesicles and/or infected skin lesions that fail to respond to oral antibiotics raise suspicion that herpes simplex may be causing the exacerbation of skin disease. Antiviral treatment for cutaneous herpes simplex infections is of critical importance in the patient with widespread atopic dermatitis, since life-threatening dissemination has been reported. A slit-lamp eye exam should be carried out in the patient with herpes infection and eye symptoms before ophthalmic steroids are used.

Infection with fungi can contribute to the severity of atopic dermatitis and should be treated with a trial of antifungal antibiotics.

Anti Histaminics

The sedative effect of hydroxyzine chloride is preferred.

SECOND LINE OF TREATMENT

- Intensive topical therapy —Step up therapy.
  —Step down therapy.
- Wet wrap technique.
- Allergy management.

Most food-allergic children outgrow their food hypersensitivity in the first few years of life. Allergy to aeroallergens are a more important trigger factor in older children and adults. Prolonged avoidance of house dust mites in sensitized atopic dermatitis patients has been found to result in reduction of their skin disease. Avoidance measures include: use of house dust mite-proof plastic encasings over pillows, mattresses and box springs; washing bedding in hot water weekly; removal of bedroom carpeting; and increasing indoor humidity levels.

UV Radiation

Natural sunlight can be beneficial to patients with atopic dermatitis. However, if the sunlight is associated with high heat or humidity, thereby triggering sweating and pruritus, it may worsen their skin disease. Broadband ultraviolet B (UVB), broadband ultraviolet A (UVA), narrow-band UVB (311 nm), UVA-1 (340-400 nm) and combined UVAB phototherapy have been reported to reduce skin disease associated with atopic dermatitis. Photochemotherapy with PUVA should be used only in patients with severe, widespread atopic dermatitis.

THIRD LINE OF TREATMENT

1. **Oral steroids**
2. **Cyclosporin-A: quick response**
   Dose:
   –5 mg/kg/day (fast tapering)
   –While tapering add phototherapy
3. **Methotrexate – 5-15 mg/m^2/ week**
4. **Azathioprine – slow action**
   Dose: 1-3 mg/kg/day
5. **Interferon**-50 mg/m² s/c for 12 weeks daily
   ↓ Bacterial infections by ↑ NK cell
6. **Intravenous Immunoglobulins**
7. **Thymopentin - immunostimulator**
   ↑ IFN levels
8. **Topical immunomodulators**
   Tacrolimus - (FK 506) macrolide
   ↓ T cell activation
   MOA- binds to FKBP-12
   Complex – (FKBP-12 + Tacrolimus + Ca +)
   ↓(Calcineurin + Calmodulin)
   Inhibits **phosphatase activity** of calcineurin
   ↓ (-ve)
   NF-AT (Nuclear factor of activated T cell) translocation
   Decrease release of IL –2,3, 4, 5, TNF alpha, INF gamma
   Dose: 0.03% (Children 2-15 years)
   0.1%, 0.03% (adults)
   Pimecrolimus (SDZ-ASM 981)
   Ascomycin derivative
   Binds to cytosolic receptor immunophilin-macrophilin
   This complex ↓ calcineurin phosphatase
   Dose: 0.6 to 1% cream
9. **Mycophenolate mofetil**
   Selectively inhibits *de novo* purine synthesis pathway of lymphocytes
   ↓ PGE_2 production from endothelial cells
   Dose: 1 gm BD oral (first 4 weeks)
   500 mg BD (next 4 weeks)
   S/E ↑ infections/GIT symp anemia
10. **Leukotriene inhibitors**
    Zafirleukast
    Monteleukast

REFERENCES

- Rook's Textbook of Dermatology D. A. Burns, S. M. Breathnach, Neil Cox, Christopher E., Griffiths 7th edn 2004.
- Fitzpatrick's Dermatology in General Medicine 6th edn 2003.
- Bieber T., Leung D.Y.M. (Eds.), *Atopic Dermatitis*, Marcel Dekker, Inc: New York 2002.

CHAPTER 8

COLLAGEN VASCULAR DISORDERS

Lupus Erythematosus

- The term Lupus Erythematosus **(LE)** was first introduced by **Cazenave** in 1851.
- Lupus = "Wolf".

Definition of LE

A group of connective tissue disorders primarily affecting women aged 20-40 years comprising a spectrum of clinical forms in which cutaneous disease may occur with/without systemic involvement.

Classification of LE

1. **DLE (Discoid LE) (Localized)**
   a. Discoid (classical)
   b. Bullous
   c. Mucosal
   d. Profundus
   e. Verrucous
   f. Tumidus
   g. Chilblain Lupus
   h. LE/LP Overlap (Lupus Planus)
2. **DDLE (Disseminated DLE)**
3. **SCLE (Subacute cutaneous LE)**
   a. Annular
   b. Papulosquamous
4. **Drug Induced SLE**
5. **Rowell's Syndrome**
6. **Neonatal LE**
7. **SLE (Systemic LE).**

GILLIAMS CLASSIFICATION OF SKIN LESIONS ASSOCIATED WITH LE

I. **LE Specific Skin Disease (CLE):** i.e. which show characteristic histological changes of LE.
   A. **Acute Cutaneous LE (ACLE)**
      1. Localized ACLE
      2. Generalized ACLE
   B. **Subacute Cutaneous LE (SCLE)**
      1. Annular SCLE
      2. Papulosquamous SCLE
   C. **Chronic Cutaneous LE (DLE)**
      1. Classic discoid LE (DLE)
         a. Localized DLE
         b. Generalized DLE
      2. Hypertrophic/verrucous DLE
      3. Lupus Profundus/Lupus panniculitis
      4. Mucosal DLE
         a. Oral
         b. Conjunctival
      5. Lupus tumidus (Urticarial plaques of LE)
      6. Chilblain LE (Chilblain lupus)
      7. Lichenoid DLE (LE/LP overlap, Lupus Planus).

II. **LE Nonspecific Skin Disease**: i.e. histology not characteristic of LE.
   A. Cutaneous Vascular disease
      1. Vasculitis
         a. Leucocytoclastic vasculitis
         b. Periarteritis nodosa like cutaneous lesions
      2. Vasculopathy
         a. Dego's disease
         b. Secondary atrophie blanche (livedo vasculitis)
      3. Periungual telangiectasia
      4. Livedo reticularis
      5. Thrombophlebitis
      6. Raynaud's phenomenon
      7. Erythromelalgia
   B. Non-Scarring Alopecia
      1. Lupus hair
      2. Telogen effluvium
      3. Alopecia areata
   C. Sclerodactyly

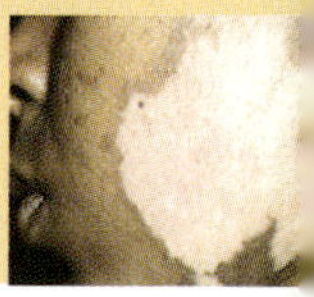

D. Rheumatoid nodules
E. Calcinosis cutis
F. LE non-specific bullous lesions
G. Urticaria
H. Papulonodular mucinosis
I. Cutis laxa/anetoderma
J. Acanthosis nigricans
K. Erythema multiforme
L. Leg ulcers
M. Lichen planus.

ETIOLOGY AND PATHOGENESIS OF LE

Epidemiological Aspects

DLE

1. Female: Male = 2: 1.
2. Peak age of onset–fourth decade in the females and slightly later in the males.

SLE

1. Female: Male = 8: 1–9: 1 (between menarche and menopause)
   And 3: 1 (in the young and older age groups).
2. Peak age of onset
   – Females = 44.2 years
   – Males = 38 years.

Etiological Factors

1. Genetic factors.
2. Immunological factors.
3. Environmental factors.

I. Genetic Factors

High concordance in monozygotic twins–65%.
Frequency of disease/autoantibodies in first degree relatives.
DLE: HLA B7, HLA B8, HLA DR2, HLA DR3, HLA DQW1
SLE: HLA DR2, HLA DR3, HLA B8, HLA A1, HLA DQ Antigens.
Frequency of **complement deficiency** C_2, C_4 (C_4A), CR1, C5–C9.
Somatic mutations occur.
There are 3 genotypes in DLE:
First genotype—3 somatic mutations affecting auto somal genes; early onset type.
Second genotype—4 mutations (1 is X linked).
Third genotype—5 mutations (1 is X linked).
– As a consequence of mutations—3 forbidden clones of lymphocytes synthesizing cellular antibodies develop in LE.

II. Environmental Factors

Ultraviolet Light – UVB and UVA
MOA:
a. Damage to DNA and production of auto antibodies to denatured DNA.
b. Increasing binding of Anti Ro, Anti La and Anti RNP to UV activated keratinocytes.
c. Alteration of cellular membrane phospholipid metabolism.
d. Increase in IL-1 released from keratinocytes and Langerhans cells.
e. Effects on suppressor T cells
   * No effect on DNA repair.

III. Miscellaneous

1. **Sex Hormones:** 20% Premenstrual flares; OCPs exacerbate. Decreasing circulating androgens in male patients.
2. **Dietary Factors:**
   - Alfa Alfa sprouts and related sprouts can trigger LE.
3. **Tobacco Exposures:**
   - Smokers have a high risk of SLE because of Lupogenic aromatic amines.
   - High risk of DLE.
   - Less responsive to anti-malarials.
4. **Infections:**
   - Bacterial DNA, Endotoxins, LPS.
   - EBV, CMV.
   - Human Retroviruses.
5. **Silicone and Heavy Metal Implants.**
6. **Drugs Exacerbating LE:**
   - Drug Induced LE is characterised by:
     – HLA DR4 genotype
     – Antihistone antibodies

Causative Drugs DLE

DLE	INH, Dapsone, Penicillamine, Griseofulvin
SCLE	ACE inhibitor, Penicillamine, NSAIDS
SLE	Hydralazine , Procainamide, Minocycline, INH, Phenytoin

PATHOGENESIS

Overview

It is a multifactorial disease with an interplay of immunological and genetic factors. The most important factor is the role of release of nuclear antigens because of enhanced apoptosis.

Model for Pathogenesis

First Phase: Susceptibility Phase–HLA and other genes.

Second Phase: Induction Phase–UV light and other triggers (Loss of self-tolerance).

Third Phase: Expansion Phase (Auto-antibody formation)–T cell expansion, Epitope spreading.

Fourth Phase: Injury Phase (Immune complex formation)–Clinically most important.

Antinuclear Antibodies: Positive in >98% cases of SLE. By Fluorescent Antibody Testing.
Significant Titres > 1: 160.

Autoantibody	*Incidence*	*Clinical significance*
ANA–Antinuclear Ab	95%	SPA repeatedly negative test makes SLE unlikely
Anti DNA – ds	70%	Most specific for active SLE and severe nephritis
Anti DNA – ss		Non-specific; found in a variety of rheumatic and non rheumatic disease
Anti Sm	30%	Specific for SLE
Anti RNP	40%	Overlap syndrome; If positive in SLE, without ANA, risk of nephritis is low
Anti–Ro (SS - A)	30%	Sjögren's, SCLE, ANA negative LE, Lupus in elderly, Neonatal lupus, C–2 deficient LE
Anti LA (SS–B)	10%	Always associated with Anti Ro; Risk for nephritis is low if positive in SLE
Antihistone	70%	Drug induced LE
Anticardiolipin	50%	Higher risk of thrombosis, higher PTT, VDRL +ve APLA syndrome
Anti ribosomal P	15%	Associated with psychosis
Anti erythrocyte	60%	Overt hemolysis
Anti lymphocyte	70%	Leukopenia
Anti neuronal	60%	In CSF, high IgG correlate with diffuse CNS lupus

ANA Patterns—Clinical Significance

Pattern	*Previous nomenctature*	*Autoantibody*	*Associated disease*
Particulate	Speckled, thready, fibrillar, reticular	Anti–RNP's Anti–Sm Anti Ro. La Anti SCL	MCTD, SLE, Scleroderma, undifferentiated connective tissue disease
Homogenous	Diffuse, solid	Antibody to DNA-histone complex	SLE, connective tissue disease
Peripheral	Shaggy, rim, membranous	Anti DNA	Active SLE (most specific), common in LE with nephritis
Speckled	True speckled, "Pepper dots"	Anti–Centromere	Scleroderma/ CREST, Raynaud's phenomenon
Nucleolar	Large discrete speckles		Scleroderma, Raynaud's phenomenon, uncommon in SLE, rare in MCTD

Skin Biopsy with DIF (Lupus Band Test Positivity)

	Lesional	*Non lesional, Sun exposed*	*Non lesional, Non sun exposed*
SLE	50 – 100%	73 – 90%	26 – 92%
SCLE	54 – 100%	18 – 100%	0 – 100%
DLE	60 – 94%	0 – 10%	0 – 10%

Pattern of Deposition: Linear, granular, shaggy.

In DLE:

Dermoepidermal junction (DEJ) = IgG, IgM (IgM>IgG)

Cytoid bodies = IgM, IgA

In SCLE:

DEJ = IgG and IgM (IgG>IgM)

Cytoid bodies = IgM, IgA

In SLE:

- DEJ: IgG, IgM, IgA, C3 (IgG>IgM)
- Cytiod bodies: IgM, IgA
- Epidermal nuclei: IgG.

Clinical Features

DLE

Definition: A relatively benign, autoimmune disorder of the skin most frequently involving the face, characterized by various sized, reddish, well-defined, scaly patches which tend to heal with atrophy, scarring and pigmentary changes.

History of Raynaud's phenomenon, chilblains, poor peripheral circulation, arthralgias, photosensitivity.

a. **Classical DLE:** Circumscribed as discoid lesions (Fig. 8.1):

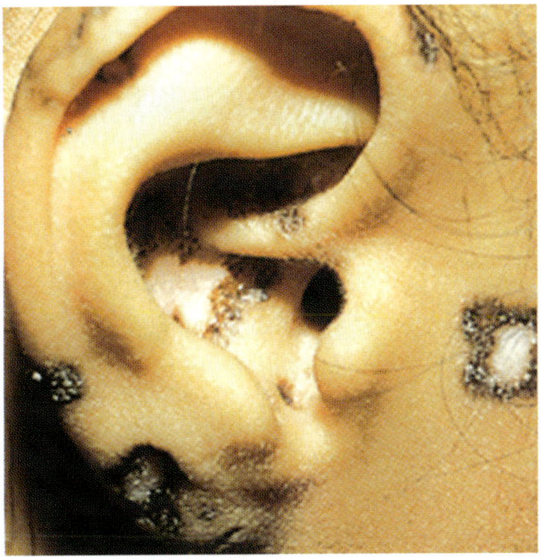

Fig. 8.1: Papules with an atrophic hypopigmented center and hyperpigmented border (chronic discoid LE)

- Most common on face.
- Scarring alopecia on scalp.
- Tin Tack Sign/Carpet Tack/Cat's Tongue Sign positive.
- Wide follicular pits in concha/triangular fossa of ear.
- Nail changes.

Histology: Epidermal atrophy, follicular plugging, basement zone degeneration, hair follicle degeneration and mucin/PAS positive basement membrane deposition.

Ancillary features—civatte bodies.

Diagnosis:

Skin biopsy.

DIF: Deposit of IgG and C3 in BMZ of involved skin in 60-80 % of cases, negative in normal uninvolved skin.

Antibody: Low titre ANA, anti SS DNA.

b. **Chilblain Lupus:** Association with antiphospholipid Antibodies; female; pregnancy.
c. **LE Profundus (Panniculitis):** Subcutaneous deep dermal nodules which heal leaving behind a depressed area. D/D: Sarcoidosis.
d. **Verrucous LE (lupus hypertrophicus et profundus).**
e. **LE–LP Overlap:** Lupus Planus–H/P shows overlapping features–lupus band is positive but DIF suggestive of LP.
f. **Rubric LP:** Hypertrophic LE + LP.
g. **Mucosal DLE:** Oral, conjunctival and genitalia involvement.
h. **Lupus Erythematosus Tumidus:** Succulent, edematous, urticarial plaques.
i. **Bullous DLE.**
j. **DLE with Annular Lesions:** lupus erythematosus gyratus in reaction to the underlying malignancy.
k. **Rowell's syndrome:** LE + Erythema multiforme like lesions, speckled type of ANA + with AntiRo, AntiLa Positivity.

DDLE

- Disseminated DLE.
- Lesions below the chin.

Sub-acute LE

The subset comprises around **10%** patients of LE.

2/3rd: Papulosquamous.

1/3rd: Annular, polycyclic.

Lesions are characteristically photosensitive and lesions occur in sun exposed parts.

Lesions heal without scarring but vitiligo like leukoderma and telengiectasias +/–.

Histology: Interface dermatitis, superficial dermatitis.

Diagnosis: Skin biopsy.

DIF: Deposit of IgG and C3 in BMZ of involved skin in 50-60 % of cases, 10-20% in normal uninvolved skin.

Auto Antibody: Low titre ANA , anti ssDNA, Autoantibodies to Ro/SS-A.

Neonatal LE

- Skin lesions of SCLE in newborns (within 1st 2 months).
- Mothers have asymptomatic LE.
- Babies affected by IgG AntiRo transplacentally.
- Heart Block: Usually third degree.
- Speckled ANA.

Drug Induced LE

HLA-DR4, Antihistone Antibodies, Slow acetylators

Male : Female = 4 : 1.

Drugs Causing

- **Antihypertensives:**
  β–Blockers = Propanolol, Atenolol, Acebutolol, Labetolol, Pindolol, Oxprenolol, Practolol.
  Others = Hydrochlorthiazide, Minoxidil, Captopril, Hydralazine, Methyldopa.
- **Antibiotics**–Cotrimoxazole, Penicillin, Streptomycin, Nitrofurantoin, Tetracyline, Sulphonamides, Minocyline, Quinine.
- **ATT**–INH, PAS.
- **Anti Fungal**–Griseofulvin.

- **Anti Epileptics**–Phenytoin, Carbamazepine, Valproate, Primidone, Ethosuximide.
- **NSAIDS**–Piroxicam, Phenylbutazone, Ibuprofen.
- Others–Chlorpromazine.
  - OCP's
  - Lithium
  - Propylthiouracil
  - Hydroxyurea
  - Sulphasalazine
  - Gold Salts
  - Clofibrate, Simvastatin
  - IFN
  - Procainamide
  - Penicillamine
  - Allopurinol.

SLE

Definition: A systemic disease characterized by the association of immunological abnormalities with pathological changes affecting a number of organ systems, in particular, skin, joints and the vasculature.

INITIAL MANIFESTATIONS

a. Articular = 58%
b. Cutaneous = 13.5%
   Systemic Fatigue, Weight loss, Menstrual irregularities (irregular in 18%, absent in 75%).

Raynaud's Phenomenon (35%)

Various skin manifestations are: Skin lesions seen in 80% patients.

1. Cutaneous erythema
2. Butterfly rash (51%)
3. Photosensitivity (63%)
4. Facial oedema
5. Bullous lesions (8%)
6. Epidermal necrolysis; Rowell's syndrome
7. Chronic discoid lesions (Fig. 8.2)
8. Urticaria
9. Hypocomplementemic vasculitis
10. Papular/nodular lesions due to mucinous deposits
11. Reticulate telangiectatic erythema
12. Nail changes
13. Gangrene of tip of fingers and toes
14. Leg ulcers
15. Erythromelalgia
16. Widespread purpura
17. Livedo reticularis
18. Atrophie blanche

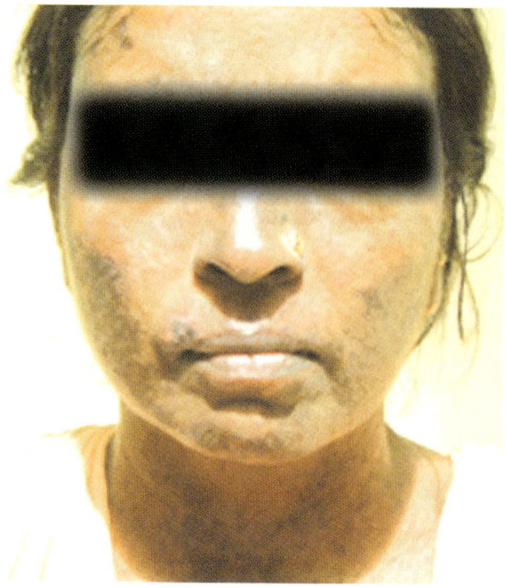

Fig. 8.2: Atrophic hypopigmented patches with peripheral hyperpigmentation (chronic discoid lupus erythematosus)

19. Chilblain lupus
20. Pigmentary disturbances.
21. Alopecia–diffuse hair loss (Fig. 8.3)
22. Lupus hair
23. Subcutaneous nodules
24. Relapsing nasal and auricular chondritis
25. Hyperkeratotic follicular erythematous papules
26. Widespread icthyosis
27. Hyperkeratosis of palms and soles
28. Bullous LE
29. Mucosal lesions: Palate, buccal, mucosa, gums, chelitis, nasal septum, genital
30. Pemphigus erythematosus.

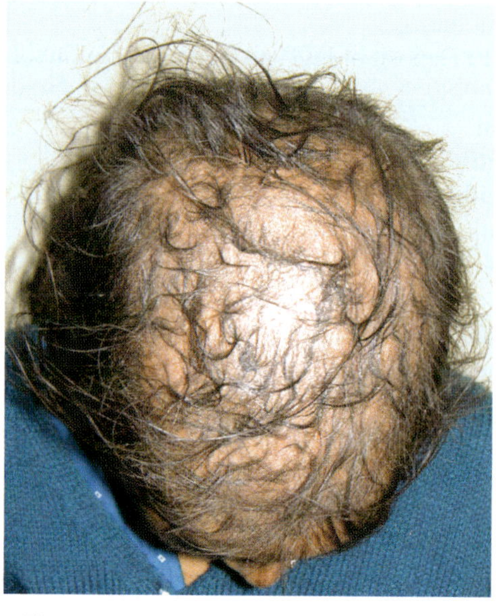

Fig. 8.3: Non-scarring alopecia of scalp

VESICOBULLOUS LESIONS IN LE

- **LE Specific**
  1. Acute Cutaneous LE
     Toxic Epidermal Necrolysis like LE
  2. Subacute Cutaneous LE
     Toxic Epidermal Necrolysis like SCLE
     Vesicobullous annular SCLE
  3. Chronic Cutaneous LE
     Bullous DLE
- **LE Non-specific**
  1. Bullous SLE
     - DH like LE non-specific skin disease.
     - EBA like LE non-specific-skin disease.
     - LE nonspecific vesicobullous eruption of SLE.
  2. Vesicobullous disorders are reported to occur in LE but relationship not well established.
     - Bullous pemphigoid.
     - Dermatitis herpetiformis.
     - Pemphigus erythematous.
     - Porphyria cutanea tarda.

Bullous SLE

- Formation of subepidermal vesicles; containing neutrophils with microabscesses and nuclear dust and fibrin at tips of dermal papillae.
- Linear deposit of IgA, IgG, IgM and C_3 at basement membrane.
- Target antigen: Type VII collagen.
- Bullous lesions: On face, neck, upper trunk–heal with milia formation.
- Treatment = Dapsone + Prednisolone.

EXTRACUTANEOUS MANIFESTATION OF SLE

1. **General:** Fever (90%), fatigue, malaise, weight loss.
2. **Musculoskeletal:** (90%)
   - Symmetric, small joint arthralgia, arthritis (non-deforming or deforming), morning stiffness.
   - Myalgia, myositis.
   - Tendonitis, Avascular (aseptic) bone necrosis.
3. **Haematologic:**
   - Anemia–Normocytic, Normochromic, Hemolytic.
   - Leukopenia–lymphopenia, granulocytopenia.
4. **Cardiopulmonary:**
   - Pleurisy, pleural effusion, aseptic pneumonitis, pulmonary hemorrhage.
   - Pericarditis, tachycardia, cardiomegaly, congestive heart failure, arrhythmias, conduction defects, coronary arteritis, libmann sacks endocarditis.
5. **Renal:** (67%)
   - Mesangial glomerulonephritis (WHO: Class II): mild proteinuria.
   - Focal proliferative glomerulonephritis (WHO: Class III): Proteinuria, hematuria, nephrotic syndrome.
   - Diffuse proliferative glomerulonephritis (WHO: Class IV): Proteinuria, hematuria, RBC casts, renal insufficiency, hypertension, nephrotic syndrome.
   - Membranous glomerulonephritis (WHO : Class V): Severe proteinuria, nephrotic syndrome.
6. **Neuropsychiatric:** (25%)
   Peripheral neuritis, neuropathy, transverse myelitis, Guillain-Barré syndrome, chorea, choreoathetosis, seizures.
   Headache (severe, migraine like).
   Brain infarcts due to cerebral arteritis.
   Organic brain syndrome–psychosis due to cerebral arteritis.
7. **Psychological depression.**
8. **Gastrointestinal:**
   Anorexia, nausea, vomiting, abdominal pain, bowel infarction/perforation (mesenteric vasculitis); Pancreatitis, peritonitis, ascites, hepatomegaly, chronic active hepatitis.
9. **Ocular:**
   Conjunctivitis, Episcleritis.
   Blindness–Due to central retinal artery occlusion; cytoid bodies, keratoconjunctivitis.
10. **Lymphatic System:** Lymphadenopathy, splenomgaly.

ACR REVISED CRITERIA FOR DIAGNOSIS OF SLE

Person will have SLE if any 4 or more out of 11 criteria are present, serially or simultaneously, during an interval of observation.

1. **Malar Rash**–fixed erythema over the malar eminences, tending to spare the nasolabial folds (Fig. 8.4).

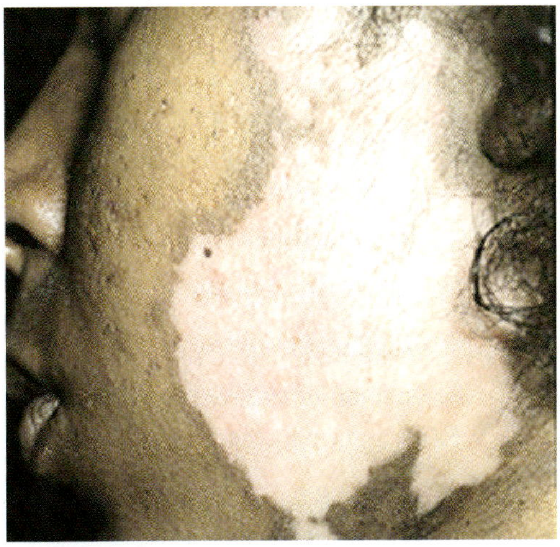

Fig. 8.4: Malar rash with hypopigmentation

2. **Discoid Rash**–Erythematous raised patches with keratotic scaling, atrophic scarring.
3. **Photosensitivity**–Unusual reaction to sunlight.
4. **Oral Ulcers**–Oral/Nasopharyngeal; usually painless, observed by physican.
5. **Arthritis**–Non-erosive arthritis involving 2 or more peripheral joints, tenderness, swelling or effusion.
6. **Serositis**–Pleuritis: pericarditis: ECG changes, rub, pericardial effusion.
7. **Renal Disorder:**
   a. Persistent Proteinuria—0.5g/day or greater than 3+ Cellular Casts–Red cell, Hb, granular, tubular, mixed.
8. **Neurological Disorder:** Seizures – in the absence of offending drugs or known metabolic derangements e.g. uremia.
   Psychosis–In the absence of offending drug/metabolic derangements.
9. **Haematological Disorder:**
   - Hemolytic anemia with reticulocytosis.
   - Leukopenia <4,000/μl on 2 or more occasions.
   - Lymphopenia <1,500/μl on 2 or more occasions.
   - Thrombocytopenia <100,000/μl on 2 or more occasions/in absence of offending drugs.
10. **Immunological Disorders:**
    a. Anti – DNA (dsDNA)
    b. Anti Sm
    c. Antiphospholipid Antibodies:
       I. Increasing IgG/IgM anticardiolipin antibodies.
       II. Positive result of anticoagulant test.
       III. False positive STS at least for 6 months.
11. **Antinuclear Antibody**–An abnormal titre by Immunofluorescence and absence of drug Induced Lupus Syndrome.
    The ARA criteria were again revised in 1998 and LE cell test removed.

APPROACH TOWARDS A PATIENT WITH SLE

1. History.
2. Physical Examination.
3. Complete Blood Counts: Hb, TLC, DLC, P/C +PTT – for hemolytic anemia, leukopenia, lymphopenia, thrombocytopenia.
4. Erythrocyte sedimentation rate: Elevated.
5. Haematocrit.
6. Direct Coombs Test.
7. Urinanalysis: For albuminuria, red cells and casts.
8. KFT–serum creatinine to assess renal status.
9. VDRL/WR (Wasserman reaction): Biological false positive.
10. Antinuclear Antibody (ANA) and RA factor.
11. Antibody:
    - Anti Sm Antibody.
    - Anti–dsDNA.
    - Anti Ro.
    - Anti histones.
    - Anti thyroid antibodies; gastric parietal cell cytoplasmic antibodies.
    - Antiphosphoslipid antibodies: Lupus anticoagulant.
12. Complement levels: Decrease in C3, C4 levels, C2 levels.
13. Skin biopsy:
    a. Histopathology
    b. Direct immunofluorescence.
14. Miscellaneous:
    - Cryogubulins – positive in 10% of patients with SLE.
    - Cold agglutinins – positive in 6% cases.
    - B2-macroglobulins; Serum interferons – indicators of disease activity in SLE.
    - Serum C reactive proteins – elevated slightly in SLE.
    - Australia Antigen: Can be seen in 25% patients of SLE antibodies.
    - T cell Counts – decrease; B counts cell – Normal
    - Kidney biospy.
    - Other tests can be done to assess **disease activity:**
      – Soluble IL-2 Receptor levels in serum
      – Serum ICAM
      – Serum TNF–α
      – IL–10 in serum
      – Serum heat shock proteins
      – Urinary neopterin levels
      – Urinary IL–6 levels.

TREATMENT OF LE

General Measures

- It is an episodic disease, therefore tailor treatment according to patient.
- Maintain morale.
- Bed rest: During severe exacerbations.
- Protection from sunlight: Broad brimmed hats, tight weave clothing, sunscreens with SPF > 15 UV blocking films.
- Avoid artificial sources of UV light.
- Low fat diet: Marine oil eicosapentaenoic acid (20g/d).

Topical Therapy

Local Glucocorticoids

- Triamcinolone acetonide (face)(0.1%)
- Clobetasol propionate (0.05%)
- Betamethasone dipropionate (0.05%)
  *Twice weekly BD application f/b 2 weeks rest.

Intralesional Glucocorticoids

- Triamcinolone acetonide 2.5–5 mg/ml with a 30 G needle; infiltrate the active border.
- Useful only if limited lesions.

SYSTEMIC THERAPY IN LE (Table 8.1)

First Line:
- Hydroxychloroquine
- Hydroxychloroquine + Quinacrine
- Chloroquine + Quinacrine.

Second Line:
- Dapsone
- Retinoids
- Isotretinoin
- Etretinate
- Acitretin
- Thalidomide

Third Line:
- Clofazimine
- Gold

Fourth Line:
- Systemic Glucocorticoids
  – Oral prednisolone
  – Pulse I/V methylprednisolone.
- Azathioprine
- Methotrexate
- Cyclophosphamide.
- Sulphasalazine
- Phenytoin
- Danazol
- Dehydroepiandrosterone
- Cytosine arabinoside
- Cyclosporine
- Chlorambucil
- Immunotherapy
  – High dose I/V globulin
  – CD_4 T cell depleting monoclonal antibody
- Phototherapy (UVA-1)
- Plasmapheresis
- Levamisole
- Mycophenolate mofetil.

Glucocorticoids

- Regimen 1: Daily Oral Short acting steroid (methyl prednisolone) 1-2 mg/kg daily.
- Regimen 2: I/V methylprednisdone 500-1000 mg everyday for 3-5 days; then 1-1.5 mg/kg/day of oral prednisolone.
- Regimen 3: 1 or 2+ other immunosuppressant (Table 8.2).

Indications for Steroids

1. Vasculitis.
2. Severe dermatitis of SCLE.
3. Polyarthritis.
4. Polyserosits.
5. Myocarditis.
6. Lupus pneumonitis.
7. Glomerulonephritis–proliferative type.
8. Hemolytic anemia.
9. Thrombocytopenia.
10. Diffuse CNS syndrome.
11. Severe cognitive defects.
12. Myopathies.
13. Peripheral neuropathies.
14. Lupus crisis–high fever and prostration.

Table 8.1

Agent	*Initial dose*	*Maintenance dose*	*Response*	*Toxicities*
Hydroxy Chloroquine	400-600 mg/day	100–400 mg/day	Dermatitis, arthralgias, arthritis, oral ulcers, fatigue	Retinal damage, corneal deposit, rashes, alopecia, peripheral neuropathy, cardiomyopathy, nausea, anorexia, diarrhoea, psychosis
Chloroquine	500-1000 mg/d	500 mg daily or A/D	- do -	Most toxic for retina
Quinacrine	100 mg/day	50-100 mg/day	Fatigue	Aplastic anemia, Yellow pigmentation of skin; no retinal damage
Dapsone	25 mg BD	25 mg/day	Dermatitis	Methemoglobunemia, Sulfhemoglobunemia, Hemolytic anemia, GI intolerance
Etretinate	1mg/kg/day		0.25–0.5 mg/kg/day	Dermatitis hemolysis in G6PD deficient ht., Hyperlipidemia, Cheilitis

Table 8.2

Drug	*Initial dose*	*Maintenance*	*Advantages*	*Toxicities*
Azathioprine Requires 6-12 months to work well	1-3 mg/kg/d	1-2 mg/kg/d	Less flares Less renal scarring Less glucocorticid dose req.	Bone marrow suppression Leukopenia Infections Malignancies Infertility Nausea
Cyclophosphamide Requires 2-16 weeks to work well	1-3 mg/kg/d orally or 8 –20 mg/kg/I/V once a month + MESNA	0.5-2 mg/kg/day orally or 8-20 mg/kg I/V every 4 – 12 weeks + MESNA	More effective than Azathioprine	Nausea Leukopenia Infections Malignancies Cystitis Infertility Menopuase Alopecia

- **Neonatal LE:** Topical corticosteroids + Implantation of pacemaker.
- **SLE in Pregnancy:** If evidence of heart block/ then–Dexamethasone 4 mg/day + I/V gamma globulins.
- **Antiphospholipid Syndrome:** Warfarin, Aspirin: Offer protection.

Discoid Lupus Erythematosus

1. Apply superpotent topical steroids to the lesions twice daily.
2. Use sunscreens:
   - If the patient responds, continue the treatment, emphasizing the need for year-round photoprotection.
   - If the patient fails to respond and there are fewer than *10 lesions*, consider intralesional triamcinolone acetonide 5-10 mg/mL to the active lesions.
   - If there are *more than 10 lesions*, or there is active scalp/face disease, consider in this order:
     a. Hydroxychloroquine 200 mg twice daily.
     b. Chloroquine 250 mg daily.
     c. The combination of one of the above with quinacrine 100 mg daily.
     d. Isotretinoin 40-80 mg daily.
     e. Thalidomide 50-100 mg daily to start and increasing to as much as 400 mg if the response is inadequate.
     f. The addition of a systemic immunosuppressive agent such as azathioprine 50-100 mg daily, or mycophenolate mofeteil 2-3 g per day.

Subacute Cutaneous Lupus Erythematosus (SCLE)

In patients failing to improve with topical treatments, consider in the following order:

a. Hydroxychloroquine 200 mg twice daily.
b. Chloroquine 250 mg daily.
c. The combination of one of the above with quinacrine 100 mg daily.
d. Isotretinoin 40-80 mg daily.
e. Thalidomide 50-100 mg daily to start and increasing to as much as 400 mg if not responding.
f. The addition of a systemic immunosuppressive agent such as a pulse of systemic steroids (tapered over 1-2 months), azathioprine 50-100 mg daily, or mycophenolate mofeteil 2-3 g per day.

PROGNOSIS

i. ACLE/SLE

5 years survival rate = 80-95%
10 years survival rate = 70-90%

Ominous prognostic signs:

- Hypertension
- Nephritis
- Systemic vasculitis
- CNS disease.

ii. SCLE

Intermittent recurrences of skin disease activity:

- 15% patients of SCLE will develop active SLE, including lupus nephritis.
- **Risk Factors:** Papulosquamous SCLE, high titer **ANA**, leukopenia, antibodies to dsDNA.

iii. CCLE:

DLE–risk of developing SLE 5-6.5%.
DDLE–risk of developing SLE 22%.

Risk Factors:

- DDLE.
- Males developing DLE before 40 years.
- HLA B8.
- Lab abnormalities/High ANA titres.

REFERENCES

- Therapeutic Strategies in Dermatology Timothy G. Berger, M.D. Bruce U. Wintroub, M.D.
- Rook's Textbook of Dermatology D. A. Burns, S. M. Breathnach, Neil Cox, Christopher E. Griffiths 7th edn 2004.
- Fitzpatrick's Dermatology in General Medicine 6th edn 2003.
- Lever's Histopathology of the Skin by David E Elder, Rosalie Elenitsas, Bernett L Johnson, George F Murphy 9th edn. 2004.

Scleroderma

TYPES

i. Localized.
ii. Systemic.

SYSTEMIC SCLEROSIS

Classification

1. Prescleroderma:
   - Raynaud's phenomenon + Nail fold capillary changes.
   - Digital ischemic changes.
   - Antibodies (Ab):
     - Anticentromere Ab (ACA)
     - Antitopoisomerase - I
2. Diffuse SSc:
   - Onset of skin changes within 1 year of Raynaud's phenomenon.
   - Truncal or acral involvement.
   - Visceral organ involvement.
   - Tendon friction rubs.
   - Nail fold capillary dilatation and dropout.
   - Anti Scl–70 Ab.
   - Absence of ACA.
3. Limited SSc–CREST:
   Diagnostic criterion is:
   - Raynaud's phenomenon present for years.
   - Limited skin involvement.
   - (10-15 years) Pulmonary Hypertension.
   - Calcification.
   - Telangiectasia.
   - Esophageal dysfunction.
   - ACA (70-80%).
   - Dilatation of nail fold capillaries without dropout.
4. Scleroderma sine scleroderma:
   - Raynaud's phenomenon present.
   - No skin involvement.
   - Ab to Scl – 70, ACA.
5. Mixed Connective Tissue Disease (MCTD):
   - U1-RNP positive.
   - Benign course.

ARA CRITERIA'S FOR DIAGNOSIS OF SSC

Major criteria: Scleroderma proximal to digits, affecting limbs, face, neck or trunk.

Minor criteria:

a. Sclerodactyly
b. Digital pitted scars
c. B/L pulmonary fibrosis
   1 major/2 minor.

Clinical Features

1. Cutaneous changes (Figs. 8.5 to 8.8)
   - Bound down skin
   - Facial changes
   - Digital pitted scars
   - Pulp atrophy
   - Nails
   - Telangiectasias
   - Pigmentation.
2. Calcinosis
   - Fingers
   - Male > Female (10 times).
3. Bone changes
   - Absorption of terminal phalanges
   - Erosive arthropathy.
4. GIT
   - Macroglossia
   - Esophagus

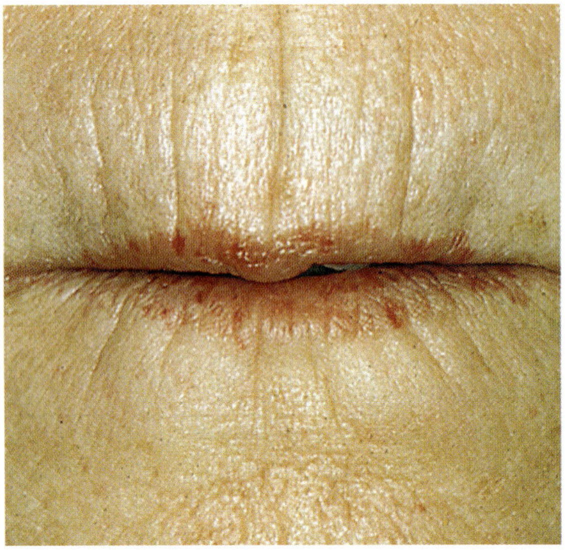

Fig. 8.5: Pinched mouth associated with pursed lips and matted telangiectases of acrosclerosis

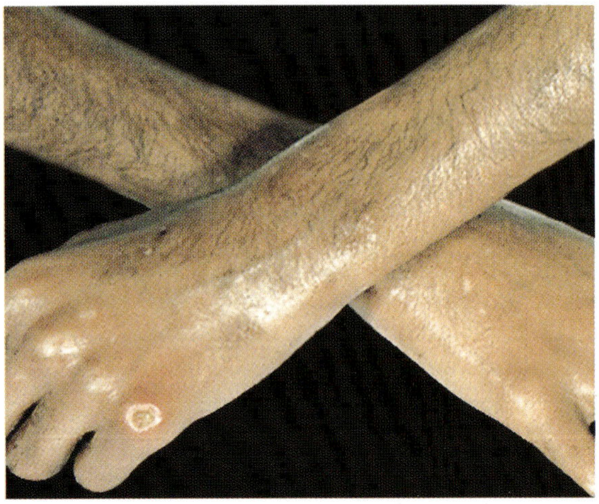

Fig. 8.6: Tight skin of arms and fingers of acrosclerosis has resulted in flexion contractures and in ulcerations of knuckles

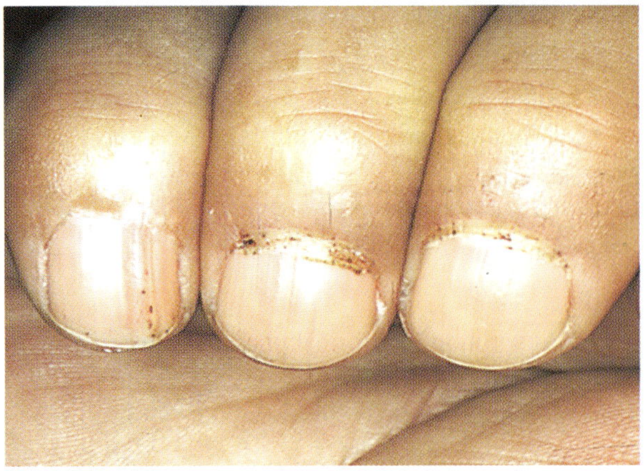

Fig. 8.7: Petechiae in the cuticle, posterior nail folds and beneath a nail plate

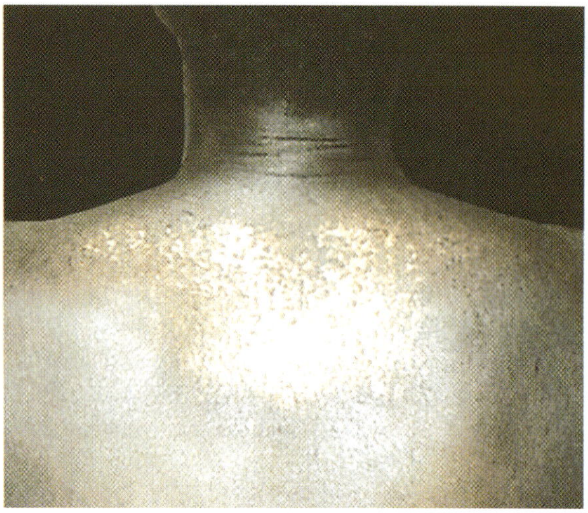

Fig. 8.8: "Salt and pepper" pattern on the chest, shoulders and neck

- Stomach
- Intestine
- Colon.

5. Lungs
   - Restrictive lung disease
   - Radiological abnormality – 40%
   - Deranged PFTs–70%
   - Recurrent episodes of pneumothorax, pleurisy, effusion or pneumonia
   - Diffuse basal interstitial fibrosis.
6. Cardiac
7. Renal–slight proteinuria (earliest)
8. Muscles
9. Tendon
10. Joints
11. Dental–thickening and calcification of periodontal ligament
12. CNS
13. Eyes.

Laboratory Investigations

Hematological:

1. Hb, TLC, DLC
   ESR raised in 50%
   Serum globulins increased
2. Biochemical profile:
   RFT–blood urea, serum creatinine, urine analysis
   LFTs
3. P.F.T.—Pulmonary Function Tests
4. Chest X-ray
5. Barium swallow
6. Endoscopy

7. False + VDRL serology—5%
8. Cold agglutunins—25%
9. LE cell–8%
10. RA factor–30%
11. **Antinuclear antibody**
    - Anticardiolipin Ab–25%
    - Anticentromere Ab–40–70% (seen in CREST)
    - Scl – 70 (Topoisomerase-1 Ab)–20% (SSC)
    - Anti –ds DNA Ab – negative
    - Antiendothelial Ab – 30%
    - Anti IgE and Antismooth muscle Ab may be found
    - Antihistone Ab–42%
    - Antinucleolar Ab–20-30%
    - Anti U1-RNP–5-10%.

ANA positivity
ANA 78% (rat liver)
97% (hep-2 cells)
Speckled/homogenous/nucleolar pattern.

Skin Biopsy

- Sclerosis, collagen increase, loss of appendages.
- DIF–IgM and C3 are found at the basement membrane and dermal vessels.

Course and Prognosis

Systemic scleroderma:
- Male—poor prognosis.
- Renal/lung involvement—poor prognosis.
- HLA B8—poor prognosis.
- Less CMI—poor prognosis.

Treatment (Table 8.3)

Symptomatic: 0.025% to 0.05% tretinoin–lessens facial tightening.
Skin ulcers:
- Surgical debridement.
- Antibiotics.
- Local nitroglycerine.

Skin Involvement

Vasodilators

1. **Ca channel blocker:**
   Nifedipine (30-60 mg daily)
   S/E–headache, flushing, edema
   Others–diltiazem, verapamil
2. Low dose Aspirin
3. Dipyridamole (400 mg daily)
4. Pentoxyphylline (400 mg TDS)

Table 8.3: Treatment of systemic sclerosis

(i) ***Raynaud phenomenon***
Nifedipine, verapamil hydrochloride
Losartan potassium
Iloprost
(ii) ***Pulmonary hypertension***
Epoprostenol
Iloprost (carboprostacyclin)
Captopril
(iii) ***Renal crises***
Captopril
Enalapril malate
Kidney dialysis
Kidney transplantation
(iv) ***Skin induration***
Immunosuppressants
Methotrexate
Cyclosporine
(v) ***Antifibrotics***
D-Penicillamine
Colchicine
Interferon gamma
Relaxin
(vi) ***Interstitial lung disease***
Cyclophosphamide

5. Losartan (Antagonist of Angiotensin II)–50 mg OD
   S/E–dry cough, muscle cramps, backpain, dizziness, insomnia
6. PGE1 (Iloprost)
   - Prologed vasodilatation
   - Less platelet aggregation
   - Promotes endothelial cell lining
   - 2 mg/kg/min I/V infusion for 8 hours × 3 days
   - Oral iloprost 50 mg BD.

Immunosuppressants

1. Mtx–15 mg to 25 mg/week for 24 weeks.
2. Cyclosporine – selectively low IL–2
   1 mg/kg/day to 5mg/kg/day–48 weeks
   S/E – nephrotoxicity.
3. Azathioprine.
4. Cyclophosphamide.
5. Extracorporeal photopheresis.
6. Antithymocyte globulin (3-5 mg/kg × 5 days).

Antifibrotic Agents

- Reduce synthesis, excretion or polymerization of collagen.
- Enhance collagenase activity.

- Neutralize (TGF-B, IL-4, 6)
  1. D–penicillamine–250 mg TDS
     S/E–BM depression/nephritic synd/GIT distress/skin reactions
  2. Colchicine–0.6 mg BD
  3. Interferon gamma
  4. Relaxin–S/c infusion–24 weeks.

SYSTEMIC INVOLVEMENT

Kidney Involvement

- ACE inhibitor
  - Captopril (12.5-50 mg)
  - Enalapril
- Kidney dialysis
- Renal transplantation.

Lung Involvement

- Cyclophosphamide alone or with low dose prednisolone
- I/V iloprost–also effective.

NEWER THERAPIES

- Minocycline–100 mg OD × 4 weeks
- Psoralen–UVA
- Oral Etretinate
- Autologous stem cell transplantation
- Thalidomide
- **Etanercept**
  Fusion protein of soluble TNF receptor linked to human immunoglobulin
  25 mg s/c, twice weekly–6 months.

MORPHOEA

Definition: Cutaneous sclerosis without systemic involvement.

Epidemiology: Female: male=4:1.

Aetiology (Localized)

- Trauma/Immobilization.
- Post BCG vaccination/vit. K injection.
- Post Varicella/ measles/B. burgdorferi infection.
- Post radiotherapy/pregnancy.
- Phenylketonuria.

Types of Localized Scleroderma

1. Plaque (classic) (Fig. 8.9)

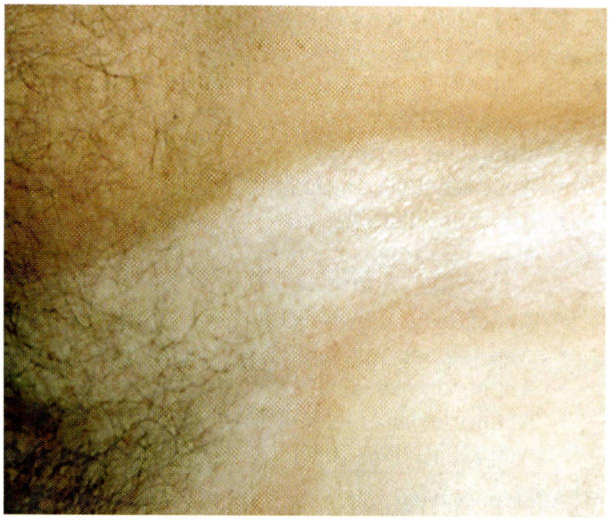

Fig. 8.9: Atrophic hypopigmented patch with hyperpigmented border of morphea

Circumscribed sclerotic plaque with ivory centre and red violet periphery (lilac ring).
- Upper trunk, breast, abdomen, thigh
- Chest wall involvement
- Raynaud's phenomenon, Telangiectasia, Visceral involvement, Radial furrowing, nail fold capillary changes–*absent.*

2. Guttate.
3. Linear.
4. Subcutaneous (Nodular/Keloidal).
5. Solitary Morphea Profunda.
6. Generalized Morphea.
7. Atrophoderma of Pasini
   - Superficial forms
   - Hyperpigmented atrophic plaques
   - Cliff drop appearance of the borders.
8. En coup de Sabre
   - Facial hemiatrophy
   - Extending to the bone
   - Overlying skin involved.

Histology

Thickening of amorphous collagen, with entrapment of adnexal structures, with eosinophilic infiltrate.

Diagnostic Approach:
- Skin biopsy.
- ANA and anti ss DNA.

Associations of Localized Scleroderma:
- Arthralgia
- Unilateral Raynaud's phenomenon

- Migraine and intermittent colicky pain
- Spinal problems
- Rib abnormalities
- Mental retardation
- Other connective tissue disorders.

Differential Diagnosis

1. Pseudo scleroderma of legs due to chronic gravitational edema and chronic scurvy (Table 8.4).

Table 8.4: Pseudoscleroderma

Edematous:
a. Scleredema
b. Scleremyxoedema.
Indurative:
1. Primary Systemic Amyloidosis
2. Porphyria cutanea tarda
3. Phenylketonuria
4. Insulin dependent DM
Atrophic:
• Acrogeria
• Werners
• LSA
• Lyme's disease.

2. Occupational scleroderma:
   a. Vinyl chloride–coldness, numbness, discolouration of fingers present
      Telangiectasia over face and difficulty in opening mouth present
      Radial furrowing and pigmentation absent
   b. Pesticides–DDT/Malathion/Parathion
   c. Organic solvents
   d. Epoxy resins
   e. Silicosis
   f. Vibration associated exposure
3. Iatrogenic (Drug induced):
   - Bleomycin/carbidopa/cisplatin
   - Cocaine/pentazocine
   - Silicon and paraffin implants
4. Toxic oil epidemic syndrome
5. Eosinophilic fascitis (Schulman's syndrome)
6. Graft Vs Host disease.

Treatment (Table 8.5)

- Topical steroids.
- Injectable steroids.
- Calcitriol and calcipotriene.
- Psoralen–UVA.
- UVA alone (340-400 nm).
- Methotrexate.
- Methotrexate + Steroids.

Table 8.5: Treatment of localized scleroderma

Morphea
Corticosteroids (topical and intralesional)
Topical calcipotriene
Linear scleroderma
Corticosteroids (intralesional for coup de sabre)
Psoralen-UV-A baths
UV-A alone (340-400 nm)
Widespread morphea
PUVA baths
UV-A alone (340-400 nm)
Oral calcitriol
Methotrexate
Methotrexate plus corticosteroids

REFERENCES

- Therapeutic Strategies in Dermatology Timothy G. Berger, M.D. Bruce U. Wintroub, M.D.
- Rook's Textbook of Dermatology D. A. Burns, S. M. Breathnach, Neil Cox, Christopher E., Griffiths, 7th edn 2004.
- Fitzpatrick's Dermatology in General Medicine, 6th edn 2003.
- Lever's Histopathology of the Skin by David E Elder, Rosalie Elenitsas, Bernett L Johnson, George F Murphy, 9th edn 2004.

Dermatomyositis

DEFINITION

A connective tissue disorder involving the skin, muscle and blood vessels.

Comprehensive Classification of Idiopathic Inflammatory Disease

1. **Dermatomyositis (DM)**
   Adult Onset
   - Classic DM
     - Classic DM alone
     - Classic DM with malignancy

- Classic DM as a part of overlap CT.
- Clinically amyopathic DM
  - Amyopathic DM
  - Hypomyopathic DM.

Juvenile Onset
- Classic DM
- Clinically amyopathic DM
  - Amyopathic DM
  - Hypomyopathic DM.

2. **Polymyositis**
   - PM alone.
   - PM as a part of overlap OT.

The Bohan Classification of Polymyositis/DM

Clinical Subgroups

1. PM (Polymyositis).
2. DM (Dermatomyositis).
3. PM or DM with malignancy.
4. Childhood DM.
5. PM/DM with Connective Tissue Disorder.

Diagnostic Criteria

1. Typical skin rash.
2. Symmetrical proximal muscle weakness with or without dysphagia or respiratory involvement.
3. Abnormal muscle, biopsy finding.
4. High skeletal muscle enzyme.
5. **Abnormal EMG**
   - Definite DM–Rash and 3 of 4 Dx Criteria.
   - Probable DM–Rash and 2 of 4 Dx Criteria.
   - Possible DM–Rash and 1 of 4 Dx Criteria.

Exclusion Criteria for Diagnosis of PM/DM

1. Peripheral nervous system or CNS involvement.
2. Sarcoidosis.
3. Active infection of muscle (Trichinella, Toxoplasma).
4. Drug/toxin related muscle injury (clofibrate, alcohol, penicillamine, aminoquinolone, antimalarial).
5. Metabolic disorders (Mac Ardle's syndrome).
6. Endocrinopathy.
7. Myasthenia Gravis.
8. Family history of muscular dystrophy.

Epidemiology

Classic DM – Age of diagnosis – 40 years (5th/6th decade)
- Cutaneous involvement occurs in 30 – 40% of adults and 95% of children with DM and PM.
- Skin precedes muscle involvement by weeks to months.
- Triggers
  - Coxsackie, Parvovirus B_{19}, EBV, AIDS, HTLV – I.
  - Silicone breast implants.
  - Collagen implants.
  - Drugs – Penicillamine.

Etiology and Pathogenesis

Key Points

- Patients with DM have a high incidence of HLA B8 and DR 3.
- Infection and UV light—inductive factors in DM—loss of self tolerance.
- Autoantibodies and autoreactive T cells—major role in tissue injury phase.
- Cell mediated myocytotoxity.
- Inflammatory cytokines—mediate metabolic muscle fatigue.
- UV causes increase in TNF alpha which induces cutaneous inflammation.

DM with Malignancy–age of diagnosis 55 years.
- High risk of malignancy seen in adult but not juvenile DM.
- Most common malignancy seen are–breast, lung, gastric, HL, NHL.

Cutaneous Manifestations

Pathognomonic

1. **Gottron's Papules** (Fig. 8.10)
   - Violaceous hue.
     Dorsal–lateral aspect of Interphalangeal/Metacarpophalangeal joints.
   - Depressed at center.

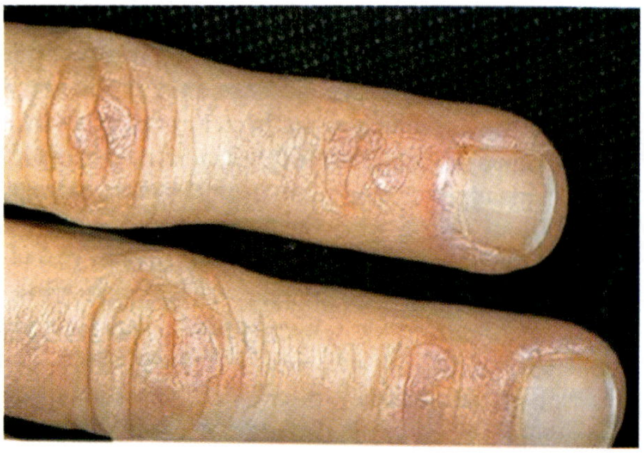

Fig. 8:10. Gottron's papules dorsal – lateral aspect of IP/MCP joint reveals papulosquamous plaque

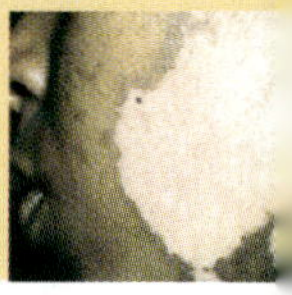

- White, atrophic appearance.
- **Histopath–**Hyperkeratosis; acanthosis, papillomatosis, high mucin.
- DIF – IgM, IgG, C3 at DEJ in 50% cases.

2. **Gottron's Sign** (Fig. 8.11)
   - Symmetric (CMVE) Confluent Macular Violaceous Erythema with/without edema overlying dorsal aspect of IP joint, MCP joint, Olecranon process, patellar or medial malleolli.

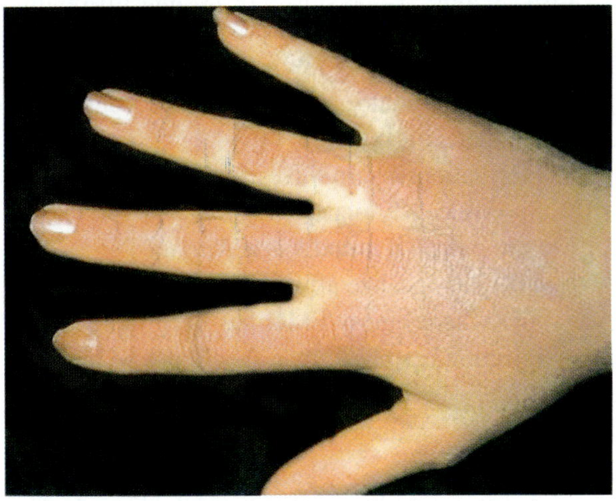

Fig. 8.11: Gottron's Sign—Confluent macular erythema over the extensor aspect and overlying and tracking over the tendons

Characteristic

1. **Heliotrope erythema:** Periorbital confluent macular erythema (30 – 60% cases).
2. **Periungual telangiectasias.**
3. **Symmetrical CMVE:**
   - Pruritic.
   - **Shawl sign—Involvement of neck and shoulders.**
   - **Holster's sign—Side of thigh.**
   - **V sign—Exposed site of neck.**
4. **Mechanic's hand (due to antisynthetase antibody)**
   - Non-pruritic.
   - Hyperkeratotic.
   - Scaling, fissuring, hyperpigmentation.
   - Bilateral and symmetrical.
   - Ulnar aspect of thumb, radial aspect of fingers.

Compatible with DM

1. Poikiloderma atrophicans vasculare (Fig. 8.12).
2. Calcinosis cutis.

Other Features of DM

1. Highly pruritic scaling scalp involvement – DM, associated with non scarring alopecia.
2. Proximal muscle weakness.

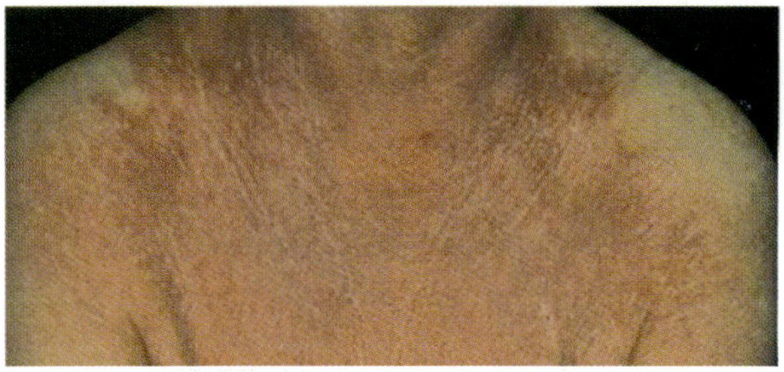

Fig. 8.12: Poikiloderma on the chest

3. Difficulty with speech and swallowing.
4. Flagellate erythema.
5. Hyperpigmentation.
6. Raynaud's phenomenon in 10%.
7. Bursitis of shoulders, hips and joint effusion.
8. Nail changes—Periungual telangiectasia.

Systemic Manifestations

1. Musculoskeletal:
   - Symmetric weakness of proximal muscles of extremities.
   - Pain or tenderness in affected muscle group (acute stage).
   - High serum muscle enzymes.
   - EMG
     - Muscle biopsy changes–can be false negative as muscle involvement is not uniform.
     - MRI is method of choice specially when there is either:
       a. Normal Muscle Enzymes
       b. Lack of proximal muscle weakness.

   Steroid Myopathy:
   - Mimics worsening of DM and PM.
   - Selective atrophy of type II muscle fibres.
   - Progressive weakness despite normal or no increase in CK values.
   - Reduction of neck flexor strength.
   - Trial by increase or decrease of steroid leading to corresponding change in muscle weakness within 2 – 8 weeks.
2. Cardiac.
3. Respiratory.
4. G.I.T.
5. Ophthalmic.
6. Internal malignancy.

AMYOPATHIC DM

Typical cutaneous manifestations of DM without clinical/ laboratory finding of muscle involvement × 6 months after onset of rash.

OVERLAP SYNDROME

- PM > DM.
- Assoc with SLE, scleroderma, PAN, Sjogren's syndrome.
- Raynaud's, polyarthritis, sclerodactyly, later myositis.
- RNP ab +, SCL 70+, antidsDNA+, ANA+, RA factor+.
- Myositis in overlap syndrome responds better to corticosteroids.

JUVENILE DM (SALIENT FEATURES)

- Two peaks 5-9 years/10-14 years (HLADR3)
  1. Higher rate of ***vasculopathy/vasculitis*** in JDM–forerunner of dystrophic calcification.
  2. 4 types of ***calcification*** in children are seen:
     a. Superficial pattern.
     b. Calcinosis circumscripta.
     c. Calcinosis universalis.
     d. Exoskeleton.
  3. In classic JDM–MRI shows edema/inflammation of skin, subcutaneous tissue, fascia.
  4. Vasculitis—Cutaneous ulceration due to **infarctive vasulopathy** and calcification is common.
  5. Distinctive feature on nail:
     - Nail folds—dilatation of capillary loops.
     - Dropout of surrounding vessels.
     - Arborized cluster of capillary loops.
  6. Low grade fever.
  7. Hypertrichosis.
  8. Lipoatrophy.
  9. Gover's sign—Patient has difficulty in standing up and has to "climb on to himself".
  10. Symmetric arthritis of large and small joints, joint contracture.

INVESTIGATIONS

Muscle Involvement

Evaluation of Patient with Myositis

1. **History:**
   a. Previous malignancy.
   b. Associated symptoms.
   c. Toxins, infections, travel, drug intake.
2. **On examination:**
   a. Dermatologic evaluation.
   b. Female–Pelvic, breast examination.
   c. Male–Rectal examination.
3. **Evaluation of muscle involvement:**
   a. Muscle enzymes
   Creatinine Kinase CK, Aldolase.
   Elevated Serum C.K. most sensitive and specific for disease activity.
   - Helpful to follow clinical course of DM/PM.
   - Corresponds with clinical status.
   - Elevated in other conditions–therefore not a specific marker for diagnosis.
   - Combination of AST level (> 50 IU/l).
   (CK)(AST) RATIO (<40).
   CK MB fraction (>2%) provide a specific and sensitive diagnostic tool to differentiate PM from other myopathies.

   b. EMG if muscle enzymes are normal differentiates neurogenic and myogenic process.
   Abnormal EMG
   – Small amplitude, short duration, polyphasic motor unit potentials.
   – Fibrillations, sharp waves, high insertional activity.
   – Spontaneously bizarre, high discharges.

   c. Muscle biopsy if *a and b are Normal*
   - MRI can localize affected area for biopsy.
   - Site where biopsy/EMG has been done or where injection has been given should not be biopsied.
   - Triceps preferred
     – **H/P** – Muscle shows fibre degeneration/regeneration.
     – Perifascicular atrophy.
     – Capillary injury.
     – Occlusive vasculopathy in childhood DM/PM.
     – Muscular immunopathology–high B cells CD_4+ cells.
4. **Skin Biopsy Evaluation:**
   - Earliest – PAS+ve thickening of basement membrane.
   - High dermal mucin.
   - Histology mimics that of LE.

   Immunohistology of skin
   – Bandlike granular deposits of IgG and complement along Dermoepidermal Junction.
   – Dermal microvessel C5 deposits.
5. **Autoantibodies**
   a. ***MSA – Myositis specific antibodies***
   - Anti – t – RNA Synthetase.
   - **Anti Mi – 2 antibody – Highly specific for classic DM.**
   - **Anti SRP**–Cardiac involvement.
   - **Anti Jo – 1 – antisynthetase syndrome.**

   b. ***NMSA – Non MSA***
   - **High ANA**–60 – 80% of classic DM.
   Titre of >1:160 indicates overlap Syndrome.
   - **Anti RNP**–Overlap of SLE and PM/DM or MCTD.
   - **Anti PM–Scl antibody**–Overlap with scleroderma.
   - **AntiKu**–Overlap of PM/DM with SLE or scleroderma.

6. **Routine Lab Studies**
   a. CBC, and urinalysis.
   b. Thyroid function.
   c. Occult blood testing.
   d. ECG.
   e. Female–Pap smear and mammography.
7. Radiological examination–CxR PFT.
8. Esophageal studies.
9. MRI, USG – Non invasive.
10. KFT with serial estimates of the 24 hours urinary creatinine provides best index of disease activity.

Treatment

General

1. Avoid excessive sun exposure, use sunscreens.
2. ***Topical Treatment.***
3. ***Systemic Treatment.***
   Topical Steroids,Tacrolimus, Sunscreens.
   Cutaneous Manifestations:
   1. Hydroxychloroquine – DOC for—cutaneous disease –200–400 mg/day.
   2. Low dose weekly methotrexate (2.5 – 30 mg/wk) for resistant disease.

   Systemic Disease
   1. Sytemic steroids–1st line treatment
      Early intervention–better prognosis.
      - **Adults – T. Prednisolone – 1 – 1.5 mg/kg/day.**
      - **Children – T. Prednisolone 1-2 mg/kg/day.** continued for 12-24 months.
      - If clinical signs, serum CPK level and 24 hours urinary creatinine does not show improvement after 2 months of prednisolone give bolus infusion of methyl prednisolone.
      - Acutely ill–I/V pulse steroids with methyl prednisolone.
      - Objective improvement in muscle strength by 3rd month of therapy–if no improvement–other immunosuppressive drugs.
   2. **Immunosupressives**
      - Methotrexate 10 – 50 mg/week) – 1st line adjuvant treatment.
      - Azathioprine (1-2 mg/kg/day).
      - Cyclophosphamide (1-2 mg/kg/day).
      - Mycophenolate (1-1.5 g/day).
   3. **Extracorporeal photo chemotherapy.**
   4. **Anti TNFa Drug:**
      - Etanercept.
      - Infliximab.
      - Thalidomide.
   5. **Treatment of Dystrophic Calcification:**
      - Aluminium hydroxide antacids.
      - Diltiazem.
      - Others–Probenecid, Potassium PABA, warfarin, EDTA, colchicine, alendronate.

THERAPEUTIC LADDER FOR DM/PM

Juvenile DM/PM

1. Oral C.S.
   - Prednisolone 2 mg/kg/day – tapered to half dose over 6 months.
   - Attempt alternate day dosing once 10 mg is reached.
2. Low dose weekly methotrexate.
3. Azathioprine.
4. Others–high dose IVIG, pulse cyclophosphamide, cyclosporine.

Adult DM/PM

1. Oral C.S.
   - Prednisone 1mg/kg/day tapered to half over 6 months.
   - Attempt alternate day dosing.
   - Usually required for 2 years.
   - Options to use pulse, split dosing.
2. Low dose weekly methotrexate.
3. Azathioprine 2-3 mg/kg/day.
4. Others–high dose IVIG, pulse cyclophosphamide, cyclosporine.

PROGNOSIS

Poor Indicators

a. Recalcitrant disease.
b. Delay in diagnosis and therapy.
c. Older age.
d. Malignancy.
e. Fever.
f. Asthenia–anorexia.
g. Pulmonary interstitial fibrosis.
h. Dysphagia.
i. Leucocytosis.
j. Anti SRP–antibody.

Good Indicators

a. Calcinosis is a good indicator.
b. Myositis with connective tissue disorder.

c. Anti-synthetase – Antibody.
d. Anti-Mi-2 – Antibody.

Cause of Death

- Respiratory infection.
- Cardiac failure.
- Malnutrition.
- Weakness/disability due to difficulty in swallowing.
- Carcinoma.
- Side effects of steroid therapy.

REFERENCES

- Therapeutic Strategies in Dermatology, Timothy G. Berger, M.D. Bruce, U. Wintroub, M.D.
- Rook's Textbook of Dermatology, D. A. Burns, S. M. Breathnach, Neil Cox, Christopher E. Griffiths, 7th edn 2004.
- Fitzpatrick's Dermatology in General Medicine, 6th edn 2003.
- Lever's Histopathology of the Skin by David E Elder, Rosalie Elenitsas, Bernett L Johnson, George F Murphy, 9th edn 2004.

CHAPTER 9

VESICULOBULLOUS DISORDERS

The vesiculobullous diseases although uncommon have a social and economic impact on the patient and the family. These are classified into **genetic** (epidermolysis bullosa) and the **acquired autoimmune** blistering disorders (pemphigus, bullous pemphigoid, dermatitis herpetiformis, chronic bullous dermatosis of childhood, epidermolysis bullosa acquisita) (Table 9.1).

Table 9.1: Classification of disorders based on histopathological level

Intra-epidermal disorders	*Dermal-epidermal junction*
Granular layer • Friction blister • Pemphigus foliaceus • Subcorneal pustular dermatosis • Staphylococcal scalded skin syndrome • Bullous impetigo ***Spinous layer*** • Eczematous dermatitis • Herpes virus infection • Familial benign pemphigus ***Suprabasal*** • Pemphigus vulgaris • Darier's disease ***Basal layer*** • Erythema multiforme • Lupus erythematosus • Lichen planus • Epidermolysis bullosa simplex	***Junctional (at the lamina lucida)*** • Junctional epidermolysis bullosa • Bullous pemphigoid ***Dermolytic (below basal lamina)*** • Epidermolysis bullosa dystrophicans • Epidermolysis bullosa acquisita • Porphyria cutanea tarda • Dermatitis herpetiformis

Intercellular-Adhesion Molecule (Fig. 9.1)

The intercellular adhesion, molecule between the keratinocytes is called cadherin. A detailed analysis reveals that the intercellular substances is composed of desmocollin and desmoglein and the component within the cell is composed primarily of desmoplakin and plakoglobin. Similarly the basement membrane zone is composed of numerous strectures (Fig. 9.2) that play a role in bullous disorders.

Classification of Pemphigus
• Pemphigus vulgaris
• Pemphigus foliaceus
• Pemphigus erythematosus (Senear Usher)
• Pemphigus vegetans (Neumann, Hallopeau)
• Fogo Selvagem: Endemic
• Drug-induced
• IgA (SCPD, Intra-epidermal type) pemphigus
• Paraneoplastic pemphigus

Pemphigus

Definition

Pemphigus, an autoimmune disease is characterized by intraepidermal blistering at various levels in the epidermis, because of disruption of the intercellular cementing substance. It is due to an autoantibody attack (IgG) on the cellular adhesion proteins (desmogleins) (Table 9.2) leading to acantholysis seen on tzanck smear (Fig. 9.3).

Epidemiology

Rare, equal in men and women, onset at 40 to 60 years of age, more common in Jewish or Mediterranean descendants.

Aetio-Pathogenesis

Antibody **IgG1 and C3** against **DG 3** (Table 9.2).

Drugs: Sulfydryl group-penicillamine, captopril, rifampicin.

Others (beta blockers, cephalosporins, penicillin and rifampicin).

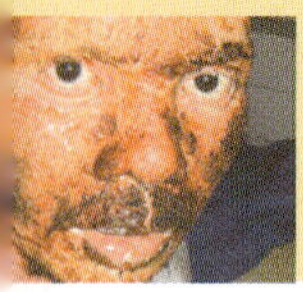

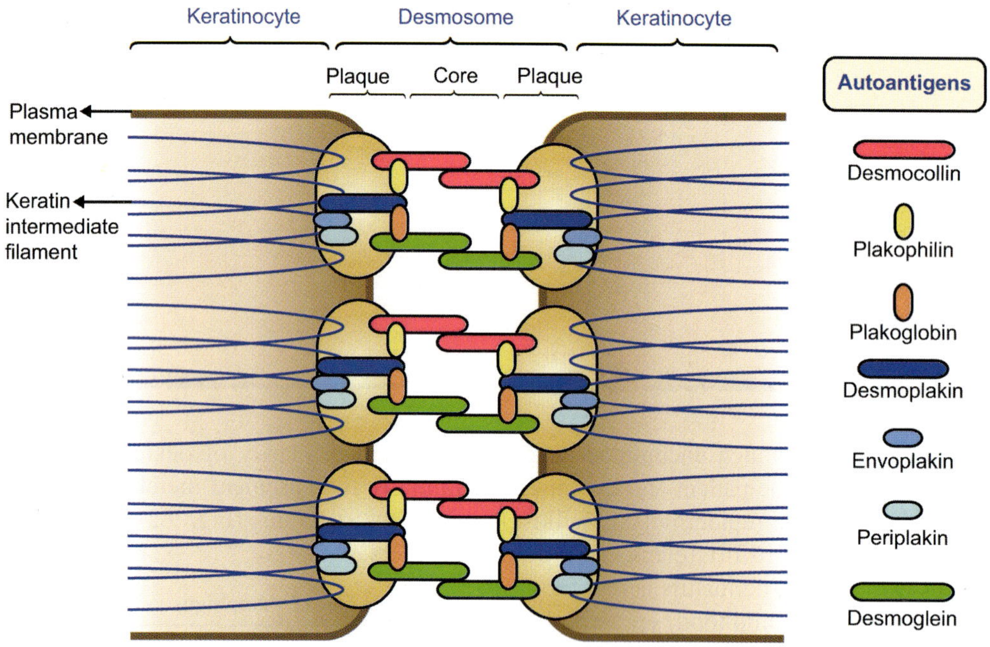

Fig. 9.1: A line diagram depicting the desmosome

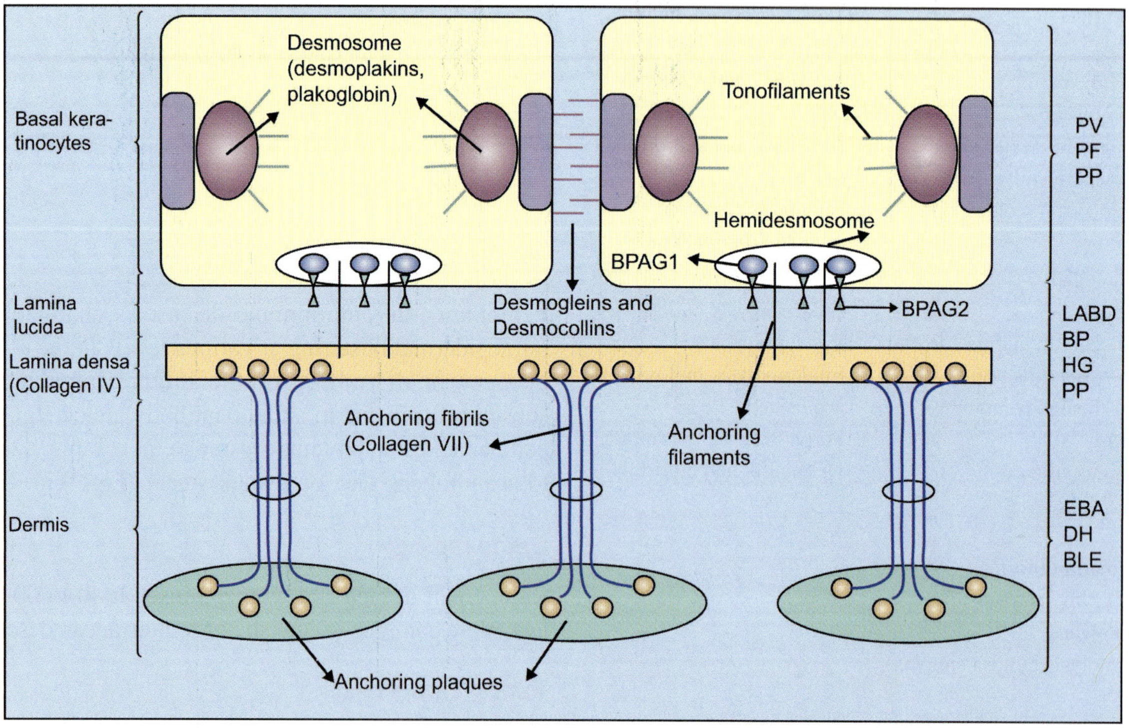

Fig. 9.2: The dermal-epidermal junction consists of the basal keratinocytes, the basement membrane and the papillary dermis with their structural and attachment molecules. Diseases are listed on the right by the location of their target antigen(s). PV = pemphigus vulgaris, PF = pemphigus foliaceus, P = paraneoplastic pemphigus, LABD = Liner IgA bullous dermatosis, BP = bullous pemphigoid, HG = herpes gestationis, EBA = epidermolysis bullosa acquisita, DH= dermatitis herpetiformis, BLE = bullous lupus erythematosus, BPAG1 and 2 = bullous pemphigoid antigens 1 and 2

Table 9.2: Antigen–Pemphigus

Variant	*Tissue antigens*
P. vulgaris	**Dsg 3, Dsg 1**, desmocollins, plakoglobin, cholinergic keratinocyte receptor (CKR- alpha9 and pemphaxin), annexins, α chain of high affinity IgE
P. vegetans	**Dsg 3, Dsg 1,** desmocollins 1 and 2
P. foliaceus	**Dsg1**,desmoplakin, periplakin, envoplakin, plakoglobin
P. herpetiformis	**Dsg 3, Dsg 1,** desmocollin
P. erythematosus	Dsg1(3),ANA, 230kDa, 190 kDa, periplakin
Drug-induced	heterogenous
IgA - SCPD type	**Desmocollins 1&2**
IgA - IEN type	**120 kDa, Dsg 1 & 3**
Atypical IgG/IgA	Desmocollins 1-3
Paraneoplastic	Envoplakin,periplakin,desmoplakin 1 & 2, BP-230,plectin, Dsg1&3,170 kDa transmembrane antigen
Endemic	Dsg 1, 3

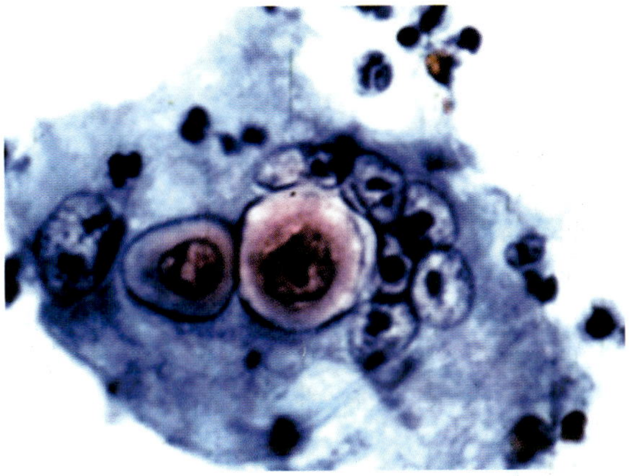

Fig. 9.3: Multiple acantholytic cells

Clinical Features (Figs. 9.4(a) to 9.4(c))

Mucosal lesions are seen in almost **all** the patients. Either the onset is with painful oral erosions (50-70%) or is involved during the course of the disease. Other mucosae involved are conjunctiva, pharynx, larynx, oesophagus, urethra, vulva and cervix.

Skin lesions are asymptomatic, **flaccid** bullae on normal or erythematous skin. The sites involved are scalp, face, trunk, axillae and groins (flexural surfaces). Rupture of bulla causes painful erosions that heal spontaneously leaving behind hyperpigmented macules. Peeling of skin takes place when tangential force is applied (**Nikolsky's** sign). Bulla spread sign (**Asboe-Hansen sign**) is also positive.

Course and Complications

Prognosis is poor without treatment but with systemic steroids, mortality has been reduced to 5-15%.

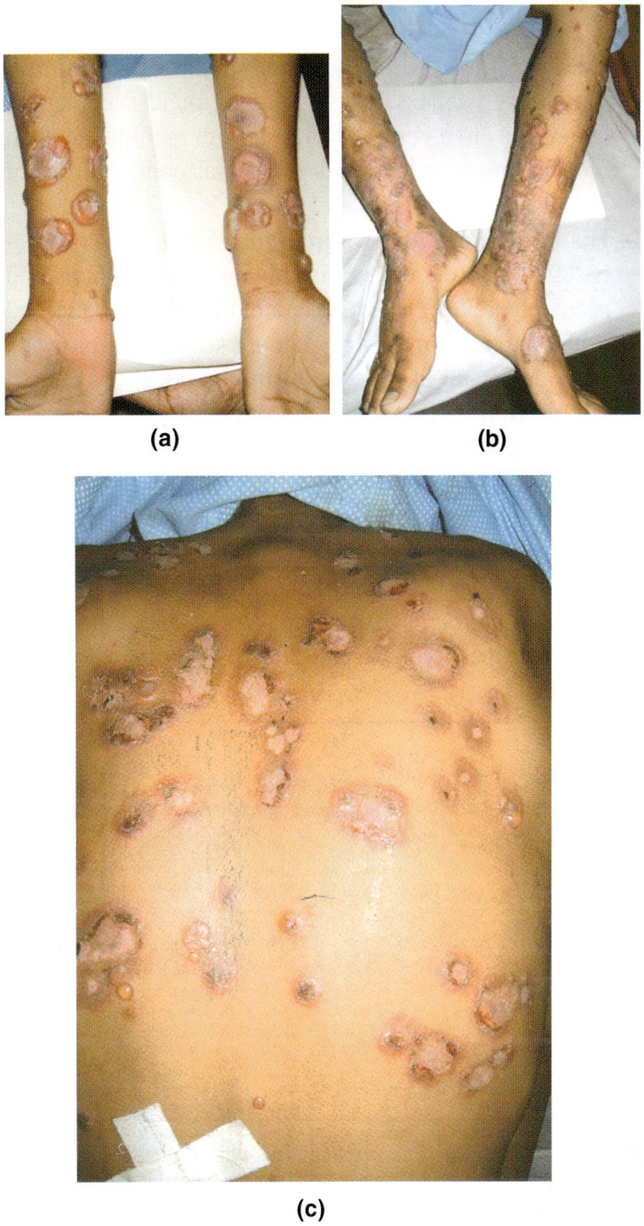

Fig. 9.4(a) to 9.4(c): Multiple erosions and flaccid bulla on the back and extremities

Even with the use of corticosteroids and other immunosuppressive agents, there is still significant morbidity and mortality associated with pemphigus vulgaris. A common cause of death is infection secondary to the immunosuppression required to treat the disease. Most deaths occur within the first few years of the disease. Unfortunately, many of the drugs used to treat this disease have serious side effects, and patients must be monitored closely for infection, renal and liver function abnormalities, electrolyte disturbances, hypertension, diabetes, anemia, and gastrointestinal bleeding.

Investigation

1. **Tzanck** smear from the floor of the blister shows acantholytic cells, which is a large, rounded epidermal cell with a large vesicular nucleus with multiple nucleoli with perinuclear halo and peripheral condensation of cytoplasm (Fig. 9.3).
2. **Histopathological examination** (Fig. 9.5): A suprabasal cleft in the epidermis containing eosinophils and acantholytic cells. The basal keratinocytes remain attached to the basement membrane but are separated from each other and stand like a '**row of tombstones**'.
3. **Direct immunofluorescence** from the lesional skin will have deposition of intercellular IgG throughout the epidermis in a '**fish-net**' pattern (IgG, IgA,C3,C1q) (Fig. 9.6).
4. **Indirect immunofluorescence** detects circulating IgG antibodies in 80-90% of the cases *whose levels correlate with disease activity* (monkey esophagus is the tissue used and the **titre correlates with activity**).
5. ELISA –Dsg1, 3.

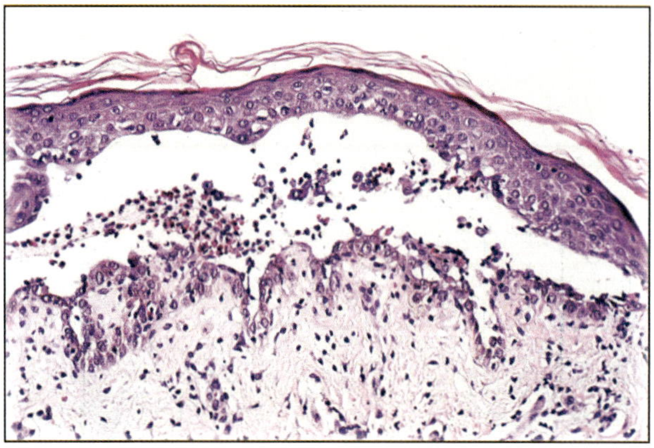

Fig. 9.5: A suprabasal split with multiple acantholytic cells with the basal layer resembling a "row of tombstones" appearance

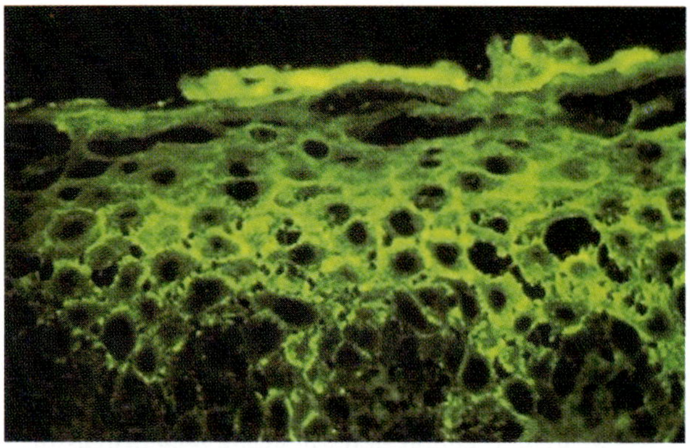

Fig. 9.6: Direct immunofluorescence reveals a characteristic fish net pattern of IgG and C3

Treatment of Pemphigus Vulgaris

Systemic steroids in a dose of 2-3 mg per kg body weight, is the drug of choice.

First Step

Treat with prednisone 60-80 mg/day.

In the case of persistent oral lesions, treat for candidiasis with oral fluconazole 150 mg once weekly.

Dental trays filled with superpotent topical steroids and worn for 4-8 hours daily may be effective for refractory gingival disease.

Subsequent Steps

1. In patients responding to the above treatment, gradually taper the systemic steroids and immunosuppressives over 3-6 months (described on page 199, 462-464).
2. The titer of the circulating autoantibody may be useful in determining response to treatment and the rate at which immunosuppressive therapy can be tapered. It should be monitored **every 6 months**, and should decrease with each measurement.

In **refractory pemphigus vulgaris**, consider the following options:

a. Increasing the dose of mycophenolate mofetil to 3 g/day.
b. Monthly pulse steroids of 1 g of methyl prednisolone daily for 3 days intravenously; or dexamethasone 100 mg daily for 3 days with cyclophosphamide 500 mg/2nd day.
c. High-dose intravenous immunoglobin 2 g/kg/month over several days.
d. Mycophenolate mofetil 2.0 g daily along with the prednisone.
e. *Daily cyclophosphamide 1-3 mg/kg/day*; or cyclophosphamide 50 mg per day in combination with monthly pulses of methyl prednisolone.
f. *Cyclophosphamide* treatment is combined with systemic steroid therapy and often pulse systemic steroid treatment in refractory cases.

Pemphigus Foliaceous (Fig. 9.7)

It is less severe than pemphigus vulgaris and is characterized by crusted, moist, scaly lesions in a **seborrheic** distribution involving scalp, face, chest and upper back. Bullous lesions may not be seen because of the superficial level of the split that may cause erosions, scaling and crusting. Oral lesions are absent.

- Antibody is IgG and is against DG1 (Desmoglein 1) (Table 9.2).
- The acantholytic cell is cuboidal in shape.

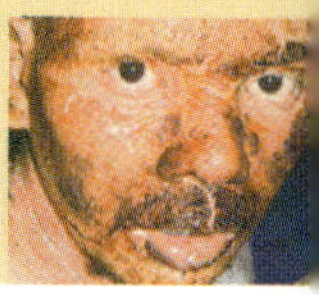

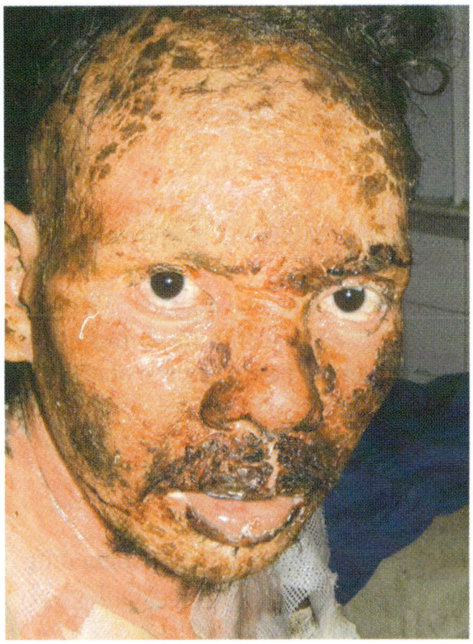

Fig. 9.7: Erosions on the face and crusting on the limbs

Treatment

Prednisone 20-40 mg/day may be used for severe flares, but chronic therapy should be avoided except in the most severe cases.

Dapsone 100-300 mg daily alone or in combination with systemic steroids may be effective in refractory cases, and should be considered as a part of a maintenance regimen.

Tetracycline 500 mg 4 times daily or doxycycline 100 mg twice daily, plus nicotinamide 500 mg 3 times daily may be considered as a steroid-sparing regimen, but response is variable.

Apply a superpotent topical steroid cream twice daily for 2-3 weeks, supplemented by intralesional injections of triamcinolone acetonide 5 mg/ml to select lesions.

Alternative Steps

If the condition is severe and refractory to the above treatments, consider adding an immunosuppressive agent, either mycophenolate mofetil 2.0-3.0 g/day, or azathioprine 100 mg/day.

Pitfalls

Drugs such as penicillamine and captopril may cause pemphigus foliaceus. These should be discontinued. Most drug-induced cases can be treated with superpotent topical steroids.

Pemphigus Erythematosus

It is a variant of pemphigus foliaceous characterized by immunological features of both pemphigus and lupus erythematosus (LE), that is, intercellular IgG & C3 in the epidermis (as in pemphigus) and in the basement membrane zone and antinuclear antibodies (as in LE). Clinically, erythematous, scaly rash over the nose and cheeks simulate LE while lesions on the trunk are similar to those in pemphigus foliaceous.

Pemphigus Vegetans

It is a clinical variant of pemphigus vulgaris characterized by vegetating lesions primarily in the flexures. Initial lesions are bullae or pustules, which rupture and progress to form vegetating plaques in the axillae and groins.

Other Variants of Pemphigus

Endemic pemphigus foliaceous (Fogo Selvagem)

It is a variant of pemphigus foliaceous, endemic to certain parts of South America and is postulated to be caused by bites of the black fly (Simuliidae). The burnt appearance and burning sensation gave the disease its name, fogo selvagem, meaning "wild fire".

Drug induced pemphigus (penicillamine, captropril, pyritinol, penicillin, rifampicin)

Commonly present as pemphigus foliaceous.

Paranoplastic pemphigus

Mucocutaneous ulcerations associated with an underlying neoplasm.

Pemphigus herpetiformis

Superficial vesicles and inflammatory papules occur in herpetiform distribution.

IgA pemphigus

Clinically it may resemble subcorneal pustular dermatosis.

Juvenile pemphigus

Pemphigus occurring in children.

Neonatal pemphigus

It is because of transplacental transfer of maternal anti-intercellular cements substance antibodies to the fetus. Blisters resolve in 2 weeks.

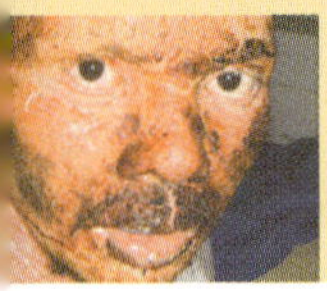

PEMPHIGOID GROUP

1. **Bullous pemphigoid**
2. **Pemphigoid gestationis**
3. **Cicatricial pemphigoid**
4. **Linear IgA disease**
5. **EB acquisita**
6. **Dermatitis herpetiformis.**

Bullous Pemphigoid (BP)

Definition

Bullous pemphigoid is an autoimmune skin disorder characterized by subepidermal blistering which results in large, tense bullae.

Epidemiology

It occurs mainly in the **elderly** and rarely in children. Onset is typically between 60 and 80 years of age. There is equal incidence in men and women, and there are no known racial or ethnic predilections It is more common than pemphigus vulgaris.

Pathogenesis

Include formation of IgG antibodies against components of the basement membrane zone (BMZ–structure which binds epidermis to the underlying dermis and mesenchyme).

Antigen: Hemidesmosome (BPAg1 and BPAg2) (Fig. 9.2).

This leads to loss of structural integrity of the BMZ due to resultant inflammation and separation of the intact epidermis from underlying dermis and forms a subepidermal cleft containing eosinophils and neutrophils.

Drug: Benzodiazepine, furosemide, penicillin, sulfasalazine.

Clinical Features (Fig. 9.8)

Lesions start as urticarial wheals, which are preceded by **itching**. It lasts for 1-3 weeks and finally **tense bullae** on **normal or erythematous skin** predominantly over flexural aspects of the limbs, lower abdomen, groins and axillae are formed. Face and scalp is relatively spared. Bullae rupture to leave erosions that heal spontaneously with postinflammatory hyperpigmentation and scarring. Nikolsky's and bulla spread sign are negative. Mucosal lesions are uncommon (20%).

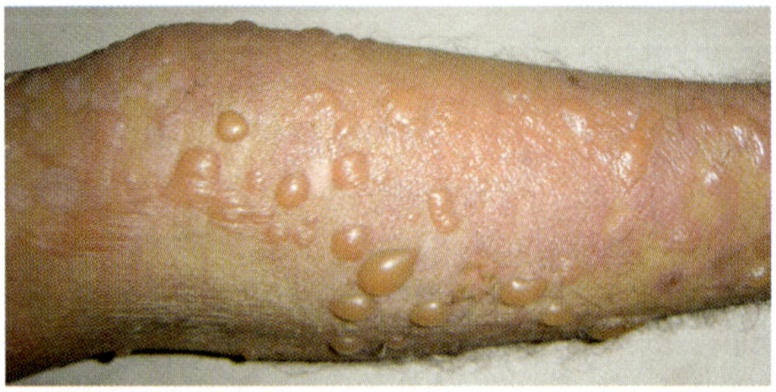

Fig. 9.8: Tense blisters overlying urticarial base over the lower limb (Bullous pemphigoid)

Prognosis

It is better than pemphigus and it runs a chronic self-limiting course. It may be fatal in the active stage in the elderly or debilitated patients. It may be associated with an underlying malignancy (gastric carcinoma commonly) and other autoimmune diseases like diabetes mellitus, rheumatoid arthritis and psoriasis.

Diagnosis

1. **Tzanck** smear—Eosinophils.
2. **Histology–Subepidermal cleft** containing eosinophils and neutrophils is seen on histopathological examination (Fig. 9.9).
3. **DIF** linear IgG (45-90%) and C3 (80-100%) deposition in the basement membrane zone (Fig. 9.10).
4. **Indirect immunofluorescence** demonstrates circulating IgG autoantibodies in most cases but unlike in pemphigus, their titers do not correlate with disease.
5. **ELISA** antibodies against BP **antigens** 180/230.

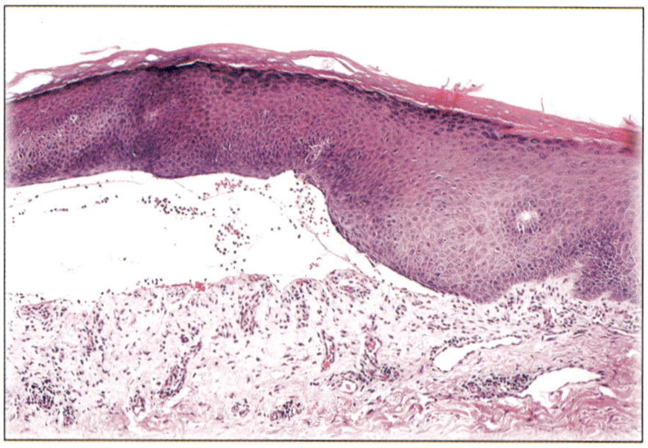

Fig. 9.9: Subepidermal blister with eosinophils

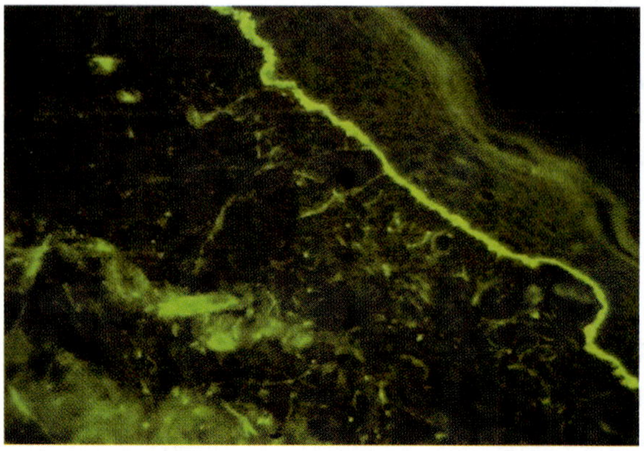

Fig. 9.10: Linear band of IgG at the BMZ

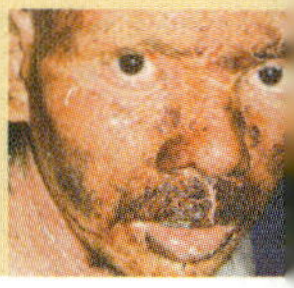

Treatment

1. Treat with oral prednisone alone at 40-60 mg/day in a single morning dose. A dramatic clinical response will be seen in 70-80% of patients after 2-3 weeks.

   Tapering* of steroids in Bullous pemphigoid by

   Decrease by 10 mg (every 2-3 weeks).

   ↓

   Decrease to 30 mg (by 2-8 weeks).

   ↓

   Decrease to 10-20 mg (over next 2-3 months).

   ↓

   Decrease to 10 mg alternate day (over 2 months).

   ↓

   Decrease by 1 mg alternate day (every 1-4 weeks).

   ↓

   STOP IT.

2. 0.05% clobetasol ointment or another superpotent topical steroid is applied to the affected areas twice daily.

Alternative*

Alternative agents may be used in patients who do not rapidly respond to systemic steroids or in patients in whom the use of systemic steroids is contraindicated.

1. If the patient has complications or side effects from prednisone, has persistent severe disease, or if sufficient clinical response is not achieved after 3 weeks, begin an immunosuppressive agent in combination with prednisone. In each case, continue the immunosuppressive agent for at **least 2 months before abandoning it as ineffective**. Once the steroid-sparing agent has begun to work, the dose of systemic steroids is gradually tapered following the protocol above. The choice of immunosuppressive agent is determined by the patient's coexistent medical conditions, the risk of complications, and the cost. *There is no evidence that one agent is superior to another.* Steroid-sparing immunosuppressives include:
   a. Mycophenolate mofetil 500 mg-1.5 mg twice daily (1.0-3.0 g daily).
   b. Azathioprine 100-150 mg/day.
   c. Methotrexate 5 mg to 25 mg once weekly as a single oral dose.
   d. Cyclophosphamide 50-150 mg/day.
2. Adjunctive measures that may be added to prednisone or prednisone plus immunosuppressive agents.
   a. Tetracycline 500 mg three or four times daily plus niacinamide 500 mg three times daily. This may be adequate alone to control mild disease or may provide additional anti-inflammatory effect without causing additional immunosuppression.

* Same principles are also applicable in pemphigus.

Cicatricial Pemphigoid

Rare, female to male ratio is 2 : 1, onset at 40 to 60 years of age.

Bullae rupture within hours leaving painful erosions that heal with scarring; most common sites are oral and conjunctival mucosa; skin involved in one third of cases, head and upper chest.

Investigation

Histology: Subepidermal blister with mixed infiltrate in fresh lesions and predominant fibroblasts in older, scarring lesions.

DIF: Linear IgG and C3 on the basement membrane,+/- IgA or IgM.

Treatment

Corticosteroids; may add dapsone for oral involvement or cyclophosphamide or azathioprine for ocular involvement; topical treatment of oral lesions with steroid gel or dexamethasone mouthwash.

Herpes Gestationis

Definition

It is autoimmune blistering disease of young women which occurs in **2nd trimester** of pregnancy or within 1st week postnatally.

Clinical Features

Clinically the onset is with severe pruritus and urticarial wheals and plaques, followed by bullous lesions in the **peri-umbilical** area, lower abdomen and thighs. Mucosal involvement is uncommon and lesions improve after delivery. **Recurrence** may occur in subsequent pregnancies, pre-menstrually or with oral contraceptive pills (OCPs). Direct immunofluorescence shows **linear C3** deposits at the BMZ with IgG in some cases.

Treatment

For mild, localized cases, prescribe a superpotent topical steroid cream (e.g., clobetasol, or betamethasone dipropionate) to be applied once or twice daily. Once the condition improves the strength of the steroid and frequency of application may be reduced.

For moderate to severe cases, begin therapy with prednisone 40-60 mg/day. Expect remission in 5-15 days. Attempt to reduce the dose by half over the next 4-6 weeks, then gradually taper the dose to the lowest possible daily or every other day dose to control symptoms and maintain the minimum daily dose of prednisone throughout pregnancy.

Large blisters may be ruptured with a sterile needle to avoid them spreading by hydrostatic pressure.

Antihistamines may help to control pruritus. Both hydroxyzine and diphenhydramine 25-50 mg 2 to 4 times daily are considered to be safe in pregnant women.

Epidermolysis Bullosa Acquisita (EBA)

It is chronic, bullous disorder of old age and sometimes difficult to differentiate from bullous pemphigoid clinically. IgG class of autoantibodies directed against collagen VII causes it. Collagen VII is the major component of the anchoring fibrils found in the subepidermal zone. There are two clinical forms. Mechanobullous type–blistering over trauma prone sites, which heals with scarring and milia formation and bullous pemphigoid (BP) like. Mucosal lesions may be seen in some patients. Bullae are often hemorrhagic.

SUB-EPIDERMAL IgA-MEDIATED DISORDER

Dermatitis Herpetiformis (DH)

Definition

Dermatitis herpetiformis is an **intensely pruritic**, chronic skin disease characterized by **papulovesicular** lesions and urticarial wheals located on the **extensor** surfaces in a symmetric distribution. The disease persists indefinitely, and is associated with a gluten-sensitive enteropathy in most patients.

Epidemiology

The incidence of dermatitis herpetiformis is 10 to 39 cases per 100,000 persons. Onset tends to be between 20 and 40 years of age but may occur at any age, including childhood, and there is a 2 : 1 preponderance for men.

Dermatitis herpetiformis is principally a disease that affects whites. It rarely occurs in Blacks or Asians.

Aetio-Pathogenesis

IgA antibody against Gliadin cross reacts to the intestinal epithelium and that reacts with an antigen in the skin **TG II**.

Clinical Features (Fig. 9.11)

The lesions of dermatitis herpetiformis usually begin as a vesicle, but may also be erythematous papules, urticarial-like wheals, excoriations, crusts, or rarely, large bullae. The lesions may be **grouped**, giving a "**herpetiform**" appearance. Once the lesions have resolved, there may be transient hyper- or hypopigmentation. The lesions are usually **intensely pruritic**, accompanied by burning and stinging. Many patients experience localized burning, stinging, and pruritus approximately eight to 12 hours before the onset of lesions, and many are able to predict an eruption. Rarely, the lesions may be asymptomatic. There is symmetric distribution along the extensor surfaces, including the elbows, knees, buttocks, shoulders, and sacral areas. Less frequently, the lesions are found on the scalp, face, hairline, and the posterior neck. Involvement of the palms and soles is rare, and mucous membrane lesions are uncommon.

Investigations

1. **Histopathological-neutrophilic microabscesses** in dermal papillae, dermal infiltration of neutrophils and eosinophils, and the formation of subepidermal vesicles. Blisters form within the lamina lucida. Dermal blood vessels may be surrounded by a lymphohistiocytic infiltrate as well.
2. **Direct immunofluorescence** reveals **granular** deposition of **IgA** in the tips of dermal papillae. In areas corresponding to IgA deposits, there may also be complement deposition (Fig. 9.12).
3. **Indirect Immunofluorescence** IgA and IgG antireticulin and antiendomysial antibodies have been detected in dermatitis herpetiformis patients' sera.

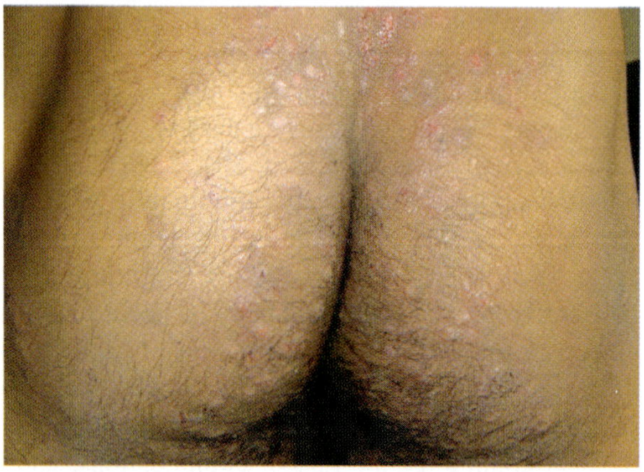

Fig. 9.11: Tense, grouped, vesicles on the buttock

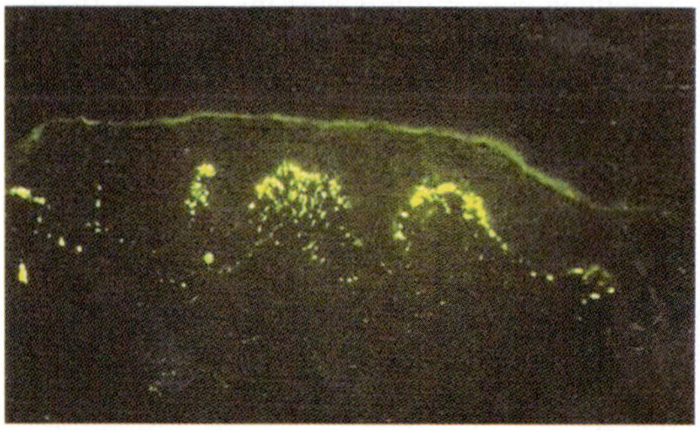

Fig. 9.12: Granular deposit of IgA in the dermal papilla

Section - 4

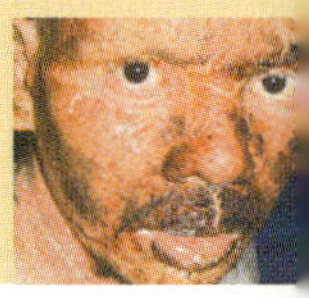

4. An increased incidence of antinuclear and antithyroid microsomal antibodies are also found in these patients.

Course and Complications

Dermatitis herpetiformis follows a prolonged course, lasting up to years. Approximately one third of patients eventually have spontaneous remission. Dermatitis herpetiformis responds well to medications and diet, and has a good prognosis.

Associated manifestations that may cause complications include the gluten-sensitive enteropathy, which can cause steatorrhea, abnormal D-xylose absorption, and anemia. There has also been an increased incidence of atrophic gastritis and achlorhydria in patients with gluten sensitivity. Reports of increased frequency of gastrointestinal lymphomas have also been noted, from which the gluten-free diet has been found to be protective. Patients with dermatitis herpetiformis have also been found to have an increased incidence of other autoimmune disorders.

Treatment

Following G6PD screening, the drug of choice is **dapsone 100 mg/day**. Expect a dramatic clinical response within 4-5 days. Reevaluate the patient after 2 weeks, and increase dapsone to 200 mg/day if clinical improvement is inadequate. Check the CBC every 2 weeks as the dose is increased.

Subsequent Steps

Continue the amount of dapsone required for clearing for 2 weeks, and then taper the drug by halving the dose every 2 weeks. Maintain the patient on the least amount of dapsone required for control of lesions. Although most patients require between 50 and 150 mg daily, some patients are controlled on significantly lower doses (25 mg dapsone per week). Once the appropriate dapsone dose is found, the CBC is checked on a 6-month basis.

Alternative Steps

1. *Sulfapyridine,* may be used in an initial dose of 1-2 g/day in patients who cannot tolerate dapsone. Taper to the minimum required dose which is usually 1.0-1.5 g/day.
2. *Combination therapy:* If partial control is obtained on maximal doses of sulfapyridine (4 g/day), a small dose of colchicines may be added (0.6 mg once or twice daily).
3. *Gluten-free diet:* Because dermatitis herpetiformis is gluten dependent, most patients will respond to a gluten-free diet. Clinical response usually requires the patient to be on a rigid gluten-free diet for 6-12 months. Although not as ideal, even partial avoidance of gluten is helpful. To obtain dietary directions, refer the patient to a dietician skilled in treating patients with celiac disease. A successful dietary regimen requires an intelligent, highly motivated patient who dines at home. Most patients who adhere to their diet will be able to reduce their medication dose by 50% or more.

While a gluten-free diet takes 6 months to have efficacy and allow reduction or discontinuation of medication, gluten exposure may be followed within hours or days by a flare of the skin lesions.

Linear IgA Dermatosis (LAD) or Chronic Bullous Disease of Childhood (CBDC) (Fig. 9.13)

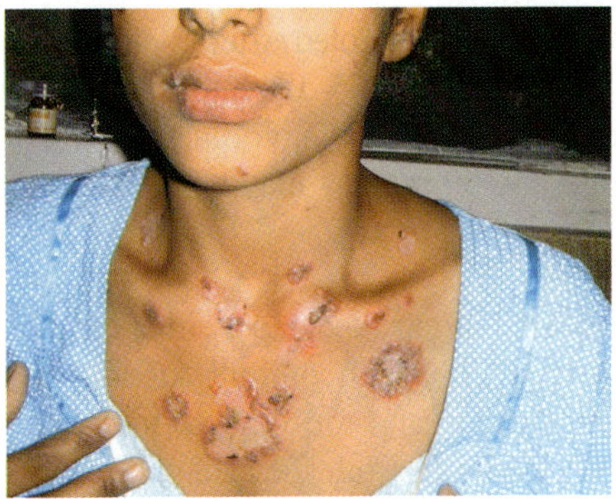

Fig. 9.13: Grouped **"ring of pearls"** appearance of blisters

Definition

Linear IgA dermatosis is a rare autoimmune bullous disorder, characterized by linear deposition of IgA along the basement membrane. Linear IgA dermatosis most commonly presents in patients older than 30 years. Chronic bullous disease of childhood occurs in young children, usually presenting in those younger than five years.

Clinical Features

The lesions of linear IgA dermatosis consist of pruritic, annular papules, vesicles, and bullae that are present in groups. There is a predilection for the extensor surfaces, with symmetric distribution. Lesions are seen on the elbows, knees and buttocks. Because of itching, excoriations will lead to the formation of crusted papules.

Chronic bullous disease of childhood presents with abrupt onset of tense bullae on an inflamed, erythematous base and is accompanied by pruritus and a burning sensation. The lesions are most frequently appear on or near the genitalia, but may also be found on other areas, including the face, especially the perioral region. Oral ulcers are noted in 50% of cases. Characteristic "**collarettes**" of blisters often form as new lesions arise in the periphery of old lesions.

In both forms of linear IgA dermatosis, **mucous membrane involvement** may occur and ranges in severity from mild oral ulcers to severe oral or conjunctival disease.

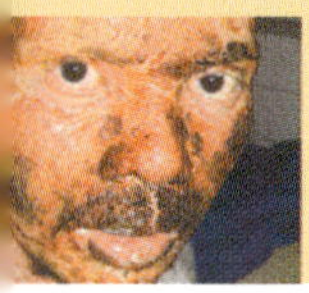

Investigation

1. **Histopathology,** in linear IgA dermatosis and chronic bullous disease of childhood, the bullae are subepidermal, with collections of **neutrophils** along the basement membrane and occasionally in the dermal papillary tips.
2. **Direct immunofluorescence,** deposition of IgA in a linear pattern is noted along the basement membrane. There may also be deposition of IgG and C3.

Treatment

1. Treat with either **dapsone** 2 mg/kg/day or sulfapyridine 35-70 mg/kg/day.
2. If no improvement is noted after 5 days, increase the dosage of either drug at 5-day intervals until an efficacious dose is reached. Sulfapyridine 200 mg to 2 g/day or dapsone 25-200 mg/day may be required.

Subsequent Steps

When the disease is controlled, taper either drug to the dose required to maintain patient comfort. Attempt to wean the patient off medication at 4- or 6-month intervals. Recheck the CBC every 2 months while the patient is receiving maintenance sulfones.

Alternative

Although most respond to sulfones, addition of corticosteroids (e.g., prednisolone) may be required to achieve control.

If control is not possible with 2 g of sulfapyridine or 200 mg of dapsone, add prednisolone 1 mg/kg/day and attempt to convert to a alternate day steroid schedule as quickly as possible.

MECHANOBULLOUS DISORDERS

Epidermolysis Bullosa

Epidermolysis bullosa (EB) also known as 'mechanobullous' disorders is characterized by blistering of the skin and mucosae at birth or soon afterwards because of mild mechanical trauma. Main types are **EB simplex** (intra-epidermal); **Junctional EB** (split through the basement membrane zone); **Dystrophic EB** (split in the subepidermal level).

EB simplex is the most common and mildest form of EB of autosomal dominant inheritance which occurs over trauma prone sites at birth or infancy and heals without scarring. Mucosae, nails and hair are normal.

Junctional EB are autosomal recessive disorders and are broadly classified into two main types, the **lethal** and **non-lethal forms**. They present at birth or soon after with severe fragility of the skin leading to extensive blistering and denudation. Orophayngeal mucosae may be severely involved. Teeth may be malformed and prematurely lost and nails may be shed.

Dystrophic EB is seen at birth or early infancy. It has either autosomal recessive or dominant inheritance. The autosomal recessive form is more severe and trauma prone sites are commonly involved. Oral involvement causes ankylogossia and oesophageal strictures. Perianal blistering, erosions and scarring lead to stenosis and fecal retention. Symblepharon, corneal erosions and opacity are seen in the eyes. Contractures and deformities (**'Mitten hands'**) are the hallmarks. Histology, electron microscopy to ascertain the level of split and structures involved antigen mapping and immunohistochemistry confirm the diagnosis. Prental DNA testing can be advised to couples at risk of having affected children.

Treatment

Establishing the Diagnosis

There is clinical overlap, so virtually all cases require electron microscopy or immunofluorescent mapping for correct diagnosis. This is critical for therapy, genetic counselling and prognosis.

Genetic Counselling

Since these diseases are inherited, genetic counselling is essential. Prenatal diagnosis via DNA testing is available for patients in whom previous pregnancies resulted in severely affected children.

1. *Family education:* Some forms of EB are devastating, and demand a significant commitment on the part of the patient, the family, and health care providers.
2. *Trauma:* Even very minor trauma induces lesions. Efforts to reduce trauma by protection and lubrication are essential to care. Nurse specialists at special EB centers are valuable in training nurses caring for EB patients, and are also key in training the family in the transition of the neonate to home care.
3. *Infection:* Healing is diminished by secondary infection of skin lesions, usually by *S. aureus* or β-hemolytic streptococci. Topical antibacterial ointments, specifically mupirocin, can be of great help, but treatment should be limited to short courses, as resistance can emerge. When obvious infection occurs, administer an oral semi-synthetic penicillin (*dicloxacillin*) or a first-generation cephalosporin. Perform cultures, as antibiotic resistance may occur.
4. *Blister care:* The normal skin forming the roof of the blister should be left on as long as possible; it is the

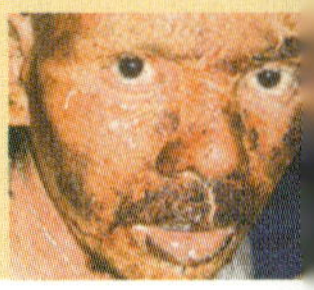

optimal biologic dressing. If the hydrostatic pressure of the fluid in the blister tends to increase its size, open the blister and drain the fluid. If a blister becomes infected, drain it and remove the roof. For open erosions, cleanse gently with saline and cover with petrolatum impregnated soft fine-mesh gauze, or alternatively, a soft silicone wound care dressing, the later left on for 7 days.

REFERENCES

- Rook's Textbook of Dermatology, D. A. Burns, S. M. Breathnach, Neil Cox , Christopher E. Griffith's, 7th edn 2004.
- Fitzpatrick's Dermatology in General Medicine, 6th edn 2003.
- Therapeutic Strategies in Dermatology, Timothy G. Berger, M.D. Bruce U. Wintroub, M.D.

CHAPTER **10**

VASCULAR DERMATOSIS

A compilation of common conditions causing clinical symptoms due to a basic defect in vasculature are enumerated.

PERNIOSIS (CHILBLAINS)

In this common, sometimes familial, condition, inflamed purple-pink swellings appear on the fingers, toes (Fig. 10.1) and rarely, ears. They arrive with winter and are induced by cold. They are painful, and itchy or burning on rewarming. Occasionally they ulcerate. Chilblains are caused by a combination of arteriolar and venular constriction, the latter predominating on rewarming with exudation of fluid into the tissues. Warm housing and clothing help.

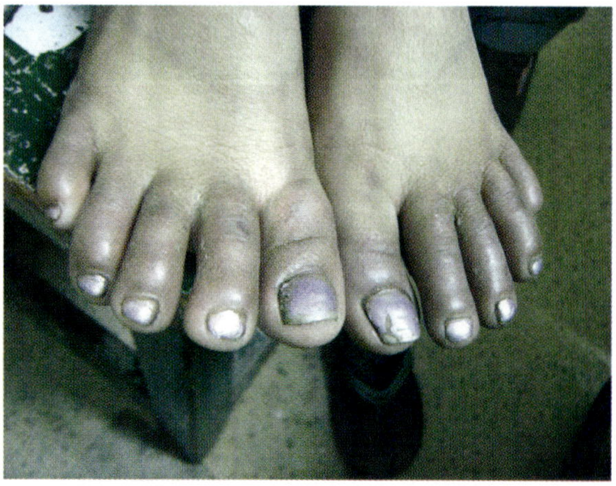

Fig. 10.1: Bilateral dusky hue of toes with itching: Chilblains

Topical remedies rarely work, but the oral calcium channel blocker nifedipine may be useful. The vasodilator nicotinamide (500 mg three times daily) may be helpful alone or in addition to calcium channel blockers.

Acrocyanosis

This type of 'poor circulation', often familial, is more common in females than males. The hands, feet, nose, ears and cheeks become blue-red and cold. The palms are often cold and clammy. The condition is caused by arteriolar constriction and dilatation of the subpapillary venous plexus, and to due cold-induced increases in blood viscosity.

Erythrocyanosis

This occurs in fat, often young women. Purple-red mottled discoloration is seen over the buttocks, thighs and lower legs. Cold provokes it and causes an unpleasant burning sensation.

Erythromelalgia

This is a rare condition in which the extremities become red, hot and painful when exposed to heat (Fig. 10.2). The condition may be idiopathic, or caused by a myeloproliferative disease (e.g., polycythaemia rubra vera or thrombocythaemia), lupus erythematosus, rheumatoid arthritis, diabetes, degenerative peripheral vascular disease or hypertension.

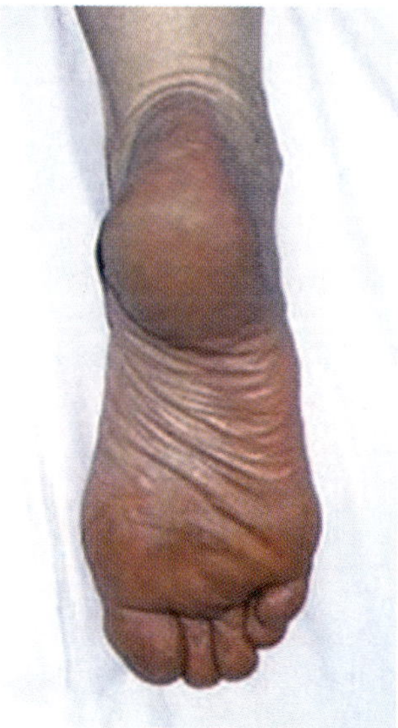

Fig. 10.2: Erythema with pain of soles

Small doses of aspirin give symptomatic relief. Alternatives include non-steroidal anti-inflammatory drugs (NSAIDs), α blockers and oxpentifylline (pentoxifylline).

Spider Naevi

These stellate telangiectases look like spiders, with legs radiating from a central, often palpable, feeding vessel. If the diagnosis is in doubt, press on the central feeding vessel with the corner of a glass slide and the entire lesion will disappear.

Spider naevi are seen frequently on the faces of normal children, and may erupt in pregnancy or be the presenting sign of liver disease, with many lesions on the upper trunk. Liver function should be checked in those with many spider naevi.

The central vessel can be destroyed by electrodessication without local anaesthesia or with a pulsed dye laser.

Livedo Reticularis

This cyanosis of the skin is net-like or marbled (Fig. 10.3) and caused by stasis in the capillaries furthest from their arterial supply: at the periphery of the inverted cone supplied by a dermal arteriole 'Cutis marmorata' is the name given to the mottling of the skin seen in many normal children. It is physiological and disappears on warming, whereas true livedo reticularis remains.

Causes of livedo reticularis

1. Autoimmune	Antiphospholipid syndrome
2. Congenital	
3. Cryopathies	Cryoglobulinaemia cold agglutininaemia
4. Connective tissue disorders	Polyarteritis, livedo vasculitis and systemic lupus erythematosus Syphilis, tuberculosis
5. Hyperviscosity states	Polycythaemia/thrombocythaemia Macroglobulinaemia
6. Idiopathic	
7. Physiological	Cutis marmorata
8. Vessel wall disease	Atherosclerosis

Erythema ab igne

This appearance is also determined by the underlying vascular network. Its reticulate pigmented erythema, with variable scaling, is caused by damage from long term exposure to local heat (open fire, hot water bottle or heating pad).

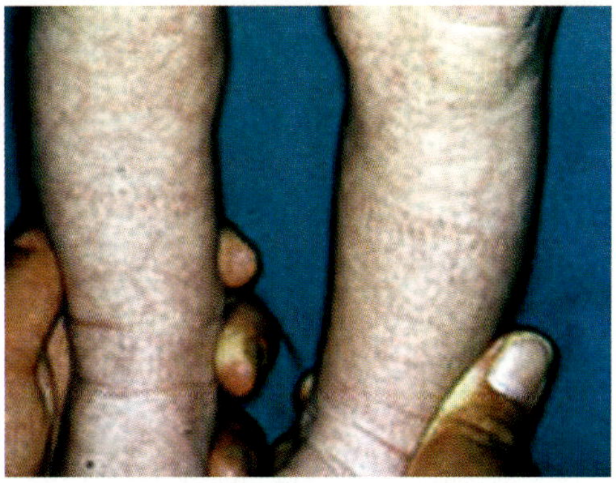

Fig. 10.3: Livedo reticularis (net-like) cyanotic (reddish blue discoloration) cutaneous discoloration surrounding pale central areas

Flushing

This transient vasodilatation of the face may spread to the neck, upper chest and, more rarely, other parts of the body. There is no sharp distinction between flushing and blushing apart from the emotional provocation of the latter.

Paroxysmal **flushing** ('hot flushes'), common at the menopause, is associated with the pulsatile release of luteinizing hormone from the pituitary, as a consequence of low circulating oestrogens and failure of normal negative feedback. However, luteinizing hormone itself cannot be responsible for flushing as this can occur after hypophysectomy. It is possible that menopausal flushing is mediated by central mechanisms involving encephalins. Hot flushes can usually be helped by oestrogen replacement.

Alcohol-induced flushing is most commonly seen in oriental people. Ethanol is broken down to acetaldehyde by alcohol dehydrogenase and acetaldehyde is metabolized to acetic acid by aldehyde dehydrogenase. Acetaldehyde accumulation is in part responsible for flushing. Oriental people not only may have a high-activity variant of alcohol dehydrogenase but also defective aldehyde dehydrogenase. Disulfiram (Antabuse) and, to a lesser extent, chlorpropamide inhibit aldehyde dehydrogenase so that some individuals taking these drugs may flush.

Causes of flushing

1. Physiological	
2. Emotional	
3. Menopausal	
4. Food:	Hot drinks, spicy foods, additives (monosodium glutamate), alcohol (especially in oriental people)

Contd.

Contd.

5. Drugs:	• Vasodilatators including nicotinic acid Bromocriptine • Calcium channel blockers including nifedipine • Disulfiram/Chlorpropamide + alcohol (diabetics)
6. Pathological:	Carcinoid tumours—with asthma and diarrhoea Phaeochromocytoma (tumor producing adrenaline)—with episodic headaches (caused by transient hypertension) and palpitations

Raynaud's Phenomenon

This is a paroxysmal pallor of the digits provoked by cold or, rarely, emotional stress. At first the top of one or more fingers becomes white. On rewarming, a painful cyanosis appears and the area turns red before the hands return to their normal colour. In severe disease the fingers lose pulp substance, ulcerate or become gangrenous, **Raynaud's disease,** often familial, is the name given when no cause can be found. However, some patients with what seems to be Raynaud's disease will later develop a connective tissue disease, usually scleroderma.

The main treatment is to protect the vulnerable digits from cold. Warm clothing reduces the need for peripheral vasoconstriction to conserve heat. Smoking should be abandoned.

Calcium channel blockers (e.g. nifedipine 10-30 mg three times daily) are the most effective agents although they work best in patients with primary Raynaud's disease. Initially it is worth giving nifedipine as a 5 mg test dose with monitoring of the blood pressure in the clinic. If this is tolerated satisfactorily the starting dosage should be 5 mg daily, increasing by 5 mg every 5 days until a therapeutic dose is achieved (e.g. 5-20 mg three times daily) or until intolerable side-effects occur.

Diltiazem (30-60 mg three times daily) is less effective than nifedipine but has fewer side-effects.

Systemic vasodilators such as nicotinic acid and thymoxamine (moxisylyte) are also worth trying.

Glycerol trinitrate ointment, applied once daily may reduce the severity and frequency of attacks and may allow reduction in the dosage of calcium channel blockers and vasodilators.

Infusions with reserpine or prostacyclin help some severe cases although occasionally sympathectomy is needed.

Causes of Raynaud's phenomenon

1. Familial	
2. Raynaud's disease	
3. Connective tissue diseases:	Systemic sclerosis, Lupus erythematosus, Mixed connective tissue disease
4. Arterial occlusion:	Thoracic outlet syndrome, Atherosclerosis, Endarteritis obliterans
5. Repeated trauma:	Pneumatic hammer/drill operators ('vibration white finger')
6. Hyperviscosity:	Polycythaemia, Macroglobulinaemia
7. Cryopathies:	Cryoglobulinaemia, Cryofibrinogenaemia, Cold agglutinaemia
8. Neurological disease:	Peripheral neuropathy, Syringomyelia
9. Toxins:	Ergot,Vinyl chloride

ERYTHEMA MULTIFORME (Table 10.1)

Erythema multiforme, as originally described by Hebra, is an uncommon, distinct disease of unknown cause characterized by red iris-shaped or **bull's eye-like** macules, papules, or bullae confined mainly to the extremities, the face, and the lips. It is accompanied by mild fever, malaise, and arthralgia. It occurs usually in children and young adults in the spring and the fall, has a duration of 2 to 4 weeks, and frequently is recurrent for several years.

The only relation between Hebra's erythema multiforme and the following diseases or syndromes is the clinical appearance of the eruption:

- **Stevens-Johnson syndrome** is a severe and rarely fatal variant of erythema multiforme. It is characterized by high fever, extensive purpura, bullae, ulcers of the mucous membranes, and, after 2 to 3 days, ulcers of the skin. It can be related to drugs and its severest form is considered by some to be the same as toxic epidermal necrolysis. It is also described as a patient **having 2 mucosa involved with loss of skin between 10-30% BSA.**
- **Toxic epidermal necrolysis** is characterized by **atypical EM lesions (purpuric and ecchymotic) with, 2 mucosa involved and loss of > 30% BSA and** is a severe, chronic, bullous disease of adults: Sulfonamides, anticonvulsant agents, allopurinol, chlormezanone, and nonsteroidal anti-inflammatory drugs.
- Erythema multiforme-like eruption is caused rather commonly as part of a herpes simplex outbreak and also in conjunction with rheumatic fever, pneumonia, meningitis, measles, coxsackievirus infection, pregna-

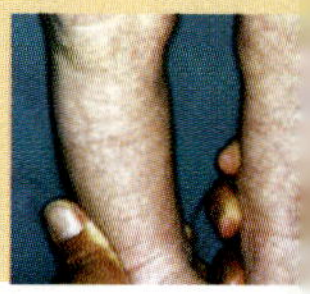

Table. 10.1: Spectrum of disorders with varying presence of characteristic skin lesions, blistering and mucous membrane involvement EM (minor), EM (major), SJS TEN

Comparison of Erythema Multiforme, Stevens-Johnson Syndrome and Toxic Epidermal Necrolysis

	Erythema Multiforme (EM)	*Stevens-Johnson Syndrome (SJS)*	*Toxic Epidermal Necrolysis (TEN)*
Lesion	• Macules/papules with central vesicles • Classic **bull's-eye** pattern of concentric light and dark rings (**target lesions**) • Bilateral and symmetric • **EM minor**—No mucosal involvement	• EM with more mucous membrane involvement and blistering • **"Atypical lesions"**-red circular patch with dark purple centre • More 'sick' (high fever) • Sheet-like epidermal detachment **in <10%** • **Nikolsky sign +**	• Severe mucous membrane involvement • **"Atypical lesions"** 50% have no target lesions • Diffuse erythema then necrosis and sheet-like epidermal datachment in **>30%**
Sites	• Mucous membrane involvement (oral, genital, conjunctival) • Extremities with face> trunk • Involvement of palms and soles	• Generalized with prominent face and trunk involvement • Palms and soles may be spared	• Generalized • Nails may also shed
Etiology	• Drug-sulfonamides, NSAIDs, anticonvulsants, penicillin, allopurinol • Infection–herpes, mycoplasma • Idiopathic->50%	• 50% are drug related • Occurs upto 1-3 weeks after drug exposure with more rapid onset upon rechallenge	• **80%** are definitely drug related • <5% are due to viral infection, immunized
Pathology/ Pathophysiology	• Perivascular PMN infiltrate, edema of upper dermis	• Cytotoxic cell-mediated attack on epidermal cells • No dermal infiltrate • Epidermal necrosis and detachments above basement membrane	• Same as Stevens-Johnson syndrome

ncy, and cancer, as well as after deep X-ray therapy, and as an allergic reaction to foods.

ERYTHEMA NODOSUM

Erythema nodosum is an uncommon reaction pattern seen mainly on the anterior tibial areas of the legs. It appears as erythematous nodules in successive crops and is preceded by fever, malaise and arthralgia.

Clinical Features

Bilateral red, tender, rather well-circumscribed nodules are seen mainly on the pretibial surface of the legs but also on the arms and the body. Later, the flat lesions may become raised, confluent, and purpuric. Only a few lesions develop at one time.

The lesions last several weeks, but the duration can be affected by therapy directed to the cause, if it is known. Relapses are related to the cause. It can be idiopathic and have a chronic course.

Aetiology

Careful clinical and laboratory examinations are necessary to determine the cause of this toxic reaction pattern. The following tests should be performed:

- Complete blood cell count.
- Erythrocyte sedimentation rate.
- Urinalysis.
- Strep tococcal screen, serum pregnancy test, angiotensin converting enzyme, tuberculin skin test.
- Serologic test for syphilis.

- Chest X-ray.
- Mantoux test.
- ASO titre.
- ANA.
- Throat swab.
- Biopsy.

Causes

- Tuberculosis.
- **Streptococcal infection** (rheumatic fever, pharyngitis, scarlet fever, arthritis).
- Fungal infection (coccidioidomycosis, trichophyton infection).
- Pregnancy.
- Sarcoidosis.
- Lymphogranuloma venereum.
- Syphilis.
- Chancroid.
- **Drugs** (contraceptive pills, sulfonamides, iodides, bromides).

It is rare in children, but when it occurs group **A β-hemolytic streptococcal** infection (which may be occult) is the most common cause. **Oral contraceptives** are a common cause in adult women.

The disorder occurs predominantly in adolescent girls and young women.

Laboratory Findings

Histopathologic examination reveals a non-specific but characteristically localized inflammatory infiltrate in the subcutaneous tissue and in and around the veins.

Differential Diagnosis

- **Erythema induratum:** Chronic vasculitis of young women that occurs on the posterior calf area and often suppurates; biopsy shows a tuberculoid-type infiltrate, usually with caseation.
- **Necrobiosis lipoidica diabeticorum:** An uncommon cutaneous manifestation of diabetes mellitus, characterized by well-defined patches of reddish-yellow atrophic skin, primarily on anterior areas of legs; the lesions can ulcerate.
- **Periarteritis nodosa:** A rare, sometimes fatal, arteritis that most often occurs in men; 25% of patients show painful subcutaneous nodules and purpura, mainly of the lower extremities. It is a multiorgan system disease; renal failure is often a component. There is a cutaneous variety (+) p-ANCA blood test.
- **Superficial thrombophlebitis migrans (Buerger's disease):** An early venous change of Buerger's disease commonly seen in male patients, with painful nodules of the anterior tibial area.
- **Nodular panniculitis or Weber-Christian disease:** Occurs mainly in obese middle-aged women; tender, indurated, subcutaneous nodules and plaques are seen, usually on the thighs and the buttocks; each crop is preceded by fever and malaise; residual atrophy and hyper-pigmentation occur.
- **Leukocytoclastic vasculitis:** Includes a constellation of diseases, such as allergic angiitis, allergic vasculitis, necrotizing vasculitis, and cutaneous systemic vasculitis. Clinically, palpable purpuric lesions are seen, most commonly on the lower part of the legs. In later stages, the lesions may become nodular, bullous, infarctive and ulcerative.

Treatment

- Treat the cause, if possible.
- Rest, local heat, and aspirin are valuable. The eruption is self-limited if the cause can be eliminated.
- Chronic cases can be disabling enough to warrant a short course of corticosteroid therapy. Some cases have benefited from naproxen, 250 mg b.i.d. (or other nonsteroidal anti-inflammatory drugs), for 2 to 4 weeks.
- Potassium iodide solution 10-15 drops increase to 45-60 drops mixed with fruit juice is known to help some idiopathic cases.

PURPURIC DERMATOSES

Purpuric lesions are caused by an extravasation of red blood cells into the skin or mucous membranes. The lesions can be distinguished from erythema and telangiectasia by the fact that purpuric lesions do not blanch under pressure applied by the finger or by a clear glass slide (diascopy) (Fig. 10.4).

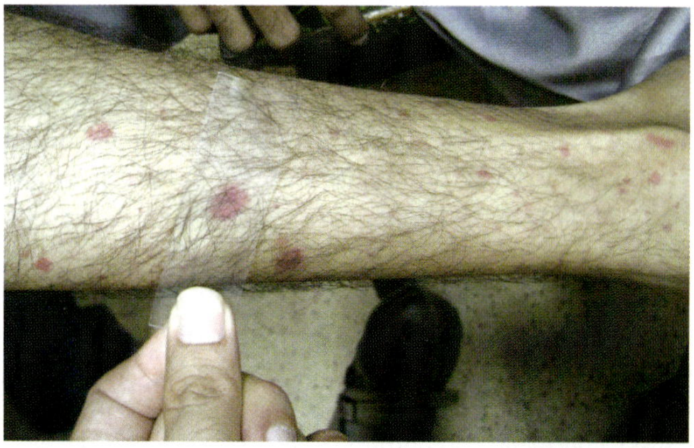

Fig. 10.4: Blanching of the lesions reveals persistence of eryhthema suggestive of purpura (diascopy)

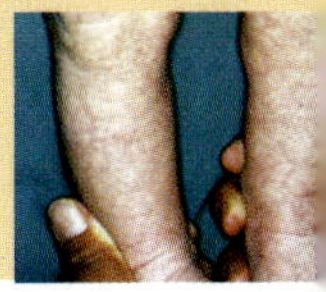

- **Petechiae** are small, superficial purpuric lesions. These are most often a sign of platelet deficiency or malfunction **(macules < 3 mm).**
- **Ecchymoses,** or bruises, are more extensive, round or irregularly shaped purpuric lesions often seen in the elderly (senile purpura), patients on chronic topical or systemic corticosteroids and patients on anticoagulants. ecchymotic (**macules > 3 mm**).
- **Hematomas** are large, deep, fluctuant, tumor-like hemorrhages into the skin.

The purpuras can be divided into the thrombocytopenic forms and the nonthrombocytopenic forms.

- **Thrombocytopenic** purpura may be idiopathic or secondary to various chronic diseases or to a drug sensitivity. The platelet count is below normal, the bleeding time is prolonged, and the clotting time is normal, but the clot does not retract normally. This form of purpura is rare.
- **Nonthrombocytopenic purpura** is more commonly seen. **Henoch-Schönlein purpura** is a form of nonthrombocytopenic purpura most commonly seen in children that is characterized by recurrent attacks of purpura accompanied by arthritis, hematuria, IgA glomerulonephritis, and gastrointestinal disorders. Approximately 75% of the time it involves skin only.

Thrombocytopenia causes petechiae, whereas abnormalities in the clotting cascade commonly cause ecchymoses. Necrotic ecchymoses are found when thrombi form in dermal vessels and lead to infarction and hemorrhage, e.g., disseminated intravascular coagulation (DIC).

The ecchymoses, or senile purpura, seen in elderly patients after minor injury are very common. Ecchymoses are also seen in patients who have been on long-term systemic corticosteroid therapy and also occur after prolonged use of the high-potency corticosteroids locally and from corticosteroid nasal inhalers. Anticoagulants make these more common.

Another common purpuric eruption is that known as stasis purpura. These lesions are associated with vascular insufficiency of the legs and occur as the early sign of this change, or they are seen around areas of stasis dermatitis or stasis ulcers. Frequently seen is a petechial drug eruption owing to the chlorothiazide diuretics. A detailed list is given below:

I. **Petechiae (non-palpable)**
  A. Hemostatically relevant thrombocytopenia (**platelet count; if less than 50,000/mm**
    1. Idiopathic thrombocytopenic purpura
    2. Thrombotic thrombocytopenic purpura (some cases)
    3. Disseminated intravascular coagulation
    4. Drug-related thrombocytopenia
      a. *Peripheral destruction:* quinidine, quinine
      b. *Marrow:* idiosyncratic or dose related
    5. Marrow infiltration, fibrosis, or failure
  B. Abnormal platelet function
    1. Congenital or hereditary platelet function defects
    2. Acquired platelet function defects (e.g., aspirin, renal or hepatic insuficiency, monoclonal gammopathy)
    3. Thrombocytosis in meloproliferative disease $(>1,000,000/mn^3)$
  C. Elevated intravascular pressure (Valsalva maneuver).
  D. Chronic pigmented purpura (occasionally palpable, caused by minimal small-vessel inflammation)

II. **Ecchymotic**
  A. Procoagulant defect (often localized to sites of minor trauma)
    1. Hemophilla
    2. Anticoagulants
    3. Disseminated intravascular coagulation
    4. Vitamin K deficiency
    5. Hepatic insufficiency with poor procoagulant synthesis
  B. Poor dermal support of vessels (usually localized to sites of minor trauma)
    1. Actinic (senile) purpura
    2. Corticosteroid therapy, topical or systemic.
    3. Scurvy
    4. Systemic amyloidosis (light chain related)
    5. Ehlers-Danlos syndrome, primarily type I, IV, VI, VIII, and X
    6. Pseudoxanthoma elasticum
  C. Other
    Benign hypergammaglobulinemic purpura of Waldenstrom (as a result of mild vessel inflammation, usually causes macular hemorrhage, but can produce palpable purpura)

III. **Palpable purpura**
  A. Classic palpable purpura
    1. Small vessel (*leukocytoclastic vasculitis*)
      a. Post-infectious, drug-induced, or idiopathic IgG, IgM immune complex vascultitis
      b. Post-infectious, drug-induced, or idiopathic IgA predo-minant vasculitis (Henoch-Schönlein purpura)
      c. Mixed cryoglobulinemia
      d. Associated with lupus, rheumatoid arthritis, Sjögren's syndrome
      e. Small vessel lesions of Wegener's, Churg-Strauss, or lymphomatoid granulomatosis
    2. Pityriasis lichenoides et varioliformis acuta (PLEVA) syndrome
    3. Erthema multiforme (some variants)
  B. Target lesions
    1. Erythema multiforme
  C. Inflammatory *retiform purpura* (usually vasculitis, both retiform morphology and prominent early erythema)
    1. IgA-predominant small vessel leukocytoclastic vasculitis (some)
    2. Syndromes of small and medium vessel leukocytoclastic vasculitis, such as rheumatic vasculitis, polyarteritis, and Wegener's granulomatosis (occasionally)

3. Some early lesions of warfarin- or heparin-induced necrosis demonstate erythema, but the tends to be at the margin of large, confluent areas of necrosis

IV. **Non-inflammatory retiform purpura** (occlusion syndromes, usually retiform morphology without early erythema)

A. Disorders of platelet plugging: Myeloproliferative thrombocytosis, heparin necrosis, rarely thrombotic thrombocytopenic purpura, paroxysmal nocturnal hemoglobinuria.
B. Diorders of cold-relation cryogelling or agglutination
C. Disorders of vessel invasive organisms: Ecthyma gangrenosum, aspergillus and other opportunistic fungi, disseminated strongyloidsis
D. Disorders of local or systemic control of coagulation inherited or acquired severe protein C or S deficiency (acquired includes some sepsis/disseminated intravascular coagulation, coumarin necrosis, some antiphospholipid antibody syndromes), antiphsopholipid antibody syndromes, some atrophic blanche.
E. Disorders of embolization: Cholestererol or oxalate emboli, atrial myxoma, crystalglobulins
F. Miscellaneous disorders: Cutaneous calciphylaxis, Dego's disease, sickle cell ulcerations.

Pigmented Purpuric Eruptions

A less common group of cases are those seen in middle-aged adults, classified under the name pigmented purpuric eruptions. They are usually asymptomatic but some cases of pigmented purpuric eruptions itch severely. The cause is unknown; most cases have a positive tourniquet test, but other bleeding tests are normal.

Clinical Features

Clinically, these patients have grouped petechial lesions that begin on the legs and extend up to the thighs, and occasionally up to the waist and onto the arms. They turn into a brown **Cayenne-pepper** nonpalpable discoloration that fades over weeks to months.

Some clinicians are able to separate these pigmented purpuric eruptions into:

- Purpura annularis telangiectodes (**Majocchi's** disease).
- Progressive pigmentary dermatosis (**Schamberg's** disease), and
- Pigmented purpuric lichenoid dermatitis (**Gougerot** and **Blum disease**).

Majocchi's disease commonly begins on the legs but slowly spreads, to become generalized (Fig. 10.5). Telangiectatic capillaries become confluent and produce annular or serpiginous lesions. The capillaries break down, causing purpuric lesions. Schamberg's disease is a slowly progressive pigmentary condition of the lower part of the legs that fades after a period of months but may recur. The Gougerot-Blum form is accompanied by severe itching and eczematous changes; otherwise it resembles Schamberg's disease.

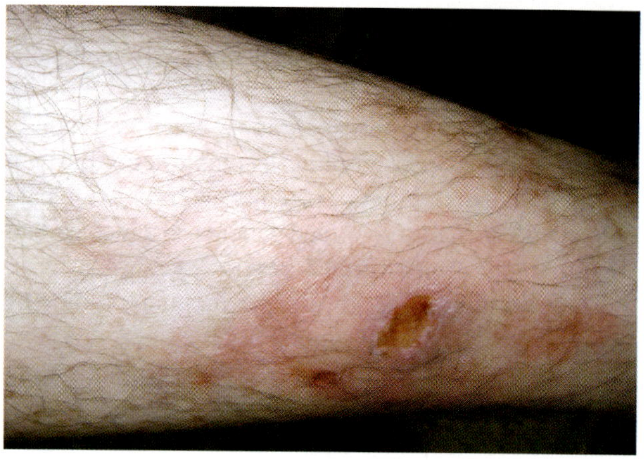

Fig. 10.5: Purpura annularis telangiectodes with ulceration

Treatment

For these pigmented purpuric eruptions, therapy may not be necessary. Occlusive dressing therapy with a corticosteroid cream can be beneficial. For resistant cases, prednisone, 10 mg, 1 to 2 tablets in the morning for 3 to 6 weeks, is indicated.

Other drugs tried are pentoxyfylline, Rutoside, oral flavanoids, PUVA, Vitamin C, griesofulvin and cyclosporine.

TELANGIECTASES

Telangiectases are abnormal dilated small blood vessels. Telangiectases are divided into **primary** forms, in which the causes are unknown, and **secondary** forms, which are related to some known disturbance. The primary telangiectases include the simple and compound hemangiomas of infants, essential telangiectasias, and spider hemangiomas. Diseases with numerous telangiectasias include:

- Cirrhosis of the liver.
- Osler-Weber-Rendu disease, which also has mucous membrane involvement.
- lupus erythematosus.
- Scleroderma.
- Dermatomyositis.
- Cutaneous polyarteritis.
- Metastatic carcinoid syndrome.
- Ataxia telangiectasia.
- Angiokeratoma corporis diffusum.
- Telangiectasia macularis eruptiva perstans, and rosacea.
- Overlying basal cell cancers.

Unilateral nevoid telangiectasia syndrome can be congenital or acquired. The acquired form appears when increased estrogen levels occur in women with puberty or pregnancy and in cirrhosis. C_3, C_4, and trigeminal dermatomes are the most common.

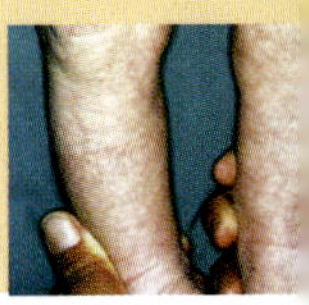

Secondary telangiectasia is very commonly seen on the fair-skinned person as a result of aging, chronic topical and systemic corticosteroid use, and chronic sun exposure. X-ray therapy and burns can also cause dilated vessels.

Treatment for the secondary telangiectasias can be accomplished quite adequately with very light electrosurgery to the vessels, which is usually tolerated without anesthesia or for many extensive lesions use of laser therapy or intense pulsed light therapy. Injectable sclerosing agents are available for therapy on the lower legs.

VASCULITIS

Inflammation of the blood vessels (vasculitis) commonly affects the skin and has numerous underlying causes. It can be cutaneous only, Gougerot and Ruiter's type, but often involves other organs, most commonly joints, kidney, and gastrointestinal tract and rarely the nervous system, eye (temporal arteritis), heart, and respiratory tract.

Aetiopathogenesis

An overview of the aetiological pathological sequence and an enumeration of the aetiological factors is given below : (Fig. 10.6)

1. Infections
   A. Hepatitis C or occasionally B, rarely hepatitis A
   B. Acute respiratory infections (viral or bracterial)
   C. Streptococcal infections and post-streptococcal diseases
   D. Bacterial endocarditis
   E. Intestinal bypass syndrome
   F. Mycobacterial diseases

II. Drugs and other ingestants: Any drug can cause vasculitis, but particularly
   A Aspirin
   B. Sulfonamides
   C. Cephalosporins
   D. Penicillins
   E. Barbiturates
   F. Amphetamines
   G. Propyithiouracil

III. Genetic: Deficiency of a component of complement

IV. Abnormal globulins
   A. Cryoglobulinemia: Essential or secondary
   B. Multiple myeloma
   C. Macroglobulinemia

V. Rheumatic diseases
   A. Systemic lupus erythematosus
   B. Rheumatoid vasculitis
   C. Dermatomyositis or polymyositis

VI. Other diseases
   A. Ulcerative colitis
   B. Lymphomas
   C. Colonic carcinoma
   D. Hairy cell leukemia
   E. Serous otitis media

VII. Idiopathic

Vasculitis classification is complex of two classification are given in Tables 10.2 and 10.3.

Clinical Features

Palpable purpura is the classic clinical appearance. Varying shades of bluish-red discoloration may be firmly indurated or difficult to feel. Lesions can be large (many centimeters) or quite small (several millimeters) with a petechial look. The dependent areas are the location where it is most commonly seen—legs on ambulatory patients, on buttocks and back in bedridden patients.

Table 10.2: Vasculitis classification (Vessel size)

Vessel size	*Types*	*Clinical picture*	*Systemic*	*Therapy*	*Prognosis*
Small vessel (venules)	Leukocytoclastic Vasculitis Churg Strauss Syndrome	Urticarial lesions, palpable purpura	Minimal	Symptomatic	Good
Small artery	Wegeners granulomatis Microscopic polyangitis Cryoglobulinemia Henoch-Schönlein purpura	Erythema nodosum-like lesions	Mild, unless associated with systemic disorders	Symptomatic	Good
Medium-sized artery	Classic PAN Kawasaki	Necrosis of major organs, livedo reticularis, purpura, mononeuritis multiplex	Severe	Steroids, cytotoxic drugs	Guarded
Large vessel	Giant cell arteritis Takayasu arteritis	Claudication, necrosis	Moderate	Steroids, cytotoxic drug	Poor

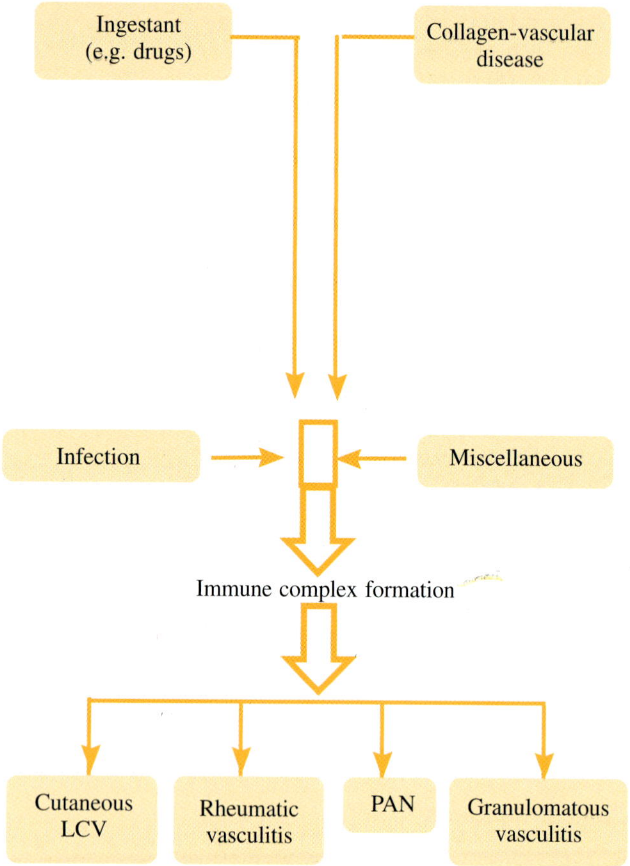

Fig. 10.6: Overview of pathogenesis

Table 10.3: Types of vasculitis

I. Leukocytoclastic vasculitis (hypersensitivity angiitis or allergic vasculitis)
   A. Idiopathic
   B. Drug induced
   C. Hypocomplementemic vasculitis (often urticarial)
   D. Essential mixed cryoglobulinemia
   E. Hyperglobulinemic purpuras **(Waldenström's macroglobulinemia)**

II. Rheumatic vasculitis
   A. Systemic lupus erythematosus
   B. Rheumatoic vasculitis
   C. Dermatomyositis

III. Granulomatous vasculitis
   A. Allergic granulomatous vasculitis (Churg-Strauss)
   B. Wegener's granulomatosis
   C. Lymphomatoid granulomatosis

IV. Polyarteritis nodosa
   A. Classic type
   B. Cutaneous type

V. Giant cell arteritis
   A. Temporal arteritis
   B. Takayasu's disease

As the vascular damage progresses, blisters, nodules, ulcers, necrosis, and gangrene may occur. Livedo reticularis is a bluish-red, netlike appearing condition that can be associated with vasculitis.

THE AMERICAN COLLEGE OF RHEUMATOLOGY CLASSIFICATION CRITERIA FOR VASCULITIS

Giant-cell (temporal) arteritis (CGA)

1. Age >50 years at onset.
2. New type of headache.
3. Abnormal temporal artery on clinical examination (Tenderness to palpation or decreased pulsation).
4. Elevated erythrocyte sedimentation rate.
5. Temporal artery biopsy showing vasculitis.

Three criteria classify CGA with sensitivity of 95. 5% and specificity of 91.2%.

Takayasu's arteritis (TA)

1. Age less than 40 years at onset.
2. Limb claudication.
3. Decreased brachial artery pulses.
4. BP >10 mm Hg difference between two arms
5. Bruits.
6. Arteriogram abnormal.

Three criteria classify TA with sensitivity of 90.5% and specificity of 97.8%.

Polyarteritis nodosa (PAN)

1. Weight loss >4 kg.
2. Livedo reticularis.
3. Testicular pain or tenderness.
4. Myalgias, myopathy or tenderness.
5. Neuropathy.
6. Hypertension (diastolic BP >90 mm Hg).
7. Renal impairment (elevated BUN or creainine).
8. Hepatitis B virus.
9. Abnormal arteriography.
10. Biopsy of artery showing PMN.

Three criteria classify PAN with sensitivity of 82.2% and specifically of 86.6%.

Wegner's granulomatosis (WG)

1. Nasal or oral inflammation.

2. Chest X-ray showing nodules, infiltrates (fixed or cavities).
3. Microscopic hematuria or red cell casts in urine.
4. Granulomatous inflammation on biopsy (within vessel wall or perivascular).

   Two criteria classify WG with sensitivity of 88.2% and specificity of 92.0%.

Churg-Strauss syndrome (CSS)

1. Asthma.
2. Eosinophilia (>10%).
3. Neuropathy.
4. Pulmonary infiltrates (nonfixed).
5. Sinusitis.
6. Extravascular eosinophils on biopsy.

   Four criteria classify CSS with sensitivity of 85% and specificity of 99.7%.

Hypersensitivity vasculitis

1. Age > 10 years onset.
2. Medications that may have precipitated event.
3. Palpable purpura.
4. Cutaneous eruption.
5. Positive biopsy results.

   Three criteria classify HSV with sensitivity of 71.0% and specificity of 83.9%.

Henoch-Schönlein purpura (HSP) (Fig. 10.7)

1. Palpable purpura.
2. Age at onset <20 years.
3. Bowel angina.
4. Vessel wall granulocytes on biopsy.

   Two criteria classify HSP with sensitivity of 87% and specificity of 88%.

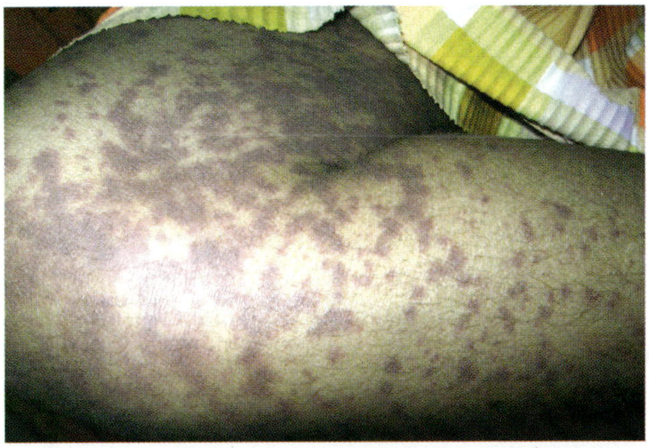

Fig. 10.7: Purpura on the lower limb in patient with preceding abdominal pain (Henoch-Schönlein purpura)

Basic Laboratory Evaluation of Vasculitis

- Urine analysis (most crucial test because early asymptomatic renal disease can be detected and progression to renal failure prevented).
- Stool screen for occult blood (stool Guaiac).
- Complete blood count with platelets and coagulation screen.
- Hypercoagulability studies may be indicated such as anticardiolipin and antiphospholipid antibodies.
- Antinuclear antibody, rheumatoid factor, liver enzymes, hepatitis screen, cryoglobulins, cryofibrinogen, and complement immunoglobulins.
- Antineutrophil cytoplasmic antibody (ANCA) that is positive in Wegener's granulomatosis (c-ANCA) and polyarteritis nodosa (p-ANCA).

Treatment

Systemic corticosteroids are the mainstay of early therapy. Corticosteroid-sparing drugs include colchicine, dapsone, azathioprine, methotrexate, cytoxan (drug of choice for Wegener's granulomatosis), intravenous gamma globulin, antimalarials, and plasmapheresis have all been used.

PRESSURE SORES

Sustained or repeated pressure on skin over bony prominences can cause ischaemia and pressure sores.

These are common in patients over 70 years old who are confined to hospital, especially those with a fractured neck of femur. The morbidity and mortality of those with deep ulcers is high.

Cause: The main factors responsible for pressure sores are as follows:

1. Prolonged immobility and recumbency (e.g. caused by paraplegia, arthritis or senility).
2. Vascular disease (e.g. atherosclerosis).
3. Neurological disease causing diminished sensation (e.g. in paraplegia).
4. Malnutrition, severe systemic disease and general debility.

Management

The following are important: Prevention: By turning recumbent patients regularly and using antipressure mattresses for susceptible patients.

1. Treatment of malnutrition and the general condition.
2. Debridement: Regular cleansing with normal saline or 0.5% aqueous silver nitrate.

3. Appropriate topical and systemic antibiotic.
4. Plastic surgical reconstruction may be indicated in the young when the ulcer is clean.

STASIS (VENOUS) DERMATITIS AND ULCERS

Stasis dermatitis is a common condition owing to impaired venous circulation in the legs of older patients. Almost all cases are associated with varicose veins, and because the tendency to develop varicosities is a familial characteristic, stasis dermatitis is also familial. The **medial malleolus** area of the ankle is the most common location. Stasis ulcers can develop in the impaired skin.

Clinical Features

Early cases of stasis dermatitis begin as a red, scaly, pruritic patch that rapidly becomes vesicular and crusted, owing to scratching and subsequent secondary infection. Bacterial infection may be responsible for the spread of the patch and the chronicity of the eruption. Edema of the affected ankle area results in a further decrease in circulation and, consequently, more infection. The lesions may be unilateral or bilateral.

Three secondary conditions can arise from untreated stasis dermatitis:

- **Infectious eczematoid dermatitis:** This can develop on the legs, the arms, and even the entire body, either slowly, or as an explosive, rapidly spreading auto-eczematous or "id" eruption.

Treatment of Stasis Dermatitis

- Prescribe rest and elevation of the leg as much as possible by lying in bed. The foot of the bed should be elevated 4 inches by placing two bricks under the legs. Attempt to elevate the leg when sitting. Avoid prolonged standing or sitting with the legs bent.
- Burrow's solution wet packs.
- An antibiotic and corticosteroid ointment mixture.

For more severe cases of stasis dermatitis with oozing, cellulitis, and pitting edema, the following treatment should be ordered, in addition:

- Hospitalization or enforced bed rest at home for the purpose of (1) applying the wet packs for longer periods of time and (2) strict rest and elevation of the leg.
- A course of an oral antibiotic.

Treatment of Stasis Ulcer

As for any chronic difficult medical problem, there are many methods touted for successful management.

- **Manage the primary problem or problems:** Attempt to remedy the obesity, make sure there is adequate nutrition, and treat systemic or other causes of the ulcer.
- **Correct the physiologic alterations:** Control the edema with adhesive flexible bandages of adequate width (4 inches wide usually) and with correct application from foot up to knee.
- **Treat contributing factors:** Control the dermatitis, itching and infection.
- **Promote healing:** Occlusion of the ulcer has been proved to accelerate healing. Unna boots, adhesive flexible bandage dressings, and polyurethane-type films have been used with success. Enzymatic granules have their proponents as well as collagen granules and granulex.
- Skin grafting may be indicated in deep, stubborn ulcers.
- Advise a multiple vitamin and mineral supplement tablet once a day, including zinc and magnesium.
- Elevate leg as much as possible lying down prone.
- **Occlusive dressing:** This is to be applied in the office. If there is a lot of drainage and debris, the frequency of dressing should be every 3 to 4 days at first, then weekly. Use a foot-rest stand for the leg. Keep a record on the size of the ulcer.
- Pentoxifylline (Trental) at a dosage of 1200 to 2400 mg and divided into three doses per day with food has been shown to be beneficial. Gastrointestinal upset is common.

No management of a venous stasis ulcer is 100% effective, but this routine with modifications is the one we use. If an ulcer is stable or decreasing in size after 4 weeks the current treatment should be continued. If it is enlarging, then alternate therapy, including surgery, should be considered.

LEG ULCER

Causes

Atherosclerotic: These ulcers are more common on the toes, dorsum of foot, heel, calf and shin, and are unrelated to perforating veins. Their edges are often sharply defined, their outline may be polycyclic and the ulcers may be deep and gangrenous. Islands of intact skin are characteristically seen within the ulcer.

Claudication may be present and peripheral pulses absent.

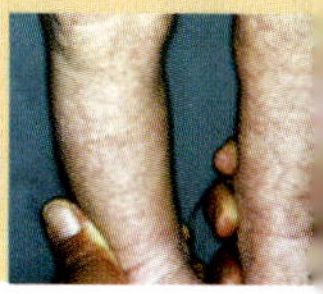

Vasculitis

These ulcers start as **painful** palpable purpuric lesions, turning into small punched-out ulcers. The involvement of larger vessels is heralded by painful nodules that may ulcerate. The intractable deep sharply demarcated ulcers of rheumatoid arthritis are caused by an underlying vasculitis.

Thrombotic Ulcers

Skin infarction, leading to ulceration, may be caused by embolism or by the increased coagulability of polycythemia or cryoglobulinemia.

Infective Ulcers

Ulcers caused by tuberculosis, leprosy, atypical mycobacteria, diphtheria and deep fungal infections, such as sporotrichosis or chromoblastomycosis, are still seen in the tropics.

Panniculitic Ulcers

These may appear at odd sites, such as the thighs, buttocks or backs of the calves. The most common types of panniculitis that ulcerate are lupus panniculitis, pancreatic panniculitis and erythema induratum.

Malignant Ulcers

Those caused by a squamous cell carcinoma are the most common, but both malignant melanomas and basal cell carcinomas can present as flat lesions, which expand, crust and ulcerate. Furthermore, squamous cell carcinoma can arise in any longstanding ulcer, whatever its cause.

Pyoderma Gangrenosum

These large and rapidly spreading ulcers may be circular or polycyclic, and have a blue, indurated, undermined or pustular margin. Pyoderma gangrenosum may complicate rheumatoid arthritis, Crohn's disease, ulcerative colitis or blood dyscrasias.

Diabetic Ulcers.

Treatment

Venous ulcers will not heal if the leg remains swollen and the patient chair-bound. Pressure bandages take priority over other measures but not for atherosclerotic ulcers with an already precarious arterial supply.

A common error is to use local treatment that is too elaborate. As a last resort, admission to hospital for elevation and intensive treatment may be needed, but the results are not encouraging; patients may stay in the ward for many months only to have their apparently well-healed ulcers breakdown rapidly when they go home.

Compression Bandages and Stockings

Compression bandaging, with the compression graduated so that it is greatest at the ankle and least at the top of the bandage, is vital for most venous ulcers; it reduces oedema and aids venous return. The bandages are applied over the ulcer dressing, from the forefoot to just below the knee.

Bandages stay on for 2-7 days at a time and are left on at night. One four-layer compression bandaging system includes a layer of orthopaedic wool, a standard crepe, the combined four layers give a 40 mmHg compression at the ankle. Once an ulcer has healed, a graduated compression stocking from toes to knee (or preferably thigh), should be prescribed, preferably at pressures of at least 35 mmHg. A foam or felt pad may be worn under the stockings to protect vulnerable areas against minor trauma.

Elevation of the affected limb, preferably above the hips, this aids venous drainage, decreases oedema and raises oxygen tension in the limb. Patients should rest with their bodies horizontal and their legs up for at least 2 hours every afternoon. The foot of the bed should be raised by at least 15 cm; it is not enough just to put a pillow under the feet.

Walking

Walking, in moderation, is beneficial, but prolonged standing or sitting with dependent legs is not.

Physiotherapy

Some physiotherapists are good at persuading venous ulcers to heal. Their secret lies in a combination of the following: leg exercises, elevation, gentle massage, ultrasound treatment to the skin around the ulcers, oedema pumps and graduated compression bandaging.

Diet

Many patients are obese and should lose weight.

Local therapy should be chosen to:

- Control or absorb the exudates.
- Reduce the pain.
- Control the odour.
- Protect the surrounding skin.
- Remove surface debris.
- Promote re-epithelialization; and
- Make optimal use of nursing time.

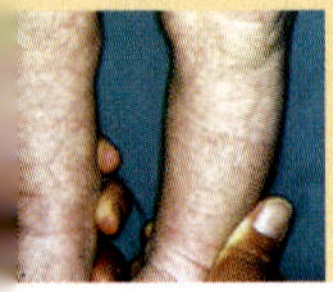

Clean Ulcers

Dressings need be changed only once or twice a week, keeping the ulcer moist. Paraffin tulle dressings, plain or impregnated with 0.5% chlorhexidine, 1% silver sulphadiazine cream, are all helpful and easy to apply. The area should be cleaned gently with arachis oil, 5% hydrogen peroxide or saline before the next dressing is applied. Sometimes immersing the whole ulcer in a tub of warm water helps to loosen or dissolve adherent crusts. The prolonged use of antiseptics may be harmful.

Infected Ulcers

These have to be cleaned and dressed more often than clean ones, sometimes even twice daily. Useful preparations include 0.5% silver nitrate, 0.25% sodium hypochlorite, 0.25% acetic acid, potassium permanganate (1 in 10000 dilution) and 5% hydrogen peroxide, all made up in aqueous solution, and applied as compresses with or without occlusion.

The main function of dextran polymer beads, and starch polymer beads within cadexomer iodine, is to absorb exudate. Although antibiotic tulles are easy to apply and are well tolerated, they should not be used for long periods as they can induce bacterial resistance and sensitize. Resistance is not such a problem with povidone-iodine, and a readily applied non-adherent dressing impregnated with this antiseptic may be useful. Surrounding eczema is helped by weak or moderate strength local steroids, which must never be put on the ulcer itself.

Oral Treatment

The following may be helpful:

Diuretics

Pressure bandaging is more important as the oedema associated with venous ulceration is largely mechanical. Diuretics will combat the oedema of cardiac failure.

Analgesics

Adequate analgesia is important. Aspirin may not be well tolerated by the elderly.

Antibiotics: Ulcers need not be 'sterilized' by local or systemic antibiotics. Short courses of systemic antibiotics should be reserved for spreading infections. Bacteriological guidance is needed.

Ferrous Sulphate and Folic Acid

For anaemia, zinc sulphate may help to promote healing, especially if the plasma zinc level is low.

Oxypentifylline (pentoxyfylline) is fibrinolytic, increases the deformability of red and white blood cells, decreases blood viscosity and diminishes platelet adhesiveness. It may speed the healing of venous ulcers if used with compression bandages.

Stanozolol: This anabolic steroid may not heal an existing ulcer more quickly, but may prevent ulceration in lipodermatosclerosis and may protect against recurrences.

DISORDERS OF THE LYMPHATICS

Lymphoedema

The skin overlying chronic lymphoedema is firm and pits poorly. Longstanding lymphoedema may lead to gross, almost furry, hyperkeratosis, as in the so-called '**mossy foot**'.

Cause

Lymphoedema may be primary or secondary. The primary forms are developmental defects, although signs may only appear in early puberty or even in adulthood. Sometimes lymphoedema involves only one leg.

Treatment

Elevation, graduated compression bandages and stockings, diuretics and the early treatment of lymphangitis or erysipelas are the cornerstones of treatment. If erysipelas recurs, long-term penicillin should be given. Surgery occasionally helps to remove an obstruction or restore drainage.

Lymphangitis

This streptococcal infection of the lymphatics may occur without any lymphoedema. A tender red line extends proximally. Penicillin flucloxacillin, cephalexin and erythromycin are usually effective.

REFERENCES

- Cherry G: The Oxford European wound healing course handbook, Oxford, Oxford University Press, 2002.
- Ghersetich I, Panconesi E: The purpuras, Int J Dermatol 1994; 33:1.
- Nussinovitch M, Prais D, *et al.*: Cutaneous manifestations of Henoch-Schönlein purpura in young children, Pediatr Dermatol 1998; 15:426-428.

CHAPTER 11

PAPULOSQUAMOUS DISORDERS

Psoriasis

DEFINITION

Psoriasis is a common inflammatory, chronic, persistent disorders that affects approximately 1-2% of population. The disease has a bimodal distribution of age of onset. Early peak of age of onset is 22 years in male and 16 years in females and the later one at 60 years in males and 57 years in females.

It affects the life cycle of skin cells. **Normal time taken for a cell to replicate is 311 hours but it is 36 hours in psoriasis. Also the normal transit time of the cell is 53 days, it reduces to 7 days in psoriasis** (Fig. 11.1).

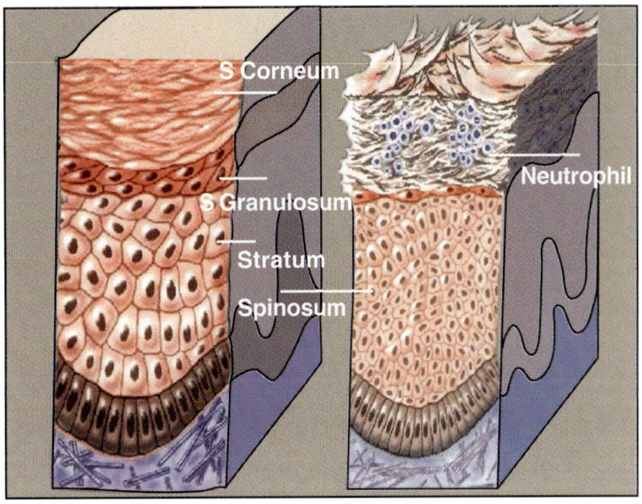

Fig. 11.1: Normal layers on the left, psoriasis on the right where the stratum corneum is disorganized, cracked and flaky/the stratum granulosum has thickened and has tremendous neutrophil accumulation/the stratum spinosum has many immature cells and is thicker

AETIOLOGY AND PATHOGENESIS

Genetic origin of psoriasis is suggested by certain HLAs like **HLA CW6** in psoriasis and **HLA B27** in generalized pustular psoriasis and psoriatic arthritis. It is considered that PSOR1, an HLA associated allele accounts for 30-50% of the causative genes of psoriasis. The others are on other sites **(chr 17,4,1,3)**.

The most widely accepted hypothesis is that there are triggering factors that activate the autoantigen in the epidermis and activate circulating T cells, that release IFN gamma, which facilitate their adhesion to the keratinocyte. The binding of activated T lymphocyte to keratinocyte releases cytokines which would cause proliferation of keratinocytes and cause vascular change and also lead to influx of cells.

There are two classes of T cells: Th1 and Th2. **Th1 release IL-2 and IFN gamma and contribute to CMI while Th2 cells release IL4,5,10 and favour humoral immunity.** The Th1 cells are proinflammatory and this is counter balanced by Th2 cells.The IFN gamma that is overexpressed in psoriasis also *increases* the levels of **Bcl-X**, which *inhibits keratinocyte apoptosis* and induces inflammatory cytokines including *TNF-alpha* (Fig. 11.2). To facilitate this the IL2 receptor CD25 is overexpressed in the T cells.

Psoriasis Triggers (Fig. 11.2)

Factors that may trigger psoriasis include:

- Infections, such as *streptococcal or candidiasis.*
- Injury to the skin, such as Isomorphic or Koebner's phenomenon, a cut or scrape, bug bite, or a severe sunburn.
- Stress.
- Cold weather.
- Smoking.
- Heavy alcohol consumption.
- Certain medications, including lithium, beta blockers, anti-malarial drugs, NSAIDS and iodides.

Two interesting phenomena occur in psoriasis. They are

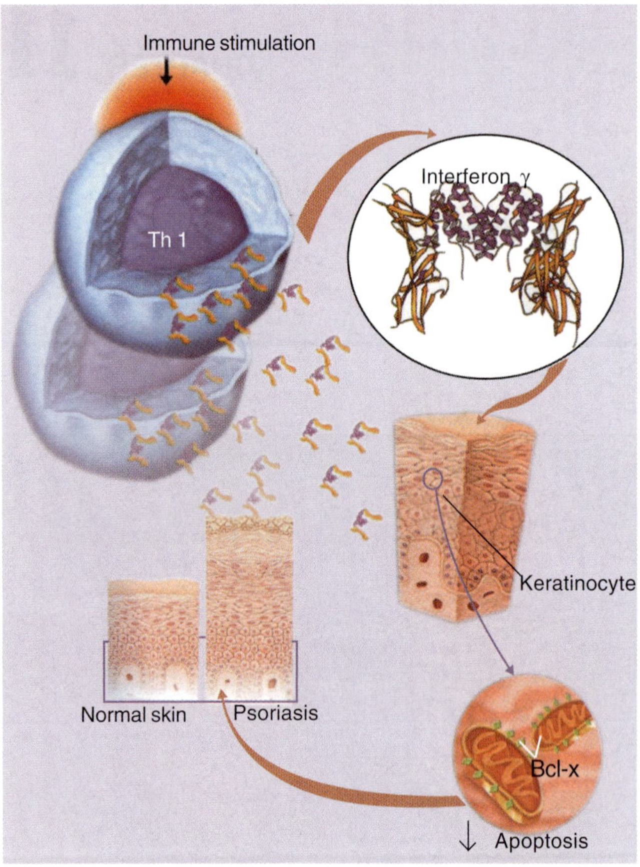

Fig. 11.2: Role and sequence of events of trigger factors in psoriasis

mutually exclusive: *Koebner* and *reverse Koebner* responses. Any form of trauma may result in psoriasis appearing in the traumatized areas which is known as Koebner phenomenon or isomorphic response. A degree of healing may occur when a psoriatic plaque is traumatized which is the reverse Koebner phenomenon. It also explains why some patients found cryotherapy is useful to suppress psoriasis.

Risk Factors (Table 11.1)

Perhaps the most significant risk factor for psoriasis is having a family history of the disease. The risk of development of psoriasis is 50% if both parents are affected and 16.4% when one parent is affected. About one in three people with psoriasis has a close relative who also has the condition. On the other hand, roughly the same proportion of people carries genes that have been linked to psoriasis yet never develop skin problems, indicating just how complex and perplexing psoriasis is.

Table 11.1: If you have psoriasis, what is the risk to

• Your unrelated neighbour?	About 2%
• Your sibling?	15-20%
• Your identical twin?	65-70%
• Your child?	25%

Other psoriasis risk factors include:

- *Other medical conditions:* HIV patients are more likely to develop psoriasis than people with healthy immune systems are. Children and young adults with recurring infections, particularly streptococcal throat, also may be at increased risk.
- *Stress:* Stress has a strong impact on immune system, high stress levels increase risk of psoriasis.
- *Obesity:* Excess weight increases risk of inverse psoriasis. In addition, plaques associated with all types of psoriasis often develop in skin creases and folds.
- *Smoking:* Smoking tobacco not only increases risk of psoriasis it also increase the severity of the disease.

Site of Predilection

The sites of predilection includes scalp, retro auricular area, knees, elbow, sacrum, external genitalia and nails.

CLINICAL FEATURES

Signs and Symptoms

Psoriasis symptoms can vary from person to person but may include one or more of the following:

- Erythematous patches of skin covered with **silvery scales** (Fig. 11.3).
- Small scaling spots (commonly seen in children).
- Dry, cracked skin that may bleed (palmoplantar psoriasis) (Fig. 11.4).
- Itching, burning or soreness.
- Thickened, pitted or ridged nails (Fig. 11.5).
- Swollen and stiff joints.

Psoriasis patches can range from a few scaly plaques to entire body surface area (erythroderma) of the body. Mild cases of psoriasis may be a nuisance. But more severe cases can be painful, disfiguring and disabling.

Most types of psoriasis go through cycles, flaring for a few weeks or months, then subsiding for a time or even going into complete remission. In most cases, however, the disease eventually returns.

Several types of psoriasis exist. These include: (Table 11.2)

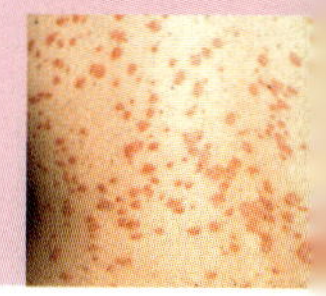

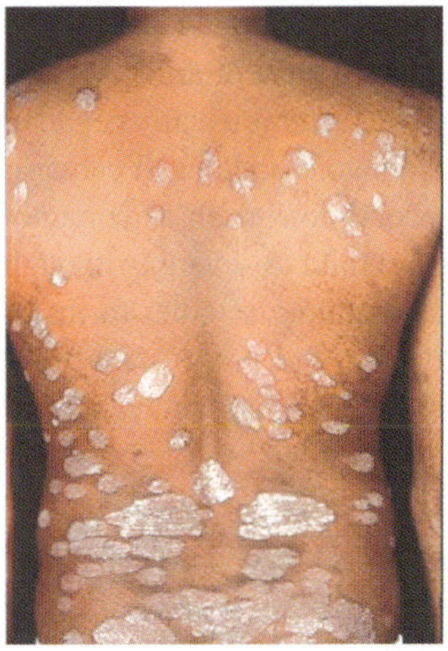

Fig. 11.3: Classic plaques of psoriasis with silvery white scales

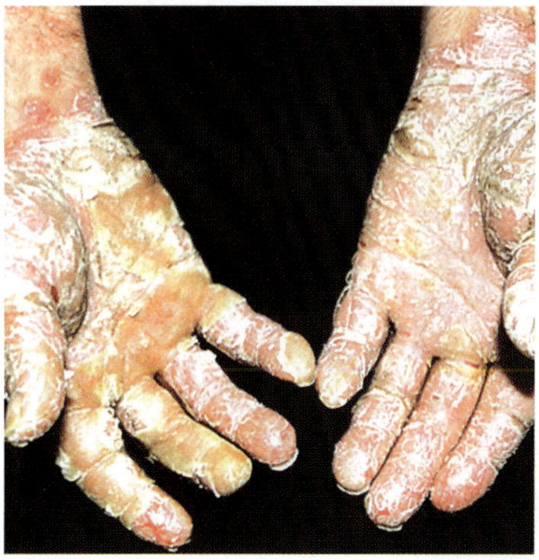

Fig. 11.4: Bilateral symmetrical erythematous plaques on palms

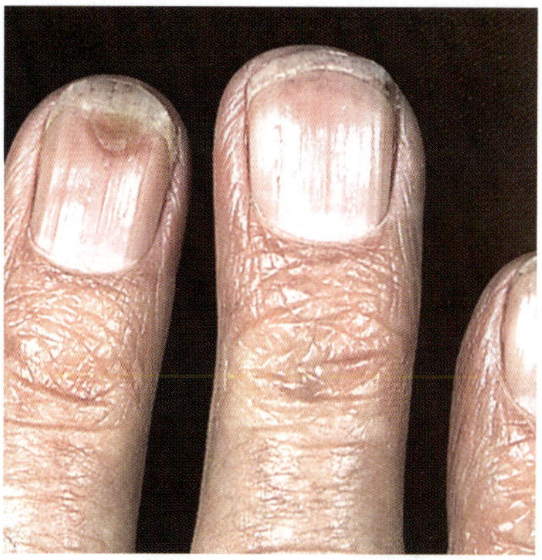

Fig. 11.5: Prominent pits of the nails and an "oil drop" sign of the nail of the fourth finger

Table 11.2: Type of psoriasis and characteristics

Type	*Characteristics, Prevalence*
Classical plaque psoriasis or psoriasis vulgaris	Dry, silver scaling patches (common psoriasis), (75%)
Guttate psoriasis	Drop-like dots, occurs after streptococcal or viral infection, (12%)
Erythrodermic psoriasis	Exfoliation of fine scales (total body "dandruff"), widespread, often accompanied by severe itching and pain, (7%)
Pustular psoriasis	Pus-filled blisters, noninfectious, fluid contains white blood cells, (2%)
Nail psoriasis	Seen on toenails and fingernails, starts as numerous pits, at times progresses to yellowing, crumbly, and thickened nail; nails may slough
Palmar/Plantar psoriasis	Erythema, thickening and peeling of the skin
Psoriatic arthritis	Inflammation, swelling, and joint destruction
Scalp psoriasis	Plaque-type lesion over the scalp
Inverse psoriasis	Smooth plaque-type lesion over the flexural surfaces

- ***Plaque psoriasis:*** The **most common** (75%) form, plaque psoriasis causes dry, red skin lesions (plaques) covered with silvery scales. The plaques itch or feel sore and may occur anywhere on the body (Fig. 11.2).
- ***Guttate psoriasis:*** It constitutes 12% of total psoriasis. This primarily affects people **younger than 30** and is usually triggered by a bacterial infection such as **streptococcal throat**. It's marked by **small, water-drop-shaped sores on the trunk, arms, legs and scalp** (Fig. 11.6).
- ***Erythrodermic psoriasis:*** The less common type constitutes 7% of total psoriasis. Erythrodermic psoriasis is the involvement of entire body surface (≥90%) with a red, scaly rash. It may be triggered by severe sunburn, by corticosteroids and other medications, or by another type of psoriasis that's poorly controlled.

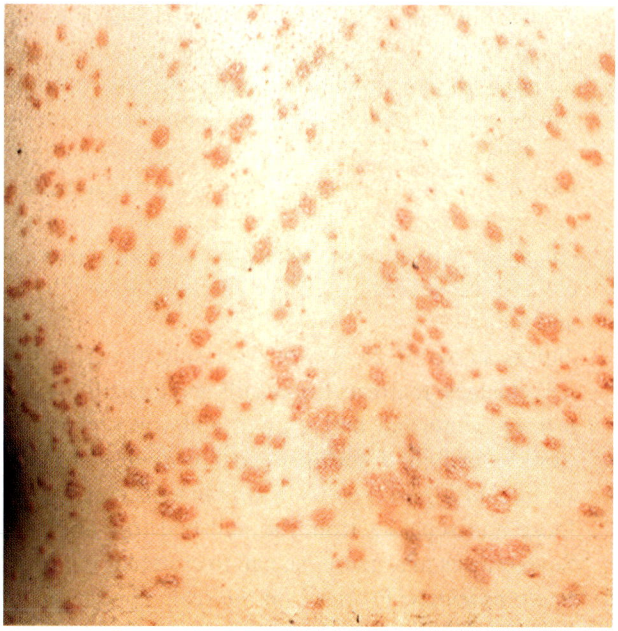

Fig. 11.6: Slightly scaly guttate (drop-sized) papules, some of which have become confluent to form plaques

- ***Pustular psoriasis:*** This rare (2%) form of psoriasis can occur in generalized **(generalized pustular psoriasis or Von Zumbusch's type)** or in localized to hands, feet (Fig. 11.7) or fingertips **(Acrodermatitis continua of Hallopeau).** It generally develops quickly,

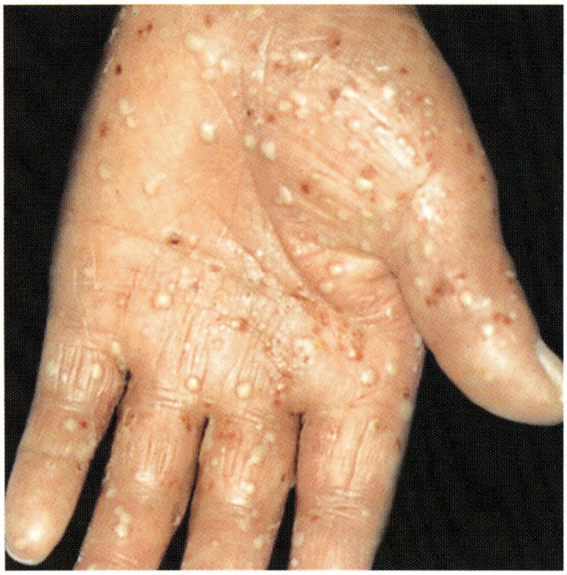

Fig. 11.7: Tiny pustules and larger pustules in company with the residuum of pustules seen here as hemorrhagic crusts

with pus-filled blisters appearing just hours after skin becomes red and tender. The blisters dry within a day or two but may reappear every few days or weeks. Occasionally, it develops from the unstable plaque psoriasis or acrodermatitis continua after inappropriate irritant therapy or withdrawal of extensive topical *steroid*.

Other triggers are topical salicylic acid, systemic iodine and rarely topical tar. *Pregnancy* can sometimes associate with the generalized pustular psoriasis (Impetigo herpetiforms). Generalized pustular psoriasis can also cause fever, chills, severe itching, weight loss and fatigue.

- ***Nail psoriasis:*** In 25-50% of psoriasis patients can have nail changes. It affects fingernails and toenails, causing ***pitting***, abnormal nail growth and waxy yellow or orange-brown discoloration *(oildrop sign)* and *subungual hyperkeratosis*. Psoriatic nails may become loose and separate from the nail bed **(onycholysis).** Severe cases may cause the nail to crumble (Fig. 11.5).
- ***Scalp psoriasis:*** Psoriasis on the scalp appears as red, itchy areas with silvery-white scales. A morphological entity consisting of plaques of **asbestos** like scaling, firmly adherent to the scalp and associated hair has been termed **pityriasis (tinea) amiantacea.**
- ***Inverse psoriasis:*** Mainly affecting the skin in the axilla, groin, under the breasts and around the genitals, inverse psoriasis causes smooth well-defined patches of red, inflamed skin. It's more common in overweight people and is worsened by friction and sweating.
- ***Psoriatic arthritis:*** In addition to inflamed, scaly skin, psoriatic arthritis causes pitted, discolored nails and the swollen, painful joints that are typical of arthritis. The serological test for rheumatoid factor is usually negative and there is absence of rheumatoid nodules. It can also lead to inflammatory eye conditions such as conjunctivitis. Symptoms range from mild to severe. Although the disease usually isn't as crippling as other forms of arthritis, it can cause stiffness and progressive joint damage that in the most serious cases may lead to permanent deformity.

  Types of Psoriatic Arthropathy: Oligoarticular asymmetrical arthritis, symmetrical involving small joints of fingers likes rheumatoid arthritis, classical distal arthropathy involving distal interphalangeal joint, destructive arthritis mutilans and psoriatic spondyloarthropathy which is similar to ankylosing spondylitis.

  The **most common** is the **asymmetrical** arthritis and the classical is **distal interphalangeal** joint involvement (Table 11.2).
- ***Palmoplantar psoriasis*:** Erythema, thickening, peeling of the skin and pustules over the palms and soles. It may often be difficult to distinguish the psoriasis from Eczema (Fig. 11.8).

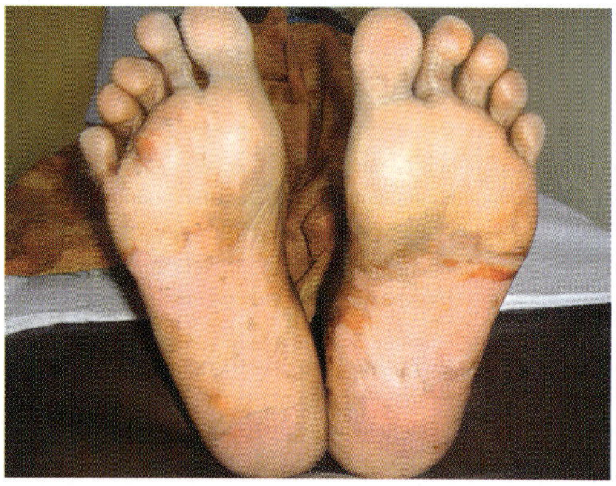

Fig. 11.8: Bilateral symmetrical erythematous plaques on soles

Severity Assessment

Mild psoriasis is defined as affecting less than 5% of the body's surface area; moderate psoriasis affects 5-10%, and severe disease affects more than 20%. However, overriding importance is the need to review the effect of psoriasis on the patient's quality of life (e.g. on social and personal interactions) and modify the treatment plan accordingly. Thus, mild psoriasis on the palms or soles frequently needs more intensive therapy than does psoriasis elsewhere. Psychosocial assessments and response to previous treatments should also be considered when selecting therapies.

INVESTIGATION

Bedside Tests

***Grattage Test*:** When the psoriatic plaque is scraped with a glass slide, the very characteristic silvery scales come out that is known as the Candle Wax/Grease Sign.

***Auspitz Sign*:** The successive removal of psoriatic scales usually reveals an underlying smooth glossy red membrane (**Berkley membrane**) with small bleeding points which appear when the thin suprapapillary epithelium is torn off.

Histopathology (Fig. 11.9)

There is parakeratosis associated with focal orthokeratosis and **Munro's microabscess formation,** near absence of the granular layer, **spongiform pustules in the Malpighian layer**, hyperplasia with elongation of rete ridges and suprapapillary epidermal thinning, mononuclear leukocyte infiltrates in the lower half of epidermis.

Dilated, tortuous papillary blood vessels almost touch the undersurface of the thinning suprapapillary epidermis and are surrounded by a mixed mononuclear and neutrophil infiltrate, as well as extravasated erythrocytes.

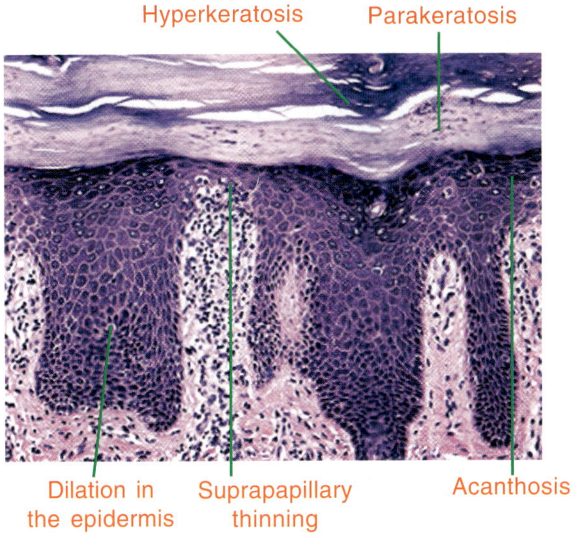

Fig. 11.9: Lymphocytes around vessels, thin rete ridges of about equal length, marked spongiosis and hyperkeratosis and parakeratosis

Treatment (Table 11.3)

Table 11.3. Treatment of choice for specific type of psoriasis

I. Plaque psoriasis or psoriasis vulgaris	Topical therapy remains the mainstay of treatment	
(a) *Less than 10% BSA* (Mild and Moderate)	1. Emollients 2. Coal tar cream 3. Vitamin D analogue	
(b) Severe plaque psoriasis or affecting ***10%-20% BSA***	1. **PUVA** 2. PUVAsol 3. Narrow band UVB	Plus topical +emollient
(c) **'Severe' psoriasis** affecting ***>20% BSA and/or PASI >12***	1. **Methotrexate** 2. Acitretin 3. Cyclosporine 4. Hydroxyurea	
II. **Erythrodermic psoriasis**	1. Methotrexate 2. Acitretin	
III. Pustular psoriasis (a) **Localized**	1. **Acitretin** 2. Methotrexate	
(b) **Generalized**	1. **Acitretin** 2. Methotrexate	
IV. Palmoplantar psoriasis	1. Topical PUVA / PUVAsol 2. Highly potent steroid and salicylic combination	
V. Psoriatic arthritis	1. Methotrexate 2. Acitretin	

Therapeutic Modalities

Many effective therapies are available for treatment of the various clinical forms of psoriasis; each is useful and may be the appropriate initial therapy in a given situation.

Topical Therapy

Numerous topical agents are available. Topical therapy alone offers excellent control for many localized forms of psoriasis.

1. **Bland emollients:** Liberal use of emollients to soften and hydrate the epidermis is a cornerstone of psoriasis therapy after soaking in warm water.
2. **Keratolytics:** These agents remove scale, soften plaques, and enhance penetration of other therapies, though they do not treat the inflammation of psoriasis. They are most effective when used after adequate hydration.
   a. Salicylic acid 2%–10% in petrolatum is applied twice daily and is allowed to remain on the lesions.
   b. Salicylic acid 6% gel, is particularly useful for hyperkeratotic lesions of palms and soles. Do not use salicylic acid on greater than 20% of the body surface area, and use caution with widespread occlusion to prevent salicylate toxicity.
3. **Topical steroids:** Topical steroids are optimally used in combination with nonsteroid agents to both increase efficacy and decrease side effects.

   Though these should be avoided in high-risk areas such as the face, groin, axillae, and other skin folds. Combination of topical steroids with calcipotriene, tazarotene, or both may increase efficacy, decrease steroid-induced atrophy, prevent irritation from the nonsteroid agents, and prevent rebound and tachyphylaxis when used sequentially.

4. **Calcipotriene:** This vitamin D-receptor agonist is an important psoriasis therapy with none of the side effects of topical steroids.

   When used regularly twice daily it can be more effective than class 2 steroids, though the efficacy is decreased by 50% when use drops to once daily.

   Perilesional irritation or facial/genital irritation may occur with calcipotriene, and there is a minute risk of hypercalcemia when use exceeds 120 g per week in adults.

   It is not stable in combination with acids such as salicylic acid, but may be ***combined immediately before use with topical steroids such as halobetasol propionate to speed response and decrease irritation.***
5. **Tazarotene:** This topical retinoid is available in gel or cream formulations in *0.05% or 0.1%* concentrations. It is used as monotherapy once daily at night to lesional skin or in a *Short contact method* applying *30 minutes* before showering. To lessen irritation, start with every other day dosing. Tazarotene is pregnancy category X and should be avoided in reproductive-age women.
6. **Tar preparations:** A great variety of tar-containing agents are available. The following is a partial listing:
   a. Crude coal tar may be compounded in 2%-10% concentrations in petrolatum and nonionic base cream. Salicylic acid or lactic acid 2%-10% may be added to provide keratolytic action.
   b. Tar-containing shampoos are useful for treatment of scalp psoriasis. Leave these shampoos on for 15 to 20 minutes in the shower daily or as needed to treat the scalp.
7. **Anthralin:** Ointment may be compounded in *0.1%-10%* concentrations. These agents may cause irritation and purple-brown staining of skin, clothes, porcelain, and furniture.

   Short-contact therapy uses anthralin cream or ointment for short periods to minimize irritation.
   a. Start with anthralin *0.25%* concentration. Use a disposable plastic glove to apply anthralin cream or ointment to lesions. Allow anthralin to remain on for 15 minutes. Shower, washing lesions with soap and water.
   b. If no irritation is noted after 1 week, increase anthralin concentration to 1%.
   c. Next, increase contact time by 15-minute increments each week to 60 minutes maximum or until mild irritation develops. Continue therapy until lesions clear.
   d. Alternatively, start with 1% anthralin applied for 5 minutes on the first day. Increase by 5 minutes every other day until 15 minutes is reached, then follow regimen above.

8. **Topical immunomodulators:** Tacrolimus ointment and pimecrolimus cream are *not* FDA approved for use in psoriasis. However, tacrolimus ointment applied twice a day has shown promise in the treatment of facial, genital, and intertriginous psoriasis.

Intralesional Therapy

Intralesional corticosteroids are useful in the therapy of localized, persistent psoriatic plaques. Upto a total of 20 mg of an insoluble corticosteroid (e.g., triamcinolone acetonide 2.5-10.0 mg/*cc*) may be injected at one visit without significant systemic effect. Give total upper limit (i.e., 20-40 mg) over a 2-month period.

1. Using a 30-gauge needle, inject 0.2-0.3 cc of triamcinolone acetonide 2.5-10.0 mg/*cc* directly into multiple, ordered sites within several lesions, including center and periphery.
2. Sites may be reinjected after 4-6 weeks.
3. Patients must be cautioned about the risk of atrophy and hypopigmentation at sites of injection.

Phototherapy

Two forms of UVB are in general use: Broadband UVB and narrowband UVB. Daily use of emollients is essential to the phototherapy regimen, and use of non-UVB absorbing lubricants such as mineral oil or petrolatum before receiving light can optimize the optical properties of skin.

Other topicals (calcipotriene, tar, tazarotene) may further increase the efficacy of UVB but should *not be applied within 2 hours* prior to phototherapy.

1. **Broadband UVB therapy (290-320 nm):** BBUVB may be administered in either an erythemogenic or suberythemogenic fashion.
   a. In **erythemogenic** UVB therapy, start UVB just below the MED. The goal is to maintain a barely perceptible erythema for 12-24 hours after each treatment. Patients are treated **three times each week (upto five times a week); 20-30 treatments will be required to clear ordinary cases.**
   b. **Suberythemogenic** therapy uses the lowest dose of UVB commensurate with clinical improvement, thus limiting total UVB exposure and avoiding light-induced burns. The initial UVB dose should be determined by skin type or 50% of the MED; subsequent doses are determined by assessment of clinical response. If lesions improve, do not increase the UVB dose. With lack of improvement or slowing of progress, gradually increase the UVB dose.
2. **Narrowband UVB therapy (310-313 nm):** The NBUVB treatment wavelength was developed to produce the best therapeutic response at suberythemogenic doses. Its

efficacy in treating psoriasis appears to be between that of broadband UVB and PUVA therapy. If using MED, initial dose is 50% of the patient's MED. Plan treatments *three times a week* (upto five times a week). Appropriately lubricate before treatment or plan to always treat clean, dry skin. *Increase dose* of NBUVB by *10%* of MED based on clinical exam (pinkness of skin, patient complaint of itch or burn). Alternatively, protocols for initial dose and incremental increases based on Fitzpatrick skin type may be used.

Photochemotherapy (PUVA)

Topical or oral administration of 8-methoxypsoralen (psoralen) and UVA radiation is the most widely accepted form of photochemotherapy (PUVA = psoralen + ultraviolet A). A more completely absorbed formulation of psoralen called methoxsalen is currently used. This therapy is effective, requiring *20-30* treatments to achieve clearing; patients may then require infrequent regular treatments to maintain clinical remissions. Shield the patient's eyes, face, and male genitalia during treatment. Instruct the patient to wear protective glasses for 12 hours following psoralen ingestion.

1. *Systemic PUVA:* Give methoxsalen *0.4-0.6 mg/kg* 1 to 2 hours before UVA exposure. Begin UVA exposure with 0.5-4.5 J/sq cm, using protocols based on the patient's degree of melanization (skin type). Treat at 2- to 3-day intervals with incremental increases of 0.5-1.0 joule as tolerated until clear.
2. *Bath PUVA:* Soak the patient for 15-30 minutes in a dilute solution (5 capsules [50 mg] methoxsalen dissolved in boiling water, then added to 100 liters of water in a bathtub) of psoralen just prior to UVA phototherapy. Benefits of bath PUVA are avoidance of the GI side effects and the risk of cataracts.
3. *Soak PUVA:* May be used for treatment of localized areas such as the hands or feet. Dissolve 10 mg methoxsalen (1 tablet) in 1 cup boiling water. Add to 2 liters of water for concentration of 0.5 mg/L. Soak hands and/or feet in psoralen solution for 30 minutes prior to UVA exposure.
4. *Paint PUVA:* Apply psoralen (0.1% methoxsalen in a petrolatum or mineral based emollient) with a cotton-tipped applicator for 30 minutes before UVA exposure. Zinc oxide can be used around the areas of treatment to protect surrounding skin. This preparation is the highest concentration of topical PUVA and can result in severe burns. Starting dose of UVA should be as low as 0.25 joules.

Pitfalls

1. Early side effects include nausea following oral psoralen administration, phototoxic erythema, pruritus, variable pigmentation, and occasional worsening of psoriasis.
2. Late side effects include skin carcinogenesis (SCC > BCC > controversial increase in melanoma), enhanced photoaging, pigmentary changes, and cataracts. To minimize these effects, shield the patient's eyes, genitals, and face during therapy, and warn the patient to wear protective glasses and sunscreen for 12 hours following psoralen ingestion.
3. While UVB phototherapy may be used in pregnant and lactating women, PUVA should be avoided in this population.

Systemic Therapy (Table 11.4)

Many systemic agents are or have been used to treat psoriasis. Methotrexate, acitretin, cyclosporine, and biologic agents are accepted forms of therapy.

Methotrexate

Methotrexate is an effective agent with well-studied efficacy and toxicity. Its use is reasonably standardized.

1. **Indications** include psoriatic erythroderma; acute pustular psoriasis; localized pustular psoriasis; psoriatic arthritis; extensive psoriasis unresponsive to other, less toxic therapies; psoriasis that interferes with quality of life; and psychologically disabling psoriasis.
2. Contraindications include decreased renal function, significantly abnormal liver function, pregnancy or anticipated pregnancy, recent or active hepatitis, cirrhosis, excessive alcohol consumption, severe leukopenia, thrombocytopenia, anemia, active peptic ulcer, active severe infectious diseases, and an unreliable patient. HIV infection is a relative contraindication.
3. Pretherapy evaluation should include history and physical examination, CBC with differential and platelet count, urinalysis, serum creatinine, BUN, LFTs, hepatitis serologies, and consideration of HIV testing and chest X-ray depending on risk factors.
4. **Therapeutic regimens:** The goal of therapy is to achieve control, rather than complete clearing, at the lowest possible dose of drug. Typical psoriasis patients respond to a dose of *15 mg per week* within a period of 6-8 weeks.
   a. *Test dose:* To eliminate hematologic idiosyncratic reactions, give oral or intramuscular methotrexate 5 mg and check a CBC after 5-7 days; do not proceed if the WBC is depressed below normal.
   b. *Divided oral dose:* Administer three doses of methotrexate 2.5-5.0 mg every 12 hours each week.
   c. *Single dose:* A test dose of 0.5-7.5 mg is given, followed by a CBC. Weekly single doses of

Table 11.4: Dosages, contraindications and precautions/monitoring for systemic treatments used for psoriasis

Treatment	*Dosage*	*Contraindications*	*Precautions and monitoring*
Photochemotherapy (PUVA)	Oral 8 MOP: 0.6 mg/kg 2h before UVA; oral 5 MOP: 1.2 mg/kg 2h before UVA	Pregnancy and lactation; cataract; age <12 years; previous cutaneous malignancy; concomitant cyclosporine or methotrexate therapy; exposure to arsenic or ionizing radiation; porphyria; photosensitivity disorders; cumulative lifetime dosage > 1500J/cm^2; hepatic impairment	Contraception; UVA eye protection; shielding of genitalia unless specific need to treat; regular skin examination for premalignant and malignant changes
Methotrexate	10-25 mg once weekly, adjusted according to response; consider dose reduction in elderly patients, commencing at 5 mg weekly in patients >65 years of age	Pregnancy and lactation; hepatitis (active or recent); cirrhosis; anemia; leukopenia; thrombocytopenia; active infectious disease; diabetes or extreme obesity; excessive alcohol consumption; renal impairment (reduce dose); immunodeficiency; interactive drugs	Contraception; avoid interacting drugs; FBC; LFT; U and E; serum creatinine; PIIINP; consider liver biopsy
Acitretin	Initially 25-30 mg daily for 2-4 weeks, adjusted according to response, usually within range 25-50 mg daily (upto a maximum 75 mg daily)	Pregnancy and lactation (or wish to conceive within 2 years of stopping treatment); severe hypercholesterolemia or hypertriglyceridemia; severe hepatic or renal impairment; concomitant methotrexate therapy	Contraception; LFT and fasting serum lipids; annual lateral X-ray of thoracic spine
Cyclosporine	Initially 2.5 mg/kg daily in two divided dosages, increasing gradually to a maximum 5 mg/kg daily if no improvement within 1 month. Initial dosage of 5 mg/kg daily justified if condition requires rapid improvement	Pregnancy and lactation; renal impairment; uncontrolled hypertension (diastolic blood pressure >95 mm Hg); previous or concomitant malignancy; concomitant radiation treatment; immunodeficiency or immunosuppression; interactive drugs; drug or alcohol abuse	Contraception; blood pressure; serum creatinine
Hydroxyurea	Initially, 500 mg twice daily (maximum 1.5 g/day)	Pregnancy and lactation; anemia; leukopenia; thrombocytopenia	Contraception; FBC; LFT (weekly during first month, then monthly)

FBC = full blood count; **LFT** = liver function tests (AST, ALT, alkaline phosphatase, γ-glutamyl transpeptidase, bilirubin, albumin); **MOP** = methoxypsoralen; **PIIINP** = amino-terminal peptide of type III procollagen; **U & E** = serum urea and electrolytes; **PUVA** = psoralens + UVA.

methotrexate 7.5-25 mg orally, or 7.5-37.5 mg intramuscularly, are appropriate. The dose should be increased on a biweekly basis in 2.5-5.0 mg increments as necessary until the disease is controlled.

5. **Monitoring of methotrexate therapy:**
   a. CBC with differential and platelets should be monitored weekly during dose escalation and at monthly intervals when the dose is stabilized. Always obtain blood counts 1 week after drug administration.
   b. Perform liver function studies every 1-2 months.
   c. Perform renal function studies every 3-4 months.
   d. Because liver damage may occur in the absence of abnormal LFTs, liver biopsy should be obtained after the first 1.5 g of methotrexate administered in patients without risk factors. Repeat biopsies should be obtained at 1.0-1.5 g intervals.
   e. Patients with risk factors for hepatic fibrosis should have a pretreatment or early treatment liver biopsy, with repeat biopsy after each 1.0 g of methotrexate.
   f. A chest X-ray should be performed yearly in patients with acute or chronic pulmonary disease to rule out methotrexate pneumonitis.
6. **Side effects of methotrexate:** Common short-term side effects are nausea, anorexia and fatigue. Nausea may respond to daily folic acid supplementation, antiemetics, or to divided dose therapy. The most concerning complications, however, are hepatic fibrosis, bone marrow suppression, and rare pneumonitis. Drug interactions, such as with trimethoprim, make methotrexate toxicity much more likely. Methotrexate is category X for pregnancy, and also should not be used in women wishing to conceive.

Acitretin

Acitretin is the only systemic retinoid currently approved

for the treatment of psoriasis. It is the main metabolite of etretinate, which has been discontinued due to an unusually long half-life. The *half-life of acitretin is 50 hours,* compared with 120 days for etretinate. Although the exact mechanism of action is unknown, acitretin likely works by binding nuclear retinoid receptors causing modulation of abnormal epithelial differentiation.

1. Acitretin is indicated as monotherapy in the treatment of **pustular and erythrodermic psoriasis**, but is best used in combination with phototherapy or other systemic agents when treating moderate to severe plaque psoriasis.
2. Acitretin should *not* be used in women of childbearing potential or in patients with uncontrolled lipid abnormalities or active hepatitis.
3. Acitretin is usually started at *25 mg daily*, and the dose titrated upto 50 mg daily as tolerated.
4. When using acitretin as monotherapy for patients with erythrodermic or pustular psoriasis, begin with a dose of *0.5 mg/kg/day* and increase to a maximum of *1.0 mg/kg/day*. The therapeutic dose may be changed at one- to three-week intervals depending on the clinical situation and side effects encountered. Dose is usually limited by the cutaneous and mucosal side effects described below.
5. Re-UVB or Re-PUVA (retinoid + UVB or PUVA) can result in tolerable doses of acitretin for patients with plaque psoriasis (10-25 mg daily), faster and more complete clearing with phototherapy, and lower cumulative doses of ultraviolet light.
6. Monitoring for acitretin should include CBC with differential, LFTs, BUN, creatinine, lipid panel, and a pregnancy test (as appropriate) at baseline, every 2 weeks during initial dose escalation, and at 1-2 months intervals once the dose is constant.
7. Common, dose-dependent side effects include cheilitis, facial dermatitis, conjunctivitis, xerosis, dry mouth, scaling, and hair loss. Systemic problems include arthralgia, hyperlipidemia, transaminase elevation, headache, teratogenicity, and a proposed association with depression and suicidal ideation.

Cyclosporine

Cyclosporine may be used to treat a variety of severe forms of psoriasis. The clinical response is often dramatic and may result in relatively rapid control of disease. Cyclosporine does, however, have potentially significant toxicity, and its use must be limited to one-year periods.

1. Cyclosporine is indicated in generalized plaque psoriasis, erythrodermic psoriasis, and psoriasis of the palms and soles in immunocompetent patients who have failed other therapies. Cyclosporine is especially useful in sudden, severe flares of disease.
2. Contraindications to cyclosporine use include renal disease, poorly controlled hypertension, severe infections, internal malignancy, immunodeficiency, pregnancy, liver disease, concomitant nephrotoxic drugs, gout, and noncompliance with medical care. Extensive history or concurrent photochemotherapy are relative contraindications.
3. Pretherapy evaluation should include a history and physical exam with special attention to the medication history. Baseline blood pressure and serum creatinine should be determined on two separate occasions and should be similar. Other baseline labs include CBC with differential, electrolytes with BUN, magnesium, uric acid, LFTs lipids, and urinalysis.
4. **Therapeutic regimens:** There are two basic approaches when using cyclosporine, and the choice of which to use depends on the severity of the disease and the speed of response required. The low dose approach is appropriate for stable, moderate to severe psoriasis, while the high dose regimen is appropriate for severe, inflammatory flares of disease or extremely resistant cases.
   a. **Low dose approach:** Start with *2.5 mg/kg/day* in a divided dose. After 1 month, increase the dose by 0.5-1.0 mg/kg/day increments every 2 weeks to a maximum of 5 mg/kg/day.
   b. **High dose approach:** Start with *4.0-5.0 mg/kg/day*. The FDA recommends a maximum dose of 4.0 mg/kg/day, but doses upto 5.0 mg/kg/day have been used). Once disease is controlled, decrease dose by 0.5-1.0 mg/kg/day, until the lowest effective dose is determined.
   c. The most common reasons to adjust the dose are increases in serum creatinine 25% above baseline and increases in blood pressure.
5. Monitoring at 2 weeks, 4 weeks, and monthly after the dose is stable should include a history and physical exam including blood pressure and new medications. Labs should include CBC, electrolytes, BUN, creatinine, magnesium, LFTs, lipids, uric acid and urinalysis.
6. The most concerning adverse effects of cyclosporine are hypertension and the dose related renal toxicity it may represent. Other side effects include nausea, headache, paresthesia, hypertrichosis, gingival hyperplasia, GI upset, and laboratory abnormalities (**elevated lipids, hypomagnesemia, hyperkalemia, and elevated uric acid**). There is concern about an increased risk of lymphoma, though this is unproven in psoriasis patients.

Hydroxyurea

Hydroxyurea is used off-label by some in combination with

other therapies, but is infrequently used as a primary agent. Give 1000-1500 mg/day in divided doses, and monitor the CBC weekly for anemia, leukopenia, and development of macrocytosis. Once the treatment dose is stable, check a CBC with differential monthly and check serum chemistry (with LFTs, BUN, Creatinine) and urinalysis every 3-6 months.

Biologic Therapies

1. **Etanercept** is a recombinant, human protein that was designed to block the proinflammatory and hyperproliferative actions of tumor necrosis factor alpha *(TNF-α)*. It is a fully human fusion protein that combines the extracellular portion to two p75 TNF-α receptors with the Fc region of a human IgG1 molecule.
   - Etanercept is approved as a 2nd line drug for the treatment of chronic, moderate to severe psoriasis, psoriatic arthritis.
   - When treating psoriasis, it is given in a dose of **50 mg** by subcutaneous injection **twice weekly** for the first **3 months** of therapy.
   - When 50 mg twice weekly for 3 months and a 50 mg/week maintenance dose is used, **46%** of psoriasis patients achieve 75% reduction in PASI score at 12 weeks, and this improvement is maintained at 24 weeks. Etanercept has been used in rheumatoid arthritis for over 5 years, and has had an impressive track record for safety.
   - The **most common** side effect is an *injection site reaction*, though discussions with patients should include the possibility of worsening *CHF* and autoantibody development and the rare reports of demyelinating disease, severe infection (such as tuberculosis, sepsis), and pancytopenia. It is important to screen prospective patients for a history of these disorders and to obtain a *tuberculosis skin* test and/or chest X-ray. This agent is category B for pregnancy.
2. **Efalizumab** is now approved for treatment of patients with chronic plaque psoriasis. It is a humanized IgG monoclonal antibody that binds to the *CD11a subunit of lymphocyte associated antigen-1 (LFA-1), thus interfering with the LFA-1/ICAM-1 association and the resultant T-cell activation and migration to the skin.*
3. **Alefacept** is a fully human receptor fusion protein, which combines the first extracellular domain of lymphocyte function associated *antigen-3 (LFA-3) with the Fc portion of human immunoglobulin 1 (IgG1)*. It is approved for treatment of chronic plaque psoriasis and is *unique* in its *remittive properties*. Alefacept binds to CD_2 on memory-effector T cells, blocking their activation and proliferation and also resulting in apoptosis.
   - Dosage is *15 mg* by intramuscular injection once per week for *12 consecutive weeks.*
   - Because alefacept decreases CD_4 T-cell count in peripheral blood, *absolute CD_4 cell counts* are monitored at baseline, then weekly during therapy. If cell counts fall below 250 cells/mm^3 for 1 week, the dose should be held. If the count remains below 250 cells/mm^3 for 4 consecutive weeks, the drug should be discontinued. A repeat course after a 3-month rest period is appropriate in patients not experiencing precipitous drops in CD_4 count.
   - Alefacept is relatively well tolerated, though patients must understand that response times are relatively slow.
   - Responders often see improvement toward the end of the 12-week injection period and continue to improve over the following 3 months. After a period of 24 weeks, approximately 33% of patients achieve 75% improvement in PASI score.
4. **Infliximab** is a chimeric (mouse-human) IgG1 monoclonal antibody directed against *TNF=α.*
   - When used for psoriasis, this drug is given *as a 5mg/kg intravenous infusion over 2-3 hours* at weeks 0, 2, 6 and every 8 weeks thereafter. Impressive and rapid responses have been seen in plaque psoriasis as well as in cases of severe variants such as generalized pustular psoriasis. Approximately 80% of patients treated achieve a 75% improvement in the PASI score by week 10, and improvement may be seen as early as 2 weeks.
   - A negative PPD is required before starting therapy with infliximab, and a full history and physical exam should be performed. Adverse effects of infliximab include infusion reactions (fever, chills or rarely hypotension, chest pain, dyspnea, anaphylaxis), neutralizing antibodies and autoantibodies, worsening of CHF, infection (including sepsis and opportunistic infections), and reactivation of latent tuberculosis.

Psoriasis Day Treatment Programs

Day treatment programs are usually based on classical Goeckerman and Ingram regimens and are best suited to hospital and psoriasis day-care settings owing to the use of messy tars and anthralin. Patients with severe, generalized psoriasis often require 4-6 weeks of therapy (5 days per week) to obtain clearance, and remissions can last months to years if regular outpatient phototherapy is maintained in conjunction with regular application of nonsteroid topical agents.

The basic tenets of **Goeckerman therapy** include repeated application of crude coal tar preparations accompanied by aggressive UVB therapy. **Ingram therapy** consists of the combined use of UVB therapy and anthralin.

Treatment of Psoriasis (Table 11.3)

Often, the approximate percent body surface area (BSA) involved is used to determine if a patient has mild/localized psoriasis or moderate-to-severe generalized psoriasis. Using the size of the patient's palm as 1%, **mild disease is roughly 5% BSA, moderate disease is 5%-10% BSA, and severe disease is >10% BSA.** However, patients with particularly disabling or visible psoriatic lesions (face, palm and sole) are often considered to have a moderate to severe case despite a lesser percentage of involved skin.

Therapy of Plaque Psoriasis

Localized Plaque Psoriasis

1. Initiate a regimen of *hydration and liberal use of emollients*. Sequential therapy with *calcipotriene and superpotent topical steroids* can yield excellent results over 2-4 weeks.
2. Recalcitrant, local lesions may be treated with intralesional corticosteroids. Lesions on the elbows and knees may benefit from this approach. Intralesional injection is particularly useful in patients who do not wish to undertake regular home, topical therapy.
3. Anthralin preparations, especially the new less staining formulations, are suitable for treatment of thick, recalcitrant plaques.
4. Ultraviolet light therapy may be given to localized, resistant lesions, such as those on the lower legs, using a light box and shielding uninvolved skin.

Generalized Plaque Psoriasis

1. **Phototherapy with UVB or NBUVB three times a week**, combined with use of a simple emollient, is safe and effective. Patient inconvenience is an issue, and response is often gratifying but takes 6-10 weeks. Some patients benefit from a home UVB light source, which may be built or purchased. Efficacy is increased by adding topical agents and/or acitretin.
2. **Photochemotherapy (PUVA)** is an effective therapy often used in patients who fail UVB alone, cannot realistically be treated with the Goeckerman regimen, and wish to avoid or cannot tolerate other systemic options. Acitretin may be added.
3. **Goeckerman regimen:** Although safe and highly effective, the patient must commit 4-6 weeks to this program and will usually be unable to work. This therapy is usually given in an outpatient day-care setting and does not require overnight hospitalization.
4. **Methotrexate** is an excellent agent for otherwise healthy patients with significant disease who are unable to comply with the Goeckerman regimen, UVB, and PUVA because of lifestyle.
5. **Biologic agents** are indicated for treatment of chronic plaque psoriasis, and the efficacy of each has been described. One of these, etanercept, is uniquely valuable, as it is indicated for patients with both psoriasis and psoriatic arthritis.
6. **Acitretin** is most useful in combination when treating patients with generalized plaque psoriasis or as a maintenance agent after control is obtained. This will allow titration of doses ranging from 10-50 mg daily, minimizing side effects such as cheilitis, dry eye, and hair loss. Acitretin should not be used in women of reproductive age.
7. **Cyclosporine** is appropriate in healthy patients with recalcitrant plaque psoriasis to gain initial control of disease. As it can only be used for one year at a time, patients must be transitioned to safer, maintenance therapy.
8. **Combination therapies** are often appropriate for patients with severe plaque psoriasis. They include:
   a. Topical agents and any systemic choice or phototherapy.
   b. Phototherapy or Goeckerman therapy plus retinoids or methotrexate. When using acitretin, start with 10-25 mg daily and adjust dose of light appropriately for iatrogenic photosensitivity. If still resistant, consider increasing to 50 mg daily. When the patient is clear, discontinue acitretin and maintain remission with outpatient phototherapy.
   c. Biologic agents in combination with other modalities are now under investigation. It is premature to recommend these approaches.
   d. There are many other combinations in use that warrant caution due to possible overlapping toxicity. These include methotrexate, cyclosporine, or biologics plus acitretin, biologics plus phototherapy, and methotrexate plus cyclosporine.

Therapy of Scalp Psoriasis

1. Shampoo for 5-20 minutes with a shampoo containing tar and/or salicylic acid on a regular or and as needed basis. A daily shampoo may be required initially, but the process may be controlled with less frequent but regular use.

2. Apply mid-high potent steroids twice daily.
3. Other:
   a. Tazarotene gel nightly.
   b. Anthralin cream 0.5% solution.

Therapy of Guttate Psoriasis

This type of psoriasis may follow streptococcal upper respiratory tract infection and may be self-limited, lasting 6-8 weeks or may signal the onset of generalized psoriasis. Obtain a throat culture and treat if streptococcus is found. Therapeutic alternatives include:
1. Therapy with bland emollients or widespread use of medium potency topical steroids (e.g. Triamcinolone ointment/cream).
2. **Broadband or narrowband UVB phototherapy.**
3. Repeated courses of antibiotics and tonsillectomy are controversial in patients with documented relationship to streptococcus.

Therapy of Erythrodermic (Exfoliative) Psoriasis

First Steps

1. If patient appears systemically ill, hospitalize the patient in a comfortably warm environment (to limit loss of body heat), and carefully monitor for sepsis and potential cardiovascular, thermoregulatory, fluid, and electrolyte problems. For otherwise healthy patients, a day treatment center may be appropriate.
2. Treat with medium strength topical corticosteroids in an ointment or cream twice a day under sauna suit occlusion if tolerated.
3. Initiate treatment with cyclosporine if there are no contraindications. Expect improvement in first week.
4. If cyclosporine not an option, consider methotrexate therapy.
5. Phototherapy, systemic steroids, and potentially irritating topical agents (tazarotene, calcipotriene, tar) should be avoided during the period of acute inflammation.

Subsequent Steps

1. When erythroderma improves, taper cyclosporine and begin the patient on the Goeckerman regimen (if available) or transition to acitretin 25-50 mg daily.
2. Maintenance therapy for psoriasis is often required following resolution of the erythrodermic episode, depending on the residual clinical morphology. This may include acitretin, phototherapy, topical agents, etc.

Alternative Steps

For patients not responding rapidly to hydration, emollients, and hospitalization, or who cannot tolerate cyclosporine or methotrexate, consider acitretin in doses of 0.5-1.0 mg/kg/day.

Pustular Psoriasis (Generalized)

First Steps

1. Hospitalize the patient, or admit the patient to day treatment center.
2. Rule out sepsis and assure normal fluid and electrolyte balance.
3. Start the patient on **acitretin 0.25-1 mg/kg/day (0.25-0.5 mg/kg is often adequate).**
4. Apply midpotency topical steroids such as triamcinolone, and occlude if tolerated.
5. Wet compresses or soothing baths may be helpful.
6. Expect significant improvement within 3-7 days.
7. Gradually taper any existing steroid therapy as the patient responds to retinoids. Abrupt discontinuance of existing topical steroid therapy may aggravate pustular flaring.

Subsequent Steps

When pustulation ceases, the following approach is reasonable:
1. Taper retinoids gradually by reducing dose weekly, unless the disorder recurs.
2. Begin patient on phototherapy or the Goeckerman regimen if available. Some patients can be controlled with PUVA or UVB in the absence of retinoids, though many patients require acitretin or methotrexate for maintenance.

Alternative Steps

1. Isotretinoin 1-2 mg/kg/day will control pustulation, but is not as effective as acitretin for long-term control. It may be chosen if a shorter half-life is important.
2. Cyclosporine or methotrexate may be used in combination with acitretin or alone if retinoids are contraindicated.

Pitfalls

1. Do not use systemic corticosteroids; if used as a last resort, pustular flare may follow as steroids are reduced.
2. Antimalarials, lithium, and beta-blockers may aggravate pustular flare and should be stopped.

Therapy of Psoriasis of the Palms and Soles (Localized Pustular Psoriasis)

Although this disorder is notoriously difficult to treat, the following alternatives are reasonable and often helpful. The goal of therapy should be control of symptoms and restoration of function. Total clearing of this process is seldom achieved.

First Steps

1. Apply superpotent topical steroids twice daily. Calcipotriene and/or tazarotene may be mixed with the steroid, and the mixture can be occluded.
2. Patients may also start by soaking palms and soles for 15-20 minutes two to three times a day in a tepid tar-containing solution (e.g., coal tar emulsion) (1-2 tbsp/qt water). After soaking, pat the hands dry and apply a superpotent topical corticosteroid or a combination regimen as above.
3. Clinical response may begin within 14-21 days. Taper therapy to the level needed to maintain control and acceptance by the patient.

Alternative Steps

If satisfactory control is not achieved, the following agents can be added to the above topical regimen:

1. Acitretin 25–50 mg daily.
2. Soak PUVA to palms and soles or soak PUVA plus acitretin (Re-PUVA).
3. Methotrexate or cyclosporine.
4. Consider use of biologic agents.

Therapy of Psoriasis of the Nails

Although psoriatic nail changes may improve in patients responding to systemic therapies such as PUVA, methotrexate, acitretin, or etanercept, local nail treatment has been relatively unsatisfactory. The following alternatives may be attempted, but they require a highly motivated patient with appropriate expectations. Consider culture for concomitant dermatophyte at outset, and treat if appropriate.

1. *First-line therapy* includes topical use of high potency corticosteroids, tazarotene gel, calcipotriene, anthralin (which may stain the skin and nails), and combinations of these agents. Medications should be applied to the proximal nail and nailfold and occluded nightly with vinyl or cotton gloves. Therapy may be required for at least 6 months before any benefit is appreciated, and atrophy of the nailfolds may develop with prolonged use of corticosteroids under occlusion.
2. *Inject* each nailfold with triamcinolone acetonide 0.1 cc (5 mg/cc). Repeat therapy after 6-8 weeks as needed if tolerated. This is extremely painful and is not tolerated by most patients.
3. Consider use of systemic agents by evaluating accompanying skin and joint disease and patient disability.

TREATMENT ALGORITHM

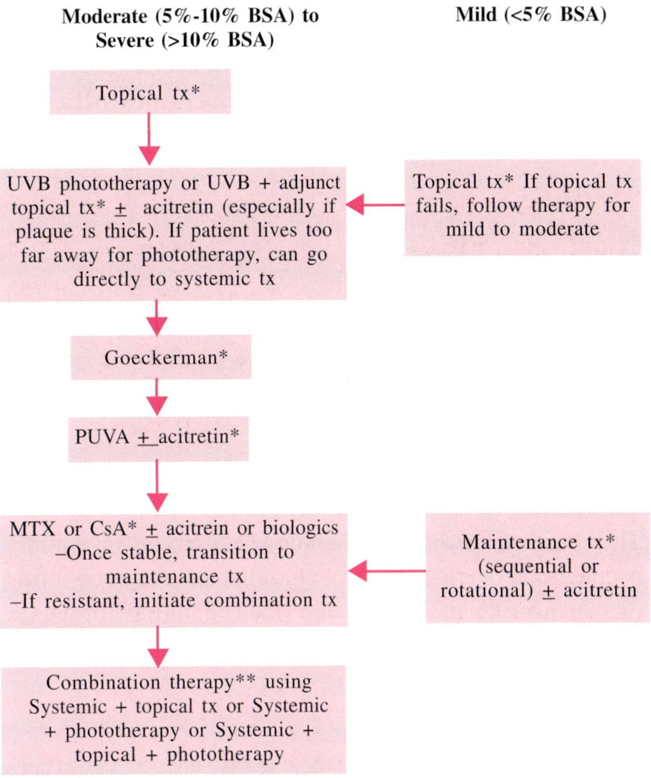

A overview of the therapeutic protocol which is a gist of the therapeutic modalities as given above is given below:

Algorithm. *Topical therapy may be added to any regimen. These algorithms may be updated as more data become available.

**Preliminary data suggest that tumor necrosis factor (TNF) inhibitors may be safe and highly effective treatments for plaque psoriasis and other biologics may be considered for patients with severe resistant disease; Abbreviations: BSA = body surface area; tx = therapy; MTX = methotrexate; CsA = cyclosporine A.

REFERENCES

- Therapeutic Strategies in Dermatology; Timothy G. Berger, M.D., Bruce U. Wintroub, M.D.
- Rook's Textbook of Dermatology; D.A. Burns, S.M. Breathnach, Neil Cox, Christopher E. Griffiths, 7th edn 2004.
- Fitzpatrick's Dermatology in General Medicine, 6th edn 2003.
- Lever's Histopathology of the Skin by David E Elder, Rosalie Elenitsas, Bernett L Johnson, George F Murphy, 9th edn. 2004.
- Lebwohl, M.G. *et al.*: Psoriasis: Treatment Options and Patient Management, National Psoriasis Foundation 2002.

Pityriasis Rubra Pilaris

The term pityriasis rubra pilaris (PRP) has been applied to a group of patients showing circumscribed follicular keratoses, palmoplantar keratoderma and erythroderma.

Varieties of PRP

Type I	Classic adult	55%
Type II	Atypical adult	5%
Type III	Classic juvenile	10%
Type IV	Circumscribed juvenile	25%
Type V	Atypical juvenile	4.5%
Type VI	HIV associated	0.5%

Etiology

The cause of the disease is unknown. A prominent finding is epidermal overactivity. Both familial and acquired forms of the disorder have been described. Familial forms are autosomal dominant.

Clinical Features

Classical PRP affects the sexes equally, and occurs at any age from early childhood to the eighth decade. There are however, two peaks: the highest incidence is between 40-60 years of age, but there is a second smaller peak in first decade.

Classical Adult Onset PRP (type I)

The eruption starts most often from the head, neck or upper trunk as erythematous scaly macules, followed by follicular papules with perifollicular erythema. Papules coalesce to form plaques. Erythema typically spreads in a **cephalocaudal** direction. The face becomes uniformly erythematous, scalp shows diffuse branny scaling. Erythroderma frequently develops. In most cases sharply demarcated islands of unaffected skin, "**island of sparing**", are present. Palms and soles become hyperkeratotic and yellow **(PRP Sandal).** The course is self-limiting (1-3 years).

Nails: Distal yellow brown discoloration, subungual hyperkeratosis, nail plate thickening, splinter hemorrhages. Pitting is minimal.

Oral cavity: Rare, diffuse whitish appearance, lacy white plaques.

Atypical Adult Onset PRP (type II)

Skin lesions are atypical, there is no well-defined cephalocaudal distribution and the tendency to erythroderma is less.

Classical Juvenile PRP (type III)

The onset is between the ages of 5-10 years; shows all the features of type 1 PRP. Again the course is self-limiting (1-2 years).

Circumscribed Juvenile PRP (type IV)

Well demarcated plaques of follicular plugging with variable degrees of erythema appear on the knees and elbows. Also known as *keratosis circumscripta.*

Atypical Juvenile Onset PRP (type V)

The morphology of the lesions are similar to type III, however the onset is earlier (at birth or first few years of life). The group overlaps with poorly defined icthyotic disorders, and there is little tendency to remit spontaneously.

Differential Diagnosis

Psoriasis

	PRP	*Psoriasis*
Age at onset	Bimodal	2nd decade
Scalp scaling	Furfuraceous	Adherent
Palmoplanter Keratoderma	Constant	Less constant
Island of sparing	Constant	Less constant
Nail changes	Pitting rare, No dystrophy	Pitting and dystrophy common
Sero -ve arthritis	Very rare	Common
Munro microabscess	Absent	Common
Response to methotrexate	Variable	Good

Diagnosis

Auspitz Sign –ve

Histopathology:

- Alternating ortho and parakeratoses oriented in vertical and horizontal directions: **checkerboard pattern.**
- Focal or confluent hypergranulosis.
- Thick suprapapillary plates.
- Acanthosis with broad short rete ridges.
- Follicular plugging, parakeratosis around follicular openings creating a **shoulder effect.**
- Dermis shows mild superficial lymphocytic infiltrate with moderate dilated blood vessels.

Treatment

Topical – emollients are the mainstay topically. Vitamin D analogues have shown some benefit.

Systemic

- Vit A.
- Methotrexate.
- Retinoids.
- Phototherapy (may cause flare of disease).

Seborrheic Dermatitis

Seborrheic dermatitis is a papulosquamous disorder patterned on the sebum-rich areas of the scalp, face and trunk. In addition to sebum, this dermatitis is linked to *Malassezia,* immunologic abnormalities, and activation of complement. It is commonly aggravated by changes in humidity, change in seasons, trauma, or emotional stress. The severity varies from mild dandruff to exfoliative erythroderma. Seborrheic dermatitis may worsen in Parkinson disease and in AIDS.

Etiopathogenesis

Seborrheic dermatitis is associated with normal levels of *Malassezia* but an abnormal immune response. The contribution of *Malassezia* may come from its lipase activity—releasing inflammatory free fatty acids—and from its ability to activate the alternative complement pathway. The *Malassezia* organisms are probably not the cause but are a cofactor linked to a T-cell depression, increased sebum levels, and an activation of the alternative complement pathway. Persons prone to this dermatitis also may have a skin-barrier dysfunction.

Clinical Features

Activity is increased in winter and early spring, with remissions commonly occurring in summer. Active phases may be complicated by secondary infection in the intertriginous areas and on the eyelids. Candidal overgrowth is common in infantile napkin dermatitis. Such children may have a diaper dermatitis variant of seborrheic dermatitis or psoriasis.

It occurs more often in association with AIDS, Parkinson and other neurological disorders, congestive heart failure, and immunosuppression in premature infants.

Skin lesions manifest as branny or greasy scaling over red, inflamed skin. A seborrheic blepharitis may occur independently.

Distribution follows the oily and hair-bearing areas of the head and the neck, such as the scalp, the forehead, the eyebrows, the lash line, the nasolabial folds, the beard, and the postauricular skin. Presternal or interscapular involvement is more common than nonscaling intertrigo of the umbilicus, axillae, inframammary and inguinal folds, perineum, or anogenital crease, which also may be present.

Two distinct truncal patterns can occasionally occur. An annular or geographic *petaloid* scaling is the most common. A rare *pityriasiform* variety can be seen on the trunk and the neck, with peripheral scaling around ovoid patches, mimicking pityriasis rosea.

Various medications may flare or induce seborrheic dermatitis. These medications include buspirone, chlorpromazine, cimetidine, ethionamide, gold, griseofulvin, haloperidol, interferon alfa, lithium, methoxsalen, methyldopa, phenothiazines, psoralens, stanozolol, thiothixene, and trioxsalen.

Treatment

Early treatment of flares is encouraged. Behavior modification techniques in reducing excoriations are especially helpful with scalp involvement.

Topical corticosteroids may hasten recurrences, may foster dependence because of a rebound effect, and are discouraged except for short-term use. Skin involvement responds to ketoconazole, naftifine, or ciclopirox creams and gels. Alternatives include calcineurin inhibitors (i.e. pimecrolimus, tacrolimus), sulfur or sulfonamide combinations, or propylene glycol. Class IV or lower corticosteroid creams, lotions, or solutions can be used for acute flares. Systemic ketoconazole, fluconazole or itraconazole may help if seborrheic dermatitis is severe or unresponsive.

Selenium sulfide (2.5%), ketoconazole, and ciclopirox shampoos may help by reducing *Malassezia* yeast scalp reservoirs.

Seborrheic blepharitis may respond to gentle cleaning of eyelashes with baby shampoo and cotton applicators.

Pityriasis Rosea

Pityriasis rosea (PR) is a mild self-limited eruption seen predominantly in adolescents and young adults during the spring and fall.

Etiopathogenesis

PR has often been considered to be a viral exanthem. Its clinical presentation supports this concept. PR has been linked to upper respiratory infections, it can cluster within families and close contacts, and it has an increased incidence in individuals who are immunocompromised. As with viral exanthems, the incidence may increase in the fall and the spring. A single outbreak tends to elicit lifelong immunity.

PR-like drug eruptions may be difficult to distinguish from non-drug-induced cases. **Medication-induced** eruptions have been reported with captopril, metronidazole, isotretinoin, penicillamine, levamisole, bismuth, gold, barbiturates, ketotifen, clonidine, aspirin, and omeprazole. A single case has been reported with terbinafine. Recently, imatinib mesylate has been implicated.

Clinical Features

The disease typically begins with a solitary macule that heralds the eruption (called the **herald spot/patch**), which is usually a salmon-colored macule. This initial lesion enlarges over a few days to become a patch with a **collarette of fine scale** just inside the well-demarcated border (Fig. 11.10).

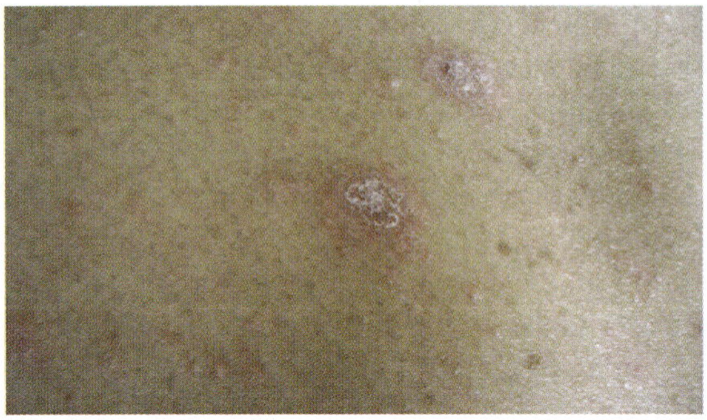

Fig. 11.10: Collarette of fine scale just inside the well demarcated border

Within the next 1-2 weeks, a generalized exanthem usually appears, although it may occur from hours to months after the herald patch. This secondary phase consists of bilateral and symmetric macules with a collarette scale oriented with their long axes along cleavage lines. This phase tends to resolve over the next 6 weeks, but variability is common.

Pruritus is common, usually of mild-to-moderate severity, and it occurs in 75% of patients.

The **herald patch** is usually a single pink patch, 2-10 cm in diameter, on the neck or the trunk with a fine collarette scale. It is observed in more than 50-70% of patients, and it may occur as multiple lesions or in atypical locations.

About 1-2 weeks after the herald patch is seen, the generalized eruption appears, although it has been known to occur from hours to 3 months later. It consists of salmon-colored macules or patches, 0.5-1.5 cm in diameter, with a collarette scale, often described as having a cigarette paper/like appearance. The long axes of the lesions are oriented in a parallel fashion along cleavage lines, giving the **classic Christmas tree pattern** (Fig 11.11). These secondary lesions most commonly occur on the trunk, the abdomen, the back, and the proximal upper extremities. Pruritus occurs in 75% of patients and is severe in 25%.

Atypical PR occurs in 20% of patients. These variations can be separated into changes in the lesions and/or their distribution. Variable distribution can be difficult to evaluate.

Variation of primary lesion	*Variation in distribution*
Classical—macular, patch	Classical – fir tree or Christmas tree pattern
Papular, urticarial	Inverse P. Rosea
Vesicular, pustular	Localized P. Rosea
Erythema multiforme like	Unilateral P. Rosea
Petechial	
Follicular	
P. Rosea giganticum	
P. Rosea circinata et marginata of Vidal	

Photosensitivity may occur, although photosensitivity is not a classic manifestation of the disease. 10% patients may show oral involvement as punctate hemorrhages, ulcers, papulovesicles, bullae, or erythematous plaques.

Treatment

The most important part of treating patients with PR is reassurance that the rash will resolve.

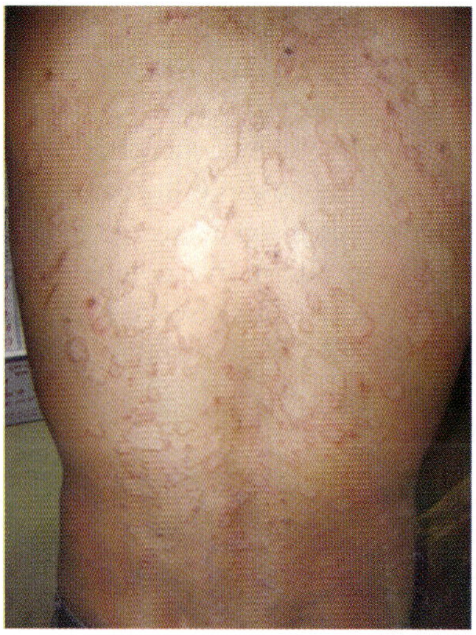

Fig. 11.11: The long axes of the lesions are oriented in a parallel fashion along cleavage lines, giving the **classic Christmas tree pattern**

- Relief of pruritus is helpful and can be accomplished by using topical steroids, oral antihistamines, topical menthol-phenol lotions, and oatmeal baths. Systemic steroids are not recommended. Although they suppress pruritus, systemic steroids do not shorten the overall disease; in fact, they may prolong or exacerbate the disease.

- Ultraviolet B (UV-B) light therapy, starting at 80% of the minimum erythrogenic dose, may rapidly relieve pruritus in resistant cases. If itching is not controlled, the dose of UV-B light should be increased by 20% until symptoms decrease.
- For vesicular PR 20 mg of dapsone twice a day.
- High-dose acyclovir (800 mg qid), Erythromycin 250 mg QID, Dapsone 20 mg BD have anecdotally been shown to have benefit, especially if instituted early in the disease course. Further trials are needed to help confirm this finding.

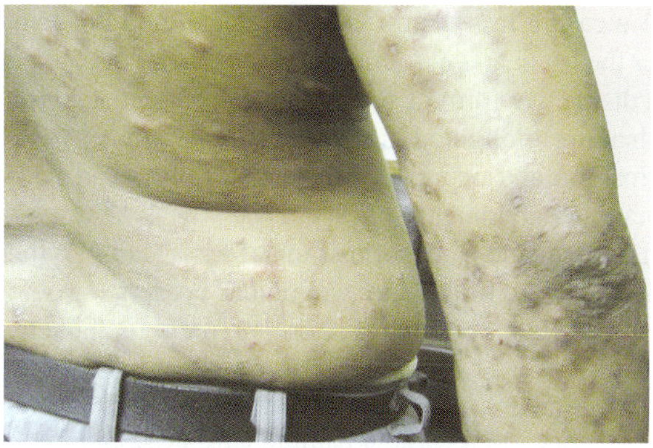

Fig. 11.12: Multiple necrotic papules (Pityriasis lichenoides et varioliformis acuta)

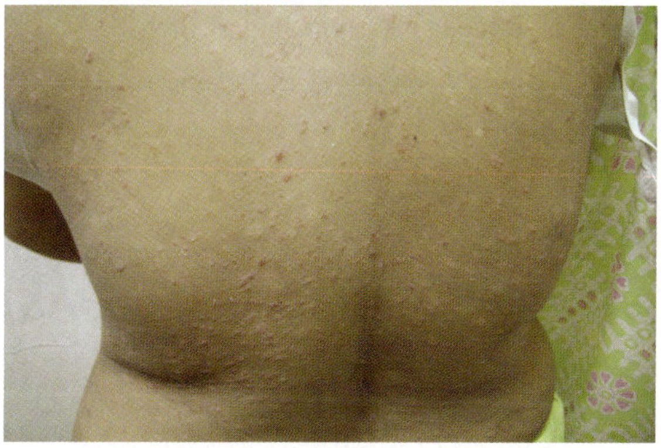

Fig. 11.13: Fine scaly papules with areas of hypopigmentation (Pityriasis lichenoides chronica)

Parapsoriasis

Parapsoriasis describes a group of cutaneous diseases that can be characterized by scaly patches or slightly elevated plaques that have a resemblance to psoriasis, hence the nomenclature. However, this description includes several inflammatory cutaneous diseases that are unrelated with respect to pathogenesis, histopathology, and response to treatment. Because of the variation in clinical presentation and a lack of a specific diagnostic finding on histopathology, a uniformly accepted definition of parapsoriasis remains lacking.

In 1902, Brocq initially described 3 major entities that fit the description:

- Pityriasis lichenoides (acuta and chronica).
- Small plaque parapsoriasis (digitate dermatoses/chronic superficial dermatitis).
- Large plaque parapsoriasis (parapsoriasis en plaque).

Pityriasis Lichenoides (Acuta Fig. 11.12 and Chronica Fig. 11.13)

Pityriasis lichenoides variants describe scaly dermatoses with necrotic papules that are clinically and histologically different from parapsoriasis. These diseases generally are benign and undergo spontaneous resolution.

Large Plaque and Small Plaque Parapsoriasis

Current terminology of parapsoriasis refers to 2 disease processes that are caused by T-cell-predominant infiltrates in the skin. These disease processes are large plaque parapsoriasis and small plaque parapsoriasis.

As the nomenclature and description of the disease spectrum under the descriptive term parapsoriasis evolved, the primary focus has been on the distinction of whether the disorder progresses to mycosis fungoides (MF) or cutaneous T-cell lymphoma (CTCL). Small plaque parapsoriasis is a benign disorder that rarely if ever progresses. Large plaque parapsoriasis is more ominous in that approximately 10% of patients progress to CTCL. Controversy exists in the classification of large plaque parapsoriasis because some think it is equivalent to the earliest stage CTCL, the patch stage.

The duration of parapsoriasis can be variable. Small plaque disease lasts several months to years and can spontaneously resolve. Large plaque disease is chronic, and treatment is recommended because it may prevent progression to CTCL.

Clinical Features

Onset of parapsoriasis is indolent. It develops from a few patches and becomes more visible over a protracted period of time. Additional lesions develop progressively in some individuals.

Lesions of small plaque parapsoriasis are well-circumscribed, slightly scaly, light salmon-colored patches that measure less than 5 cm in diameter and are scattered over the trunk and extremities (Fig. 11.14). Digitate pattern is a distinctive form of small plaque disease that consists of palisading elongated fingerlike patches that follow the dermatome and are most prominently displayed on the lateral thorax and abdomen.

Large plaque parapsoriasis manifests as faint erythematous patches with arcuate geographic borders.

- Each lesion often is greater than 6 cm in diameter.
- Lesions are scattered on the proximal extremities and the trunk.
- Lesions often show a bathing suit distribution.
- Surfaces of the lesions have a faint red-to-salmon color; show flaky thin scales; and have an atrophic, cigarette paper or tissue paper, wrinkling quality.

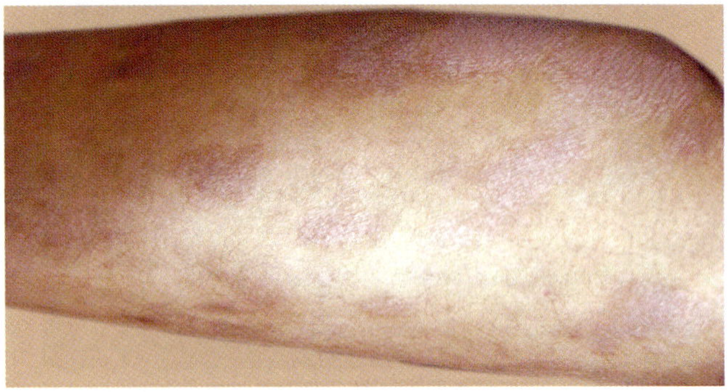

Fig. 11.14: Pigmented plaques on the limb (Parapsoriasis)

Lab Studies

Complete blood cell count with differential: A high lymphocyte count or the presence of Sézary cells suggests MF/CTCL.

Histopathology of small plaque parapsoriasis shows a mild superficial perivascular lymphocytic infiltrate with a nonspecific inflammatory infiltrate of CD_4^+ and CD_8^+ T cells. However, CD_4^+ T cells are predominant. The epidermis may show mild spongiosis, focal hyperkeratosis, scale crust, parakeratosis, and occasional exocytosis. Often the pattern is not diagnostic and is nonspecific. Lymphocytes are small and do not show atypical features.

In large plaque parapsoriasis, a superficial dermal inflammatory infiltrate consists predominantly of lymphocytes. Numerous lymphocytes abut the dermal epidermal junction and single lymphocytes can be observed in the epidermis. Lymphocytes are generally small and do not show atypical nuclei. Blood vessels are dilated, and melanophages can be present. The epidermis shows flattening of the rete ridges when epidermal atrophy is prominent on clinical examination. Acanthosis of the epidermis and irregular hyperkeratosis of the cornified layer are present. In contrast to small plaque parapsoriasis, *spongiosis is absent.*

Treatment

Parapsoriasis can be managed conservatively, based on symptoms. Often, topical treatment is effective.

Small plaque parapsoriasis usually is asymptomatic. Treatment should be based on alleviation of symptoms associated with scaliness. Patients should be reassured of the benign self-limiting nature of the disease.

- Emollients may be sufficient to treat scaliness; however, a trial of midpotency topical steroids (class 3-5) may lead to greater clinical responsiveness.
- Phototherapy is effective in treating lesions that are widely scattered. Broad- or narrow-band UV-B can be effective and can lead to remission. More recalcitrant presentations can be treated with psoralen and long-wave ultraviolet radiation (PUVA).
- Annual follow-up is recommended. An increase in the number of lesions, an increase in the size of lesions, or the development of induration or epidermal atrophy should prompt a repeat biopsy to consider a diagnosis of MF in evolution.
- Large plaque parapsoriasis should be treated because this may prevent progression to MF (CTCL).
  - Therapy includes mid- to high-potency topical steroids (class 2-4), topical nitrogen mustard, and topical carmustine (BCNU).
  - Phototherapy with either broad- or narrow-band UV-B or PUVA can be effective in inducing remission.
  - Follow-up every 6 months is recommended. Increasing number of lesions, increase in lesion size, or the development of induration or epidermal atrophy should prompt a repeat biopsy to consider a diagnosis of MF in evolution.

Erythroderma

Erythroderma or exfoliative dermatitis represents an inflammatory skin disease involving 90% or more of the skin surface, characterized by widespread reddening and scaling. It is a morphological representation of a wide variety of skin disorders.

Aetiopathogenesis

The disease is characterized by an increased rate of epidermal turnover and increased mitotic rate of the germinative cells of the epidermis. Hence there is an increased production and loss of scales from the skin surface. The total amount of scales lost per day is between **20 g and 30 g**. The total amount of protein loss in erythroderma is **10-15%** above the normal daily protein loss and this is increased in diseases like psoriasis where the protein loss is upto 25% more than normal protein loss. Such a large amount of protein loss can affect the systemic metabolism.

Causes of Erythroderma

1. **Pre-existing skin disorders:** Psoriasis, atopic dermatitis, allergic contact dermatitis, stasis dermatitis, photosensitive eczema, vesiculobullous disorders, cutaneous T-cell lymphomas.
2. **Hereditary conditions:** Ichthyosis, pityriasis rubra pilaris.
3. **Infections:** Superficial fungal infections, Norwegian scabies, HIV.
4. **Systemic diseases:** Subacute cutaneous lupus erythematosus, dermatomyositis, sarcoidosis.
5. **Internal malignancies:** Hodgkin's disease, leukemia, carcinoma of lung, fallopian tube, colon.
6. **Drugs:** Allopurinol, antimalarials, anticonvulsants, penicillin.
7. **Idiopathic:** Not known.

Clinical Features

Erythroderma commonly occurs between 41-61 years of age with a male-female ratio of 2:1 to 4:1. Neonates and infants are uncommonly involved. It is characterized by generalized erythema, oedema and scaling involving 90% or more skin surface. The body can be covered with fine flakes or large sheets of scales which can be silver or yellowish. Large scales are seen in acute cases and small ones in chronic cases. Severe pruritus can be present in erythroderma due to atopic dermatitis, allergic dermatitis or cutaneous lymphoma. Scalp involvement and hair loss is common. In the cases of erythroderma due to pre-existing dermatoses, there may be some signs of the condition such as psoriatic plaque or islands of sparing in pityriasis rubra pilaris. In neonates, ichthyosiform erythrodermas such as Collodion baby will present as a shining membrane which covers the skin surface along with ectropion and eclabium.

The systemic symptoms may vary in severity. The body temperature can be raised due to fever or due to hypothermia which is due to thermoregulatory disturbances. There is usually tachycardia and high output cardiac failure can occur as a complication. As there is an increase in loss of protein due to excessive scaling, hypoalbuminemia and peripheral and pedal oedema may be present. Per abdominal examination will reveal hepatosplenomegaly if the erythroderma is secondary to drug hypersensitivity or malignancy. Lymphadenopathy which is secondary to a widespread skin condition is also present (dermatopathic lymphadenopathy) in 50% cases.

Complications

The complications of erythroderma that can occur are sepsis, cardiac failure, adult respiratory distress syndrome, renal failure, liver failure and capillary leak syndrome, malabsorbtion, hypoalbuminemia, electrolyte imbalance.

Course

The prognosis of erythroderma will depend on the underlying cause. Drug induced erythroderma has the best prognosis once the drug is withdrawn. The erythrodermas caused by preceding dermatoses also resolve on specific treatment of the condition. Idiopathic erythroderma has an unpredictable course.

Treatment

Although erythroderma is considered a dermatological emergency, general measures and a careful monitoring by the dermatologist can help in a good recovery of the patient. Regular monitoring of pulse, temperature, respiratory rate and blood pressure as well fluid intake and output charting should be done. Adequate nutrition and local skin care are other important measures. All drugs should be withdrawn. Bland emollients, sedating antihistamines, treatment of secondary infection are general measures. Specific treatment has to be given for specific underlying dermatoses if diagnosed. Psoriatic erythroderma would require systemic treatment with PUVA therapy or metho-trexate. Oral retinoids such as acitretin would have to be considered in cases of ichthyosiform erythroderma. Treatment of internal maligncies with surgery, chemotherapy and radiotherapy is required in cases of erythroderma due to internal malignancies.

Lichen Planus

In 1869 Erasmus Wilson delineated the condition Lichen Planus. It's derived from Greek word Lichen—"tree moss". It's a common inflammatory disorder that affects skin, mucous membranes, nail and hair.

Epidemiology

The overall prevalence of lichen planus is **< 1%.** No racial predilection is observed. 2/3rd of the cases occur between the ages of 30-60 years. Males develop at an earlier age while females are affected in their fifties and sixties. No sexual predilection is evident. The development of L.P. may be affected by seasonal and environment factors with increased incidence in months of December and January or from March to July.

Genetics

Fewer than 100 cases of familial lichen planus have been reported, familial forms are more protracted, severe and present with erosive, linear or ulcerated forms or atypical features affecting young adults and children. Certain HLA haplotypes including HLAB-7, HLA-AW19-B18 and CW8. In oral lichen planus HLAB-8 is more common.

Etiology and Pathogenesis

Both CD_4+ and CD_8+ T cells are found in lesional skin of lichen planus. Preferential accumulation of CD_8^+, CD45RO (memory) in the epidermis and CD4+ and CD8+ accumulation in the dermis. The epithelial lymphocyte interaction can be divided upto 3 stages:

1. Antigen recognition.
2. Lymphocyte activation.
3. Keratinocyte apoptosis.

Clinical Features

The classical **5Ps** are **purple pruritic plane polygonal papules** present mainly on periphery. The lesions are faintly erythematous to violaceous flat topped sometimes with central umbilication. A thin transparent adherent scale atops the lesion. Fine whitish puncta or reticular network known as **Wickham striae** (Fig. 11.15) may be present. These

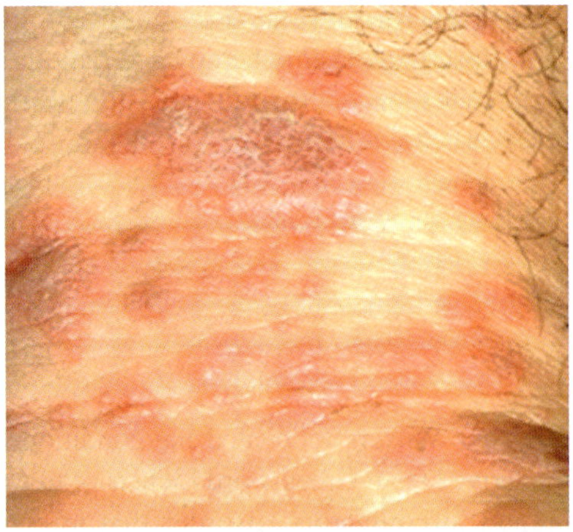

Fig. 11.15: Papules and plaques are covered by Wickham's striae on the flexor aspect of wrist

are highly characteristic. Lesions begin as macules then papules. They generally begin from the extremities and bilateral symmetrical flexures are preferentially involved. Lesions are quite pruritic generally proportional to extent of involvement. Lesions of oral mucosa (erosive lesions) are extremely painful. Scratching/injury may induce **Koebner's** phenomena. Lesions heal with hyperpigmentation usually.

Clinical Variants

Based on:

1. Configuration.
2. Morphologic appearance
3. Site of involvement.

1. **Based on Configuration**
   a. **Annular**
      Occur in 10% cases (Fig. 11.16).
      A. Formed by clustered papules with central clearing especially seen over scrotum.
      B. Larger lesions become peripherally hyperpigmented and clear centrally.
   b. **Linear:**
      A. Spontaneous, isolated eruption on extremities or face.
      B. Trauma.
      C. Zosteriform pattern.

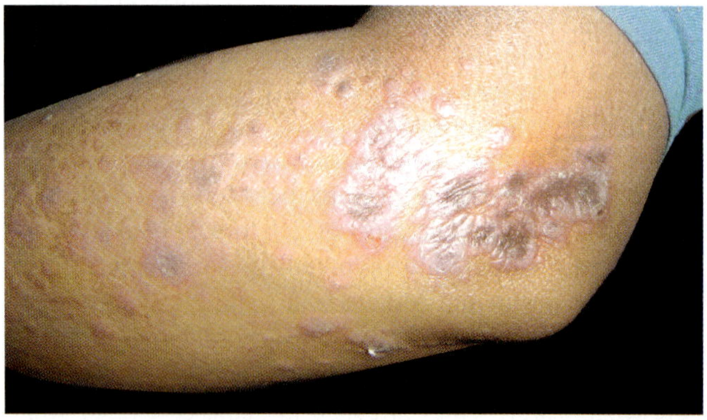

Fig. 11.16: Annular arrangement of violaceous papules

2. **Based on Morphology**
   a. **Hypertrophic** also known as **Lichen planus verrucosa** (Fig. 11.17), occurs on extremities esp. shins and interphalangeal joints. Thick, elevated, purplish and hyperkeratotic; heal with scar and hypo and hyperpigmentation usually associated.
   b. **Atrophic:** Well demarcated whitish blue papules or plaques with central superficial atrophy. Lesions may show erythema and are present over lower extremities and trunk.
   c. **Vesiculobullous:** Rare variant characterized by bulla which appear on extremities, may arise on papules/ normal skin.

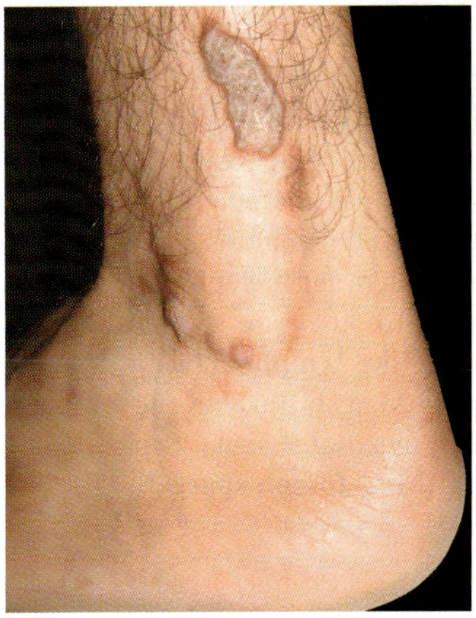

Fig. 11.17: Raised lichenified plaque on lower limb (Lichen planus hypertrophicus)

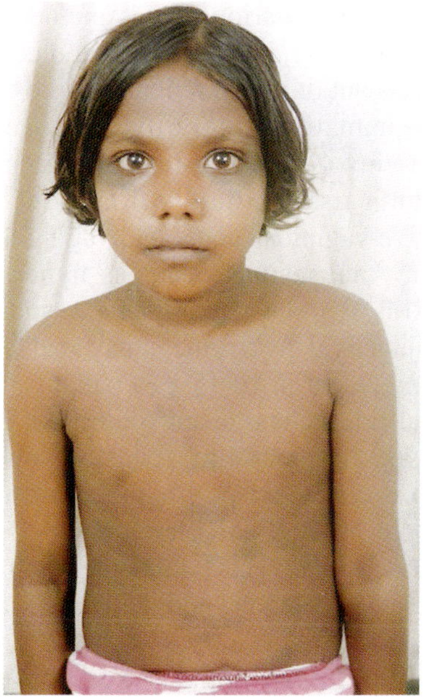

Fig. 11.18: Flat pigmented macules on face and trunk (Lichen planus pigmentosus)

d. **Erosive and ulcerative:** Present as chronic bulla or ulceration of feet, usually painful may lead to scarring associated with changes in toe nails and scalp. May be associated with erosion of oral mucosa or esophagus.

e. **Follicular** keratotic papules or plaques seen over trunk, medial aspect of proximal extremities, scalp—**cicatricial alopecia**. The triad of follicular L.P. of skin and (or scalp), multifocal cicatricial alopecia and non-cicatricial alopecia on axillary and pubic areas is called **(Graham Little Piccardi syndrome).**

f. **Lichen planus pigmentosus:** Hyperpigmented dark brown macules in sunexposed areas and flexures (Fig. 11.18).

g. **Actinic lichen planus:** Lichen planus subtropicus (lichen melanodermatosis), common in spring and summer over the exposed areas of face, dorsum of hands and nape of neck (Fig. 11.19).
   - Pruritus is minimal.
   - Hyperpigmented papules with rolled up edge showing well defined border and *a perilesional halo*.

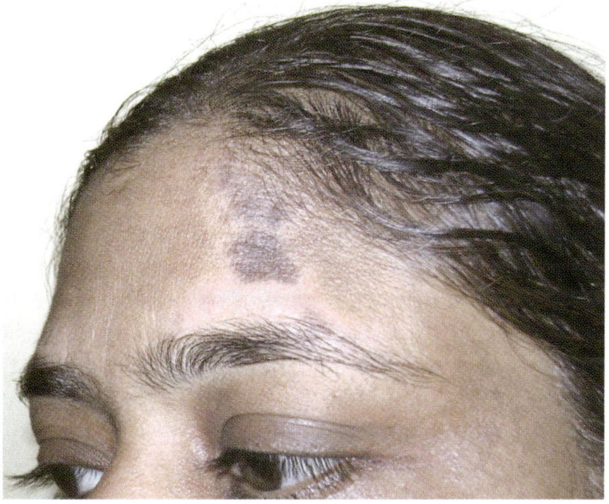

Fig. 11.19: Violaceous macule surrounded by hypopigmented zone (Lichen planus actinicus)

3. **Based on Site of Involvement**

a. *Lichen planus of scalp:* It's more common in females. May be associated with cutaneous, nail or mucous membrane involvement. Perifollicular erythema and acuminate follicular plugs are characteristic. These are usually observed in the periphery of alopecia patches.

b. *Mucosal* (Fig. 11.20): LP affects mucosa of mouth, vagina, esophagus, conjunctiva, urethra, anus, nose and larynx. Oral involvement occurs in 60-70% of

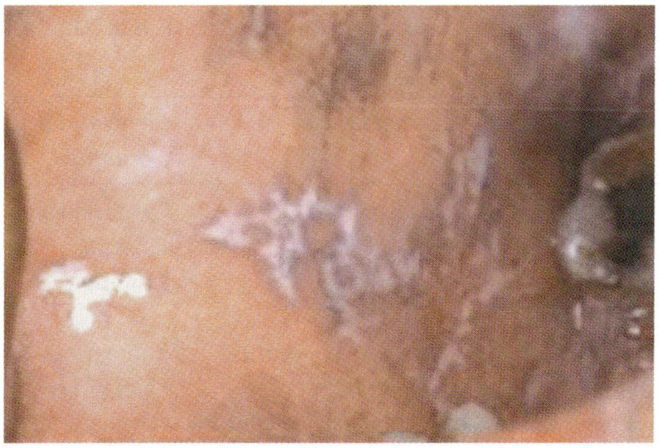

Fig. 11.20: Oral reticular pattern with "Wickham's striae"

patient of L.P. The various types include reticular, plaque like, atrophic, papular, erosive ulcerative and bullous forms out of which reticular is most common form. Desquamative gingivitis may occur. Male genitalia are involved in 25% cases especially glans and presents as annular lesions. In females, desquamative vaginitis occurs and vaginal adhesions may occur. Anal lesions occur as hyperkeratosis, leukokeratosis, fissuring vulvo-gingival syndrome may occur. Conjunctival involvement may lead to scarring.

c. *L.P. of nails:* Occur in 10-15% of patients. Thinning, longitudinal ridging and distal splitting of nail plate, onycholysis, longitudinal striation, anonychia. **pterygium** is characteristic finding. **Tenting or pup tent sign** (elevation of nail plate) may be present.

d. *Inverse lichen planus:* This is characterized by reddish brown discrete papules and nodules in axilla and groin areas.

e. *Palmoplantar lichen planus:* Very pruritic erythematous scaly plaques with or without hyperkeratosis are characteristic.

Special Forms

1. *LP-LE overlap:* Atrophic patches with hypopigmentation or/and livid red to blue colour with telangiectasia and minimal scaling are characteristic. Lesions mainly occur on extremities. The patients may be positive for ANA.
2. *Lichen planus pemphigoides:* Characterized by development of tense bullae atop lesions of lichen planus or de novo.
3. *Keratosis lichenoides chronica* (Nekam's disease) characterized by violaceous papular or nodular lesions arranged in a reticular pattern on dorsum hands or feet, extremities and buttocks. May be associated with seborrheic dermatitis of scalp, face, neck. May be very resistant to treatment.
4. *Lichenoid drug eruption:* Drugs may induce lichenoid eruption photodistributed.
   E.g.: 5-fluorouracil, carbamazepine, chlorpromazine tetracycline in oral mucosa.
   E.g.: Allopurinol, ACE inhibitors, Gold, Ketconazole.

	Lichen planus *Vs*	*Lichenoid drug eruption*
Lesions	Smaller	Large and scaly
Wickhams stria	Present	Absent
Residual hyperpigmentation	Possible	Common
Predilection	Flexural, extremities	Sunexposed areas
Mucous membrane	Common	Uncommon
Cytoid in granular	Uncommon	Common
Parakeratosis	-do-	-do-

Pathology

Two major pathological findings are:

1. **Basal epidermal keratinocyte damage**.
2. Lichenoid interface lymphocytic reaction.

Epidermal changes include: Hyperkeratosis, **wedge shaped** areas of hypergranulosis, elongation of rete ridges with **saw tooth** pattern and multiple-apoptotic cells or colloid hyaline **(civatte)** bodies are seen at dermal epidermal junction. **Band like lymphocytic infiltrate** around the papillary dermis. Many histiocytes and few plasma cells are seen (except in mucosal lesions). Separation of epidermis in small clefts **(Max Joseph spaces)**.

DIF (Direct Immunofluorescence)

Apoptotic cell at Dermoepidermal junction stain with IgM and occasionally with IgG/IgA Shaggy deposition of fibrinogen at D-E junction Majority of cellular infiltrate by immunocytochemical studies are T-lymphocytes.

Differential Diagnosis

1. Psoriasis.
2. Seborrheic dermatitis.
3. Secondary syphilis.
4. Granuloma annulare.
5. Lichen simplex chronicus.
6. Prurigo nodularis.
7. Lichen nitidus/spinulosus.
8. Paraneoplastic pemphigus.

Oral Mucosa

A. **General measures:** Good oral hygiene, replacement of gold or amalgam.

B. **Topical steroids:** 1st line. Use of occlusion e.g. orabase may provide protection and sustained contact e.g. fluocinonide 0.1% adhesive gel may be used. Simultaneous use of chlorhexidine and anticandidiasis medications may be useful.

Tacrolimus 0.10% or 0.03%

Pimecrolimus 1%

Cyclosporine (100 mg/ml) 5 ml TDS (Swish and spit).

Systemic Agents

- **Systemic glucocorticoids** are useful in erosive oral and vulvovaginal lichen planus. Dose of 30-80 mg/d tapered over 3-6 weeks shows benefit.

- **Etretinate** used at 75 mg/d shows improvement in erosive L.P.

Cutaneous Lichen Planus

1. Topical steroids.

   Intralesional—for hypertrophic, oral and L.P. of nails.

   Regression occurs after 3-4 months.
2. Systemic steroids (30-80 mg/d for 4-6 weeks with gradual tapering over 4-6 weeks) useful in lichen-planopilaris, patients with flare, patient in early stage of evolution.
3. *Retinoids:* Used because of their antiinflammatory activity. 30 mg/d of acetretin for 8 weeks provides symptomatic relief.
4. Photochemotherapy—PUVA is especially useful for generalized lichen planus, used in conjunction with oral steroids. Both oral PUVA and baths are effective.
5. Immunosuppressive agents e.g. systemic cyclosporine which causes clearance of rash in 4-6 weeks. Azathroprine may be used in recalcitrant, generalised disease and LP pemphigoides.
6. Other drugs used for treating lichen planus include Dapsone, antimalarial, INFα a 2b, thalidomide, metronidazole. Low molecular weight heparin (3 mg weekly). Rarely ulcerative disease may require skin grafting.

Course with Prognosis

Chronic relapsing course over many years.

Duration varies according to extent, site and morphology of lesions. Longer for mucosal and hypertrophic variants and lichen plano-pilaris.

Relapses occur in 15-20% patients (usually at same site). Malignant transformation occurs in 1-2%.

REFERENCES

- Fitzpatrick's Dermatology in General Medicine, 6th edn 2003.
- Lever's Histopathology of the Skin by David E Elder, Rosalie Elenitsas, Bernett L Johnson, George F Murphy, 9th edn 2004.

CHAPTER **12**

PHOTODERMATOLOGY

Photobiology is the study of effects of UV and visible light on living matter while Photodermatology is the study of these effects on skin.

Sunlight comprises a spectrum of EM waves in increasing order of wavelength as follows (Fig. 12.1):
Electrical waves > Radio waves > Infrared rays >
Visible spectrum > UV rays > X-ray and cosmic rays.

- Solar spectrum reaching the earth's surface consists of UVR > 290 nm, the visible spectrum (400-760 nm) and IR rays (760-1800 nm).

ULTRAVIOLET RANGE (200-400 nm)

UVA: 320-400 nm

- Also called as long wave UVR or near UVR.
- Comprises 90-95% of UVR reaching earth.

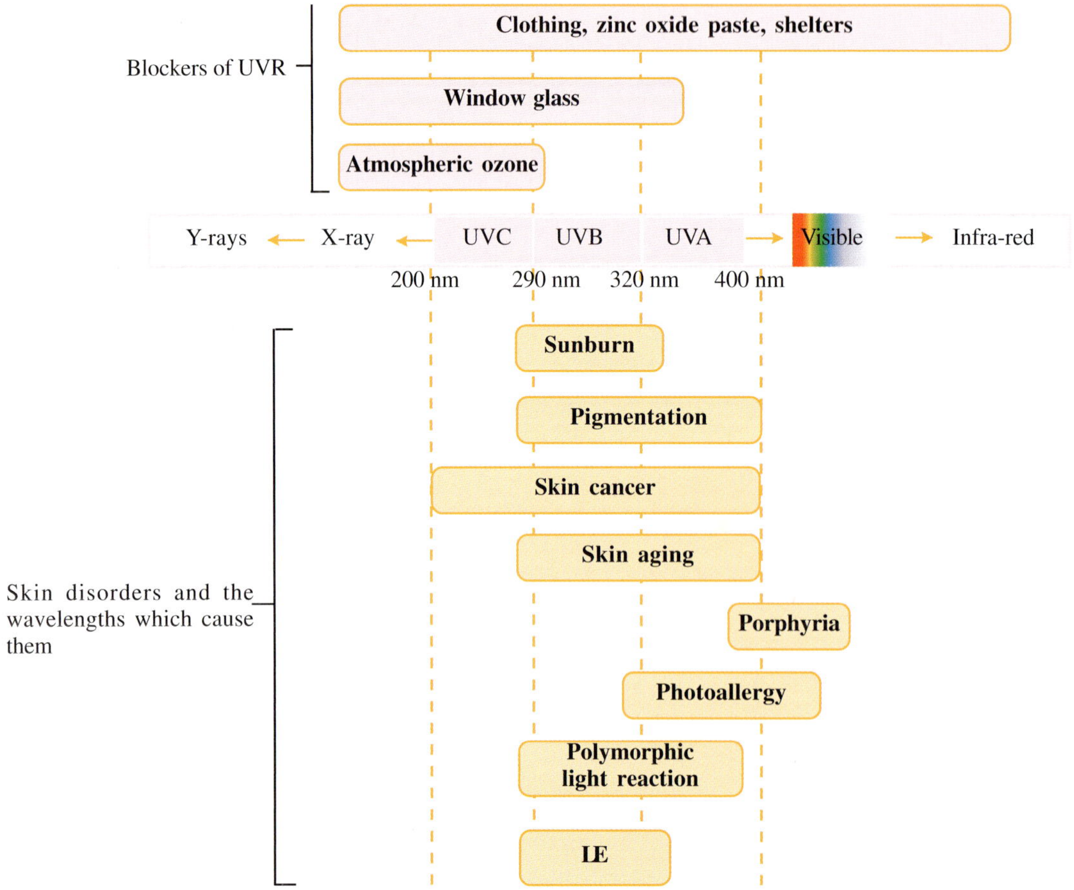

Fig. 12.1: Spectrum of UV/Visible light and the effects thereon

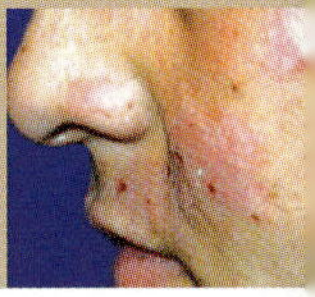

- Penetrates deeply in dermis.
- Causes both immediate and delayed tanning with or without erythema; also causes photo-aging; photo-sensitization and immunosuppression.
- Divided into UVA-1 (340-400 nm)
  UVA-2 (320-340 nm).
- UVA1 is less erythemogenic and melanogenic than UVA-2.

UVB: 290-320 nm

- Also called as mid-UVR, sunburn radiation or solar erythema band.
- Comprises 5-10% of UVR reaching the earth.
- More potent and harmful.
- Principal cause of sunburns and skin cancers.
- Most biological activity at 308 nm.

UVC: 100-290 nm

- Also called as short UVR or far UVR.
- Erythemogenic, mutagenic and carcinogenic to lab animals.
- Absent at earth's surface because of its absorption and filtration by oxygen and ozone layer.

SKIN PHOTOTYPES (SPT)

- Six SPTs based on an individual genetically determined sunburning and tanning tendency following exposure to UV radiation.
- Helps in determination of safe but effective dose regimen for phototherapy and photo-chemotherapy.
- Also determines individual's susceptibility to photo-aging and skin cancer.

Type	*Definition*	*Description*
I	Always burns but never tans	Pale skin, red hair, freckles
II	Usually burns, sometimes tans	Fair skin
III	May burn, usually tans	Darker skin
IV	Rarely burns, always tans	Mediterranean
V	Moderate constitutional pigmentation	Latin American, Middle Eastern
VI	Marked constitutional pigmentation	Black

LIGHT ABSORPTION IN THE SKIN

- Shorter wavelengths of UVB – epidermis.
- Longer wavelengths of UVB – mid-dermis.
- UVA, visible light and IR rays – subcutaneous tissue.

EFFECTS OF UVR ON SKIN

EARLY EFFECTS

1. Sunburn

- Inflammatory response to excessive exposure to sunlight.
- Clinically characterised by erythema, pain, warmth, swelling.
- Minimal erythema dose (MED): The minimum amount of UV radiation of a wavelength required to produce barely perceptible erythema well defined margins.
- UVB is 1000 times more potent in causing erythema.

Erythemogenic Response

- UVC—short lasting pink erythema.
- UVB—red erythema, starts in 3-5 hours; peaks at 20-24 hours, fades in 72-96 hours.
- UVA—deep red; starts **earlier** with a peak at 8-12 hours and fades earlier in 20-30 hours.

2. Tanning – 2 Phases

i. Immediate pigment darkening (IPD)/**Meirowsky** phenomenon:
   - Grayish.
   - Appears in seconds of exposure to 20-120 KJ/m^2 of UVA.
   - Last for a few minutes to hours.
   - Results from photo-oxidative darkening and cellular redistribution of epidermal melanin.

ii. Delayed tanning:
   - Appears after 48-72 hours, lasts for days to weeks.
   - Neomelanogenesis stimulated by UVB and UVA.
   - Mechanism: Increased tyrosinase activation
     - Increase in size and arborization of melanocytes.
     - Activation of quiescent melanocytes.

3. Hyperplasia of Skin

- UVB or UVC (not UVA) exposure for hours to days.
- Persists for 1-2 months.
- Increase in rate of cell mitosis and synthesis of DNA, RNA and proteins.
- Epidermis and dermis esp. stratum corneum thicken 2-4 times.

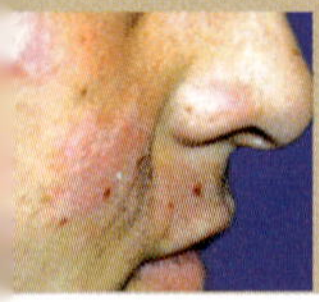

4. Immunological Changes

- Altered epidermal Langerhan's cell morphology and function.
- Increase in non-Langerhan's APC + circulating suppressor T cells.
- Modified antigen presentation.
- Enhanced immunological suppression.
  – Suppression of DTH.
- Suppression of contact hypersensitivity.
- Increased risk of skin cancer.

5. Vitamin-D Synthesis.

LATE EFFECTS

1. Pseudoporphyria

Regular exposure to predominantly UVA for weeks to months causes cutaneous blistering, increased fragility and superficial atrophic scarring.

2. Photoaging/Dermatoheliosis

- Mottled pigmentation, telangiectasias, comedones and freckles.
- Fibroelastolytic papulosis.
- Actinic elastotic plaque.
- Elastotic nodules of ear.
- Poikiloderma of civatte.
- Cutis rhomboidalis nuchae.
- Favre-Racouchot syndrome.
- Actinic comedonal plaque.
- Also increase in skin fragility and actinic purpura.

Histologically, accumulation of amorphous, basophilic degenerated elastic tissue in epidermis known as elastotic degeneration.

3. Photocarcinogenesis

Abnormal responses to ultraviolet radiation (UVR) exposure can be broadly categorized into four groups:

i. Acquired idiopathic, probably immunologic photodermatoses.
ii. DNA repair-defective photodermatoses.
iii. Photosensitization by exogenous drugs or chemicals.
iv. Dermatoses exacerbated by UVR.

The first group, the idiopathic, probably immunologic photodermatoses, and the last, the photoexacerbated dermatoses are discussed below.

POLYMORPHIC LIGHT ERUPTION

Clinical Features

Small itchy red papulovesicles or eczematous plaques arise from 2 hours to 5 days, most commonly at 24 hours, after exposure to UVR. The eruption is itchy and usually confined to sun-exposed areas remembering that some UVR passes through thin clothing.

The disorder tends to recur each spring after UVR exposure. Tanning protects some patients so that if the initial exposures are limited, few or no symptoms occur later.

PMLE has many morphologic variants, while any combination of these is also possible. Thus, papular, papulovesicular, plaque, vesiculobullous, eczematous, insect bite-like, and erythema multiform-like variants have been described, relating mostly to the clinical severity of the disorder and its site. Rarely, only pruritus may occur.

Such subdivisions do not apparently relate to differences in disease pathogenesis.

The papular form, of either large or small separate or confluent lesions (generally tending to be in clusters), is the most common, followed by the papulovesicular and plaque variants; the others are rare.

Differing morphologies may also occur at different skin sites in the same patient; thus, diffuse facial erythema and swelling, for example, may accompany typical papular lesions at other sites. Juvenile spring eruption, that affects mainly boys, apparently represents an extreme example of this phenomenon.

Treatment

Sunscreens should be used. Protective clothing, such as widebrimmed hats, long-sleeved shirts and long trousers, is helpful. In some patients, a 4-week PUVA course in the late spring can create, enough pigmentation, confer protection for the rest of the season. Moderately potent topical steroids usually improve the eruption. Hydroxychloroquine may be effective when used over the sunny season.

ACTINIC PRURIGO

This is clinically distinct from a polymorphic light eruption although its cause may be the same.

Papules, crusts and excoriations arise on sun-exposed areas and sometimes also on other sites (Fig. 12.2). Lesions may persist through the winter.

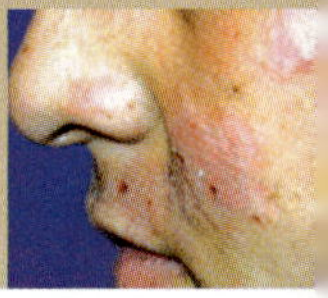

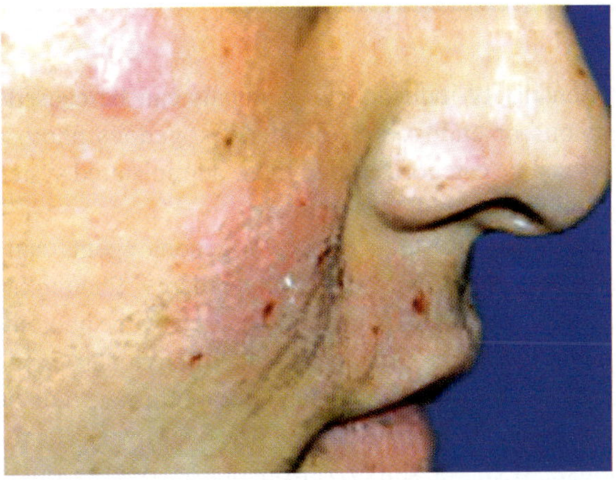

Fig. 12.2: Papulovesicle on the face of a child (Actinic prurigo)

HYDROA VACCINIFORME

Hydroa vacciniforme (HV) is a very rare photodermatosis of unknown etiology that principally starts in childhood. It is characterized by recurrent crops of papulovesicles or vesicles most commonly on the face and the dorsa of the hands but other sun-exposed areas of the skin may also be involved. The vesicles resolve with *pock-like scarring.*

Clinical Features

Erythema with a burning or itching sensation, and sometimes with associated swelling, begins within hours of sufficient sun exposure in light-exposed skin areas, particularly on the face and the hands. This is followed by the appearance of symmetrically scattered tender papules within 24 hours. These generally later become vesicular, umbilicated, and, on occasion, confluent and hemorrhagic. Within a few weeks, crusting followed by detachment of the lesions leaves permanent, depressed, hypopigmented scars. Vesicles and bullae, as well as the scars, resemble the lesions of vaccinia.

Treatment

The treatment of HV consists of restriction of sun exposure and use of broad-spectrum sunscreens. Occasionally, antimalarials have been helpful, but their true value remains to be established. Similar observations have been made with beta-carotene. As in polymorphic light eruption, prophylactic phototherapy with narrowband UVB or PUVA may be helpful, particularly the latter, although it should be administered with care to avoid exacerbations.

SOLAR URTICARIA

Solar urticaria (SU) is a rare but severely disabling, photosensitive disease in which UVR or visible radiation leads to whealing of some or all exposed skin.

Pathogenesis

SU is due to an immediate type I hypersensitivity response to a cutaneous or circulating photoallergen generated from a precursor after the absorption of light energy. Both a circulating photoallergen and reaginic antibodies have been demonstrated.

Clinical Features

SU is slightly more common in females, usually beginning between 10 and 50 years of age and persisting indefinitely, occasionally slowly worsening or gradually improving. Within 5 to 10 min of sun exposure, patients experience itching, erythema, and patchy or confluent whealing, which resolves generally with sun avoidance within 1 to 2 hours; very rarely.

Treatment

High-protection-factor sunscreens and appropriate clothing cover may be useful in UVB-sensitive subjects, but are much less effective in those sensitive to UVA and particularly visible light. However, nonsedating H 1 antihistamines may help significantly, increasing the minimum whealing dose tenfold or more. The addition of H 2 blockers rarely may offer a slight further advantage. In many patients chronically exposed skin, such as on the face and the hands, becomes tolerant. Based on this observation, therefore, patients with SU can be treated with repeated artificial UV exposures; this can be done with narrowband UVB, broadband UVB, UVA alone, a combination of UVB and UVA, and even visible light. The major disadvantage of phototherapy is that the tolerance obtained usually lasts only a few days, although a more lasting effect is obtained with PUVA, the protection provided lasting several weeks.

CHRONIC ACTINIC DERMATITIS

Chronic actinic dermatitis is a persistent photosensitivity disorder in which patients respond abnormally to UVA, UVB, and sometimes to visible irradiation. The disorder is pruritic, and results in thick, lichenified photodistributed plaques (Fig. 12.3). It may develop in persons with polymorphous light eruption or in those who have had a photosensitive drug eruption (from either a topical or systemic photosensitizer). CAD may occur in persons with dark skin (skin types 4, 5, 6) who are unaccustomed to being photosensitive.

Course

These patients may be exquisitely sensitive to UVR.They are usually middle-aged or elderly men who react after the slightest exposure, even through window glass or from

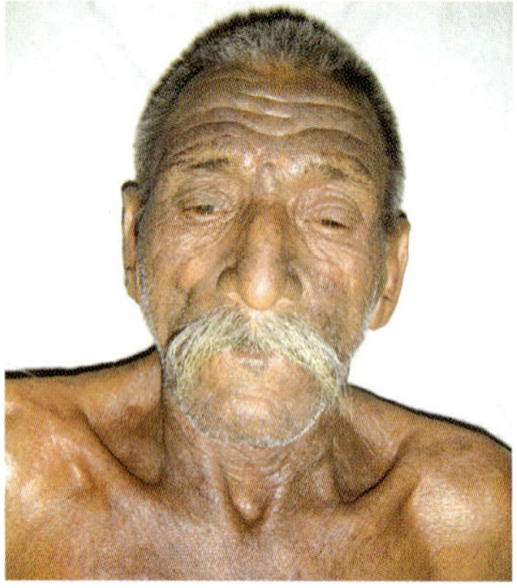

Fig. 12.3: Thick lichenified appearance on the face: chronic actinic dermatitis

fluorescent lights. Affected individuals also become allergic to a range of contact allergens, especially oleoresins in some plants (e.g. chrysanthemums).

Differential Diagnosis

Airborne allergic contact dermatitis may be confused, but does not require sunlight. Sometimes the diagnosis is difficult as exposure both to sunlight and to the airborne allergen occurs only out of doors. Airborne allergic contact dermatitis also affects sites which sunlight is less likely to reach, such as under the chin (Fig. 12.3). A continuing drug photoallergy, a polymorphic light eruption (see below) or eczema as a result of some other cause must also be considered.

Histology shows a dense lymphocytic infiltrate and sometimes atypical lymphocytes suggestive of a lymphoma, but the disorder seldom becomes malignant.

Investigations

Persistent light reaction can be confirmed experimentally by exposing uninvolved skin to UVA or UVB. Patch tests and photopatch tests help to distinguish between photoallergy and airborne allergic contact dermatitis, and the action spectrum may point to a certain drug. This sort of testing is difficult, and should be carried out only in specialist centres.

Treatment

Usually cared for by specialists, these patients need extreme measures to protect their skin from UVR.These include protective clothing and frequent applications of combined UVA and UVB blocking agents. Patients must protect themselves from UVR coming through windows or from fluorescent lights. Some can only go out at night.

As even the most potent topical steroids are often ineffective, systemic steroids or immunosuppressants (e.g. azathioprine) may be needed for long periods.

PHOTOSENSITIVITY REACTIONS

Photosensitivity induced by chemicals can be caused by exogenous or endogenous agents. Exogenous photosensitizers can be categorized into those administered systemically and agents applied topically.

Photosensitivity induced by exogenous agents can be divided into phototoxicity and photoallergy. Phototoxicity is the result of a direct tissue injury caused by the phototoxic agent and radiation; it can occur in all individuals exposed to adequate doses of the agent and the appropriate radiation. In contrast, photoallergy is a type IV delayed hypersensitivity response; it has a sensitization phase, occurs only in sensitized individuals, and requires only a minimal concentration of the photoallergen.

Phototoxicity

Basic photochemical laws require a drug to absorb UVR to cause such a reaction. Most drugs mentioned below absorb UVA as well as UVB, and so window glass, protective against sunburn, does not protect against most phototoxic drug reactions.

- Amiodarone
- Chlorpropamide
- Nalidixic acid
- Oral contraceptives
- Phenothiazines
- Psoralens
- Quinidine
- Sulphonamides
- Tetracyclines
- Thiazides

These reactions are not immunological. Everyone exposed to enough of the drug, and to enough UVR, will develop the reaction. Contact with psoralens in plants can cause a localized phototoxic dermatitis (phyto photodermatitis). These areas burn and may blister, leaving pigmentation in linear streaks and bizarre patterns.

Clinical Features

Tenderness and redness occur only in areas exposed both to sufficient drug and to sufficient UVR.

Differential Diagnosis

Photoallergic reactions are difficult to distinguish; the more so as the same drugs can often cause both photoallergic and phototoxic reactions. The main differences between phototoxicity and photoallergy are shown below:

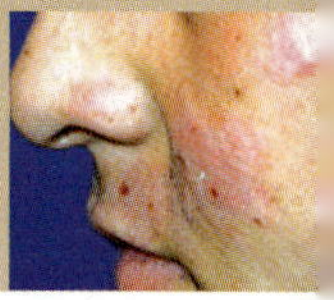

Phototoxicity	*Photoallergy*
Erythematous and smooth (may blister)	Eczematous and rough (may weep)
Immediate onset	Delayed onset (when immunity develops may not occur on first exposure)
Hurts	Itches
Photopatch testing negative	Photopatch testing positive

Photoallergy

Drugs, topical or systemic, and chemicals on the skin, can interact with UVR and cause immunological reactions.

UVR converts an immunologically inactive form of a drug into an antigenic molecule. An immunological reaction, analogous to allergic contact dermatitis, is induced if the antigen remains in the skin or is formed there on subsequent exposure to the drug and UVR. Many of the same drugs that cause phototoxic reactions can also cause photoallergic ones.

Clinical Features

Photoallergy is often similar to phototoxicity. The areas exposed to UVR become inflamed, but the reaction is more likely to be *eczematous*. The eruption will be on exposed areas such as the hands, the V of the neck, the nose, the chin and the forehead. There is also a tendency to spare the upper lip under the nose, the eyelids and the submental region (Fig. 12.4).

Often the eruption does not occur on the first exposure to ultraviolet, but only after a second or further exposures. A lag phase of one or more weeks is needed to induce an immune response.

The original lesions are red patches, plaques, vesicles or bullae, which usually become eczematous. They tend to resolve when either the drug or the exposure to UVR is stopped, but this may take several weeks.

Investigations to Diagnose Photosensitive Disorders

Photopatch testing by an expert can confirm the diagnosis.

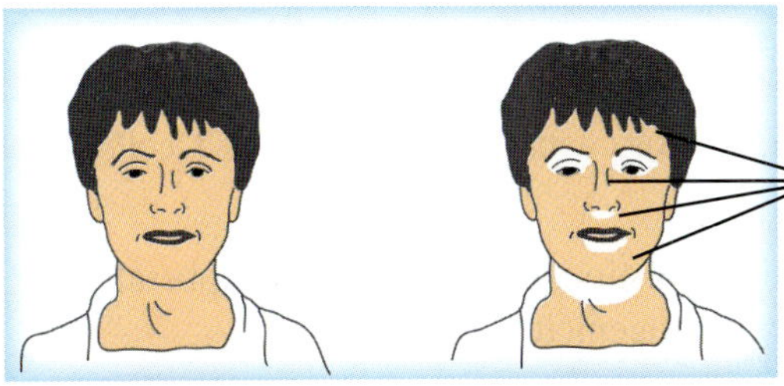

Fig. 12.4: Difference between airborne allergy and photosensitivity

An acute photo allergic contact dermatitis is then elicited. A control patch, not irradiated, rules out ordinary allergic contact dermatitis.

Other Investigations

1. ANA, SSA (Ro), SSB (La) Antibody titers.
2. Porphyrin levels (blood/urine/stool).
3. Histology
   - **PMLE**–Perivascular lymphocytic infiltrate with dermal infiltrate.
   - **Hydroa Vacciniforme**–Intra epidermal vesiculation with epidermal necrosis.
   - **Actinic Prurigo**–Lichenification and epithelial hyperplasia with dermal edema.
   - **Chronic actinic dermatitis**—Epidermal spongiosis lymphoid epidermotropism, Pautrier microabscess heavy lymphoid dermal infiltrate.

PHOTO TESTING

Photopatch testing is a well-established method to use for identifying phototoxic or photoallergic substances. It should be performed whenever a phototoxic reaction or photoallergic contact dermatitis is suspected. Diseases of the CAD spectrum are also indications for testing. In the latter, contact sensitivity may also be noted to airborne allergens such as plant oleoresins, which may have an inducing or exacerbating role in CAD.

Photopatch Test

Test materials are applied to the back in a duplicate set, one for irradiation, the other as a control.

- Patches to be irradiated are left on the skin for 24 hours; control patches are applied for either 24 or 48 hours.
- Nonirradiated patches are used as controls to exclude nonphotoinduced plain contact sensitivity.
- Test sites are evaluated before and immediately after irradiation as well as 24, 48 and 72 hours later.
- Control sites are read shortly after removal of the patches as well as 24 and 48 hours later.

Interpretation of Photopatch Test

	Reading at irradiated site	*Non irradiated site*	*Result*
1.	O	O	Normal
2.	Positive	Negative	Photoallergic dermatitis
3.	Positive	Positive (Equal intensity)	Contact allergic dermatitis
4.	Positive (More intense)	Positive	Both

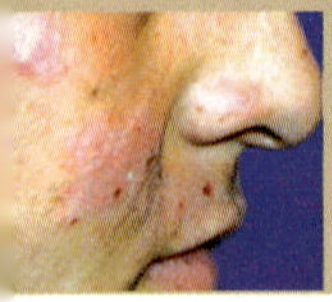

Photo Test Responses

Disease	*Spectrum Abn. findings*	*Frequency*
Actinic prurigo	UVA > UVB	Sometimes
CAD	UVB+UVA ± VL	Always
Drug induced	UVA >UVB	Frequent
Hydroa vacciniforme	UVA > UVB	Sometimes
Photoallergic CD	UVA + UVB	Frequent
PMLE	UVA > UVB	Sometimes
Solar urticaria	UVB + UVA + VL	Frequent

PRINCIPLES OF PHOTO PROTECTION

1. **Avoid or Minimize Sun Exposure.**
2. **Usage of Sun Blocking Tools – Clothes/Cap/ Umbrella.**
3. **Beware of Reflecting Surfaces – Sand/Water/ Snow.**
4. **Conduct Periodic Skin Examination.**
5. **Beware of Photosensitive Drugs.**
6. **Sunscreens.**

a. Physical

Reflect and scatter sunlight (UVA + UVB) + VL
e.g., Titanium dioxide, MgO, Mg silicate, ZnO, Fe^2O^3, Kaolin, Red petrolatum.
Advantages:
- Visible (easy to apply).
- UVA+UVB.
- Photoallergy (Rare).

Disadvantages:
- Cosmetic: Most are non-water soluble.
- ↑ Acne/folliculitis.

b. Chemical

Aromatic compounds containing benzene ring which absorb photons of light energy.

UVA blockers:
a. Dibenzoylmethanes (Avobenzone).
b. Anthranilates.

UVB blockers:
a. PABA.
b. Cinnamates.
c. Salicylates.
d. Camphor derivatives.

UVA+UVB:
a. Benzophenones (Dioxybenzone/Oxybenzone).
b. Physical (Mechanical sunscreens).

7. Tanning Lotion

DHA (Dihydroxyacetone) → 3-5% DHA
(4-5) Applications produce a golden brown color.
↓ Penetration of UVA and visible light.

8. Anti Oxidants

- Polypodium leucotomas/silyburn marianum.
- Aloe extracts.
- Vit. C (Ascorbic acid) blocks UVA.
- Vit. E (tocopherol) blocks UVB.

B-Carotene: Especially in EPP and other porphyrias.
- 120 to 180 mg/day adult dose.
- Causes yellowing of skin (carotenoderma).
- Photoprotection over a period of 4-6 weeks.

9. Nicotinamide (Vit. B_3)

- Dose–3 gm/day × 2 weeks.
- C/I–Hypersensitivity, deranged liver function, peptic ulcer disease.
- MOA– Blocks the formation of kynurenic acid.

10. Anti Histamines

- H1. Blockers–Cetrizine/Fexofenadine/Loratidine Desloratidine.
- H2. Blockers–Ranitidine.

11. Anti Malarials

- MOA–Interferes with prostaglandin synthesis.
  –Blocks chemotaxis.
  –Inhibition of superoxide production.
  –Bind to DNA.
- Chloroquine–250-500-mg/ day.
- Hydroxychloroquine–200-400 mg/day.
- Total dose should not exceed 200 gm.
- C/I–hypersensitivity/psoriasis/retinal and visual field changes.

12. Thalidomide—Non Responsive Cases

- Immunomodulatory action on a sub set of T cells.
- Dose–200 mg/day.
- S/E–Sedation/constipation/weight gain/peripheral neuropathy/teratogenicity.

13. Azathioprine

- Dose 0.8 to 2-5 mg/kg/day for 3 months.

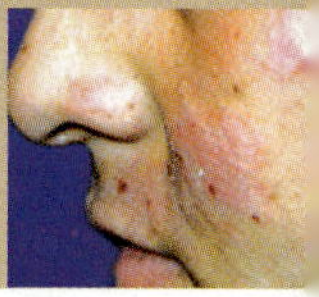

- Only in recalcitrant cases.
- Remission upto 4-12 months.
- S/E–Immunosuppression.
- Pancytopenia/infections/hypersensitivity syndrome.

14. Cyclosporine

- Recalcitrant cases.
- 3-3.5 mg/kg/day for 3-5 months.

15. Phototherapy–UVA/PUVA/Narrow Band UVB.

REFERENCES

- Rook's Textbook of Dermatology; D. A. Burns, S. M. Breathnach, Neil Cox, Christopher E., Griffith's 7th edn 2004.
- Fitzpatrick's Dermatology in General Medicine, 6th edn 2003.
- Photoaging of human skin, Photodermatology, Photoimmunology and Photomedicine 2000; 16, 239-244.
- Epstein, J.H. (1999): Phototoxicity and photoallergy, Seminars in Cutaneous Medicine and Surgery 18,274-284.
- Krutman, J., Hönigsmann, H., Elmets, C.A. and Berg-Stresser, P.R. (2001): Dermatological Phototherapy and Photodiagnostic Methods, Springer, Berlin.

CHAPTER 13

METABOLIC DISORDERS

AMYLOIDOSIS

Amyloid is a group of disorders characterized by deposition of abnormal tissue proteins in a fibrillar form with β-pleated sheet configuration.

The deposits also contain serum amyloid P, which is a globulin similar to C-reactive protein. The clinical pattern varies depending on the type of fibrillar protein and its localization.

The main types of amyloid proteins of dermatologic relevance are as follows:

- Amyloid fibrils derived from immunoglobulin light chains, known as amyloid L (**AL**). This occurs in primary systemic amyloidosis or in systemic myeloma-associated amyloidosis. Less commonly, immunoglobulin heavy chains (AH) constitute the amyloid protein in these types of amyloidosis. Nodular amyloid (of the skin or at other internal sites) also contains AL.
- Amyloid derived from serum amyloid A precursor protein, this type being termed amyloid A (**AA**). AA occurs secondary to a wide variety of chronic inflammatory disorders, such as tuberculosis, rheumatoid and other chronic arthritis, bronchiectasis, some lymphomas, and chronic venous ulceration. AA occurs in familial Mediterranean fever and other periodic fevers, as well as in familial cold urticaria and Muckle Wells' syndrome (a familial disorder with urticaria and deafness).
- Amyloid derived from **altered keratin**—this occurs in several skin tumors, such as basal cell carcinoma and Bowen's disease, and in benign lesions, such as seborrheic keratoses and porokeratosis, but is rarely prominent clinically. It is probably also the amyloid type in macular amyloidosis and lichen amyloidosis, in which scratching may play a part in disrupting keratinocytes.

Clinical Features

Cutaneous involvement in different types of amyloidosis is listed in Table 13.1 below:

Table 13.1: Cutaneous involvement in amyloidosis

Clinical type	*Amyloid*	*Skin findings protein*
Primary cutaneous amyloidosis		
i. Macular amyloidosis	Keratin	Rippled pigmentation, usually trunk.
ii. Lichen amyloidosis	Keratin	Lichenoid papules, usually legs.
iii. Nodular amyloidosis	Amyloid L (AL)	Usually solitary, yellowish brown, sometimes rather translucent nodule.
Secondary cutaneous amyloidosis		
Related to localized lesions	Keratin	Amyloid may be present in numerous lesions, including basal cell carcinoma, nevi, seborrheic keratosis, porokeratosis.
Systemic amyloidosis		
i. Primary systemic (AL) amyloidosis and myeloma-associated amyloidosis	Mainly AL/	Skin Findings in about 30-40% **macroglossia**. **Purpura:** Especially at areas of minor trauma (includes 'pinch purpura'), or periorbital (raccoon sign) if increased vascular pressure by coughing. **Plaques:** Due to skin infiltration; waxy yellowish or purpuric, often papular or cobblestoned plaque. **Others:** Bullae, sclerodermoid plaques, paronychia or nail dystrophy.
ii. Reactive amyloidosis **(amyloid A, AA).**	AA	Skin findings are rare, although the diagnosis may often be made by subcutaneous fat aspirate for histologic examination. There may be features of a chronic skin disorder that has led to reactive amyloidosis, for example psoriasis, scleroderma, lupus erythematosus, hidradenitis suppurativa.
iii. Hereditary forms	AA	Familial Mediterranean fever may cause urticaria-like skin lesions; Muckle-Wells' syndrome is familial urticaria and deafness (Note: There are many other hereditary amyloidoses in which other amyloid proteins are involved).

i. **Lichen amyloidosis** presents as small, brown, keratotic papules on the shins (Fig. 13.1).
ii. **Macular amyloidosis** is the most common. It usually affects the upper back and presents as *rippled brown lines*. It may be associated with chronic itch and scratching or rubbing, for example in notalgia paresthetica (Figs. 13.2 and 13.3).
iii. **Nodular amyloid** occurs mainly in older patients, and consists of one or several reddish brown nodules that appear mainly on the face and extremities. Most nodular amyloid is probably due to a polyclonal reactive process of AL fibrils, but some patients have a monoclonal gammopathy or urinary Bence Jones protein.

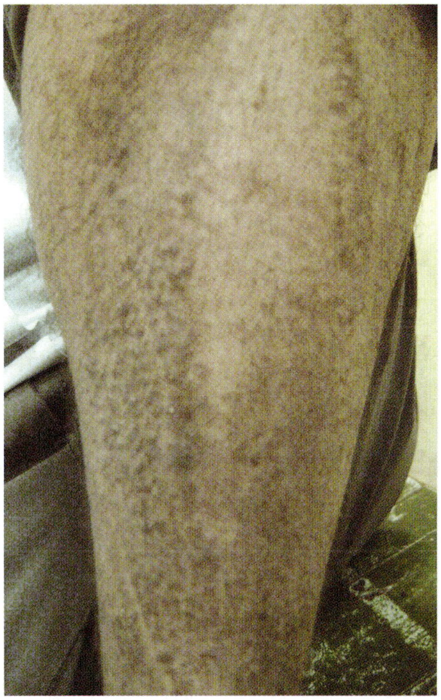

Fig. 13.1: Biphasic amyloidosis with nodules, papules and macules

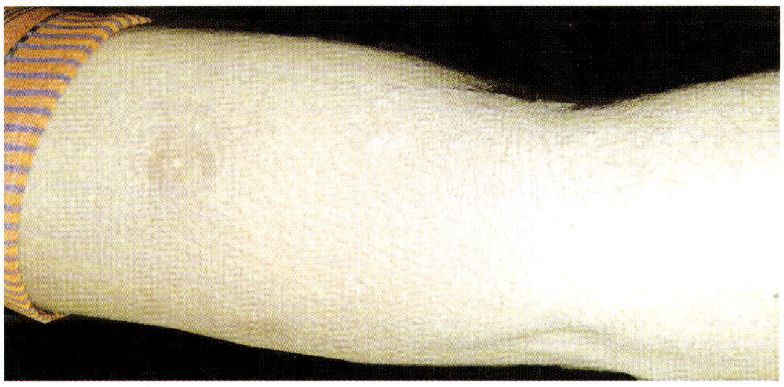

Fig. 13.2: Macular amyloidosis with rippled pattern

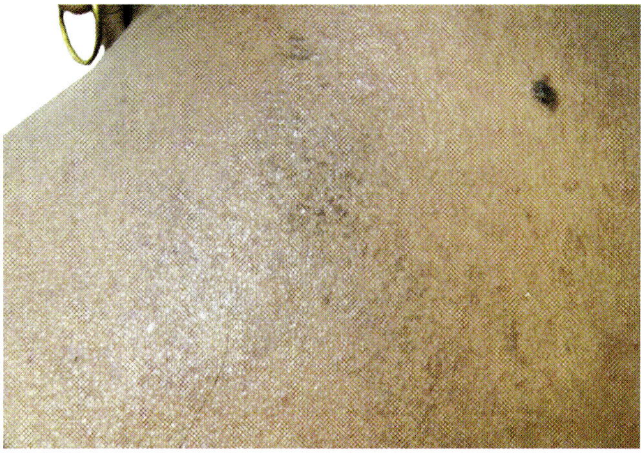

Fig. 13.3: Back involvement in a female

Differential Diagnosis

- *Nodular amyloidosis*—Differential includes primary skin tumors, such as basal cell carcinoma; granulomatous diseases, such as granuloma annulare or sarcoidosis; xanthomas; granuloma faciale (a vasculitis); and skin lymphoma.
- *Lichen amyloidosis*—Most likely to be confused with simple lichenification; lichen planus and lichen myxedematosus (papular lesions) are possible differentials.
- *Macular amyloidosis*—Other causes of rippled hyperpig-mentation include lichenification, notalgia paresthetica, and the so-called atopic dirty neck. The last in particular has the same rippled pigmented appearance as in macular amyloidosis.

Treatment

Systemic amyloidosis is treated with a variety of chemotherapeutic agents, particularly melphalan, to control the underlying plasma cell dyscrasia, together with symptomatic treatment of complications such as cardiac failure.

Localized nodular amyloid is generally treated surgically by excision, curettage or laser.

Lichen Amyloidosis—Can be treated by colchicine and cyclophosphamide.

THE PORPHYRIAS (Fig. 13.4)

There are at least seven enzymes in the metabolic pathway that leads to the synthesis of haem. There are also seven different types of porphyrias, each being caused by a deficiency of one of these enzymes, and each having its own characteristic pattern of accumulation of porphyrin and porphyrin precursors.

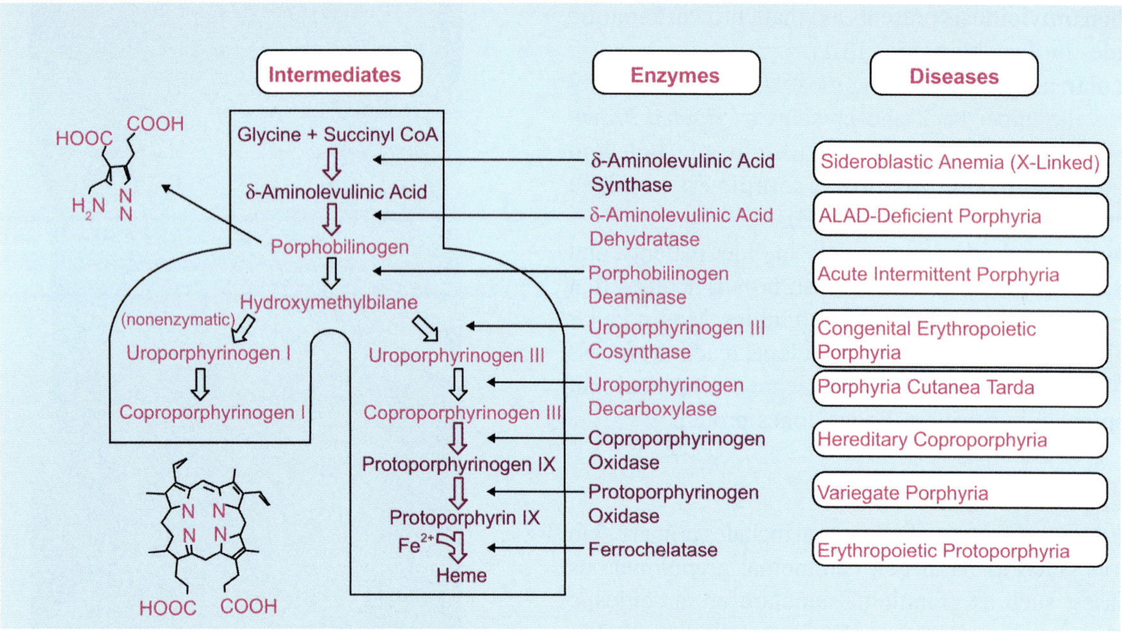

Fig. 13.4: Pathway of heme synthesis

Some of these cause the photosensitivity (to ultraviolet radiation of wavelength 400 nm, which is capable of penetrating through window glass) that is the cardinal feature of the cutaneous porphyrias.

Congenital Erythropoietic Porphyria

Rare, Gunthers disease.

Enzyme *uroporphyrinogen cosynthase*, and inherited as an autosomal recessive trait.

Clinical Features

Severe photosensitivity is noted soon after birth, and leads to blistering, scarring and mutilation of the exposed parts, which become increasingly hairy. The urine is pink and the teeth are brown, although fluorescing red under Wood's light.

Haemolytic anaemia is present.

Erythrohepatic Protoporphyria

(Erythropoietic Protoporphyria)

Common, autosomal dominant condition, caused by mutations in the *ferrochelatase gene*.

Clinical Features

A less severe photosensitivity develops during childhood. A burning sensation occurs within minutes of exposure to sunlight. Soon the skin becomes swollen and crusted vesicles sometimes appear, leading to pitted scars. Liver disease and gallstones occur.

Treatment

In addition to sun avoidance and the use of sunscreens, beta carotene may be given orally.

Cutaneous Hepatic Porphyria

(Porphyria Cutanea Tarda)

A *sporadic type* (accounting for 80% of cases) and a type inherited as an *autosomal dominant* trait (20%).

Low hepatic uroporphyrinogen decarboxylase activity.

Types

Sporadic type: Men, rarely in women, who have damaged their livers by drinking too much alcohol but may also occur in women taking oestrogens. Recently it has been shown that some cases are caused by a previous hepatitis C virus infection.

Clinical Features

Blisters, erosions and milia form on the *exposed* parts of the face, and on the backs of the hands, in response to sunlight or to minor trauma.

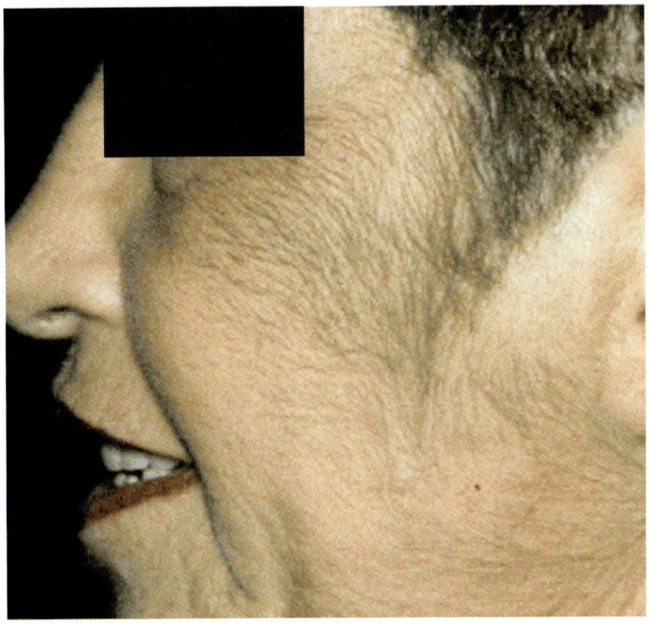

Fig. 13.5: Hypertrichosis in a case of PCT

These areas become scarred and *hairy* (Fig. 13.5).

The urine is *pink* and fluoresces a bright coral-pink under Wood's light as a result of excessive uroporphyrins.

Treatment

Treatment is based on avoiding alcohol and oestrogens, but other measures are usually needed too, including regular venesection or very low dose hydroxychloroquine therapy (e.g. 100 mg twice weekly) under specialist supervision. Higher doses cause toxic hepatitis in these patients.

Acute Intermittent Porphyria–Autosomal Dominant

Occurs due to mutations of the porphobilinogen deaminase gene.

- Skin lesions *do not occur.*
- Attacks of abdominal pain, accompanied by neuropsychiatric symptoms and the passage of dark urine, are sometimes triggered by drugs (especially barbiturates, griseofulvin, oestrogens and sulphonamides).

Variegate Porphyria

Autosomal dominant mutations of the protoporphyrinogen oxidase gene, is particularly common in South Africa.

Clinical Features

It shares the skin features of porphyria cutanea tarda and the systemic symptoms and drug provocation of acute intermittent porphyria.

Pseudoporphyria

This term is used when skin changes like those of cutaneous hepatic porphyria occur without an underlying abnormality of porphyrin metabolism. It is seen in a few patients on haemodialysis, and can be induced by some drugs notably frusemide (furosemide) and non-steroidal anti-inflammatory drugs.

MUCINOSES

1. **Myxoedema:** Characterised by the puffy hands and face of patients with hypothyroidism.
2. **Pretibial myxoedema:** Pink or flesh-coloured mucinous plaques are seen on the lower shins, together with marked exophthalmos, in some patients with hyperthyroidism. They may also occur after the thyroid abnormality has been treated.
3. **Scleromyxoedema:** A diffuse thickening and papulation of the skin may occur in connection with an immunoglobulin G (IgG) monoclonal paraproteinaemia.
4. **Follicular mucinosis:** In this condition, the infiltrated plaques show loss of hair. Some cases are associated with a lymphoma.

DISORDERS OF AMINO ACID METABOLISM

Phenylketonuria

1 in 25000

Autosomal recessive trait, the abnormal gene lying on chromosome region 12q22-q24, and is caused by a deficiency of the liver enzyme *phenylalanine hydroxylase*, which catalyses the hydroxylation of phenylalanine to tyrosine. This leads to the accumulation of phenylalanine, phenylpyruvic acid and their metabolites.

Affected individuals have *fair skin and hair*. They often develop *eczema*, usually of atopic type, and may be photosensitive. The accumulation of phenylalanine and its metabolites damages the brain during the phase of rapid development just before and just after birth. *Mental* retardation, epilepsy and extrapyramidal manifestations such as athetosis and mental retardation may then occur.

Alkaptonuria

A recessively inherited disorder, based on a *homogentisic acid oxidase deficiency*, *dark urine* may be seen in childhood, and in adult life *pigment may* be deposited in various places including the ears and sclera. Arthropathy may occur.

Hartnup Disease

Reabsorption disturbance for neutral amino acids, *pellagra* like skin lesions.

Homocystinuria

- Cystathionine synthetase deficiency.
- Livedo reticularis, facial erythema, marfanoid habitus, atrophic scar, sparse hair.

Richner Hanhart Syndrone

- Tyrosinase aminotransferase deficiency.
- Palmoplantar hyperkeratosis.

DEFECT IN LIPID METABOLISM

Xanthomas

General Aspects, Etiology and Pathogenesis

This group of disorders is characterized by deposition of abnormal lipid in the skin. At some sites, such as the eyelids *(xanthelasma)*, this is often in the context of *normal* serum lipid levels. However, *xanthomas* at other sites are usually a manifestation **of systemic hyperlipidemias.**

In many cases, xanthomas occur in patients with a hereditary predisposition (primary), although there may be environmental interaction (diet, alcohol, etc.). The **primary hyperlipidemias** were classified types I–V (World Health Organization classification, Fredericksen classification) but are now classified as follows (World Health Organization classification in square brackets).

- Hypercholesterolemia (familial and polygenic types) [IIa, IIb].
- Combined hypercholesterolemia [IIa, IIb].
- Remnant particle disease (dysbetalipidemia) [III].
- Hypertriglyceridemia (familial hypertriglyceridemia [IV]. and familial combined hypertriglyceridemia [V]).
- Chylomicronemia [I]; and
- Unclassified high-density lipoprotein abnormalities.

Secondary hyperlipidemias may be due to cholestasis, hypothyroidism, diabetes, nephrotic syndrome, renal failure, monoclonal gammopathy, or drugs. Most drug-induced hyperlipidemia does not cause dermatologic features, but olanzapine has been implicated as a cause of eruptive xanthomas due to hypertriglyceridemia; dermatologists also need to be aware of hyperlipidemia due to use of oral retinoids. Cholesterol and triglyceride are the most relevant lipids, but abnormal levels of other sterols may also be dermatologically relevant, for example elevated cholestanol in cerebrotendinous xanthomatosis.

Note that some lesions that carry the name xanthoma are actually correctly classified as histiocytoses (e.g. xanthoma disseminatum or necrobiotic xanthogranuloma) and are discussed briefly later.

Clinical Features

Xanthomas are usually clinically apparent from their yellow color. The main patterns are summarized in Table 13.2.

Treatment

In the majority of cases, in which there is an underlying hyperlipidemia, treatment is by dietary correction, drugs such as statins, and correction of other cardiac risk factors such as smoking and hypertension. Some xanthomas, especially eruptive lesions, will regress as serum lipid levels are corrected. Local treatment, such as excision, is occasionally required for xanthomas at difficult sites. Xanthelasmas may be treated with a variety of destructive modalities, such as trichloroacetic acid, electrocautery, excision and laser.

MISCELLANEOUS DISORDERS

Gout

Etiology and Pathogenesis

Gout is a disorder in which excessive urate is deposited in the tissues. This may occur for a variety of reasons, including a familial tendency, failure of excretion (e.g. chronic renal failure), or excessive purine load (e.g. from breakdown of damaged cells during chemotherapy).

Clinical Features

Gout primarily affects the joints, causing severe acute pain. However, in chronic gout there may be development of cutaneous nodules known as tophi. These affect primarily the fingers and the ears. They are hard, yellowish white subcutaneous nodules.

Fabry's Disease (Angiokeratoma Corporis Diffusum)

A deficiency of the enzyme α-galactosidase A is found in this sex-linked disorder (chromosome region Xq21.3–22); abnormal amounts of glycolipid are deposited in many tissues as a result.

Table 13.2: The main patterns of xanthomas and their differential diagnosis

Pattern	*Lipid abnormality*	*Clinical features*	*Differential diagnosis*
Tendon xanthomas	Mainly in type II or III hyperlipoproteinemia, associated with diabetes mellitus, hypothyroidism, obstructive liver disease. Tendon xanthomas also occur, with neurologic deficit, in cerebrotendinous xanthomatosis.	Usually most apparent on hands and ankles, over the extensor *tendons* (Fig. 13.6).	Confused with rheumatoid nodules or giant cell tumor of tendon sheath, less often with lipomas.
Tuberous xanthomas	Occur in type III or type II hyperlipoproteinemia.	Often occur on *elbows* or *knees* (Fig. 13.6).	May be confused with localized neurofibromas (but tuberous xanthomas are usually symmetric) or with uncommon conditions such as erythema elevatum diutinum (a chronic vasculitis that causes fibrotic nodules, often on elbows or knees).
Plane xanthomas	Depends on site. Antecubital and finger web plane xanthomas occur in type II hyperlipoproteinemia. Hand and foot involvement occurs in cholestasis. See also specific types discussed below (palmar crease, xanthelasma, normolipemic type).	*Antecubital* and *finger* webs; hands and feet, becoming generalized.	Antecubital pattern might be confused with lichenification, erythrasma, tinea. Broader areas of plane xanthoma on the neck or larger flexures, or more widespread lesions, may resemble pseudoxanthoma elasticum or the rare xanthelasmoid variant of mastocytosis.
Palmar crease xanthomas (xanthoma striatum palmare)	Almost diagnostic of *type III* hyperlipoproteinemia.	Occur in the *palmar creases.*	Occasionally confused with carotenemia, but this does not localize to the creases.
Eruptive xanthomas	Occur due to marked elevation of *triglyceride* levels (occurs in type I, IV and V hyperlipoproteinemia), associated with diabetes mellitus hypothyroidism and pancreatitis.	Tiny spots, *eruptive pattern*; typically occur on the buttocks but may be generalized.	May be confused with folliculitis, diffuse pattern granuloma annulare, or with some histiocytoses.
Xanthelasma palpebrum	A significant minority (about 25%) of patients have hyperlipidemia, usually type II.	Occur on the eyelids (Fig. 13.7).	Nodular elastoidosis, a disorder of elderly sun-damaged skin that occurs predominantly on the cheeks and in the vicinity of the eyes (but which is also characterized by comedones). Sebaceous hyperplasia lesions are more circular, usually not on eyelids. Syringomas occur on eyelids but are more discrete small skin-colored lesions. Necrobiotic xanthogranuloma (a histiocytosis associated with paraproteinemia) often produces lesions around the eyes but is usually more destructive.
Normolipemic plane xanthomatosis	None	Sheets of small yellowish papules; strongly associated with paraproteinemia or myeloma; also linked with acquired type of C1 esterase inhibitor deficiency.	Differential includes several of the histiocytoses, but the diagnosis is usually apparent from the yellow color of the xanthomatosis lesions. Plane xanthomas associated with hyperlipoproteinemia are usually much more localized.

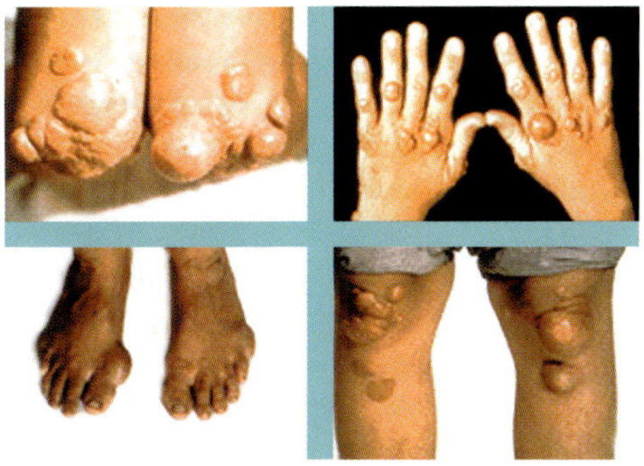

Fig. 13.6: Tuberous and tendinous xanthoma

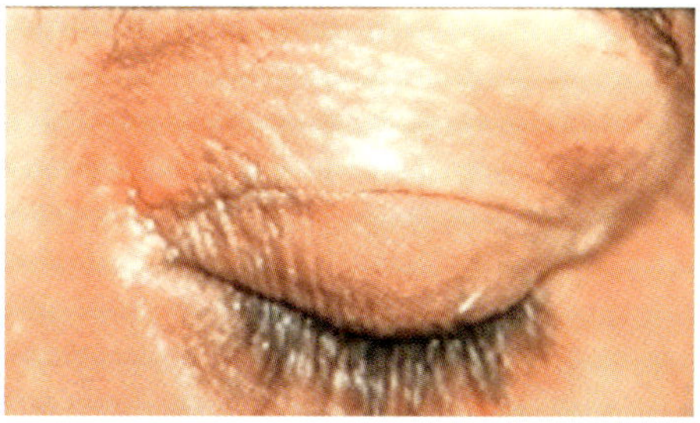

Fig. 13.7: Xanthelasma palpebrum

Skin lesions are grouped, almost black, small telangiectatic papules especially around the umbilicus and pelvis. Progressive renal failure occurs in adult life. Most patients have attacks of excruciating unexplained pain in their hands. Some female carriers have skin changes, although these are usually less obvious than those of affected males. Similar skin lesions may be seen in lysosomal storage disorders such as fucosidosis.

REFERENCES

- Rook's Textbook of Dermatology, D. A. Burns, S. M. Breathnach, Neil Cox, Christopher E., Griffiths 7th edn 2004.
- Fitzpatrick's Dermatology in General Medicine, 6th edn 2003.

CHAPTER **14**

GENETICS AND GENODERMATOSES

NOMENCLATURE

Genodermatoses: Refer to disorders due to alteration in the function of a single gene.

Familial: The clustering of a disorder with relatives affected more than predicted by the population prevalence of the condition.

Inherited: The transmission of genetic variants from one generation to the next.

Congenital: The character is present at birth but not necessarily genetically determined or familial.

FAMILIAL MULTIPLE TUMOR SYNDROMES

1. **The Neurofibromatoses (NF)**

   These comprise several distinct genetic disorders that lead to the formation of tumors surrounding nerves and a variety of other pathological features. Riccardi has proposed a classification of NF that includes 7 different types and an eight category for cases "not otherwise specified". However, the National Institute of Health (NIH) consensus conference classification classifies NF only into NF1 and NF2, which it believes could be clearly defined.

   Neurofibromatosis Type 1 [Von Recklinghausen's (NF)].

INTRODUCTION

It is an AD disorder with 100% penetrance by the age of 5 years. The gene causing it has a high rate of mutation and approximately 50% patients have no family history. Its prevalence is 1:2500-3000 births.

Pathogenesis

The NF1 gene is located on **chromosome 17** and is *a tumor suppressor gene encoding neurofibromis*. The mutation of this gene thus leads to multiple tumors seen in this condition.

Pathology

- Cutaneous neurofibromas are derived from peripheral nerves and their supporting structures, including neurilemmal cells. Ultramicroscopically, they are seen to consist of arborizing Schwann cells in collagenous interstitial tissue. Mitotic activity is low. The tumor is not locally invasive. Mast cells are seen scattered throughout the tumor.
- **Plexiform neurofibromas**, however, are locally invasive, growing within and along the nerve, enlarging the nerve fascicles and elongating each fascicle. This growth causes the fascicles to twist on themselves, eventually creating a lesion resembling a tangle of worms.
- **Café-au-lait** macules show focal hyperpigmentation in the basal layer of the epidermis. There is an increase in the number of melanocytes with an increased number of melanin giant granules.

Clinical Features (Table 14.1)

Diagnostic Features: A diagnosis of NF-1, according to the National Institute of Health consensus development

Table 14.1: NIH criterion

1. Six or more café au-lait (CAL) macules greater than 5 mm in prepubertal patients and greater than 15 mm in postpubertal patients;
2. Two or more neurofibromas of any type, or one plexiform neurofibroma;
3. Axillary or inguinal freckling;
4. Optic nerve glioma;
5. Two or more Lisch nodules (iris hamartomas);
6. A distinctive osseus lesion such as sphenoid wing dysplasia or cortical thinning of long bones, with or without pseudoarthrosis; and
7. A first degree relative with NF-1 based on the preceding criteria.

   2 or more–Diagnostic

- **(Most common benign tumor is a neurofibroma**

  Lisch nodules—appear by 6 years.

  Most common types of malignant tumors are neurofibrosarcoma and optic nerve gliomas).

conference statement, is based on 2 or more of the following criteria:

i. Six or more café-au-lait macules **(CALMs) > 5** mm in greatest diameter in prepubertal individuals and > 15 mm in postpubertal individuals. Café-au-lait macules are the first disease manifestations to appear. They are sharply defined, uniformly pigmented, light brown macules with regular edges (Fig. 14.1).

ii. Two or more **neurofibromas** of any type or 1 plexiform neurofibroma. These develop usually in the 2nd or 3rd decade. They are soft, almost gelatinous, nodules which, when pressed, tend to vaginate into the subcutaneous tissue ("**Button** Holing"). There is an increase in their size and number during pregnancy with partial regression after delivery. Plexiform neurofibromas have a characteristic **"bag of worms"** feel when palpated (Fig. 14.2).

iii. Freckling in the axillary or inguinal **regions (Crowe's sign)**. Freckling can also be seen in other specific areas like the submammary areas in females and around base of the neck. They resemble CALMs but are smaller and appear later than them (Fig. 14.3).

iv. Optic glioma.

v. Two or more **Lisch Nodules**. Lisch nodules are hamartomas of iris which are asymptomatic. They are diagnosed on slit-lamp examination as smooth dome-shaped lesions with very distinct edges. They appear during childhood, after CALM but before neurofibromas.

vi. A distinctive osseous lesion such as sphenoid dysplasia or thinning of the long bone cortex with or without pseudoarthrosis.

vii. A first degree relative with NF1 by the above criteria. **Other skin changes** include bronzing of the skin and juvenile Xanthogranulomas. Kyphoscoliosis, lordosis, short stature, spina bifida, macrocephaly, ribbon ribs and scalloping of vertebrae are some of the *bony changes* seen in NF-1. 1.5-15% neurofibromas may develop sarcomatous changes. Juvenile Xanthogranulomas in NF1 may be associated with juvenile CML.

viii. Other tumors associated include pheochro-mocytoma, Wilm's tumour, Rhabdomyosarcoma and retinoblastoma.

Differential Diagnosis

CALMs are seen in:

- 10-20% normal individuals (but are usually <6 in number.
- McCune Albright syndrome.

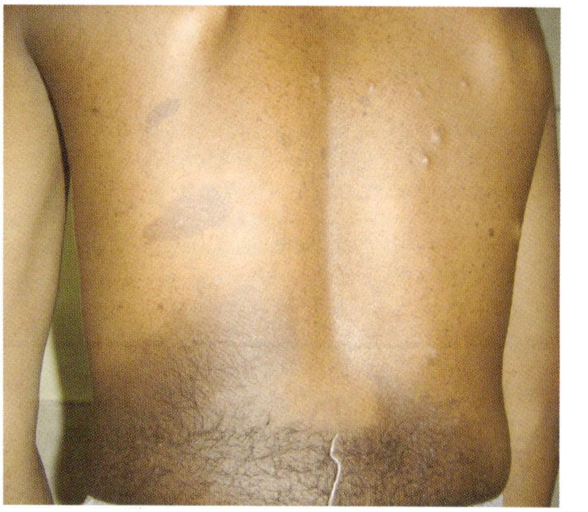

Fig. 14.1: Multiple CALM, neurofibroma on the back

Fig. 14.2: Soft, pedunculated papules–neurofibromata on the back

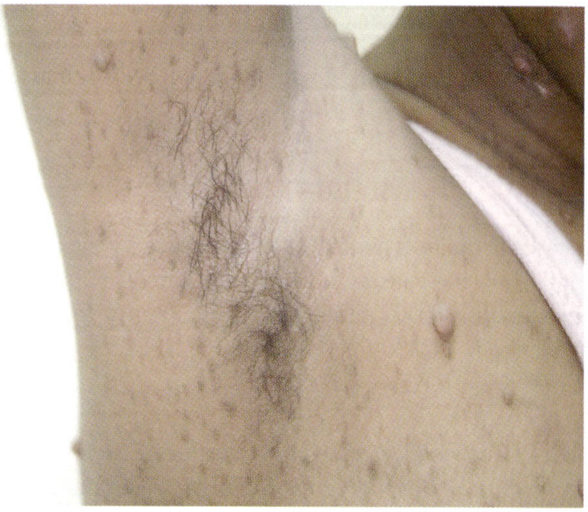

Fig. 14.3: Pigmented macule on the axilla–Crowe's sign

- Ring Chromosome syndrome.
- DNA repair syndrome e.g. Ataxia telangiectasia.

Neurofibromas may be confused with multiple lipomatosis occasionally.

Diagnosis

Diagnosis is based on clinical criteria. Identification of the NF1 gene means that prenatal diagnosis is now possible with > 95% accuracy in families. However, this is not an option for approximately 50% of cases who represent new mutations.

Treatment

Treatment is symptomatic only. The disfiguring lesions can be excised or treated with carbon dioxide laser. Surgery is also indicated when an increase in size and pain suggests possible malignant change. Routine follow up every 6-12 months is advisable.

Genetic counselling is of utmost importance. Patients should be informed that 50% of their children may be affected.

NEUROFIBROMATOSIS TYPE 2 (NF-2)

Introduction

It is also known as bilateral acoustic neurofibromatosis and accounts for 3% of all cases of NF.

Pathogenesis

The NF 2 gene, located on chromosome 22, encodes a protein called Schwannin, which is important in the linking of cytoskeletal proteins to membranes. Its incidence is 1 in 40,000 to 50,000 births.

Clinical Features

NF 2 is characterized by bilateral vestibular schwannomas (acoustic neuromas), as well as other CNS tumors of meningeal and glial orgin. Café-au-lait macules and cutaneous neurofibromas may be occasionally present in fewer numbers.

Diagnostic Features

1. Bilateral vestibular schwannomas, either proven histologically or seen by MRI with gadolinium enhancement.
2. A parent, sibling or offspring with NF2 and either:
   a. Unilateral vestibular schwannoma; or
   b. One of the following—meningioma, glioma, schwannoma, posterior subcapsular opacities, cerebral calcification.
3. Unilateral vestibular schwannoma and one of the following: meningioma, glioma, schwannoma, posterior subcapsular lenticular opacities, cerebral calcification.
4. Multiple meningioma (2 or more) and one of the following: glioma, neurofibroma, schwannoma, posterior subcapsular lenticular opacities, cerebral calcification.

The first symptoms of NF2 usually relate to the acoustic neuromas and consist of deafness, with or without associated vertigo and tinnitus. Symptomatic in early adult life (average age 22.6 years).

Diagnosis

It is recommended that annual clinical screening of at risk individuals is performed from early childhood including skin and ophthalmological examinations. Annual 'acoustic screen' MRI should be performed from the age of 15 years.

TUBEROUS SCLEROSIS COMPLEX (TSC)

Introduction

It is a genetic autosomal dominantly inherited condition with hamartoma formation in multiple organs. It is also known as Bourneville's disease and **epiloia** (Epilepsy + low intelligence + Adenoma sebaceum) and **Pringle's disease.**

Pathogenesis

Two genes have been identified associated with TSC, the first gene locus (TSC1) has been mapped to chromosome. Its protein products, hamartin, is a tumor suppressor protein. Protein product for TSC2, tuberin, has also been isolated. TSC2 is located on chromosome 16p13. Tuberin is also a tumor suppressor gene, and its mutations lead to excessive hamartomas formation. There is no significant difference in the phenotype of TSC between those families linking to TSC 1 or TSC 2.

CLINICAL FEATURES (Table 14.2)

Major Features

1. **Facial angiofibromas** or forehead plaque. The angiofibromas are firm discrete red-brown telangiectatic papules 1-10 mm over the area from the nasolabial furrows to the cheeks and chin (Fig. 14.4).

Table 14.2

Diagnostic criteria (Tuberous Sclerosis Association)

- **Major features (Definitive diagnosis of TSC requires two major features) OR 1 major and 2 minor.**
  - Facial angiofibromas or forehead plaque.
  - Non-traumatic ungual or periungual fibroma.
  - Shagreen patch (connective tissue nevus).

Contd.

Contd.

- Multiple retinal nodular hamartomas (phakomas).
- Cortical tuber.
- Calcified subependymal nodule.
- Subependymal giant cell astrocytoma.
- Cardiac rhabdomyoma, single or multiple.
- Lymphangiomyomatosis and/or Renal angiomyolipoma.

• **Suggestive features**

- Hypomelanotic macules - Ash leaf.
- Multiple randomly distributed pits in dental enamel.
- Hamartomatous rectal polyps.
- Bone cysts.
- Gingival fibromas.
- Multiple renal cysts.
- Skin tags.
- Positive family history.

(Earliest detectable abnormalities—hypopigmented macules and rhabdomyomas.

Central nervous system lesions—cortical hamartomas (tubers), focal cortical dysplasia, subependymal nodule, subependymal giant cell astrocytoma.

Renal involvement—Angiomyolipomas.

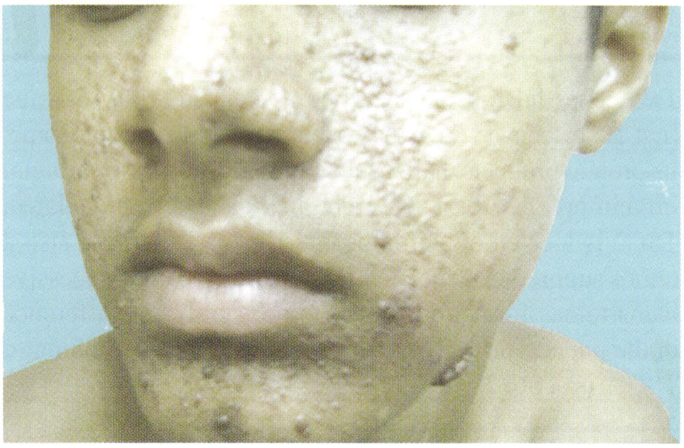

Fig. 14.4: Characterised raised papules—on the face—adenoma sebaceum

Diagnosis

Identification of ash leaf macules under Wood's light, in the presence of unexplained epilepsy, retinal phacomas, or radiologically or electroencephalographic findings or a positive family history will help establish the diagnosis.

Definite TSC = 2 major or 1 major + 2 suggestive

Probable TSC = 1 major + 1 suggestive

Possible TSC = 1 major or 2 or more suggestive.

2. Non-traumatic irregular or periungual fibroma. Also known as **Koenen's** tumor. They appear at or after **puberty** as smooth, firm flesh colored excrescences from the nail folds (Fig. 14.5).

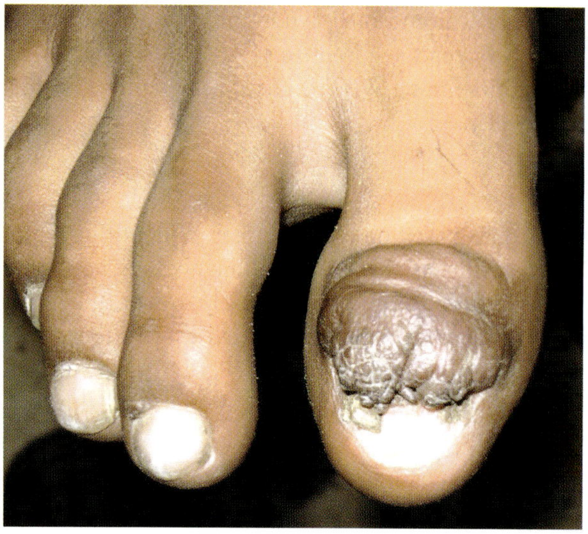

Fig. 14.5: Periungual tumor—Koenens' tumor

3. **Shagreen** patch (connective tissue naevus). It is an irregularly thickened, slightly elevated skin colored plaque, most common in the lumbosacral region (Fig. 14.6).
4. Multiple retinal nodular hamartomas.
5. **Cortical tuber.**
6. Subependymal nodule.
7. Subependymal giant cell astrocytoma.
8. Cardiac rhabdomyoma, single or multiple.
9. Lymphangiomyomatosis and/or nasal angiomyolipoma.
10. Hypomelanotic ash leaf macules **(more than 3)**. They are white 1-3 cm big macules which can be detected by Wood's light few years before other signs of TSC develop (Fig. 14.7).

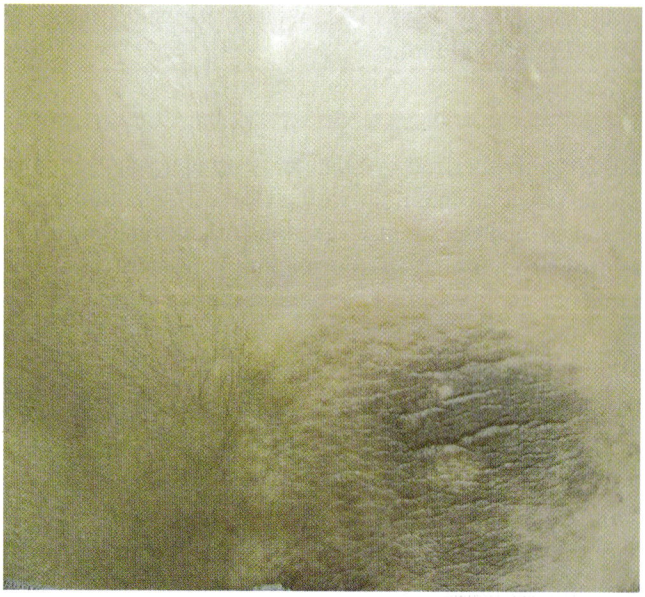

Fig. 14.6: Shagreen patch on the back

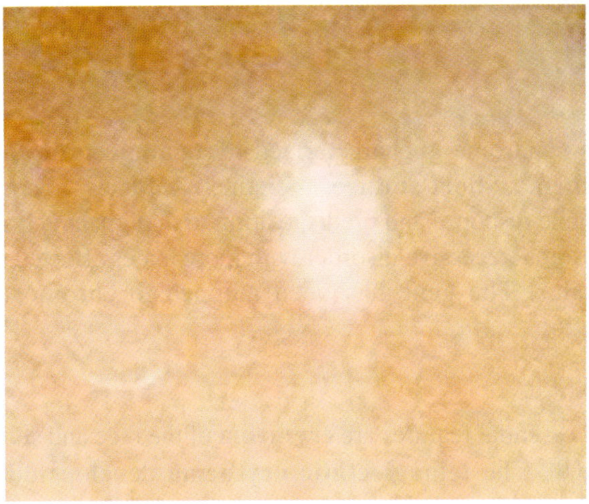

Fig. 14.7: Ash leaf macule on the back

Treatment

Cosmetically disfiguring angiofibromas can be improved with pulsed dye vascular laser (585 nm). The more nodular lesion can be treated with the carbon dioxide laser. Genetic counselling is important and all patients should be informed of the possibility of 50% of their offspring inheriting the disease. Prenatal diagnosis can be performed in 65% cases who represent sporadic new mutations.

GARDNER'S SYNDROME

Introduction

It is a multiple tumours syndrome comprising multiple epidermoid cysts, fibrous tissue tumours, osteomas and polyposis of the colon. It is an autosomal dominant disorder with variable expressivity. The gene for this syndrome is located on chromosome 5 near the bands 5q21-22. It is now thought that Gardner's syndrome is caused by mutations in the APC (adenomatosus polyposis coli) gene.

Clinical Features

- **Epidermoid cysts:** May be numerous and are usually irregularly distributed on the face, scalp and extremities. They are present in almost all cases.
- **Fibromas:** Are less frequent. They are usually poorly localised tumors in incisional scars of the abdomen, but may occur at other sites.
- **Osteomas:** Develop mainly in the maxilla, mandible and sphenoid bones, but also in other bones of the skull and, less frequently, in the bones. They present in half of the cases.
- **Polyposis of colon or rectum:** Usually arise in the second decade and is present in about 50% by the age of 20 years. Malignant change may occur in upto 40% patients by the age of 40 years.
- **Lipomas** and **leiomyomas** may also occur in some patients.

Diagnosis

In patients with multiple epidermoid or sebaceous cysts a detailed history and clinical and radiological examination for osteomas and other dermal tumors is warranted. The cutaneous lesions are an important indicator of possible asymptomatic polyposis.

COWDEN'S SYNDROME

Introduction

This is a rare syndrome, also called multiple hamartoma syndrome, in which multiple hamartomatous lesions of ectodermal, endodermal and mesodermal origins are associated with a predisposition to malignant tumors, especially of the breast. Inheritance is autosomal dominant with variable expressivity.

Clinical Features

Mucosal and Cutaneous Papillomas and Fibromas: Multiple tumors may be present on the skin and on the labial and buccal mucosa, sometimes even extending to the larynx.

Massive hyperplasia of the breast tissue may occur. One third of the female patients may develop breast carcinomas.

Thyroid Adenomas and Goitre: Thyroid carcinoma has also been reported.

SYNDROMES ASSOCIATED WITH DNA INSTABILITY

XERODERMA PIGMENTOSUM (XP)

Introduction

It is a rare autosomal recessive disorder characterized by photosensitivity, pigmentary changes, premature skin aging, neoplasia and abnormal DNA repair.

The fibroblasts from these patients lack the capacity to repair UV radiation induced DNA damage due to a defect in the nucleotide excision repair of UV photoproducts.

Clinical Features (Fig. 14.8)

The child is born normal. The symptoms first appear between 6 months and 3 years in the majority of cases. Most

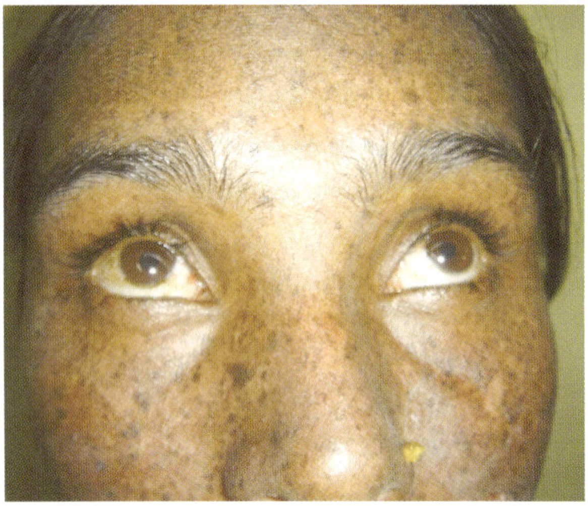

Fig. 14.8: Lentigines, freckles, seborrheic and actinic keratosis with xerosis on the face

cases beginning early in childhood have reached the tumor stage by the age of 20 years.

Freckling and increasing **dryness** on exposed areas are the earliest manifestations with shades of macules ranging from light to dark brown. They progressively increase in number with **telangiactasia** interspersed among them. Later, white atrophic macules also appear.

The first malignant tumors may develop as early as 3rd **or 4th year. Basal cell carcinoma** is common in these patients, though squamous cell carcinoma also occurs.

XP is often fatal by the age of 20 years with two thirds of patients dying by this age.

Most patients also develop ocular involvement in form of photophobia—Ectropion and destruction of the lower eyelid may occur with symblepharon formation. Pigmentation of conjunctiva, corneal opacities and epitheliomas of lids, conjunctiva or cornea may occur.

Treatment

The most important part of treatment is strict avoidance of sunlight. Clothing, hats and sunscreen should be advised to patients.

Early excision of all tumors is essential. Topical 5-fluorouracil may be useful for early or premalignant lesions. Sometimes plastic surgery and grafting may be required of large areas. Oral retinoids can be tried as prophylactic therapy to reduce the occurrence of skin cancers.

Ocular complications may be treated with artificial tears, soft contact lenses or even corneal transplant.

Recently a microbial enzyme **T4 endonuclease V** applied regularly as a topical liposome lotion has been tried. This enzyme is able to bypass the defect in XP cells. It has been seen to reduce the onset of both basal cell carcinomas and actinic keratoses.

BLOOM'S SYNDROME

Introduction

This syndrome is characterized by **telangiectatic facial erythema, short stature,** a distinctive **facies,** abnormal immune response and predisposition to malignancy. It is an autosomal recessive disorder with more males affected than females. The gene has been mapped to chromosome 15q 26.

Clinical Features

The essential features are **erythema** of the face and stunted growth. The **telangiectatic erythema** develops during infancy as macules or plaques, most numerous on the 'butterfly' area of the nose and cheeks. Photosensitivity is usual and may provoke even bullae on the lips.

The facies is characteristic with a narrow, slender, delicate facies with a prominent nose. The build is slender and the skull dolichocephalic.

Other associated features include café-au-lait macules, abnormalities of digits, congenital heart disease, high pitched voice, high arched palate and an annular pancreas. Testicular atrophy is common.

The mortality from neoplastic disease, especially acute leukemia, is significantly increased. Other reported malignancies include B-cell lymphoma and Wilm's tumor.

COCKAYNE'S SYNDROME

Introduction

It is an autosomal recessive syndrome characterized by short **stature, mental deficiency, photosensitivity, disproportionately large** hands, feet and ears, ocular defects and extensive demyelination. Unlike XP, the global nucleotide excision repair (NER) process occurs normally but the cells are defective in an important subpathway of NER. Thus, the skin fibroblasts are abnormally sensitive to UV irradiation.

Clinical Features

The child is usually normal in appearance in the first year, when facial erythema starts developing in the 'butterfly' area of the face after exposure to sunlight. Repeated exacerbations eventually produce a mottled reticulate pigmentation and atrophic scars giving the patient a prematurely senile appearance. The disproportionately large hands and feet are often blue and cold. The association of these features with large protruding ears has been compared to **'Mickey Mouse facies'.**

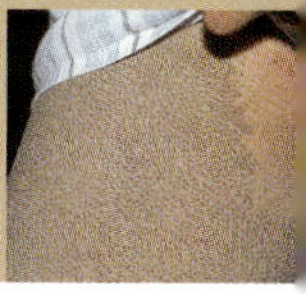

Physical and mental development are greatly retarded. Progressive loss of vision and hearing is usual.

HYPOMELANOSIS OF ITO

Streaks and whorls of hypopigmentation appearing within the first year of life are characteristic. Chromosomal **mosaicism** and translocations may occur. Because a small percentage of patients with incontinentia pigmenti (IP) may later develop hypopigmented linear and whorled lesions, the diagnosis of IP should only be made in the absence of preceding inflammation or pigmented macules (Fig. 14.9).

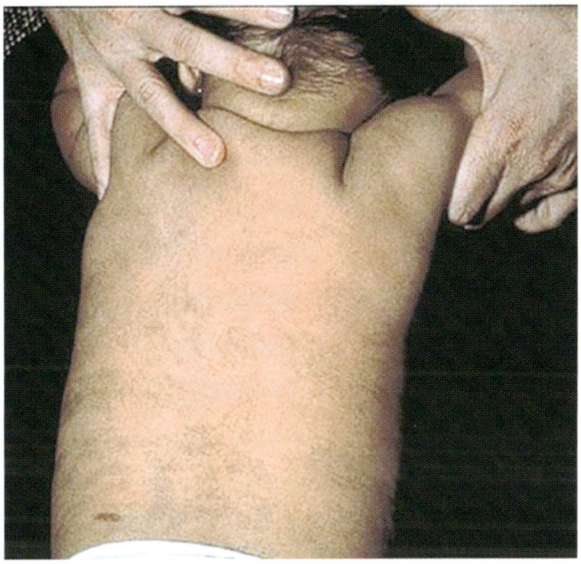

Fig. 14.9: Whorled hypomelanotic macules on the trunk

FOCAL DERMAL HYPOPLASIA

Introduction (Fig. 14.10)

Focal dermal hypoplasia (FDH), also known as Goltz syndrome, results in various defects of the dermis. Most patients are female (approximately 88%), supporting the hypothesis of X-linked dominant inheritance which is usually (but not always) lethal in males.

Clinical

Congenital linear streaks of telangiectasia and atrophy; soft, reddish-yellow nodules (fat herniations); and raspberry papillomas of the genitalia or elsewhere are characteristic of FDH. Linear hypo and hyperpigmented streaks occur, following Blaschko's lines. Skeletal abnormalities such as syndactyly, polydactyly, and absence of digits occur. Vertical stripes on the metaphyses of long bones (osteopathia striata) are characteristic.

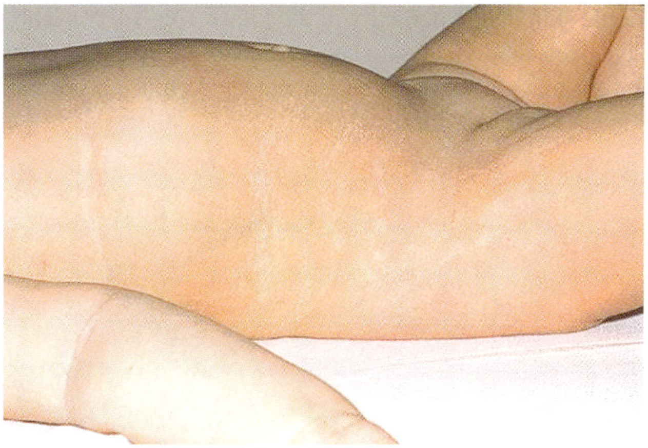

Fig. 14.10: Papular outgrowths in a whorled pattern

PEUTZ-JEGHERS SYNDROME

Peutz-Jeghers syndrome is an autosomal dominantly inherited condition which combines **cutaneous lentigines and intestinal polyps**. The gastrointestinal polyps develop from the gastroesophageal junction to the anus, with the small bowel, especially **the jejunum**, most commonly affected. Pigmented macules develop in infancy or early childhood on the lips and buccal mucosa (Fig. 14.11). Pigmented macules of the palm, fingers and soles also occur.

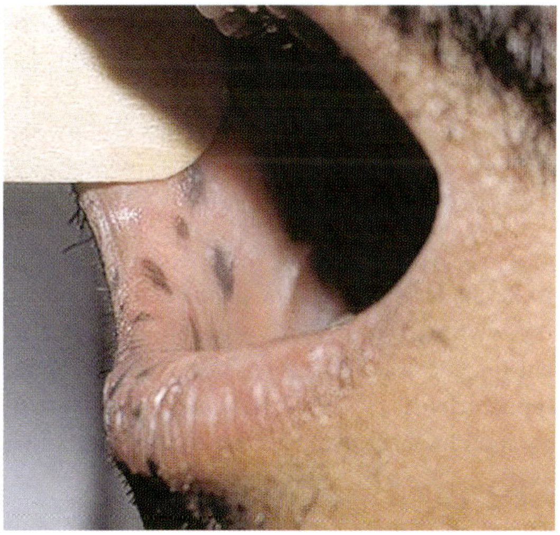

Fig. 14.11: Pigmented macules in the oral mucosa

Pachyonychia Congenita

Pachyonychia congenita (PC) is an autosomal dominant condition associated with very characteristic thickened nails.

Ehlers-Danlos Syndromes

The Ehlers-Danlos syndromes form a group of disorders with the main abnormality including hyperextensible and fragile skin and hyperlaxity of the joints (Fig. 14.12). They have been subdivided into approximately 10 different types and for many of these a specific defect in collagen production has been identified.

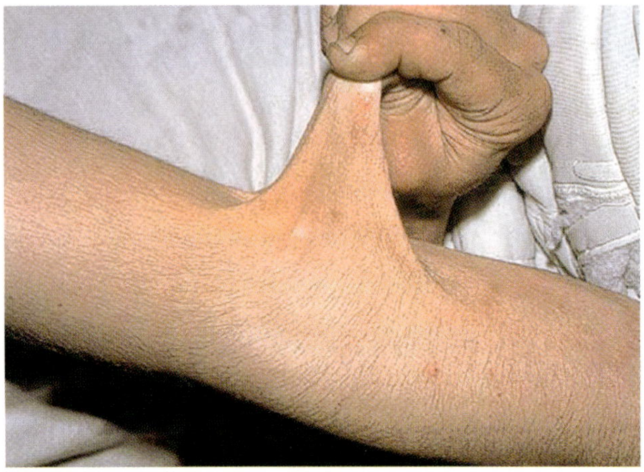

Fig. 14.12: Hyperextensible skin

PALMOPLANTAR KERATODERMA

The term palmoplantar keratoderma describes a group of conditions in which the keratin layer of the palms and soles is greatly thickened.

Adult Onset, Idiopathic

Palmoplantar keratoderma (PPK) without any family history may occur in adults, often with onset in the 40–60 age group. In women, the term **keratoderma climactericum** has been used.

Unna-Thost Syndrome

Uniform keratoderma covers the palms and soles in Unna-Thost syndrome. This relatively common autosomal dominant disease usually begins in the first 6 months of life. **Hyperhidrosis,** mental retardation, acro-osteolysis, clubbing and clinodactyly have been associated.

Epidermolytic Hyperkeratosis

This is diffuse palmoplantar keratoderma inherited in an autosomal dominant fashion, which shows epidermolytic hyperkeratosis on biopsy. It is also called epidermolytic palmoplantar keratoderma of vorner.

Greither Syndrome

PPK (autosomal dominant inheritance) that **extends onto the dorsa** of the hands and feet is characteristic. Onset is in infancy and the severity may increase in the adult years. The elbows and knees are commonly involved. It is clinically similar to mal de meleda but differs in its inheritance and tends to be milder.

Punctate Keratoderma

Discrete, keratotic papules, limited to the palms, soles, and volar aspects of the fingers occur in punctate keratoderma. These changes typically occur at puberty, but may have a later onset. Inheritance is autosomal dominant or sporadic.

Keratosis Palmaris Striata

Linear hyperkeratosis occurring in the first or second decade is characteristic.

Mal de Meleda Syndrome

(Autosomal Recessive)

Diffuse distribution **(transgradiens) with malodor and hyperhidrosis** occurs in mal de meleda syndrome.

Olmsted Syndrome

Periorificial red, scaly plaques, a mutilating, congenital palmoplantar keratoderma, nail dystrophy and scattered keratotic papules.

Papillon-Lefèvre Syndrome

In a child, palmoplantar keratoderma in a glove-and-stocking distribution (**transgradiens**), as in mal de meleda, associated with **periodontopathy** and loss of teeth, is characteristic.

Richner-Hanhart Syndrome

Tender, hyperkeratotic papules and plaques on the palms and soles are characteristic of Richner-Hanhart syndrome, also known as tyrosinemia type II. The pain may be significant enough to necessitate crawling or walking with crutches. Bilateral keratitis occurs and may lead to corneal ulceration or opacities (onset of ocular symptoms: 2 weeks to 8 years).

Acquired Palmoplantar Keratoderma: Syphilis, Psoriasis, LP, PRP, Reiters, Darier's, Scabies, LE.

DARIER'S DISEASE

Important Points: Non-immune, Involves seborrheic areas, dyskeratosis (corps ronds and grains) on histopathology.

Introduction

Darier's disease, also known as keratosis follicularis, is a disorder of keratinization. The causative gene has been localized to chromosome 12 (SERCA channels ATP2A2).

Clinical (Fig. 14.13)

Patients present with scaly, waxy, greasy papules in the seborrheic areas. It very commonly involves the chest but may occur anywhere. A **cobblestone-like** pattern on the palate and **longitudinal red/white** streaks of the nails occur. It often worsens in the summer and may be aggravated by heat or sunlight. Onset is usually in adolescence with an autosomal dominant inheritance pattern.

Treatment

Excesses of sun exposure, heat and humidity should be avoided. Tretinoin 0.1% cream under occlusion or a potent topical steroid may be tried. **Oral retinoids** (both isotretinoin and acitretin) are usually highly effective.

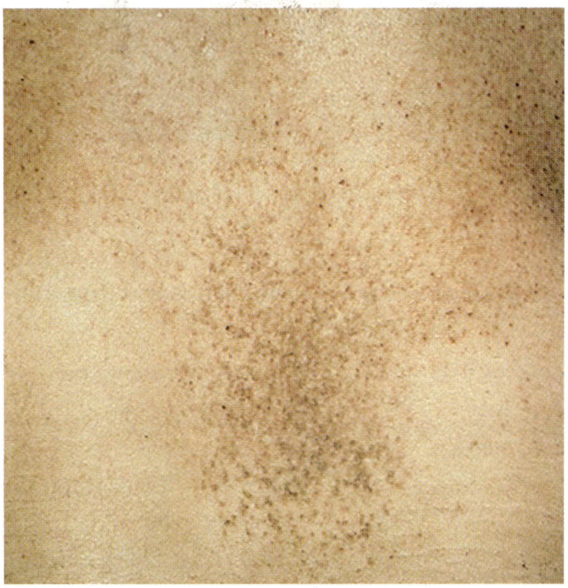

Fig. 14.13: Keratotic papules on chest (Darier's disease)

HAILEY-HAILEY DISEASE

Important Points: Non-immune, flexural involvement, increases in humidity, Histopathology shows **Dilapidated brick wall** appearance.

Introduction

Patients with Hailey-Hailey disease, also known as benign familial pemphigus, have a skin defect that leads to erosions and crusting in the flexural areas. Inheritance is autosomal dominant, ATP2C1 gene on chromosome 3 with a positive family history in 70% of the patients.

Clinical (Fig. 14.14)

In Hailey-Hailey disease 'wet tissue-paper' erosions or erythematous plaques are found symmetrically in the axillae and groin, where the skin surfaces oppose each other. On the neck and back, red, scaly annular lesions or plaques, with a scaly or vesicular border, occur. Onset is in adolescence and young adulthood. Exacerbations may occur in the summer and may occur with the menses in women. Secondary infection may occur from bacteria, *candida*, or herpes.

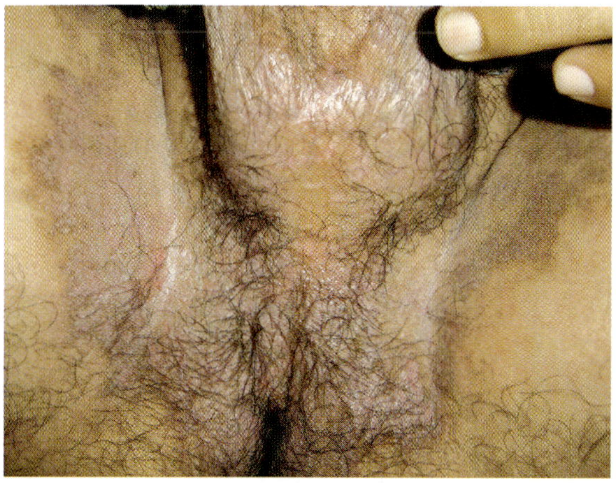

Fig. 14.14: Maceration, erosions, crusts in groin (Hailey-Hailey disease)

Treatment

Heat, sweat and friction should be avoided. Weight loss is beneficial in the obese. Oral antibiotics (e.g. erythromycin, tetracycline, or dicloxacillin) combined with topical, medium-potency steroids are often effective. Class I topical steroids may occasionally be needed. Long-term remission has been obtained with dermabrasion or CO_2 laser vaporization. In older women with menstrual flaring of the disease, hysterectomy with bilateral oophorectomy has been done.

ICHTHYOSES

The ichthyoses represent a group of disorders in which the horny layer of the skin does not desquamate normally. Hyperkeratotic scaly skin results.

- Ichthyosis vulgaris.
- X-linked ichthyosis.
- Epidermolytic hyperkeratosis.
- Lamellar ichthyosis.
- Non-bullous CIE.
- Collodion baby/harlequin fetus.

Collodion Baby

A newborn infant covered with *oiled parchment-like shiny* skin is characteristic. The condition is not a single disease but a clinical finding. It may resolve spontaneously or evolve into various diseases, including lamellar ichthyosis and congenital ichthyosiform erythroderma. Morbidity and mortality may occur secondary to impaired barrier function.

Complications include infection, dehydration, and hypernatremia. Heat regulation may also be impaired (both hyper- and hypothermia).

Intensive care, close temperature regulation, incubator, fluid status, and an emollient three times a day are important. The newborn may need intravenous fluids due to significant fluid loss.

Non-bullous Congenital Ichthyosiform Erythroderma

- Mode of inheritance — Autosomal **recessive**
- Incidence — 1: 300,000
- Fine white scales — Over the legs
Entire body with erythroderma
Large plate like scale
- Biopsy — Lipid droplets and abnormal **lamellar bodies**

The skin is diffusely erythematous with fine scaling in this variant of autosomal recessive ichthyosis. Elevated ***n*-alkanes** in the scales are thought to be a marker of this disease, although evidence suggests that the *n*-alkanes are of exogenous origin.

Treatment

Acitretin has been used and calcipotriene has shown a beneficial effect.

Ichthyosis Vulgaris (Fig. 14.15)

- Age of onset : 3 to 12 months
- Sex : M=F
- Mode of inheritance : Autosomal **dominant**
- Pathogenesis : **Absence of filaggrin**
- Incidence : 1: 250 to 1: 2000
- Atopy : 50%

Severe xerosis and fine, white scaling, with onset in the first few months of life, are characteristic. In comparison to the other ichthyoses, the skin changes of ichthyosis vulgaris are mild. The disease is worse in the winter, worse on the legs, and may worsen with age. Inheritance is autosomal dominant with variable expression within the family. An important feature histologically is an absence of the granular layer.

Treatment

Use of emollients and keratolytics is usually sufficient treatment. Ammonium lactate (12% lotion) or urea are often effective.

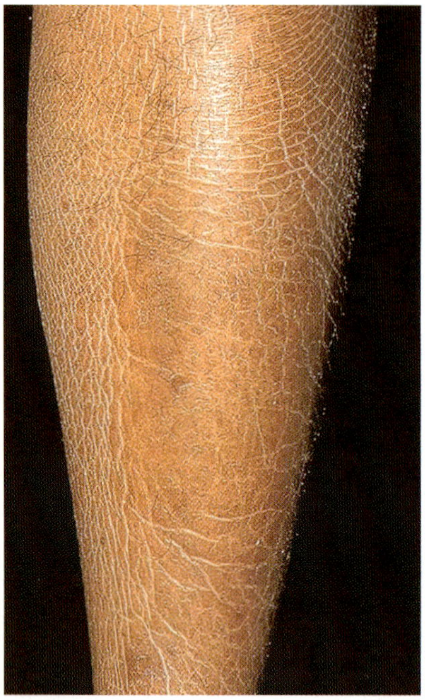

Fig. 14.15: Fish like scales on the leg (Ichthyosis vulgaris)

Lamellar Ichthyosis (Fig. 14.16)

- Age of onset : Birth (or) shortly thereafter
- Sex : M=F
- Mode of inheritance : Autosomal **recessive**
- Gene locus : 14q11
- Incidence : <1:3000
- Genetic defect : Mutations—**Transglutaminase 1 enzyme** gene.

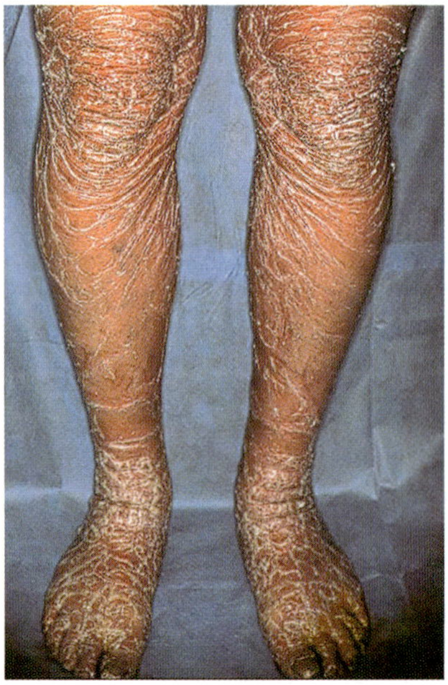

Fig. 14.16: Large scales on lower limb (Lamellar ichthyosis)

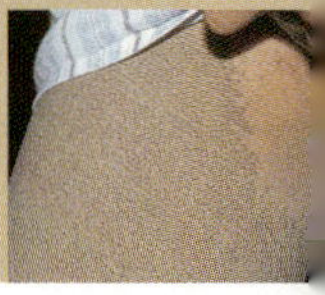

Absent transglutaminase expression has been found in several patients. Transglutaminase is an enzyme that catalyzes the cross-linking of precursor proteins such as involucrin. Lamellar ichthyosis often presents as a collodion baby at birth. Ectropion and palmoplantar keratoderma are frequently present.

Treatment

Retinoids are dramatically helpful in treating this disorder (e.g. acitretin, 35 mg/day) but side-effects limit their long-term use.

X-linked Recessive Ichthyosis (Fig. 14.17)

- Age of onset : Birth or infancy
- Sex : Male
- Mode of inheritance : X-linked recessive
- Gene locus : Xp22-32
- Genetic defect : **Steroid sulfatase** deficiency
- Incidence : 1:2000 to 1: 6000

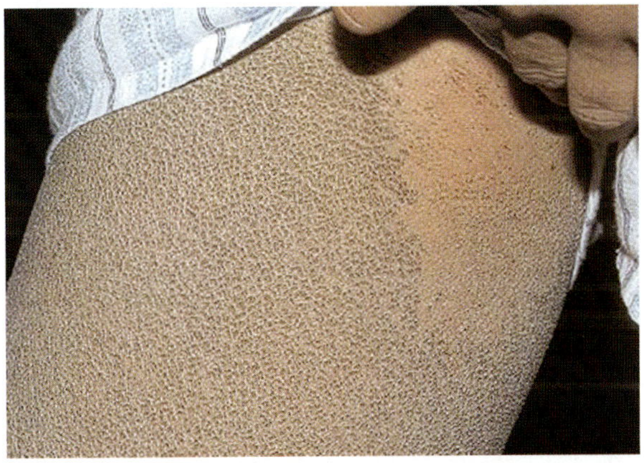

Fig. 14.17: Dark scales on back

The scales are *larger, darker* and *thicker* in RXLI. *Corneal opacities* may be found. Cryptorchidism and testicular cancer unassociated with cryptorchidism may occur. RXLI often spares the flexures. Males are affected although carrier females may exhibit mild features as well as failure to go into labor spontaneously.

Treatment

Emollients and keratolytics are used, including ammonium lactate (12% lotion). Oral retinoids (e.g. acitretin) have been used.

EPIDERMOLYTIC-HYPERKERATOSIS (BULLOUS ICHTHYOSIFORM ERYTHRODERMA) (Fig. 14.18)

- Age of onset : Birth (or) shortly thereafter
- Sex : M=F
- Mode of inheritance : Autosomal **Dominant** (Sporadic)
- Incidence : Very rare
- Genetic defect : Mutations of gene encoding **K1/K10**

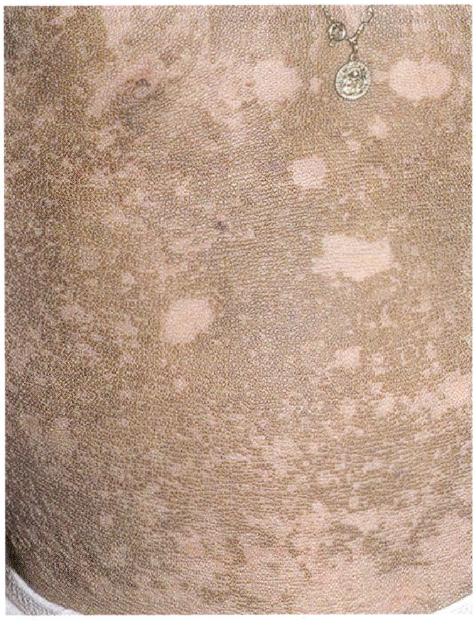

Fig. 14.18: Focal areas of skin loss with diffuse scales (Epidermolytic hyperkeratosis)

REFERENCES

- Gomez MR, Sampson JR, Whittemore VH: Tuberous Sclerosis Complex (3rd edition), Oxford University Press, 1999.
- Roach ES, Di Mario FJ, Kandt RS, Northrup H: Tuberous Sclerosis Consensus Conference: Recommendations for Diagnostic Evaluation, J Child Neurology 14 (1999) 401-407.
- Cohen BA: Pediatric Dermatology, 2nd edn., London: Mosby, 1999.
- Harper J: Inherited Skin Disorders, The Genodermatoses, Oxford: Butterworth Heinemann, 1996.
- Levy ML (ed): Pediatric dermatology, Dermatol Clin 1998; 16: 649-861.
- Moss C, Savin J: Dermatology and the New Genetics, Oxford: Blackwell Science, 1995.
- Siegfried EC, Frasier LD, Part III: Pediatric Skin Disease, In Paller (ed), Advances in Dermatology, Mosby, 1997: 12; 139-21.

CHAPTER **15**

PIGMENTARY DISORDERS

Tyrosine, formed in the liver by hydroxylation of the essential amino acid phenylalanine under the influences of phenylalanine hydroxylase, is the substrate for the reactions that occur in melanocytes.

These are the only cells in the epidermis to contain tyrosinase (dopa oxidase), the rate-limiting enzyme in melano genesis.This copper-dependent enzyme converts tyrosine to melanin. Dopa is formed by the oxidation of tyrosine, and further enzymic action leads to the formation of dopaquinone (Fig. 15.1).

Eumelanins, **brown** or **black** pigments, are then formed by polymerization.

Phaeomelanins and trichochromes, the pigments in **red** hair, are synthesized in a similar way, except that cysteine reacts with dopaquinone and is incorporated into the subsequent polymers (Fig. 15.1).

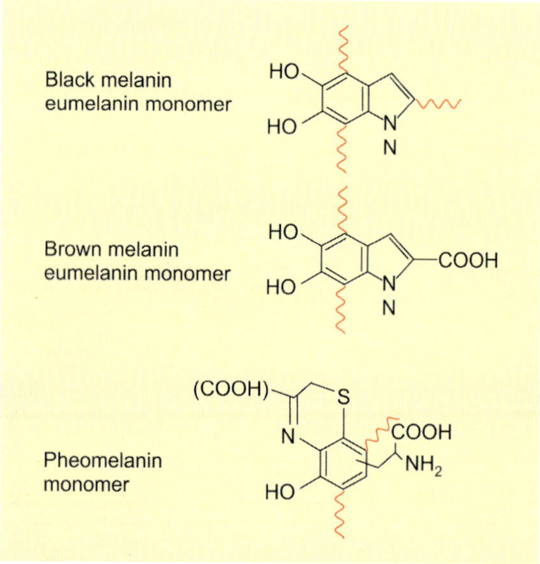

Fig. 15.1

Table15.1: Common hypopigmented birthmarks		
Clinical Condition	*Features*	*Association*
Ash leaf macule	Lance ovate on the trunk > 1 is indicative of tuberous sclerosis	Present at birth in 70-90 % of tuberous sclerosis
Mosaic hypopigmentation Nevus depigmentosus, hypomelanosis of Ito	Hypopigmented macules in a dermatomal fashion or along the Blaschko lines	Association, when extensive with mental retardation, seizures and ocular abnormalities
Nevus anemicus	Sharp, patch on the trunk surrouneded by vasodilatation, blanching on diascopy	
Piebaldism	Poorly defined, depigmented macules on the trunk, extremities inside which there are macules of pigmented skin, spares the hand feet, white forelock of hair is characteristic	**Woolf Syndrome:** Neurologic deficitswith piebaldism **Waardenburg's Syndrome:** Heterochromia of irides, hearing defect

Melanin is made within melanosomes. Negroids are not black because they have more melanocytes than caucasoids, but because their melanocytes produce more and larger melanosomes, which are broken down less rapidly in the melanosome complexes and are more diffusely distributed.

MELANOCYTOPENIC DISORDERS

- Failure of migration of melanoblasts to the skin (Piebaldism, Waardenburg's syndrome (WS).
- Failure of differentiation and/or survival of melanoblasts into melanocytes (Piebaldism, WS).
- Failure of mitotic division of melanocytes (vitiligo).

Melanopenic Disorders

- Defect of synthesis of ***functional tyrosinase* (albinism)** (Fig 15.2).
- Failure of biogenesis of melanosomal matrix.
- Defect in tyrosinase transport.
- Failure of normal melanosome formation [**tuberous sclerosis, Chédiak-Higashi syndrome** (CHS)].
- Failure of ***melanization of melanosomes* (albinism, hypomelanosis of Ito, idiopathic guttate hypomelanosis, tinea versicolor).**
- Defective ***transport or transfer of melanosomes*** [CHS, **pityriasis alba, postinflammatory hypomelanosis,** Griscelli's syndrome (GS)].

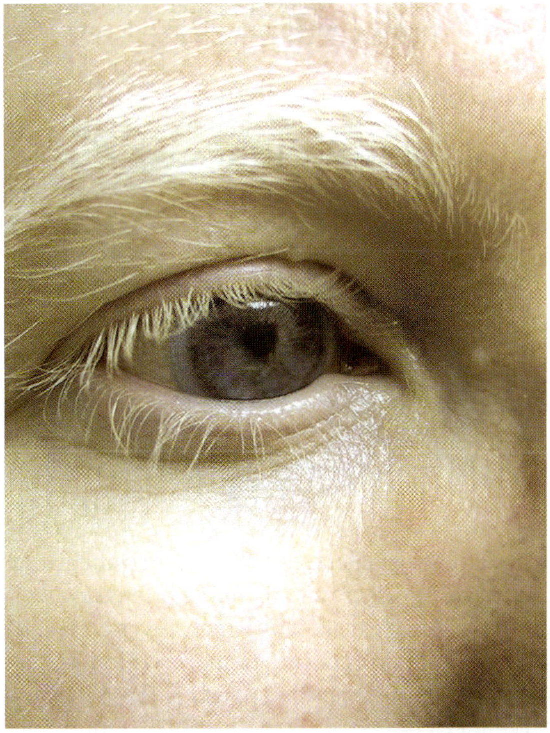

Fig. 15.2: An albino with complete absence of pigment in the skin, iris and eyebrow

- Alteration in ***degradation of melanosomes*** (CHS, **nevus depigmentosus, pityriasis alba, postinflammatory hypomelanosis,** tinea versicolor).

Miscellaneous Causes Unrelated to Melanin

Nevus anemicus, Bier's spots, Woronoff ring.

MELANOCYTOPENIC DISORDERS

Piebaldism

These patients often have a **white forelock** (Fig. 15.3) of hair and patches of depigmentation lying symmetrically on the limbs, trunk and central part of the face, especially the chin. The condition is present at birth and is inherited as an autosomal dominant trait. A genetic abnormality in mice (dominant white spotting) provided the clue that allowed the human piebaldism gene to be mapped to chromosome 4q12, where the KIT protooncogene lies.

Melanocytes are absent from the hypopigmented areas. The depigmentation, often mistaken for vitiligo, may improve with age. There is no effective treatment.

Waardenburg's Syndrome

It includes *piebaldism* (with a white forelock in 20% of cases), *hypertelorism*, a prominent *inner third* of the eyebrows, irides of different colour and *deafness.*

White Hair

Melanocytes in hair bulbs become less active with age and white hair (canities) is a universal sign of aging.

Early greying of the hair is seen in the rare premature aging syndromes, such as Werner's syndrome, and in autoimmune conditions such as pernicious anaemia, thyroid disorders and Addison's disease.

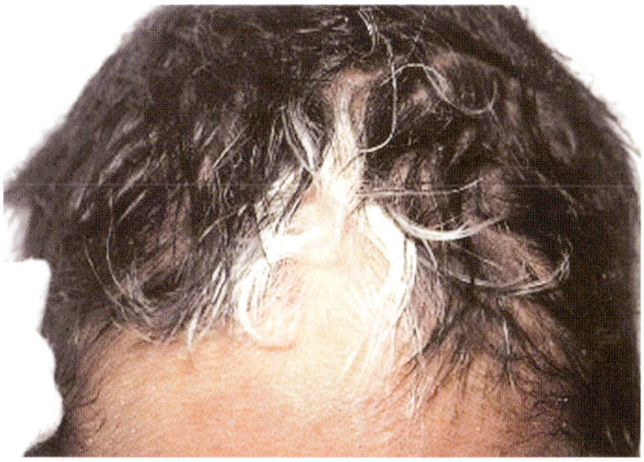

Fig. 15.3: A white forelock of hair

Vitiligo

Introduction

Vitiligo is an acquired, and very rarely congenital, form of hypopigmentation or depigmentation in which pigment production is reduced or halted. This may be due to autoimmune destruction of melanocytes, peroxidative damage to melanocytes or metabolic derangements within the melanocyte which interfere with melanin synthesis. These various pathogenic mechanisms may all result in the same outcome, *i.e.*, cellular death of the melanocyte, whether by apoptosis or oncosis-type programmed cell death pathways.

Clinical Features

Clinically, lesions appear as macules or patches of hypopigmentation and depigmentation symmetrically over the bony prominences, in the intertriginous location and periorificially. In addition, sites like the oral mucosa are often involved silently (15.4).

Leukotrichia may be notable in these patients and may include overly vitiliginous patches or represent inherent weakness of pigment production in the hairs.

Vitiligo presents in a variety of ways.

Generalized

- Vulgaris
- Universalis
- Acrofacial

Generalized and Acrofacial type present with hypopigmented or depigmented patches symmetrically located periorificially and often involving the joints and bony prominences.

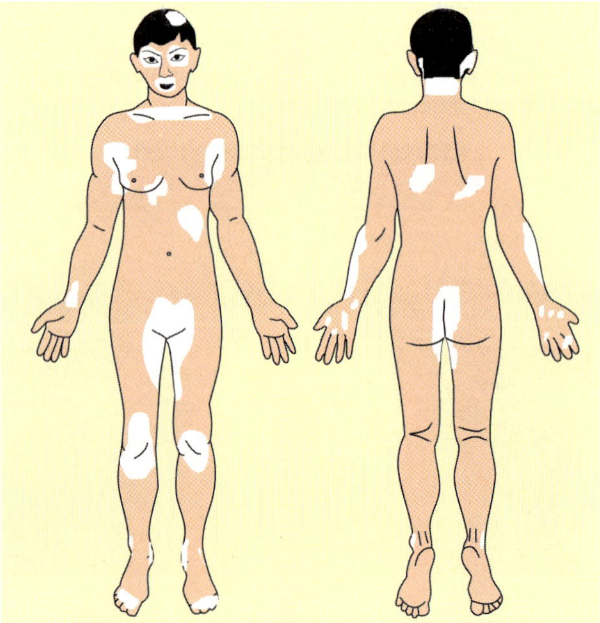

Fig. 15.4: Sites of involvement of vitiligo

Localized Vitiligo

- Focal
- Segmental
- Mucosal

Localized Vitiligo, which usually has a good clinical prognosis, of which **Segmental Vitiligo** is a subtype that follows a broad pattern of Blaschko's lines. In all, 87% of segmental cases will occur before the age of 30 years. Segmental vitiligo of the body is the only type of localized disease that was deemed difficult to repigment historically; however, facial segmental disease in children has a 94% response rate to topical tacrolimus.

Trichrome Vitiligo is an unusual variant in which there are 3 zones fully depigmented, hypopigmented and normal colour, representing absent melanocyte activity, reduced melanocyte activity and normal melanocyte activity, respectively. This type responds well to medical therapy.

Incidence and Prevalence

Most subtypes of vitiligo are inherited through a multifactorial genetic modality; however, universal vitiligo appears to have an environmental trigger. Though this trigger has not been elucidated, autoimmune diatheses and exposure to environmental toxins, such as dyes, are suspected in universal disease. Because hair dyes and strong irritants can initiate or worsen disease, patients are cautioned to proceed with gentle hair processing where possible.

Toluenediamine sulfate and paraphenylenediamine have both been reported to induce leukoderma (Contact leukoderma).

A *family history of autoimmune diseases,* especially thyroiditis, are often found in children with vitiligo.

Vitiligo patients should also be evaluated for pernicious anemia and diabetes mellitus through a blood count and fasting glucose. Other systemic illnesses can be tested for on a case-by-case basis and include polycystic ovaries, Addison's disease, rheumatoid arthritis and the presence of a circulating antinuclear antibody, which can sensitize to ultraviolet therapy or may be induced by psoralens and ultraviolet A (PUVA).

Treatment (Table 15.2)

Nondermatological Interventions

Nondermatological interventions such as cosmetics are very helpful in hiding disease and should be offered to all patients in the form of thick make-ups which cover completely for special occasions and self-tanners which reduce the cosmetic deficit and can be applied a few times a week. Self-tanners contain *dihyrdoacetone*, which causes a chemical reaction in the stratum corneum to impart a tanned appearance.

SECTION - 6

Table 15.2: Common therapies available for vitiligo vulgaris

Calcineurin inhibitors (*e.g.*, tacrolimus) with or without ultraviolet light*
Calcipotriene with or without topical corticosteroids*
Excimer laser (308 nm)*
Intralesional corticosteroids
Khellin with or without ultraviolet light
Melagnina
Narrowband UVB with or without topical therapy*
Pseudocatalase
Psoralens and UVA (with or without calcipotriene)*
Pulsed oral corticosteroids
Topical corticosteroids*
Vitamins*

* The most effective therapies.

Dermatological Treatment

Therapies are dually based, *i.e.*, often an antiinflammatory or antioxidant therapy are paired with a therapy intended to promote pigmentation.

Antiinflammatory therapies include corticosteroids and immunomodulators.

Antioxidants include calcipotriene, pseudocatalase and vitamins.

Repigmentation therapy include ultraviolet light and calcipotriene.

While PUVA was the standard of repigmentation for many years, it has been replaced in safety and efficacy with the kinder and gentler narrowband ultraviolet B (NB-UVB), which is described below. In addition, the clinical concern of disease stabilization is an important consideration. Progressive disease can be stabilized with NB-UVB light or oral corticosteroids, the latter of which may have considerable side effects. As no therapy is effective universally, cycling of therapies is required to achieve maximum repigmentation.

Topical Corticosteroids

Topical corticosteroids have been the mainstay of therapy for vitiligo for decades. Repigmentation rates vary from study to study. The first two characteristics (head and neck disease and dark skin type) appear to be associated with superior response to therapy. Preparations of high potency topical corticosteroids may show results as quickly as 2 months however, a 3-4 months trial is more consistent with repigmentation patterns.

Topical Calcineurin Inhibitors

Topical corticosteroid side effects in vitiligo are generally temporary, and these products tend to be very well tolerated even in small children. Usage on large body surface area should be weighed against the possible risk of systemic absorption.

Tacrolimus is far safer for eyelids, intertriginous and genital vitiligo, as tacrolimus will not induce atrophy of the treated skin, nor glaucoma. Furthermore, clinical results can be seen in as rapidly as 2 months but are enhanced by extending application time to at least 3 months.

Combination Therapy

When topical corticosteroids have been used with limited or no success, combination of the corticosteroids with topical calcipotriene can be used effectively.

Phototherapy

NB-UVB, a 311nm ultraviolet light source, recently has come into the spotlight for phototherapy Similar to PUVA, lesions on the face and trunk responded better than the extremities. Overall NB-UVB has demonstrated a better safety profile.

Excimer laser is a xenon chloride laser that emits a 308 nm coherent light that causes repigmentation of vitiliginous lesions, similarly to NB-UVB through emission of ultraviolet light.

Vitamins

The use of antioxidant vitamins in high doses is not recommended universally. However, for patients on NB-UVB, with pernicious anemia, teenagers and those with rapidly expanding disease, antioxidant vitamin supplementation with folic acid and vitamin B_{12} may be warranted.

One will note that no therapy mentioned has universal success at repigmenting patients. This is an unfortunate reality of therapy for vitiligo.

A summary of the international guideline on management is given below: (Fig. 15.5)

MELANOPENIC DISORDERS

Oculocutaneous Albinism

In this condition, little or no melanin is made either in the skin and eyes (oculocutaneous albinism) or in the eyes alone.

Types

Two main types: Tyrosinase-negative and tyrosinase-positive. The tyrosinase gene lies on chromosome 11q14-q21.

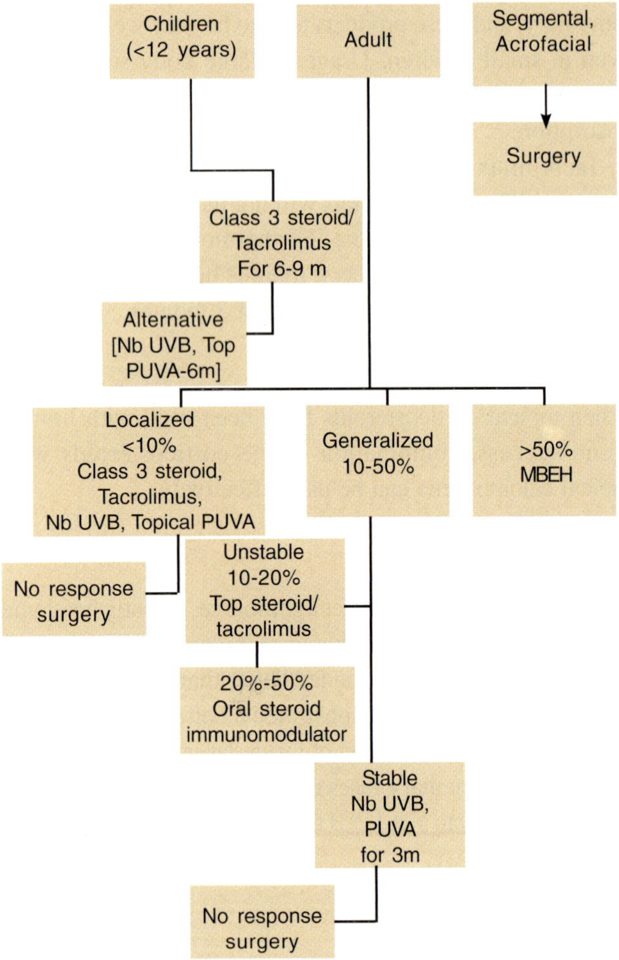

Fig. 15.5: International guidelines on management of vitiligo
Nb UVB=Narrow Band UVB (311nm)
PUVA= Psoralen+UVA
MBEH=Monobenzyl ether of hydroquinone

Clinical Features

The whole skin is white and pigment is also lacking in the hair, iris and retina (Fig 15.2). Albinos have poor sight, photophobia and a rotatory nystagmus.

As they grow older, tyrosinase-positive albinos gain a little pigment in their skin, iris and hair. Negroid skin becomes yellow-brown and the hair becomes yellow. Albinos may also develop freckles. Sunburn is common on unprotected skin. As melanocytes are present, albinos have non-pigmented melanocytic naevi and may develop amelanotic malignant melanomas.

Other related disorders are given in Table 15.3.

Table: 15.3: Syndromes associated with generalized hypopigmentation at birth

Syndrome	*Associated findings*
Angleman Syndrome	Abnormal facies, developmental delay, mental retardation, neurologic abnormalities, ocular abnormalities
Albinism	Strabismus, decreased visual acuity
Cross Syndrome	Mental retardation, spastic diplegia, ocular abnormalities
Chediak-Higashi Syndrome	Silver-gray hair, recurrent infection, seizures, pancytopenia, lymphoreticular malignancies
Griscelli Syndrome	Silver-gray hair, T-and B-cell immunodeficiency, recurrent pyogenic infections, hepatosplenomegaly, neutropenia, thrombocytopenia
Hermansky-Pudlak Syndrome	Bleeding diathesis, visual abnormalities, pulmonary fibrosis, inflammatory bowel disease
Prader-Willi[a] Syndrome	Neonatal hypotonia, hyperphagia, developmental delay, mental retardation, ocular abnormalities
Ziprkowski-Margolis Syndrome	Heterochromic irides, congenital nerve deafness, mutism

a. Skin pigment dilution present, not true depigmentation.

HYPOMELANOSIS AND CUTANEOUS MOSAICISM

Hypomelanosis of Ito

This disorder is also termed incontinentia pigmenti achromians or pigmentary mosaicism of the Ito type.

It is characterized by randomly distributed hypomelanotic macules with a bizarre whorled configuration. They consist of bilateral or unilateral streaks corresponding to the lines of Blaschko (Fig. 15.6).

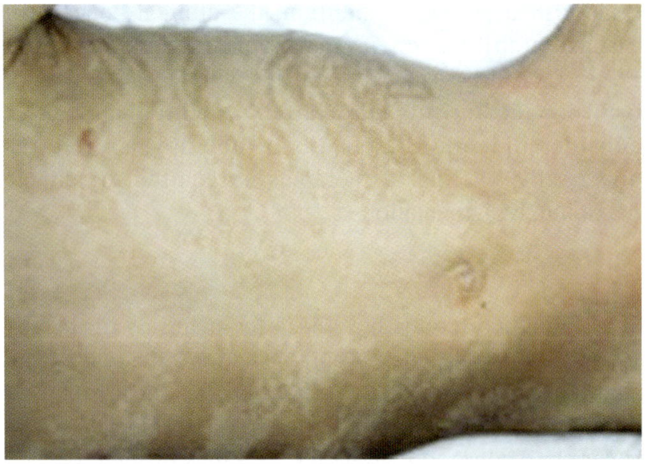

Fig. 15.6: Bilateral streaks corresponding to the lines of Blaschko

Other types of pigmentary patterns such as a checker-board arrangement likewise have been described. HI is often associated with extracutaneous anomalies (75 percent). They include *CNS abnormalities* (seizures, mental or motor retardation, microcephaly, hypotony, hyperkinesias, ataxia, and deafness), *ophthalmologic abnormalities* (ptosis, nonclosure of the upper lid, symblepharon, dacryostenosis, strabismus, nystagmus, corneal opacification, cataracts, myopia, amblyopia, microphthalmia, iridal heterochromia, scleral melanosis, patchy hypopigmented fundi, and retinal degeneration), *enamel* changes and other dental defects, and *skeletal* defects (short stature, pectus carinatum or excavatum, scoliosis, syndactyly, polydactyly, brachydactyly, clinodactyly, asymmetry of limbs, and facial asymmetry). HI is a cutaneous sign of many different forms of genomic mosaicism. Histologic and ultrastructural studies show rounded melanocytes with reduced or absent dendrites and slightly decreased epidermal melanin pigmentation.

Nevus Depigmentosus (ND)

ND occurs equally among males and females and can affect any ethnic group.

Three clinical forms of ND are described: *An isolated, circular or rectangular macule or, a dermatomal or quasi-dermatomal pattern or a systematized* (unilateral whorls or streaks) (Fig. 15.7) form.

The hypomelanotic lesion remains **stable** throughout life. ND typically does *not cross the midline*.

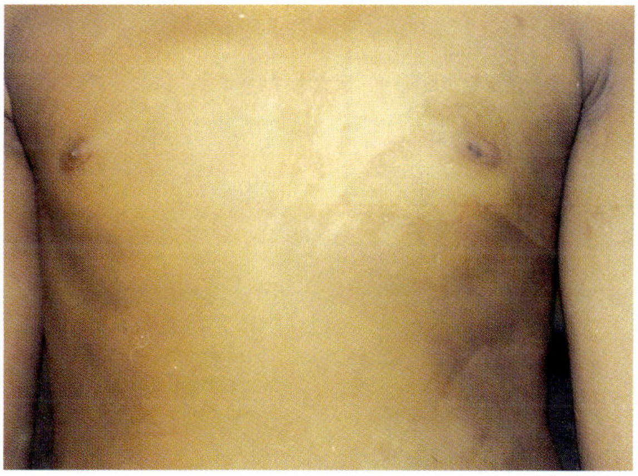

Fig. 15.7: Unilateral streaks of pigmentary loss

INCONTINENTIA PIGMENTI (IP)

IP is a syndrome characterized by skin lesions that are arranged in a linear pattern. This uncommon X-linked dominant disorder, generally lethal in males, has three stages: vesiculobullous, verrucous, and hyperpigmented. However, in about 13 percent there is a fourth stage, that of swirls of hypopigmentation, consisting of atrophic hypo or amelanotic bands of streaks that fail to tan with sun exposure. In addition, these lesions are hypohydrotic and hairless.

PITYRIASIS ALBA

Pityriasis alba is a common hypomelanosis that occurs in all races, although it is considered more common, perhaps just more obvious, in blacks.

Clinical Features

Pityriasis alba is generally a disorder of young children and affects males and females equally. The typical macule is pale pink or light brown with very indistinct margins. The subtle erythema fades over weeks to leave an off-white to tan-white macule with a powdery scale. Pityriasis alba is probably an eczematous dermatosis with hypomelanosis resulting from postinflammatory changes and ultraviolet screening effects of the hyperkeratotic and parakeratotic epidermis.

The condition is self-limited. Topical glucocorticoids are useful. PUVA has been found to be effective for extensive pityriasis alba.

POSTINFLAMMATORY HYPOPIGMENTATION

A variety of inflammatory conditions may disrupt the pigmentary system enough to leave a hypopigmented patch. The color usually returns over several months if the inciting condition has resolved.

Clinical

A hypopigmented (not depigmented) spot remains in the site of a prior inflammatory process.

Treatment

Once the precipitating disease has resolved, normalization of pigmentation should soon follow (e.g. in 1-2 months). It must be emphasized, however, that any residual activity of the precipitating disease (e.g. xerosis, eczema and psoriasis) should be sought and, if present, treated. Any dry skin should be treated with emollient cream once or twice daily. Lotions, with their high water content, are less effective. If any erythema suggesting persistent inflammation is present, a topical steroid should be prescribed. For young children with pityriasis alba of the face, hydrocortisone (1% cream) is effective.

PROGRESSIVE MACULAR HYPOMELANOSIS

Periodically, a patient will present with patchy hypopigmentation on the trunk that resembles pityriasis versicolor but that lacks erythema and scale, and is resistant to antifungal treatment. It has been proposed that the *P. acnes* secretes a factor that interferes with melanogenesis.

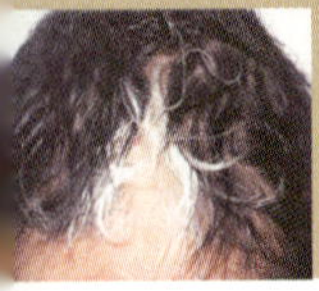

IDIOPATHIC GUTTATE HYPOMELANOSIS

Complete loss of pigment in tiny macules occurs in idiopathic guttate hypomelanosis. Multiple white macules, usually 1-4 mm in diameter, symmetrically distributed on the outer forearms or extensor legs, are characteristic. These lesions are benign and no treatment is necessary. Cryotherapy or intralesional triamcinolone has been used.

OTHER MISCELLANEOUS DISORDERS

Nevus Anemicus

This entity is a pharmacologic nevus; unlike melanocytic disorders, pressure over the lesion with a glass slide causes the lesion to become inapparent; nevus anemicus becomes invisible under the Wood's lamp but becomes more prominent after rubbing, which induces vasodilatation only in the adjacent uninvolved skin.

Bier Spots

Bier spots are small, light macules usually found on the arms and legs of young adults. The intervening skin may seem erythematous but blanches with pressure so that the light macules disappear. This is a benign physiologic vascular anomaly of no significance.

Woronoff's Ring

Woronoff's ring is a hypomelanotic ring surrounding psoriatic lesions under treatment secondary to vascular rather than melanin-related changes.

Pigmentary Demarcation Lines

Pigmentary demarcation lines most commonly occur in dark-skinned patients. The most common ones are those that appear as an abrupt transition between lighter and darker skin on the anterior portion of the upper arms. A similar change may occur on the posterior legs. In both, the darker skin is lateral and the lighter skin is medial.

Disorders of Hyperpigmentation

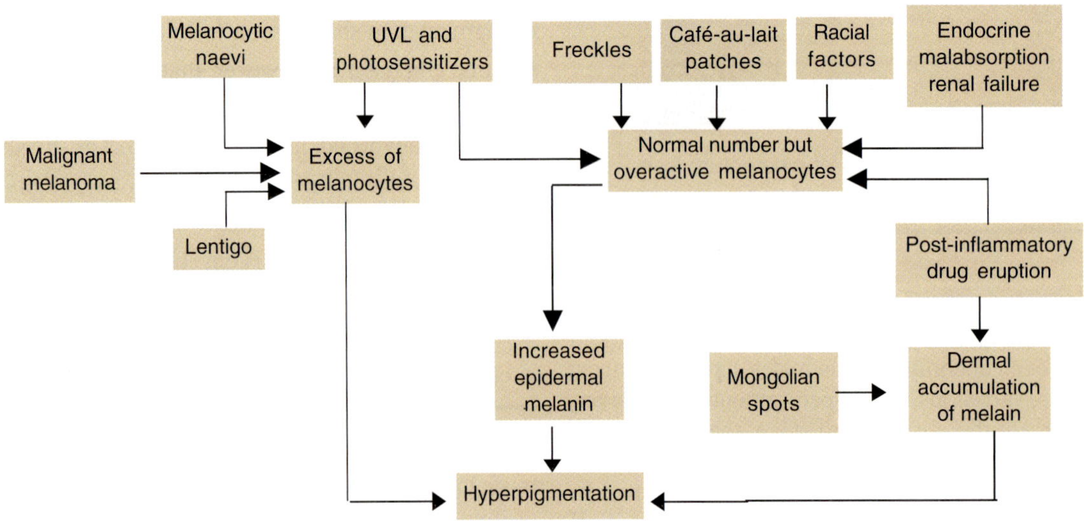

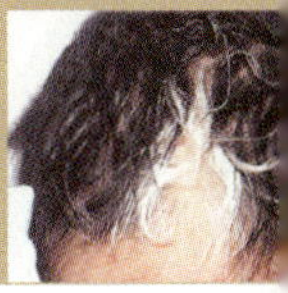

Disorders of hyperpigmentation can be classified in various ways one of which is by its description and by diagnosis Table 15.4.

Table: 15.4: Hyperpigmented birthmarks

Condition	*Clinical Feature*	*Examples*
Cafe-au-lait macule	Increased epidemal melanin, enlarge in proportion to body growth. Increase in surface hair	Neurofibromatosis (coast of california), Albright's (coast of Maine, respect midline), Watson's, Ring chromosome 2
Nevus spilus	Seen on the trunk with a overlying speckled appearance of lentigines with underlying light brown patch	
Nevus of Ito	Ito: Irregular patch on the supraclavicular area which is Blue brown in colour and may follow the line of Blaschko on trunk	Glaucoma and melanoma reported in nevus of Ota
Nevus of Ota	Similar one found around the eye	
Nevoid hypermelanosis	Swirls that are along the lines of Blaschko with a Sharp midline cutoff	Chromosomal mosaicism

CLASSIFICATION OF HYPERPIGMENTATION DISORDERS

Epidermal

- **Melanocytotic**: Lentigines.
- **Melanotic**: Freckles (Figs. 15.8, 15.9), CALM, Beckers Nevus, N. Spilus, Melasma, Endocrine causes, reticular disorders.

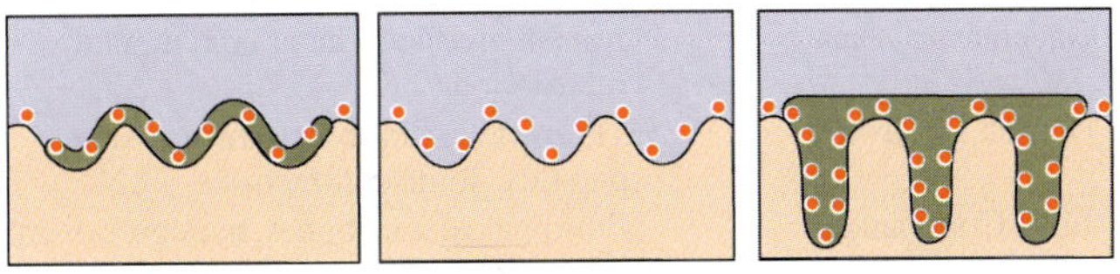

Fig. 15.8

Dermal

- **Melanocytotic:** Mongolian spot, Nevus of Ota/Ito.
- **Melanotic**: Incontinentia Pigmenti, FDE (Fixed drug Eruption), Hemochromatosis, Riehl's Melanosis, EDP (Erythema dyschromicum perstans).

Non Melanin

Alkaptonuria, Ochronosis, Drug.

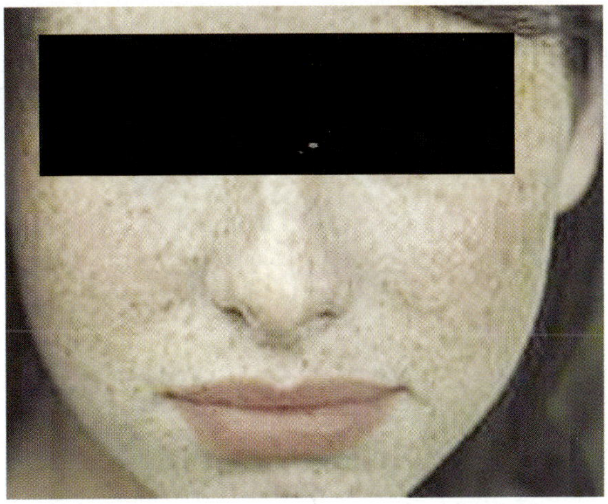

Fig. 15.9: Multiple light brown freckles

MELANOCYTOTIC EPIDERMAL HYPERMELANOSIS

Lentigo (Fig. 15.8)

Simple and senile lentigines look alike. They are light or dark brown macules, ranging from 1 mm to 1 cm across. Although usually discrete, they may have an irregular outline.

1. **Senile or solar lentigines** are common after middle age on the backs of the hands (**'liver spots'**) and on the face. In contrast to freckles, lentigines have increased numbers of melanocytes. Treatment is usually unnecessary but melanin-specific high energy lasers (e.g. pigmented lesion dye laser, 510 nm; Q-switched ruby laser, 694 nm; Q-switched alexandrite laser, 755 nm) are extremely useful.
2. **Peutz-Jeghers syndrome:** Profuse lentigines are seen on and around the lips in this autosomal dominant condition. Scattered lentigines also occur on the buccal mucosa, gums, hard palate, hands and feet. The syndrome is important because of its association with polyposis of the small intestine, which may lead to recurrent intussusception and, rarely, to malignant transformation of the polyps.
3. **Cronkhite-Canada syndrome:** This consists of multiple lentigines on the backs of the hands and a more diffuse pigmentation of the palms and volar aspects of the fingers. It may also associate with gastrointestinal polyposis. Alopecia and nail abnormalities complete the rare but characteristic clinical picture.
4. **LEOPARD syndrome:** This is an acronym for generalized **lentiginosis** associated with cardiac abnormalities demonstrated by **ECG,** Endocrine hyperpigmentation, Addison's disease. Hyperpigmentation caused by the overproduction of ACTH is often striking. It may be generalized or limited to the skin folds, creases of the palms, scars and the buccal mucosa.

Other syndromes associated with lentigines are given in Table 15.5.

Table 15.5: Syndromes associated with multiple lentigines

Syndrome	*Features*
LEOPARD	Lentigines, ECG abnormalities, ocular hypertelorism, pulmonic stenosis, abnormal genitalia, growth retardation, deafness (LEOPARD)
Peutz-Jeghers	Periorificial, mucosal, and acral lentigines; gastrointestinal polyposis
Carney[a]	Myxomas, spotty pigmentation, endocrine hyperactivity
NAME[a]	Nevi, atrial myxomas, myxoid neurofibromas, ephelides (NAME)
LAMB[a]	Lentigines, atrial myxomas, mucocutaneous myxomas, blue nevi /(LAMB)
Xeroderma pigmentosa	Lentigines, basal cell CA, squamous cell, melanoma, UV light sensitivity

a. NAME and LAMB syndromes are now considered variants of Carney syndrome.

MELANOTIC EPIDERMAL HYPERMELANOSES

Freckles (Ephelides)—Melanotic

Freckles are so common that to describe them seems unnecessary. They are seen most often in the red-haired or blond person as sharply demarcated light brown-ginger macules, usually less than 5 mm in diameter (Fig. 15.9). They multiply and become darker with sun exposure.

Increased melanin is seen in the basal layer of the epidermis without any increase in the number of melanocytes, and without elongation of the rete ridges. No treatment is necessary.

CAFÉ-AU-LAIT MACULES

Café-au-lait macules (CALMs) are discrete, uniformly pale brown, well-circumscribed, less than one to several centimeter large macules. They are characterized by serrated or irregular margins (Fig. 15.10). **Isolated CALMs** occur in upto **10 to 20 percent** of the normal population. Their size usually ranges from 5 to 15 mm in adults. Ninety-eight percent of normal young adults who have CALMs have fewer **than three.**

The main disorder is Neurofibromatosis (Page 275).

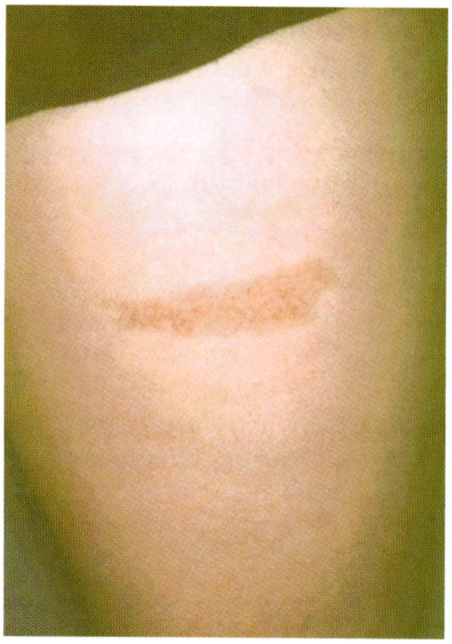

Fig. 15.10: Solitary CALM

McCune-Albright Syndrome

McCune-Albright syndrome also known as Albright's syndrome, is characterized in its complete form by the triad of bone lesions termed **polyostotic fibrous dysplasia,** a hyperfunctioning **endocrine system, and cutaneous lesions** of light-brown pigmentation.

Other associated disorders are given in Table 15.6.

Table 15.6: Diseases associated with multiple café-au-lait spots

Disease	*Major features*
Ataxia telangiectasia	Progressive ataxia, lymphoreticular malignancy
Bannayan-Riley-Ruvalcaba syndrome	Macrosomia, megalencephaly, lipomas, intestinal polyps
Basal cell nevus syndrome	Multiple basal cell epitheliomas, jaw cysts, skeletal anomalies
Bloom syndrome	Short stature, photosensitivity, chromosome breaks, malignancy
Fanconi's anemia	Limb anomalies, renal anomalies, pancytopenia
Gaucher's disease	Jewish predilection, ataxia, mental retardation
Hunter syndrome	Thickened skin, coarse facies, skin papules, joint contractures
Jaffe-Companacci	Fibromas of long bones, hypogonadism, mental retardation, ocular/cardiac anomalies
Maffucci syndrome	Venous malformations, enchondromas
McCune-Albright syndrome	Polyostotic fibrous dysplasia, precocious puberty
Multiple lentigines syndrome	Multiple lentigines, hypertelorism, pulmonic stenosis
Multiple mucosal neuroma syndrome	Mucosal neuromas, thyroid carcinoma, pheochromocytoma, parathyroid adenoma, dysautonomia
Neurofibromatosis	Neurofibromas, central nervous system tumors, iris hamartomas, axillary freckles, skeletal anomalies

Contd.

Contd.

Russell-Silver syndrome	Short stature, asymmetry, limb anomalies
Tuberous sclerosis	White macules, multiple hamartomas, central nervous system anomalies
Watson syndrome	Pulmonic stenosis, axillary freckles, low intelligence.

BECKER'S NEVUS

Becker's nevus is a common/acquired focal epidermal melanotic hypermelanosis. The reported incidence in males is 1 in 200, much less in females. The nevus typically appears at about the time of puberty as a unilateral, several centimeters large, hyperpigmented, irregular patch. It involves the upper part of the trunk, especially the shoulder, submammary area and back (Fig. 15.11).

The color, most often light brown, is uniform and rarely fades over time. The jagged margins are sharply demarcated. Although the lesion is macular, there is a palpable quality, particularly in the center. A variable amount of hypertrichosis occurs. Tissue hypoplasia, such as shortening of an arm or reduced breast development, rarely may underlie Becker's nevus. Spina bifida also has been associated. In addition to epidermal melanotic hyperpigmentation, histology shows acanthosis, papillomatosis, thickening of the dermis, and smooth muscle hyperplasia. Becker's nevus is considered as an organoid nevus with epidermal melanocytic and dermal components.

Nevus Spilus/Speckled Lentiginous Nevus

Nevus spilus/speckled lentiginous nevus (NS/SLN) presents as a circumscribed, usually lightly pigmented macule containing scattered, usually more darkly pigmented spots (Fig. 15.12).The Greek root spilos means "spot", hence the term of nevus spilus. NS/SLN can appear on any area of the body. Background pigmentation in NS/SLN is often 3 to 6 cm in diameter, but it can vary from 1 to over 60 cm.

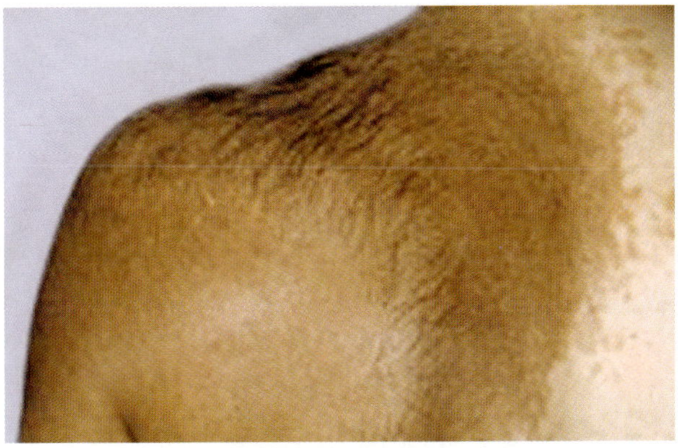

Fig. 15.11: Single becker's nevus with serrated margins with increased hair growth

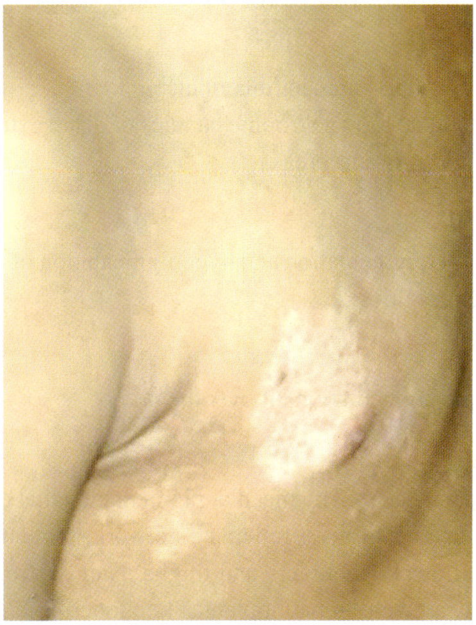

Fig. 15.12: Nevus spilus

OTHER MELANOTIC EPIDERMAL HYPERMELANOSES

Cushing's Syndrome

Increased ACTH production may cause a picture like that of Addison's disease. The hyperpigmentation may become even more marked after adrenalectomy **(Nelson's syndrome).**

Chronic Renal Failure

The hyperpigmentation of chronic renal failure and of patients on haemodialysis is caused by an increase in levels of pituitary melanotrophic peptides, normally cleared by the kidney.

Nutritional Hyperpigmentation

Any severe wasting disease, such as malabsorption, AIDS, tuberculosis or cancer, may be accompanied by diffuse hyperpigmentation. Kwashiorkor presents a mixed picture of generalized hypopigmentation and patchy postinflammatory hyperpigmentation, and in this condition the hair is red-brown or grey.

PUNCTATE AND RETICULATE PIGMENTATION DISORDERS

Reticulate Acropigmentation of Kitamura (Figs. 15.15 - 15.17)

- Autosomal dominant inheritance.
- Reticulate brown atrophic papules of distal extremities, palmar pits and breaks.

Acropigmentation of Dohi

Acral hyperpigmentation and hypopigmentation of the face, trunk, extremities.

Dyschromatosis Universalis Hereditaria

Reticulate pigmentation all over the body.

Dermatophathia Pigmentosa Reticularis

This is characterized by macular pigmentation that develops in infancy and forms a reticulate network, particularly on the trunk, neck, shoulders and thighs. Nail dystrophy and alopecia, as well as palmoplantar keratoderma have been described.

Dowling Degos Disease

Reticulate Pigmentation in the Flexures.
A detailed summary is provided in Table 15.7.

Table 15.7: Punctate and reticulate pigmentation disorders

Disease	*Major feature*
Cantu syndrome	Punctate brown macules of the feet, face forearms; palmoplantar hyperkeratosis
Dermatopathia pigmentosa Reticularis	Reticulated pigment of trunk, extremities; loss of nails; hypohidrosis; alopecia; atrophy of skin over elbows, kness
Dowling-Degos disease	Autosomal dominant, progressive symmetric brown macules, comedone-like follicular papules
Acropigmentation of Dohi	Acral location
Franceschetti–Jadassohn	Punctate pigment over waist, axilla, neck; hypohidrosis; palmoplantar keratosis; tooth, nail anomalies
Kitamura	Autosomal-dominant disorder, reticulated brown atrophic papules of distal extermities, palmar pits and breaks
Haber syndrome	Facial erythema, telangiectasia, black keratotic papules of the axilla, neck, torso

DERMAL HYPERPIGMENTATION

1. Dermal **melanocytotic** hyperpigmentation, that is, melanin formed in dermal melanocytes.
2. Dermal **melanotic** hyperpigmentation, that is, melanin formed in the epidermis by epidermal melanocytes and transferred to the dermis.
3. **Nonmelanin** dermal pigmentation, attributed to pigment other than melanin deposited in the dermis.

CIRCUMSCRIBED DERMAL MELANOCYTOTIC DISORDERS

Mongolian spots or congenital dermal melanocytosis: The term Mongolian spot, or congenital dermal melanocytosis (CDM), applies to specific blue-gray macules. CDM is almost always located on the lumbosacral skin or on the buttocks (Fig. 15.13). The lesions are macular with distinct margins and blue-black in color, although with variations in intensity.

In typical CDM, the dermal melanocytes appear microscopically at the fetal age of 3 months, and the pigmentation appears at the fetal age of 7 months. The natural course of CDM is to disappear in childhood.

Nevus of Ota (Oculodermal melanocytosis): Nevus of Ota is usually congenital but may appear in early childhood

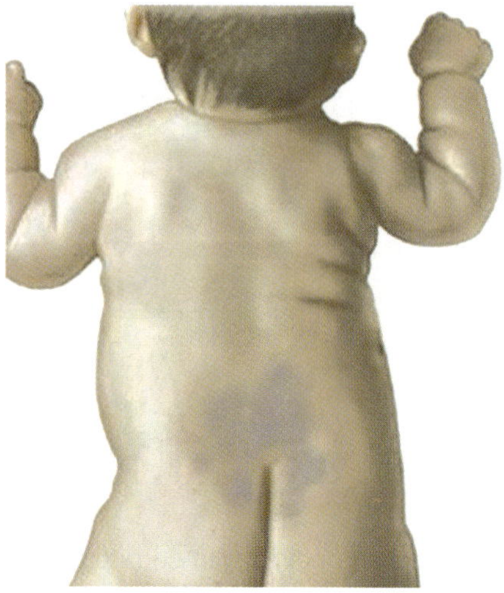

Fig. 15.13: Classic location of Mongolian spot

or in puberty. It is usually characterized by unilateral, flat, blue-black or slate-gray macules intermingled with small, flat, brown spots occurring most characteristically in the skin innervated by the first and second branches of the trigeminal nerve. Oral mucosa, conjunctivae, and tympanic membranes may be involved. Hyperpig-mentation in the involved areas of cornea, sclera (Fig. 15.14), iris, optic nerve, fundus, extraocular muscles, retrobulbar fat, and periosteum may occur. Similar involvement may be located on the hard palate, pharynx, nasal mucosa, buccal mucosa, and tympanic membrane of the involved side.

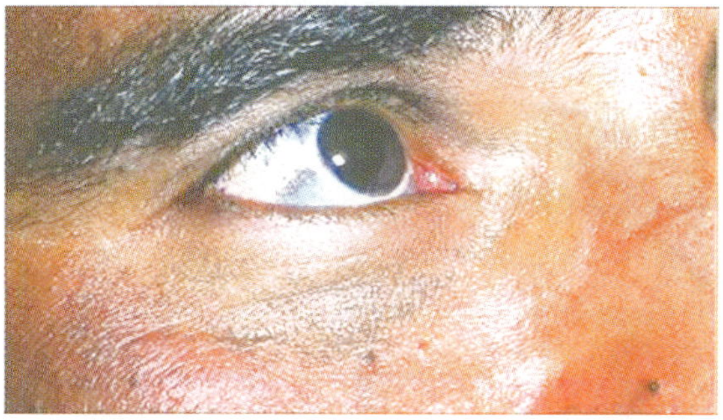

Fig. 15.14: Nevus of ota involving the eye

Course and Treatment

Nevus of Ota does not improve with time. There have been a large number of reported cases of melanoma development in nevus of Ota, but less in Indian population. Selective photothermolysis with the Q-switched ruby laser/Nd:YAG is a safe and effective treatment. Multiple treatments increase the response rate.

Acquired circumscribed dermal facial melanocytosis or Hori's nevus, is characterized by blue-brown macules that occur bilaterally on the forehead, temples, eyelids, malar areas, nasal alae, and nasal root of middle-aged Japanese women. These macules are clinically very similar to classic nevus of Ota. The lesions usually are noted in the fourth or fifth decade of life and do not extend to ocular or mucosal surfaces.

Nevus of Ito: Initially described by Ito in 1954, nevus of Ito is analogous to nevus of Ota and may in fact coexist in the same patient. With nevus of Ito, the cutaneous involvement occurs in the distribution of the lateral supraclavicular and lateral brachial nerves. Except for the fact that the involvement is more diffuse and less mottled, the pigmentary change is the same as that of the nevus of Ota.

DERMAL MELANOTIC DISORDERS

Macular Amyloidosis: The macular variety of amyloidosis is characterized by brownish-gray, reticulated pigmentation that may or may not be associated with pruritus.

Fixed Drug Eruption: This is a reddish brown to slate-gray cutaneous macule that may be localized or generalized. The most typical cases flare repeatedly in the same area following ingestion or injection of a particular medication. The initial phase of erythema, edema, and/or desquamation may be followed by a spontaneously resolving vesiculo-bullous eruption and finally by hyperpigmentation.

NON MELANOTIC DISORDERS

Widespread/Diffuse Dermal Melanoses Related to Drugs

Numerous medications have been implicated in diffuse blue-gray coloration of the skin; in some cases these represent drug bound to melanin and in others drug alone. Particularly implicated has been long-term use of *chlorpromazine, other phenothiazines, hydrochlorthiazide, and minocycline*. This blue-gray coloration may involve any normally sun-exposed area but occurs especially on the forehead, malar eminences and nose. Although the initial color is brown, repeated sun exposure leads to a slate-gray or violaceous hue.

Nonmelanin Dermal Hyperpigmentation

Drugs, heavy metals, and other exogenous agents may deposit in the dermis to give rise to a blue-gray pigmentation that clinically mimics dermal melanosis. Drugs that may lead to dermal pigmentation include minocycline, hydroquinone, and antimalarials. Heavy metals include mercury, silver, bismuth, arsenic, gold and lead.

Ochronosis, or alkaptonuria, is one disease entity that gives rise to nonmelanin ceruloderma.

Ceruloderma Due to Ochronosis: Clinically **alkaptonuria**, or ochronosis, presents as faint, uniform blue or blue-gray color of the pinnae, tip of the nose, sclera, costochondral junctions, axillae, and overlying extensor tendons of the hands. A butterfly pattern on the face, involvement of the axillae and genitalia, and uncommonly, diffuse involvement may occur. The facial pigmentation actually may result from myriads of circumscribed blue macules. Fingernails may be affected, nevi may darken, the sclerae may have pigment granules, and the tympanic membranes may be involved.

Pigmentation Due to Heavy Metals

Argyria results from deposition of silver in the skin to give rise to blue to slate-gray coloration, particularly in sun-exposed areas.

Arsenic gives a bronze color, prominent on the trunk; melanin is also implicated.

Bismuth and lead may both give generalized pigmentation and a gingival pigment line. Bismuth also may pigment the conjunctivae and oral mucosa; small granules are found in the papillary and reticular dermis.

Chrysoderma is a rare consequence of parenteral gold administration and is prominent around the eyes and in sun-exposed areas.

Nonmelanin Pigmentation Due to Drugs: Chloroquine, if taken for protracted periods of time, may be associated with ceruloderma, particularly on the shins. Clofazimine may cause both increased basilar melanin and brown pigment in dermal macrophages. Clinically, however, clofazimine-induced discoloration appears orange red. Hydroxyurea may cause ceruloderma of the back and pressure points.

FACIAL MELANOSIS

ACQUIRED

1. Melasma (Page 269)

CONGENITAL/GENETIC

1. Nevus of Ota
2. Beckers Nevus
3. Others
   – Melanocytic Nevus

2. Dermatoses

- Acne.
- L planus actinicus.
- Atopic dermatitis.
- Contact dermatitis, ABCD (Air borne contact dermatitis).
- PMLE (Polymorphic light eruption).
- Drug eruption.
- Amyloidosis.
- XP (Xeroderma pigmentosa).
- Reticulate pattern.

3. Genodermatoses

- Xeroderma pigmentosa.
- Reticulate pattern.
- Kitamura Figs. 15.15,15.16 and 15.17.
- Acropigmentation of Dohi.
- Dyschromatosis universalis hereditaria.

4. Syndromes/Spl. Conditions

- Erythema dyschromicum perstans (EDP).
- Riehl's melanosis.
- Tar/Occupational melanosis.
- Berloque dermatitis.
- Poikiloderma of civatte.
- Erythromelanosis follicularis faciei et colli.
- Erythrose peribuccale pigmentaire of Brocq.

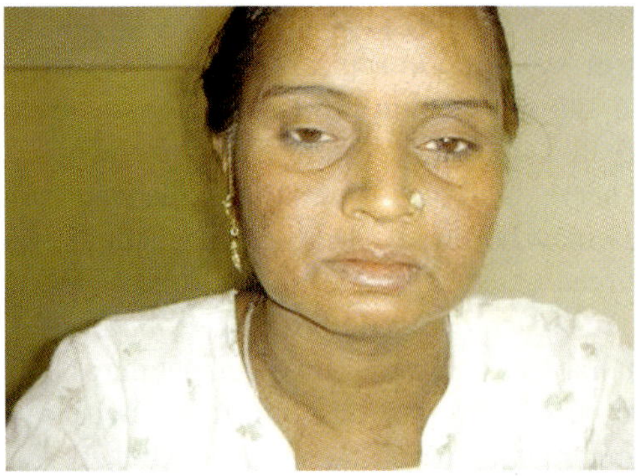

Fig. 15.15: Reticulate pigmentation on the face

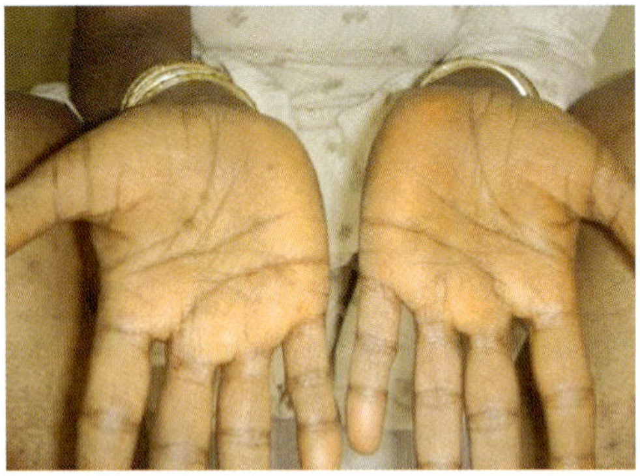

Fig. 15.16: Palmar pits and break in dermatoglyphics

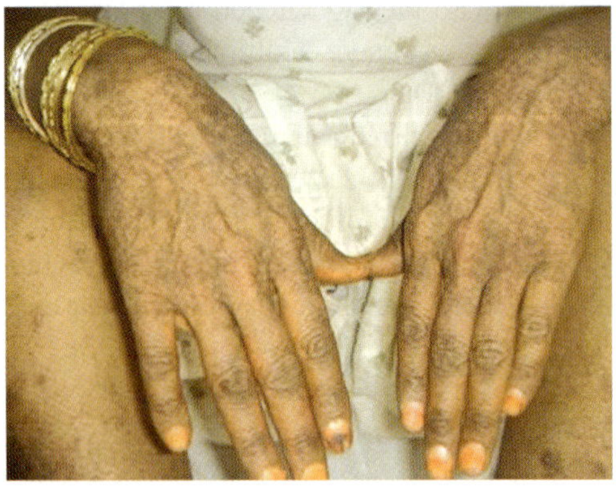

Fig. 15.17: Reticulate pigmentation on the extremities

5. Collagen Vascular Disorders

Collagen Vascular Diseases

Scleroderma: Pigmentation may be intense and diffuse or of Addisonian type, but without mucous membrane involvement.

- Dermatomyositis and systemic lupus erythematosus may be accompanied by hyperpigmentation.

- Pigmentation occasionally observed in rheumatoid arthritis and Still's disease.

6. Endocrinal

Hyperthyroidism

- 10% patients have pigmentary abnormalities.

Addisonian Pattern

- Eyelids are occasionally conspicuously pigmented.
- Mucous membrane is uncommon and pigmentation of nipples and genital skin is less striking.

7. Malignancy

Neoplastic Diseases

- Ectopic ACTH syndrome, oat-cell carcinoma of the bronchus, pigmentation is usual (distinct MSH-like compound).
- Acanthosis nigricans is associated usually with an internal malignancy, almost invariably an adenocarcinoma.
- Slaty-blue color, melanoma (Addisonian type).

8. Drugs

- *Chlorpromazine*: causes purple pigmentation or slate colored pigmentation.
- *Chloroquine*: causes bluish-black hyperpigmentation.
- *Estrogens*: cause skin melanosis.
- *Other drugs* such as phenothiazine, antipyrine, tetracycline cause skin pigmentation.
- *Bismuth*: causes gum hyperpigmentation.
- *Silver*: causes metallic blue pigmentation.
- Cyclophosphamide.
- Busulfan.
- Methotrexate.
- Dactinomycin.
- 5-FU.
- OC (Oral contraceptives).
- CQ (Chloroquine).
- Clofazimine.
- PUVA.
- Minocycline.
- Psychotropic agents.
- Silver.
- Gold.
- Arsenic.
- Topical hydroquinone causes exogenous ochronosis.

9. Miscellaneous

Hematological

- Hyperpigmentation of the skin occurs in **vitamin B_{12} deficiency**.
- The pigmentation often has a rather *dappled and mottled appearance*, and particularly affects the face, hands and feet.
- Hemolytic anemia, hypermelanosis and hemosiderosis may develop on the lower legs.

10. Hypermelanosis Associated with Other Diseases

Diseases of the Nervous System

- Schilder's disease.
- Schizophrenia, emotional stress, Parkinsonism, hepatolenticular degeneration and in ependymomas.

Hemochromatosis

- Pigmentation, *bronzed or slaty-gray in color*.
- Exposed skin but later it is generalized.
- The diagnosis should be suspected when pigmentation of this pattern occurs in middle-aged men.
- Enlarged liver and diabetes.
- Confirmed by the high level of serum iron.

Hepatic Cirrhosis

- A diffuse hypermelanosis is seen in patients with liver cirrhosis.
- Lichen planus may be associated with primary biliary cirrhosis and as lesions resolve they leave slaty-brown hypermelanotic macules.
- Malabsorption diseases such as Gaucher's and Niemann-Pick disease.

Chronic Infections

Malaria, Kala-azar, Schistosomiasis and Tuberculosis.

FACIAL MELANOSIS

Melasma

Melasma is an acquired hyperpigmentation disorder characterized by "moth-eaten" tan or brownish macules and patches that occur on the sun-exposed areas of the skin. When melasma is associated with pregnancy it is called chloasma or "mask of pregnancy".

Etiology

- Idiopathic.
- Sun exposure.
- Genetic predisposition.
- Pregnancy.
- Oral contraceptives.
- Ovarian dysfunctions (elevated levels of LH, FSH and estradiol).
- Thyroid dysfunctions.
- Antiseizure drugs (phenytoin).
- Cosmetics containing perfumes.

Clinical Features (Figs. 15.18 to 15.20)

- Clinical features of melasma usually evolve rapidly, especially after UV exposure. Lesions are uniformly light to dark brown, often symmetric, and three clinical patterns can be distinguished: Centrofacial (Fig. 15.18), Malar (Fig. 15.19), Mandibular (Fig. 15.20).

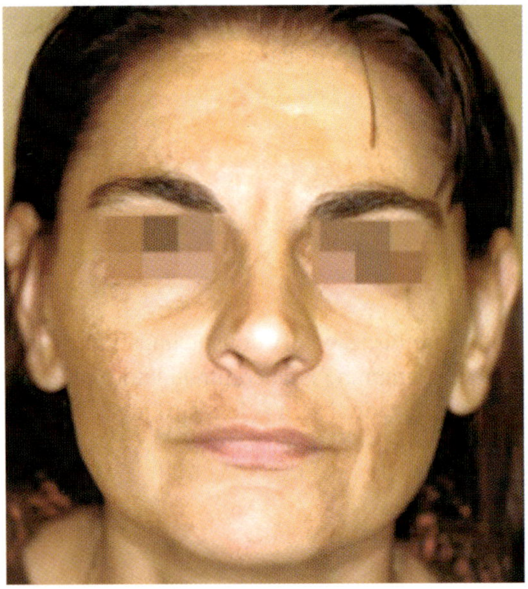

Fig. 15.18: Centrofacial

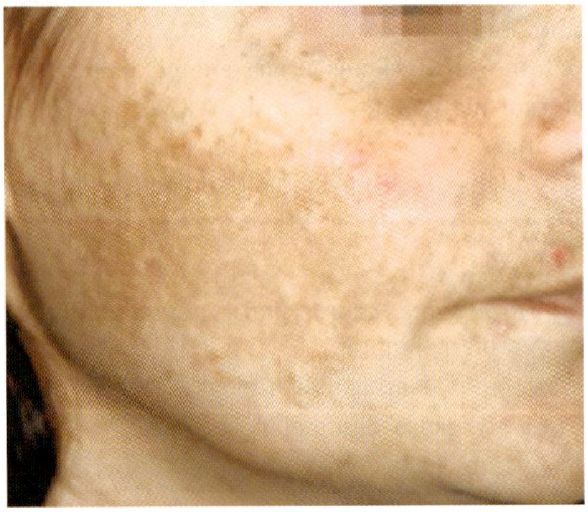

Fig. 15.19: Malar

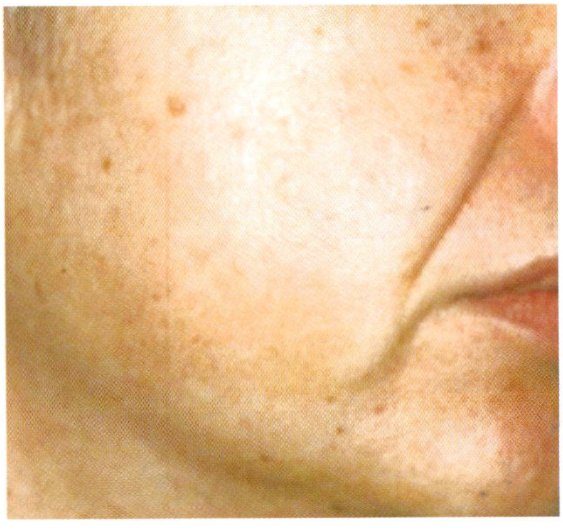

Fig. 15.20: Mandibular

THERAPY

Objectives of therapy are:

- To slow the proliferation and growth of melanocytes.
- To inhibit the formation and promote the destruction of melanosomes.

  It is commonly accepted that epidermal melasma is more responsive to therapy due to its superficial distribution.

Treatment Options are:

- Broad-spectrum sunscreens (SPF of 30 and above + UVA filters).
- Topical depigmenting agents:
  - **Tyrosinase inhibitors** (hydroquinone, azelaic acid, kojic acid).
  - **Antioxidants** (magnesium, ascorbic acid, alpha-tocopherol).
  - **Melanogenesis inhibitors** (retinoic acid, benzoic acid).
  - **Exfoliants** (AHA: glycolic acid, BHA: salicylic acid).
- Chemical peels:
  - Superficial (15-20% TCA, 50-70% glycolic acid, 25% salicylic acid).
  - Medium (resorcinol, 50% pyruvic acid).

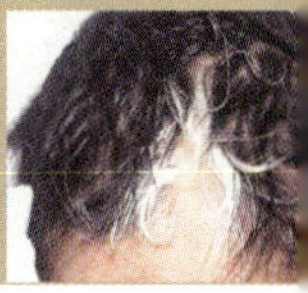

- Combined chemical peels (25% salicylic acid + 10% TCA gel).
- Laser therapy.
- Cryotherapy.

Hydroquinone

The most commonly used bleaching agent, hydroquinone is a phenolic derivative available at concentrations that may vary from 2 to 5%. Sometimes, for short course therapy, it can be prescribed at concentration of 10%. It has to be applied once a day, usually nightly. It inhibits tyrosinase and consequently melanin synthesis. Side-effects include irritant and allergic contact dermatitis, nail discoloration, post-inflammatory hyperpigmentation and ochronosis. Due to these side effects, 2% concentration is the safer concentration.

Hydroquinone is usually more effective when utilized in combination with other agents such as topical retinoids alone or topical retinoids and topical steroids.

0.1% tretinoin	5% hydroquinone	0.1% dexamethasone
0.1% tretinoin	5% hydroquinone	1% hydrocortisone
0.05% tretinoin	4% hydroquinone	0.01% fluocinolone acetonide

Azelaic Acid

Azelaic acid is a non-phenolic derivative used at concentration of 10-20% twice a day to treat melasma with minimal side effects (allergic reactions). It acts to disturb the tyrosinase synthesis and can be used as a bleaching agent in patients sensitive to hydroquinone. Better results are obtained if a glycolic acid cream is applied sequentially to azelaic acid treatment.

Kojic Acid

Kojic acid is a fungal metabolite known to inhibit tyrosinase and used to treat melasma at concentration of 2-4% twice a day. The stability is one of its advantages if compared with hydroquinone.

Unfortunately, it is considered to have a high sensitizing potential.

Other topical bleaching agents include arbutin, licorice, unsaturated fatty acids, soy extracts, serine protease inhibitors, ellagic acid and resveratrol.

Retinoic Acid (Tretinoin)

Generally used at a concentration of 0.05-0.1% with minimal side effects (erythema and desquamation), retinoic acid has to be applied once a day, usually nightly. It does not suppress melanogenesis, but accelerates epidermal turnover.

Chemical Peels

- Superficial peeling – 25% salicylic acid, glycolic acid 20-30%.
- Combined peeling with 25% Salicylic acid and 10% TCA.
- Medium peeling with 50% pyruvic acid.

Patients should undergo a superficial peeling every 2 weeks or a medium peeling every month. With a medium chemical peel, the application of the solution must be reduced in time in order to avoid overpeel.

It is important that, 3 weeks before starting peeling treatment and 10 days after each treatment, the patient does the following routine:

In the morning:

- Wash skin with an alpha-hydroxy acid containing cleanser.
- Apply a UVA/UVB sunscreen.
- Wear a hat and avoid sun exposure.

In the evening:

- Wash with an alpha-hydroxy acid containing cleanser.
- Apply a product with a combination of hydroquinone and kojic acid once every 2 days.
- Apply a topical retinoid once every 2 days.

SYNDROMES/SPECIAL CONDITIONS

1. Riehl's Melanosis

- Tar derivatives in cosmetics, geraniol, lemon oil, fragrances are suspect etiological factors.
- Brownish grey pigmentation.
- Develops quite rapidly, more intense on the forehead and temples.
- May extend to the chest, neck and scalp, and occasionally involves hands and forearms.

Treatment

Avoid Cosmetics, Use Sunscreens

- May improve over months (6 months-2 years) if offending contact stopped.
- Cosmetic camouflage may be suggested.

2. Erythema Dyschromicum Perstans

- Described by RAMIREZ.

Probable Causes

- Paraphenylenediamine hair dyes.
- Whipworm infestation.
- Contact with optical whiteners.

Clinical Features

- Early—*string like* erythematous border.
- Torso, extremities, and/or face, symmetrical arrangement.
- Slate gray to blue-brown pigmentation.
- Mild pruritus to asymptomatic.
- Late-hypopigmented halo around macules.

Treatment

- No standard effective therapy.
- 1 lac IU Vitamin A daily × 15 days, rest period of 15 days—10 such cycles.
- Clofazimine 50 mg -100 mg daily.
- Q-switched ruby laser.

3. Lichen Planus Pigmentosus

- India and Middle East.
- Also been called Toxic melanosis.
- Site: Sun exposed, flexural folds.
- Exacerbations and incomplete remissions.
- H/P may be similar to lichen planus with lichenoid changes.

Treatment

Top steroids, keratolytics, 10% DMSO, griseofulvin, prednisolone, etretinate, chloroquine have been tried.

4. Poikiloderma of Civatte

- Middle-aged women.
- Milder forms–common, patients often do not seek medical advice.

Etiology

- Photodynamic substances in cosmetics—important factor.
- An unknown endocrine factor or aging.

Clinical Features

- Reddish brown, reticulate pigmentation with telangiectasia and atrophy.
- Irregular, symmetrical patches on the lateral cheeks and the sides of the neck.
- No effective treatment.

5. Erythrose Peribuccale Pigmentaire of Brocq

- More in women.

Etiology

- Cosmetics, endocrine factors.
- Reddish brown pigmentation around the mouth, spares a narrow perioral ring.
- May extend up the centre of the face to the forehead, over the angles of the jaw and the temples.
- Erythema and pigmentation may fluctuate.

Treatment

Hydroquinone, kojic acid, glycolic acid, tretinoin, superficial peels, resurfacing lasers.

6. Toxic Melanosis/Occupational Melanosis

- Seen in workers handling coal-tar products—pitch, asphalt and creosote or mineral oils.
- Photodynamic action of anthracene, phenanthrene etc. (probable cause).
- Diffuse melanosis of exposed skin.
- Develops slowly after prolonged exposure associated with atrophy, telangiectasia, lichenoid papules and follicular keratosis. Keratoses and epitheliomas may subsequently form.

7. Berloque Dermatitis

- **E/P:** 5-methoxypsoralen (bergapten) in bergamot oil in perfumes (Eau de Cologne).
- Individual susceptibility.
- Hot, humid conditions favour absorption.
- **C/F:** Deep-brown pigmentation follows the pattern formed by the trickle of the droplets of perfume over the skin from their points of application.
- Fades after weeks or months.

REFERENCES

- Schachner L, Hansen R: Pediatric Dermatology, 2nd edn 2003.
- Fitzpatrick's Dermatology in General Medicine, 6th edn 2003.
- Kovacs, S.O.: *Vitiligo,* J Am Acad Dermatol 1998, 38: 647-66.
- Halder, R.M., Grimes, P.E., Cowan, C.A., Enterline, J.A., Chakrabarti, S.G., Kenney, J.A.: *Childhood vitiligo*, J Am Acad Dermatol 1987, 16: 948-54.
- Lee, A.Y., Youm, Y.H., Kim, N.H., Yang, H., Choi, W.I: *Keratinocytes in the depigmented epidermis of vitiligo are more vulnerable to trauma (suction) than keratinocytes in the normally pigmented epidermis, resulting in their apoptosis.* Br J Dermatol 2004, 151: 995-1003.
- Hann, S.K., Kim, Y.S., Yoo, J.H., Chun, Y.S.: *Clinical and histopathologic characteristics of trichrome vitiligo*, J Am Acad Dermatol 2000, 42: 589-96.
- Grimes, P.E., Soriano, T., Dytoc, M.T.: *Topical tacrolimus for repigmentation of vitiligo*, J Am Acad Dermatol 2002, 47: 789-91.
- Montes, L.F., Diaz, M.L., Lajous, J., Garcia, N.J.: *Folic acid and vitamin B_{12} in vitiligo: A nutritional approach*, Cutis 1992, 50: 39-42.
- Grimes PE (1995) Melasma. Arch Dermatol 131 :1453-1457.
- Antonella Tosti, Pearl E. Grimes, Maria Pia De Padova (Eds.): Color Atlas of Chemical Peels, Springer Velag 2003.

CHAPTER **16**

TUMORS OF THE SKIN

CLASSIFICATION

Classification of Tumors of the Skin

Tumors of the Surface Epidermis

1. **Linear epidermal nevus.**
2. **Benign tumors:** Defined as neoplasms that probably arise from arrested embryonal cells.
   a. Seborrheic keratosis.
   b. Pedunculated fibroma (skin tag, fibroepithelial polyp, acrochordons).
   c. Cysts:
      i. Epidermal cyst.
      ii. Trichilemmal (pilar or sebaceous cyst).
      iii. Steatocystoma multiplex.
      iv. Milium.
      v. Dermoid cyst.
      vi. Mucous cyst.
   d. Clear cell acanthoma.
   e. Warty dyskeratoma.
   f. Keratoacanthoma.
3. **Precancerous tumors:**
   a. Actinic keratosis and cutaneous horn.
   b. Arsenical keratosis.
   c. Leukoplakia.
   d. Porokeratosis.
4. **Carcinoma:**
   a. Squamous cell carcinoma.
   b. Basal cell carcinoma.
   c. Bowen's disease and erythroplasia of Queyrat.
   d. Paget's disease.
   e. Carcinoma of the skin.

Tumors of the Epidermal Appendages

Numerous other types benign and malignant, usually classified by appendage of origin:

1. Sebaceous nevi.
2. Adenoma sebaceum.
3. Sebaceous hyperplasia.
4. Sebaceous adenoma.
5. Apocrine adenomas, *Syringocystadenoma papilliferum, Hidradenoma papilliferum.*
6. Eccrine syringofibroadenoma (ESFA).
7. Apocrine epitheliomas, Syringoma, Cylindroma.
8. Hair epitheliomas: Trichoepithelioma, *Piloma-trixoma.*
9. Eccrine epitheliomas: Eccrine spiradenoma, Clear cell hidradenoma, Eccrine poroma.

Mesodermal Tumors

Tumors of Fibrous Tissue

a. Histiocytoma and dermatofibroma.
b. Keloid.
c. Fibrosarcomas.

Tumors of Mucoid Tissue

a. Myxoma.
b. Myxosarcoma.
c. Synovial cyst of the skin.

Tumors of Fatty Tissue

a. Nevus lipomatosus superficialis.
b. Lipoma.
c. Hibernoma.
d. Liposarcoma.
e. Malignant hibernoma.

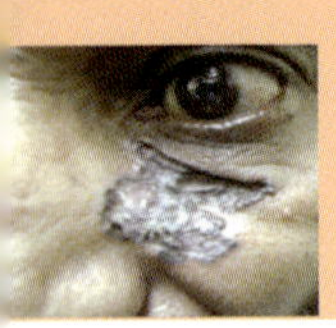

Tumors of Nerve Tissue and Mesodermal Nerve Sheath Cells

a. Neuroma.
b. Neurofibroma.
c. Neurilemoma.
d. Granular cell schwannoma.

Tumors of Muscular Tissue

a. Leiomyoma.
b. Leiomyosarcoma.
c. Multiple leiomyomas.

Tumors of Osseous Tissue

Osteoma cutis.

Tumors of Cartilaginous Tissue

Nodular chondrodermatitis of the ear.

Tumors of Vascular Tissue

Hemangiomas:

- Granuloma pyogenicum.
- Osler's disease.
- Lymphangioma.
- Glomus tumor.
- Hemangiopericytoma.
- Kaposi's sarcoma.
- Hemangioendothelioma.
- Postmastectomy lymphangiosarcoma (Stewart-Treves syndrome).
- Glomangiomas.

Nevus Cell Tumors

Melanocytic Nevi

a. Junctional (active) nevus.
b. Compound nevus.
c. Intradermal (resting) nevus.
d. Dysplastic nevus syndrome.

Lentigines

Malignant Melanoma

Lymphoma and Myelosis

a. Monomorphous Group—NHL.
b. Polymorphous Group—HL, MF.
c. Myelosis Leukemia.
d. Pseudolymphoma of Spiegler—Fendt.

LINEAR EPIDERMAL NEVUS

A rather common tumor usually present at birth, consisting of single or multiple lesions in various forms that give rise to several clinical designations, such as hard nevus, nevus verrucous (Fig. 16.1), nevus unius lateral, and when systematized (more generalized), ichthyosis hystrix. No nevus cells are present.

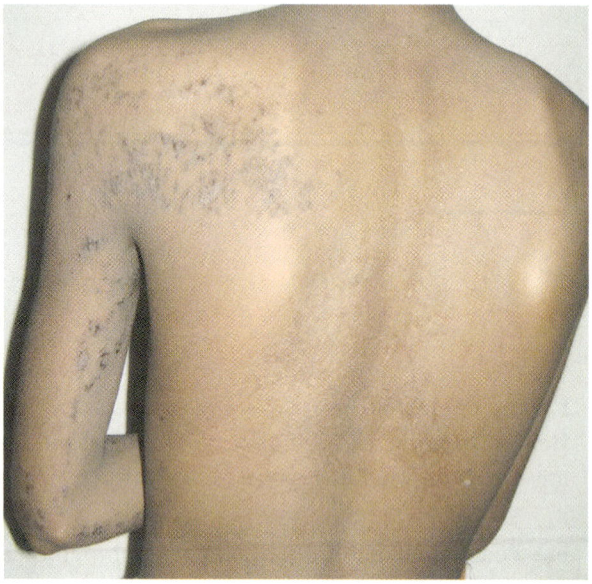

Fig. 16.1: Linear verrucous papules

SEBORRHEIC KERATOSIS

Dermatosis papulosa nigra is a form of seborrheic keratosis that occur on the face, mainly in women. These small, black, multiple tumors can be removed, but there is the possibility of causing keloids or hypopigmentation.

Stucco keratoses are numerous white 1 to 3 mm seborrheic keratoses mainly over feet, ankles and lower legs.

A very large seborrheic keratosis is sometimes referred to as a *melanoacanthoma.*

Clinical Features

The color may be flesh-colored, tan, brown, or coal black. They are usually oval in shape, elevated, and have a greasy, warty sensation to touch. White, brown, or black pinhead-sized keratotic areas called pseudohorn cysts are commonly seen within this tumor. There is an appearance of being superficial and "stuck on" the skin (Figs. 16.2 and 16.3). Pruritus is common and sudden appearance may occur. Numerous lesions coming on rapidly can be a marker of underlying cancer **(sign of Leser-Trélat).**

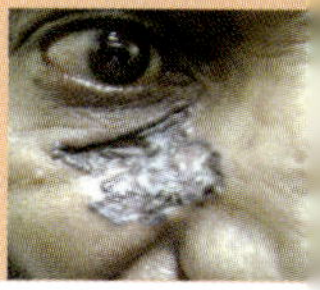

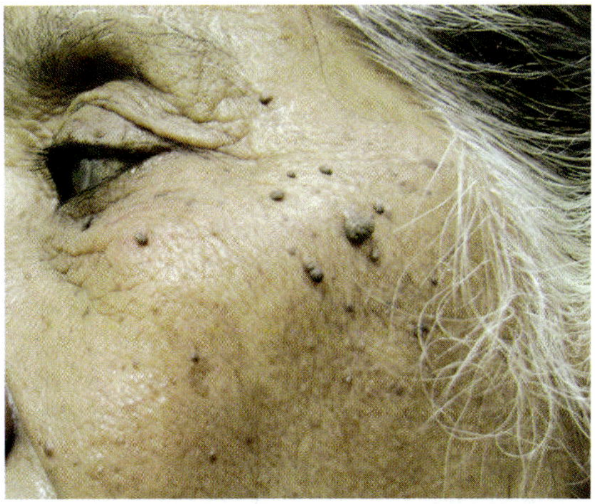

Fig. 16.2: Multiple, verrucous, papule and plaque on the face (Seborrheic keratoses)

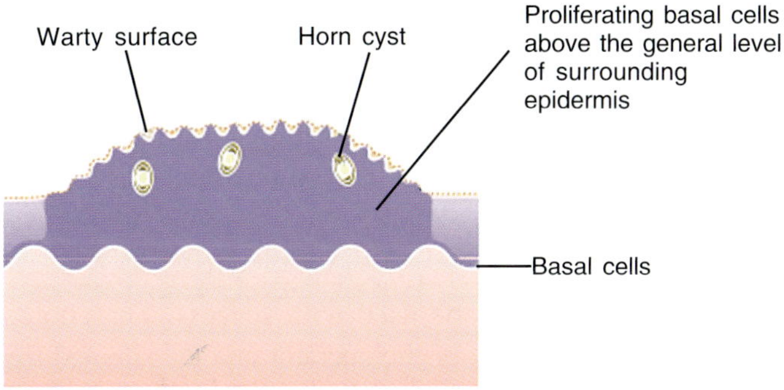

Fig. 16.3: Histology of seborrheic keratosis

Site

The lesions appear on the face, neck, scalp, back, and upper chest, and less frequently on arms, legs, and the lower part of the trunk.

The differential diagnosis is given in Table 16.1.

Table 16.1: Differential diagnosis of keratoses

Parameter	*Actinic or senile keratosis*	*Seborrheic keratosis*
Appearance	Flat, brownish, reddish, or tan scale firmly attached to skin, poorly demarcated	Greasy, elevated, brown, black, flesh-colored, warty scale and can be easily scratched away at times, 'stuck on', well demarcated
Location	Sun-exposed areas	Face, back
Complexion	Blue eyes, light hair, dry skin	Brown eyes, dark hair, oily skin
Symptoms	Some burning and stinging	Occasional itching
Precancerous	Yes	No
Cause	Sun	Inherited

Treatment

- An adequate form of therapy is curettage, with or without local anesthesia, followed by a light application of trichloroacetic acid. The resulting fine atrophic scar will hardly be noticeable in several months.
- Electrosurgery can be used, but this usually requires anesthesia.
- Liquid nitrogen freezing therapy works well, if available. It is the therapy of choice of most dermatologists. Do not freeze excessively.
- Laser therapy has been used recently by some authors.

PEDUNCULATED FIBROMAS (SKIN TAGS, ACROCHORDONS)

Multiple skin tags are common on the neck and the axillae of middle-aged, usually obese, men and women (Fig.16.4). The indications for removal are two-fold: cosmetic, as desired and requested by the patient, and to prevent the irritation and the secondary infection of the pedicle that frequently develops from trauma of a collar, necklace, or other article of clothing. It may be part of metabolic syndrome.

Clinical Features

Pedunculated pinhead-sized to pea-sized soft tumors of normal skin color or darker are seen. The base may be inflamed from injury and the lesion may thrombose and turn black if twisted. This can cause alarm in the patient.

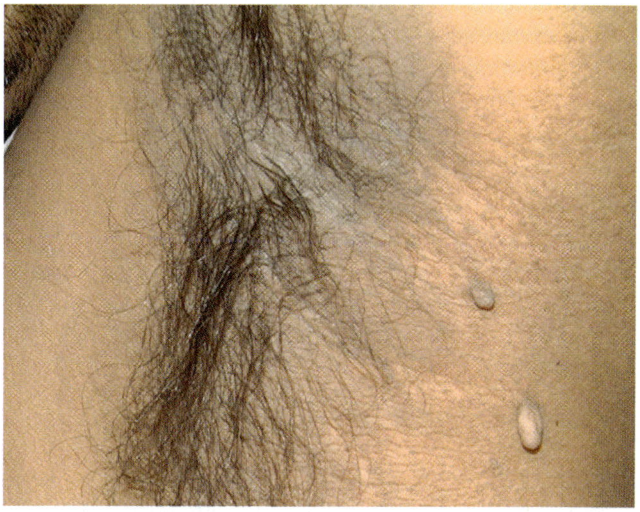

Fig. 16.4: Multiple pedunculated, soft, papules (skin tags)

Treatment

This could be done by electrosurgery. Without anesthesia, gently grab the small tumor in a thumb forceps and stretch the pedicle. Touch this pedicle with the electrosurgery needle and turn on the current for a split second. The tumor separates from the skin, and no bleeding occurs. The site heals in 4 to 7 days. For very small lesions, a short spark with the electrosurgical needle suffices. Scissor excision with or without local anesthetic is commonly done.

CYSTS

1. Epidermal cyst.
2. Trichilemmal, pilar or sebaceous cyst.
3. Steatocystoma multiplex: A dominantly inherited condition with small, moderately firm, cystic nodules adherent to the overlying skin, which on incision yield an oily fluid.
4. Milium.
5. Dermoid cyst.
6. Mucous retention cyst.

An **epidermal cyst** has a wall composed of true epidermis and probably originates from an invagination of the epidermis into the dermis and subsequent detachment from the epidermis, or it can originate spontaneously. The most common locations for epidermal cysts are the face, ears, neck, back and scalp, where tumors of varying size can be found. A central pore may be seen over the surface.

Trichilemmal cysts, formerly known as wens and pilar or sebaceous cysts, are less common than epidermal cysts, occur mainly on the scalp, usually are multiple, and show an autosomal-dominant inheritance. The sac wall is thick, smooth, and whitish and can be quite easily enucleated.

Milia are very common, white, pinhead-sized, firm lesions that are seen on the face (Fig. 16.5). They are formed by proliferation of epithelial buds following trauma to the skin (dermabrasion for acne scars), following certain dermatoses (pemphigus, epidermolysis bullosa, and acute contact dermatitis), or from no apparent cause.

Steatocystoma multiplex: A dominantly inherited condition with small, moderately firm, cystic nodules adherent to the overlying skin, which on incision yield an oily fluid.

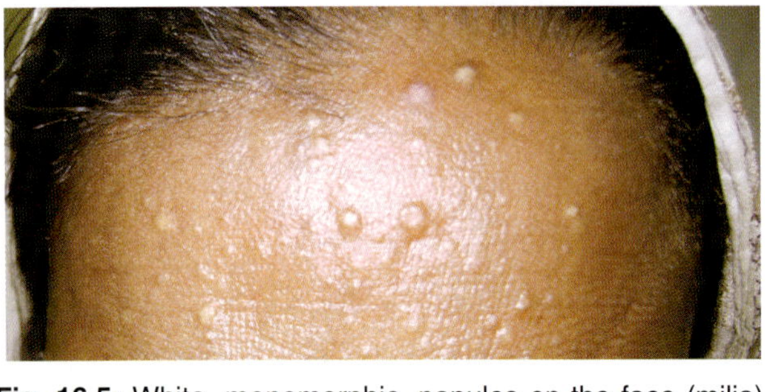

Fig. 16.5: White, monomorphic, papules on the face (milia)

Differential Diagnosis of Epidermal and Trichilemmal Cysts

- **Lipoma:** Difficult to differentiate clinically; more firm, no central pore, lobulated; no cheesy material extrudes on incision; removal is by complete excision or by liposuction; clinically similar to hibernoma.
- **Dermoid cyst:** Clinically similar; can also be found internally; usually a solitary skin tumor; histologically, contains hairs, eccrine glands, and sebaceous glands.
- **Mucous cysts:** Translucent pea-sized or smaller lesions on the lips, treated by cutting off top of the lesion and carefully lightly cauterizing the base with a silver nitrate stick or light electrosurgery; laser therapy can also be used.
- **Synovial cysts (myxoid cysts) of the skin:** Globoid, translucent, pea-sized swellings around the joints of fingers and toes that drain a syrupy clear liquid and is most common at base of nail on proximal nail fold.

Treatment of Epidermal and Trichilemmal Cysts

Several methods can be used with success. The choice depends on the ability of the operator and the site and the number of cysts. Cysts can regrow after even the best surgical care, because of incomplete removal of the sac.

Treatment of Milia

- Simple incision of the small tumors with a scalpel or a needle and expression of the contents by a comedone extractor is sufficient.
- Another procedure is to remove the top of the milia lightly with electrodesiccation.
- An 11 Bard Parker blade can be used to open the top and then an acne stylette used to express the contents.

CLEAR CELL ACANTHOMA

A rare, usually single, slightly elevated, flat, pale red, **scaling nodule** less than 2 cm in diameter, nearly always located on the lower extremities. Rare, benign tumor; mostly as single sharply demarcated, dome-shaped papule or nodule of the epidermis with a characteristic collerette of scale and a crusted surface.

WARTY DYSKERATOMA

A solitary warty lesion with a central keratotic plug, most

commonly seen on the scalp, face and neck. Histology is characteristic.

KERATOACANTHOMA

Characterized by a chronic nodule with a central crater filled with horny, hyperkeratotic material (Figs. 16.6).

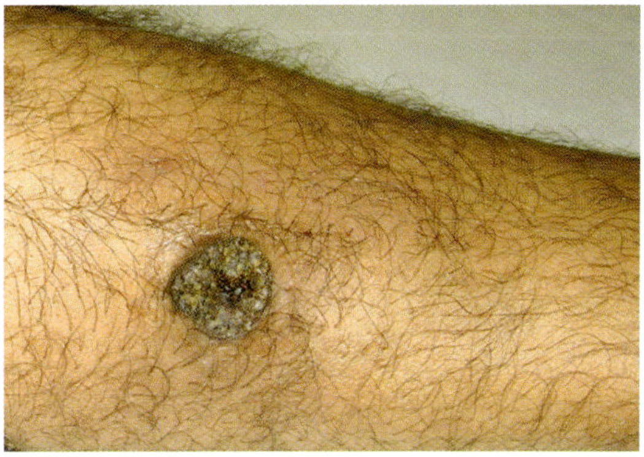

Fig. 16.6: Single nodule with central crater with horny material

PRECANCEROUS TUMORS

Precancerous types of tumors include actinic keratosis and cutaneous horn, arsenical keratosis and leukoplakia.

Arsenical Keratosis

Prolonged ingestion of inorganic arsenic (e.g., Fowler's solution, **Asiatic pills**, well water that is high in arsenic) can result in the formation many years later of small, punctate keratotic lesions, mainly seen on the palms and the soles. Progression to a squamous cell carcinoma can occur but is unusual. These patients have an increased risk of underlying solid malignancies.

Treatment

Small arsenical keratoses can be removed by electrosurgery; larger lesions can be excised and skin grafted if necessary.

Leukoplakia

A flat, whitish plaque occurs localized to the mucous membranes of lips, mouth, vulva and vagina. Single or multiple lesions may be present.

Course

Progression to squamous cell carcinoma occurs in 20% to 30% of chronic cases. Squamous cell cancer of the mucous membrane is more aggressive.

Cause

Smoking, sunlight, ethanol ingestion, chewing tobacco, snuff, and chronic irritation are the important factors in the development of leukoplakia. Recurrent actinic cheilitis may precede leukoplakia of the lips. The vulvar form may develop from presenile or senile atrophy of this area.

Differential Diagnosis

- **Lichen planus:** A lacy network of whitish lesions, mainly on the sides of the buccal cavity; when on lips, it may clinically resemble leukoplakia; lichen planus elsewhere on body; biopsy is often indicated; ulcerative lichen planus in the oral mucous membranes may have an increased risk of squamous cell carcinoma.
- **Pressure calluses from teeth or dentures:** Evidence of irritation; differentiation may be possible only by biopsy.
- **On the vulva, lichen sclerosus et atrophicus or kraurosis vulvae:** No induration, as in leukoplakia of this area; can extend onto skin of inguinal folds and perianal region; pruritus may or may not be present and can be severe with dyspareunia; biopsy is helpful; upto 5% of lichen sclerosis et atrophicus may develop a squamous cell cancer.

Treatment

- The lesion should be examined carefully. Perform a biopsy on any questionable area that shows inflammation and induration. If a squamous cell carcinoma is present, the patient should receive surgical or radiation therapy.
- Advise against use of tobacco products. The seriousness of continued smoking or other use of tobacco must be pointed out to the patient. Many early cases of leukoplakia disappear when smoking is stopped.
- Eliminate any chronic irritation from teeth or dentures.
- Protect the lips from sunlight with a sunscreen stick.
- Electrosurgery, preceded by local anesthesia, is excellent for small, persistent areas of leukoplakia. The coagulating current is effective. Healing is usually rapid. Laser therapy or a surgical lip shave are used by some dermatologists.
- Liquid nitrogen freezing is also effective.
- If alcohol abuse is present, cessation is advisable. Topical 5FU can be used.

Actinic Keratosis

Actinic keratosis is a common skin lesion of light-complexioned older persons that occurs on the skin surfaces exposed to sunlight. A small percentage of these lesions develop into squamous cell carcinomas (approximately 5-10%).

Clinical Features

Lesions are usually multiple, flat or slightly elevated, pink, brownish or tan colored, scaly and adherent, measuring up to 1.5 cm in diameter, and often arising on an ill-defined base. There is a dark variant called a superficial pigmented actinic keratosis (SPAK). Individual lesions may become confluent. A cutaneous horn may be a proliferative, hyperkeratotic form of actinic keratosis that resembles a horn. A cutaneous horn can also originate from a seborrheic keratosis, wart, squamous cell carcinoma, basal cell carcinoma, keratoacanthoma, and most commonly an actinic keratosis. If a biopsy is done, enough of the base of the lesion must be removed to obtain an accurate histologic diagnosis.

The lesion begins as a faint red, slightly scaly patch that enlarges slowly, peripherally and deeply, over many years. A sudden spurt of growth, increased thickness, or surrounding induration could indicate a change to a squamous cell carcinoma.

Treatment

Surgical Method

Liquid nitrogen, if available, applied very lightly to the lesion is an effective and rapid method of removal. This is the therapy of choice.

Curettage, followed by destruction of the base by acid or electrosurgery, is satisfactory. Local anesthesia is usually necessary. Firmly scrape the lesion with the dermal curette, which removes the mushy, scaly keratosis and exposes the more fibrous normal skin. Experience provides the necessary **"feel"** of abnormal versus normal tissue.

Medical Therapy

Fluorouracil Method

For the patient with multiple superficial actinic keratoses, fluorouracil therapy is effective and eliminates for some months or years the early damaged epidermal cells. The medication is applied twice a day for only 2 to 4 consecutive days of each week, for a total duration of 3 or 4 months of therapy. To lessen the erythema topical steroid may be needed to be applied.

Imiquimod can be used twice a day for 2 weeks or as a pulse therapy three times a week for 3 months.

EPITHELIOMAS AND CARCINOMAS

Basal Cell Carcinoma

Basal cell carcinoma is the most common malignancy of the skin fortunately, a basal cell epithelioma is almost never a metastasizing tumor, and the cure rate can be close to 100% if these lesions are treated early and adequately.

Clinical Features

There are four clinical types of basal cell carcinoma:

- Noduloulcerative.
- Pigmented.
- Fibrosing (sclerosing, morphea-like).
- Superficial spreading.

Noduloulcerative basal cell carcinoma is the *most common* type. It begins as a small waxy nodule that enlarges slowly over the years. A central depression usually forms that eventually progresses into an ulcer surrounded by a pearly or waxy border. The surface of the nodular component has a few telangiectatic vessels, which are highly characteristic. Upon stretching the skin, a gray translucent appearance may aid in diagnosis.

The pigmented type is similar to the noduloulcerative form, with the addition of brown or black pigmentation (Fig. 16.7). The pigmentation may be in the form of small (1-2 m) dots over the tumor surface.

The fibrosing type is extremely slow growing, is usually seen on the face, and consists of a whitish, scarred plaque with an ill-defined border, which rarely becomes ulcerated. This type is difficult to treat since borders are difficult to determine.

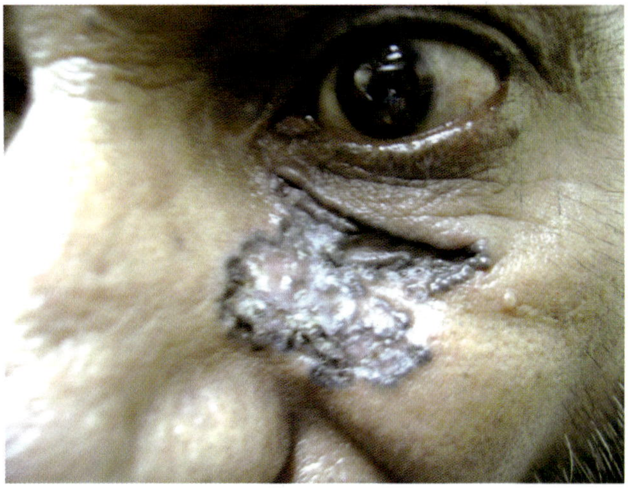

Fig. 16.7: Pigmented BCC

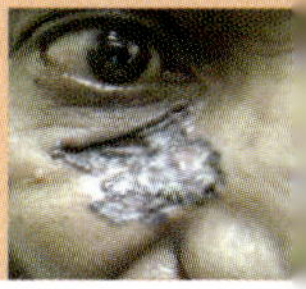

The superficial form may be single or multiple, is usually seen on the back and the chest, and is characterized by slowly enlarging red, scaly areas that, on careful examination, reveal a nodular border with telangiectatic vessels. A healed atrophic center may be present. Ulceration is superficial when it develops. The classic histology is depicted below (Fig. 16.8).

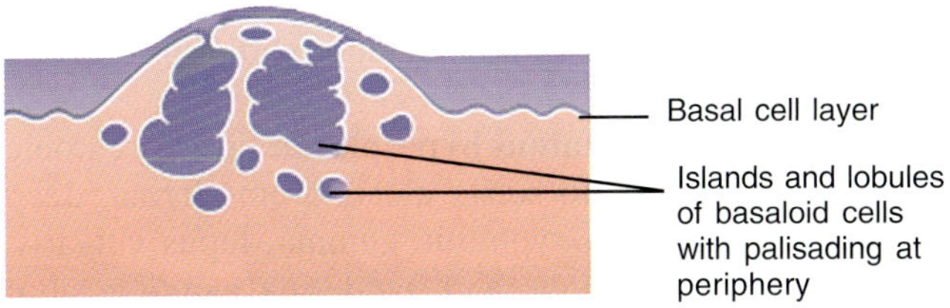

Fig. 16.8: Histology of BCC

Sites

Over 90% of the basal cell carcinomas occur on the head and the neck, with the trunk next in frequency. On the trunk and extremities the tumors may appear pink and flat without ulcerations. These tumors are rarely found on the palms or the soles.

Course

The tumor is very slow growing, but sudden rapid growth periods do occur. Bleeding is common. Destructive forms of this tumor can invade cartilage, bone, blood vessels, or large areas of skin surface and result in death. There are rare reports of metastasizing basal cell carcinomas; these are usually very large tumors.

Etiology

Basal cell carcinomas develop most frequently on the areas of the skin exposed to sunlight and in blond or red-haired persons. Trauma and overexposure to radium and X-radiation can cause basal cell carcinomas. Long-term ingestion of inorganic arsenic can lead to formation of superficial basal cell carcinomas. It can be part of the basal cell nevus syndrome. Most authors believe that a basal cell tumor is a carcinoma of the basal cells of the epidermis.

Differential Diagnosis

- **Squamous cell carcinoma:** More rapid growth, firm, scaly papule or nodule, more inflammation, no pearly telangiectatic border; biopsy is necessary.
- **Sebaceous hyperplasias:** Very common, with a central cell and fine telangiectasia, but on stretching the skin appears slightly yellow or orange and sebaceous gland lobules may be seen.
- Keratoacanthomas.
- Sebaceous adenomas.
- Large comedones.
- Warts.
- Nevi.
- Small cysts.
- Scarring from injury or radiation.

Superficial basal cell carcinomas can resemble lesions of psoriasis, seborrheic dermatitis, lupus vulgaris and Bowen's disease.

If multiple basal cell carcinomas are found, one should consider the **basal cell nevus syndrome.** This is a rare, hereditary condition characterized by multiple genetically determined basal cell carcinomas, cysts of the jaws, peculiar pits of the hands and feet, and developmental anomalies of the ribs, spine and skull.

Treatment

- Surgical excision of a basal cell carcinoma is the only method of treatment that should not be attempted by the physician who only occasionally is confronted with these tumors.
- The patient should return for a checkup on a definite schedule, such as in 4 months, then every 6 months for four visits, then yearly, for a total of 5 years. Ten-year follow-up is being suggested by some authors.
- Topical imiquimod (5% cream) is an available option for superficial lesions. Typical courses of therapy would be a thin **coat b.i.d.** Mondays, Wednesdays and Fridays for 3 months. Because of inflammation, rest periods of a week or two may have to be initiated and repeat therapy may be necessary. This is a popular treatment in superficial lesions where scarring is to be avoided.

Treatment of recurrent, deeply ulcerated, fibrosing, or large superficial basal cell carcinomas should be in the domain of the competent dermatologist, surgeon, or radiologist. **Mohs'-type surgery** for these more difficult lesions is microscopically controlled and, unless the tumor is massive, results in a very high cure rate.

SQUAMOUS CELL CARCINOMA

This rather common skin malignancy can arise primarily or from an actinic keratosis or leukoplakia. The grade of malignancy and metastasizing ability varies histologically from grade I (low, well differentiated) to grade IV (high, poor differentiated).

Clinical Features

The most common clinical feature is a rapidly growing nodule that soon develops a central ulcer and an indurated raised border with some surrounding redness. This type of lesion is the most malignant. The least malignant form has the clinical appearance of a warty, piled-up growth, which may not ulcerate. However, it is important to realize that the grade of malignancy can vary in the same tumor from one section to another, particularly in the larger lesions. This variation demonstrates the value of multiple histologic sections. The histology is given below (Fig. 16.9):

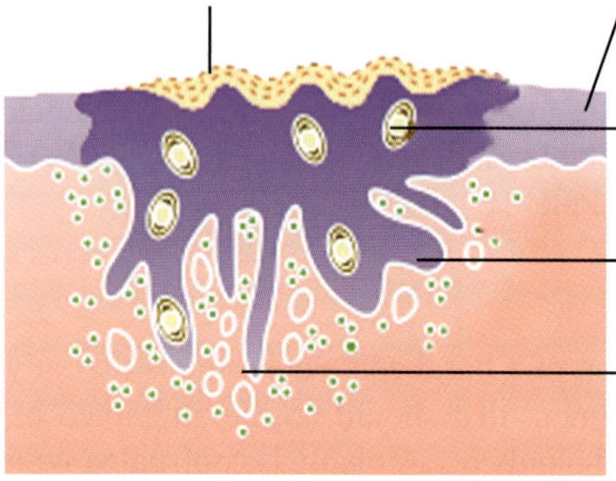

Fig. 16.9: Histology of SCC

Distribution

The lesion can occur on any area of the skin and mucous membrane but most commonly on the face, particularly the lower lip and ears, tongue, and dorsa of the hands. Chronic trauma associated with certain occupations can lead to formation of this cancer on unusual sites. Any chronic ulcer can develop a squamous cell carcinoma.

Course

The course varies with the grade of malignancy of the tumor. Lymph node metastases (4% to 5% incidence) may occur early in the development of the tumor or may never occur. The cure rate can be very high when the lesions are treated early and with the best indicated modality.

Causes

As in basal cell carcinomas, many factors contribute to provide the soil for growth of a squamous cell carcinoma.

- Hereditarily determined type of skin.
- Age of patient (elderly).
- Trauma from chemicals (tars, oils), heat, wind, sunlight, X-radiation, psoralen plus long wave ultraviolet light (PUVA) therapy and severe burns.
- Skin diseases that form scars, such as discoid lupus erythematosus, lupus vulgaris, burns (Majocchi granuloma) and chronic ulcers.
- Ingestion of inorganic arsenic.
- In the natural course of xeroderma pigmentosum.

Immunosuppressed patients, such as organ transplant patients and patients with the acquired immunodeficiency syndrome, have an increased incidence of basal cell and squamous cell carcinoma.

Differential Diagnosis

- **Basal cell carcinoma:** Slower growth, pearly border with telangiectasis, less inflammation; biopsy may be necessary to differentiate.
- **Actinic keratosis:** Slow-growing, flat, pink, constantly peeling, scaly lesions; no induration; little surrounding erythema.
- **Pseudoepitheliomatous hyperplasia:** Primary chronic lesion, such as old stasis ulcer, bromoderma, deep mycotic infection, syphilitic gumma, lupus vulgaris, basal cell carcinoma, and pyoderma gangrenosum; differentiation is often impossible clinically and very difficult histologically.
- **Keratoacanthoma:** Very fast-growing single or, more rarely, multiple lesions; clinically, this is a firm, raised, symmetric nodule with a central crater; it should be studied histologically; it may disappear spontaneously. On the other hand, a few keratoacanthomas can be highly destructive locally. Histologically, a keratoacanthoma can be difficult to distinguish from a squamous cell carcinoma. Rapid growth over days to weeks is the most distinguishing clinical characteristic.

Treatment

Because of the rapid locally invasive nature of squamous cell carcinomas, intensive surgical or radiation therapy, or both, is indicated. A discussion of such procedures is beyond the scope of this text.

Bowen's disease and erythroplasia of Queyrat: Bowen's disease is a single red scaly lesion with a sharp but irregular border that grows slowly by peripheral extension. Histologically, it is an intraepidermal squamous cell carcinoma. Erythroplasia of Queyrat represents Bowen's disease of the mucous membranes and occurs on the glans penis and rarely on the vulva. The lesion has a bright red, velvety surface.

Paget's disease: A unilateral scaly red lesion resembling a dermatitis, usually present on the female nipple, but the lesion can be extramammary. The early lesion on the nipple is an intraductal carcinoma that also involves the mammary ducts and deeper connective tissue. In the perirectal area it can be associated with underlying bowel cancer.

TUMORS OF THE EPIDERMAL APPENDAGES

Sebaceous Tumors

Nevus sebaceous (Jadassohn): Seen on the scalp or face as a single lesion present from birth, slightly raised, firm, hairless, yellowish coloured with furrowed surface. Basal

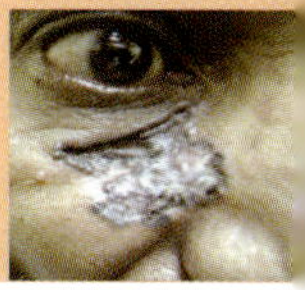

cell and squamous cell carcinomas can develop within these growths in approximately 10% of cases.

Adenoma sebaceum (Pringle's disease): Part of a triad of epilepsy, mental deficiency, and the skin lesions of adenoma sebaceum. This is called tuberous sclerosis. The skin lesions occur on the face and consist of yellowish brown, papular, nodular lesions with telangiectasia. Histopathology shows an angiofibroma.

Sebaceous hyperplasia: Very common on the face in older persons and consists of one or several small, yellowish, translucent, slightly **umbilicated nodules** (Fig. 16.10).

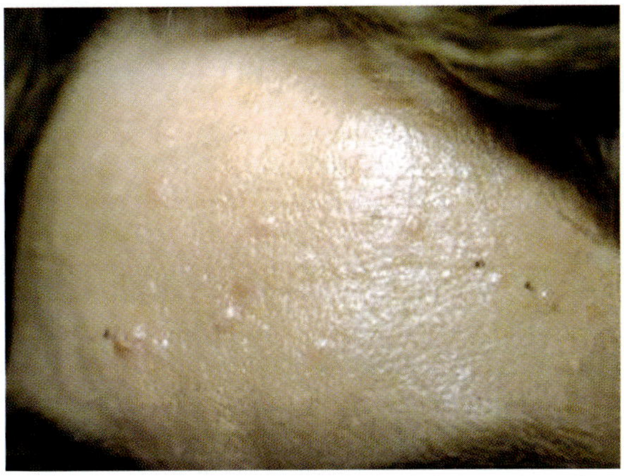

Fig. 16.10: Several small, yellowish, translucent, slightly umbilicated nodules (Sebaceous hyperplasia)

Fordyce's disease: A rather common condition of pinpoint-sized yellowish lesions of the vermilion border of the lips or the oral mucosa that represent ectopic sebaceous glands.

Sebaceous adenoma: A very rare solitary tumor of the face or the scalp, smooth, firm, elevated, often slightly pedunculated, and measuring less than 1 cm in diameter; may be associated with an adenocarcinoma of the bowel (Muir-Torre syndrome).

APOCRINE TUMORS AND ECCRINE TUMORS

- **Syringocystadenoma papilliferum:** This adenoma of the apocrine ducts appears as a single verrucous plaque, usually seen on the scalp. Basal cell epitheliomatous change occasionally does occur and may arise in sebaceous nevi.
- **Hidradenoma papilliferum:** This adenoma of the apocrine glands occurs almost exclusively on the labia majora and the perineum of women as a single, intracutaneous, benign tumor covered by normal epidermis.
- **Eccrine syringofibroadenoma (ESFA):** Solitary or multiple nodules.
  Reactive ESFA associated with inflammatory or neoplastic dermatoses usually seen on the lower extremities and easily confused with squamous cell carcinoma.
- **Syringoma:** This is characterized by the appearance of pinhead-sized soft, yellowish polygonal papules at the age of puberty in women, developing around the eyelids (Fig. 16.11).
- **Cylindroma:** These appear as numerous smooth, rounded tumors of various size on the scalp in adults and resemble bunches of grapes or tomatoes. These tumors may cover the entire scalp like a turban and are then referred to as **turban tumors**. It can be multiple and autosomal dominant with associated trichoepitheliomas and eccrine spiradenomas.

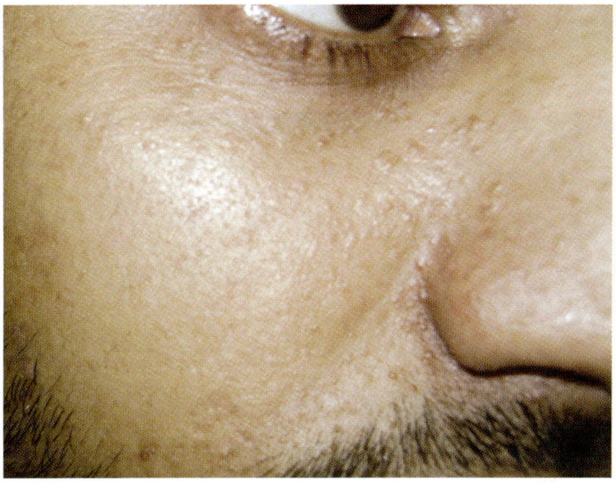

Fig. 16.11: Periocular polygonal papules

HAIR TUMORS

- **Trichoepithelioma:** Also known as epithelioma adenoides cysticum and multiple benign cystic epithelioma when multiple. This begins at the age of puberty, frequently on a hereditary basis, and is characterized by the presence of numerous pinhead to peasized, rounded, yellowish or pink nodules on the face and occasionally on the upper trunk (Fig. 16.12). May also appear as a single lesion that can be confused with a basal cell cancer histologically.
- **Calcifying epithelioma of malherbe or pilomatricoma:** Hard, nodular, nondescript 0.5 to 1.0 cm tumors especially on the scalp and face (Fig. 16.13). Malignant degeneration is very rare. There is a perforating form.
- **Microcystic adnexal carcinoma:** Relatively rare often extensive and invasive with perineural invasion. Upto 25% misdiagnosed on initial biopsy. Slow growing and 5 to 10 years follow-up is needed. Mohs surgery may be the best therapy.

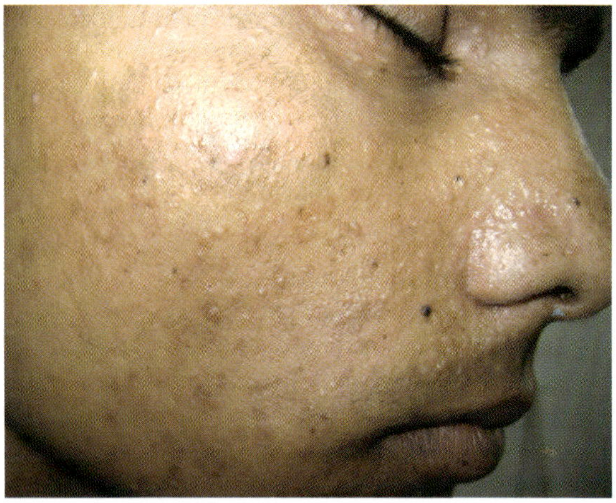

Fig. 16.12: Skin colored papules on the face and the nasolabial fold (Trichoepithelioma)

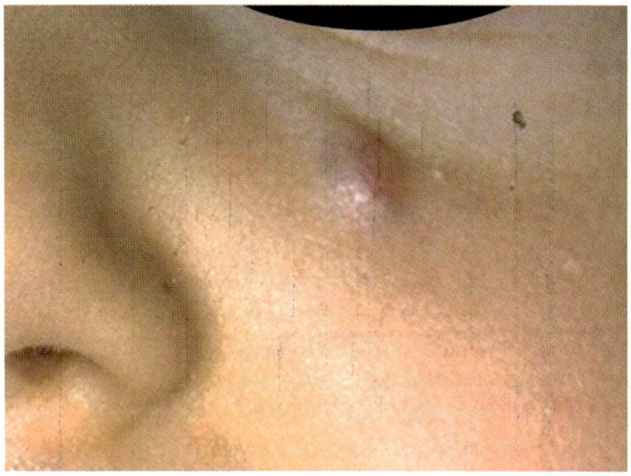

Fig. 16.13: Bluish firm nodule (Pilomatricoma)

ECCRINE TUMORS

- **Eccrine spiradenoma:** A rare, usually solitary, intradermal, firm, tender nodule.
- **Clear cell hidradenoma:** A rare, well-circumscribed, often encapsulated tumor of dermis and subcutaneous tissue.
- **Eccrine poroma:** This occurs as an asymptomatic solitary tumor on the soles and the palms.

MESODERMAL TUMORS

- Tumors of fibrous tissue.

Histiocytoma and Dermatofibroma

Histiocytomas and dermatofibromas are common, usually single, flat or only slightly elevated, reddish, or brownish nodules, less than 1 cm in size, that occur mainly on the extremities (Fig. 16.14). These tumors have a characteristic clinical appearance and firm button like feel that establishes the diagnosis. They often dimple when firm pressure is applied from both sides. They occur in adults and are nonsymptomatic and unchanging.

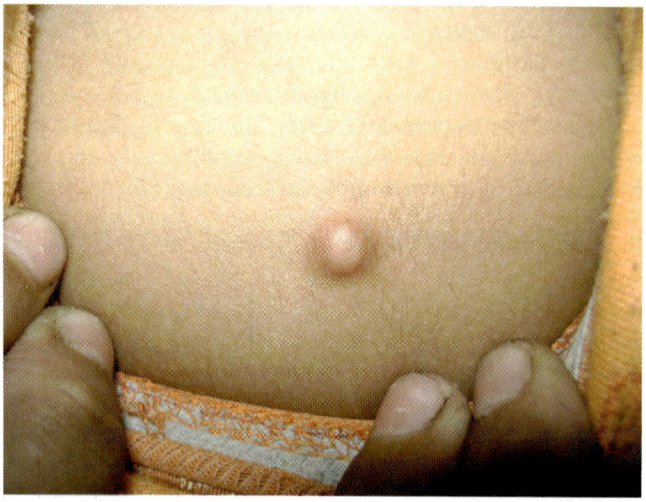

Fig. 16.14: Firm, brownish nodules on the chest (Dermatofibroma)

The histologic picture varies with the age of the lesion. The younger lesions are called histiocytomas, the older ones dermatofibromas. If the nodule contains many blood vessels, it is histologically labelled a sclerosing hemangioma.

Treatment

No treatment is indicated. If there is any doubt as to the diagnosis, surgical excision and histologic examination are indicated.

For the female patient who shaves her legs and has this lesion, liquid nitrogen applied to the papule flattens it.

Keloid

A keloid is a tumor resulting from an abnormal overgrowth of fibrous tissue following injury in certain predisposed persons (Fig. 16.15). Unusual configurations can occur, depending on the site, extent, and variety of the trauma. The back and the upper chest areas are especially prone to this proliferation.

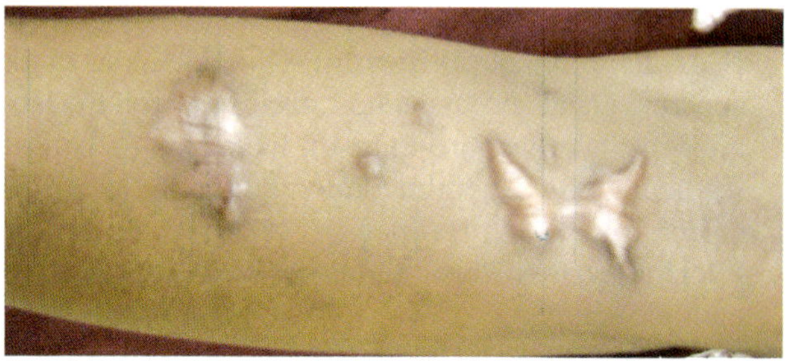

Fig. 16.15: Keloid following a trauma

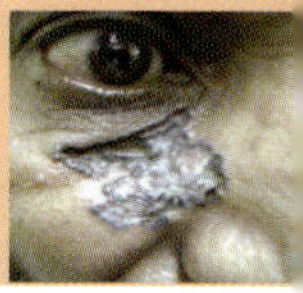

Differential Diagnosis

- **Hypertrophic sacar:** Initially same clinically and histologically as a keloid; flattens spontaneously in most cases after 1 or several years and does not extend beyond the original site of trauma.

Treatment

Therapy is unsatisfactory. Intralesional corticosteroids after cryospray or massaging with a corticosteroid ointment for 60 seconds daily after bath or shower can be tried. Occasionally, combined procedures using excision on laser and intralesional corticosteroid injections or interferon α-2b injections have been successful. Silicone sheeting therapy has its advocates. Excision should be done cautiously because recurrence of a larger tumor may occur. If removal is done, intralesional corticosteroids should be used to attempt to prevent a recurrence.

FIBROSARCOMAS

- **True fibrosarcoma:** A rare tumor that starts most commonly in the subcutaneous fat, grows rapidly, causes the overlying skin to appear purplish, and finally ulcerates.
- **Dermatofibrosarcoma protuberans:** A tumor that grows slowly in the corium and spreads by the development of adjoining reddish or bluish nodules that may coalesce to form a plaque that can eventually ulcerate. Margins are very difficult to evaluate making recurrence common. Mohs' surgery and positive CD34 immuno-histochemical staining are helpful.

TUMORS OF MUCOID TISSUE

1. **Myxoma:** Clinically seen as fairly well circumscribed, rather soft intracutaneous tumors with normal overlying epidermis.
2. **Myxosarcoma:** Subcutaneous tumors that eventually ulcerate the skin.
3. Synovial cyst of the skin.

TUMORS OF FATTY TISSUE

- **Nevus lipomatosus superficialis:** A rare, circumscribed nodular lesion, usually in the gluteal area.
- **Lipoma:** A rather common tumor that can be multiple or single, lobulated, of varying size, and in the subcutaneous tissue.
- **Hibernoma:** A form of lipoma composed of embryonic type of fat cells.
- Liposarcoma.
- Malignant hibernoma.

Tumors of Nerve Tissue and Mesodermal Nerve Sheath Cells

- **Neuroma:** Rare, single or multiple small reddish or brown nodules that are usually tender as well as painful.
- **Neurofibroma:** Benign flesh-colored soft tumor that is frequently single, but when multiple it is associated with neurofibromatosis; when very large it is called a plexiform neuroma. Can have sarcomatous degeneration.
- **Neurofibromatosis:** Also known as von Recklinghausen's disease, this hereditary disease classically consists of pigmented patches (café-au-lait spots), pedunculated skin tumors, and nerve tumors. All of these lesions may not be present in a particular case.
- Neurilemoma.
- **Granular cell schwannoma or myoblastoma:** From neural sheath cells, this appears usually as a solitary tumor of the tongue, the skin, or the subcutaneous tissue. Also, multiple, nodular, or plaque like.

TUMORS OF MUSCULAR TISSUE

- **Leiomyoma:** Solitary leiomyomas may be found on the extremities and on the scrotum, whereas multiple leiomyomas occur on the back and elsewhere as pinhead to peasized, brown or bluish, firm, elevated nodules. Both forms are painful and sensitive to pressure, particularly as they enlarge. They may have a butterfly shape.
- **Leiomyosarcoma:** Very rare.

TUMORS OF OSSEOUS TISSUE

- **Osteoma cutis.**
  Primary: The primary form of osteoma cutis develops from embryonal cell rests; these may be single or multiple.
  Secondary: Secondary bone formation may occur as a form of tissue degeneration in tumors, in scar tissue (such as acne), in scleroderma lesions (see CREST syndrome), and in various granulomas.

TUMORS OF CARTILAGINOUS TISSUE

- **Nodular chondrodermatitis of the ear:** A painful, benign, hyperkeratotic nodule, usually on the inner rim of the helix of the ear of elderly men. Trauma may be the inciting cause. Often awakens the patient at night when pressure applied. Can treat by excision or sometimes intralesional corticosteroids.

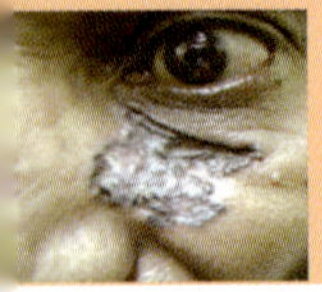

TUMORS OF VASCULAR TISSUE

1. Hemangioma.
2. **Granuloma pyogenicum:** This is a rather common (especially in pregnancy on gums) end result of an injury to the skin that may or may not have been apparent. Vascular proliferation, with or without infection, produces a small red tumor that bleeds easily. It is to be differentiated from a malignant melanoma. Biopsy and mild electrocoagulation are curative.
3. **Lymphangioma:** A superficial form, lymphangioma circumscriptum (Fig. 16.16), appears as a group of thin-walled vesicles on the skin surface, whereas the deeper variety, lymphangioma cavernosum, causes a poorly defined enlargement of the affected area, such as the lip or the tongue. Large lymphatic cisternae may underlie apparently superficial tumors.
4. **Glomus tumor:** A rather unusual small, deep-seated, red or purplish nodule that is tender and may produce severe paroxysmal pains. The solitary lesion is usually seen under a nail plate, on the fingertips, or elsewhere on the body and may erode underlying bone.
5. Hemangiopericytoma.
6. **Kaposi's sarcoma (multiple idiopathic hemorrhagic sarcoma):** Kaposi's sarcoma-associated herpes virus (HHV8) is associated with all forms. Most commonly seen on the feet and the ankles as multiple bluish red or dark brown nodules and plaques associated with visceral lesions (Fig. 16.17). It is most prevalent in elderly men of Mediterranean or Jewish origin.
7. Postmastectomy lymphangiosarcoma (Stewart-Treves syndrome).
8. **Glomangiomas:** Large dilated vessels lined with glomus cells as in a glomus tumor but are larger tumors that mimic large venous malformations clinically. Deep blue or purple, poorly compressible and usually on the face. They can be large, disfiguring, inherited as an autosomal dominant.

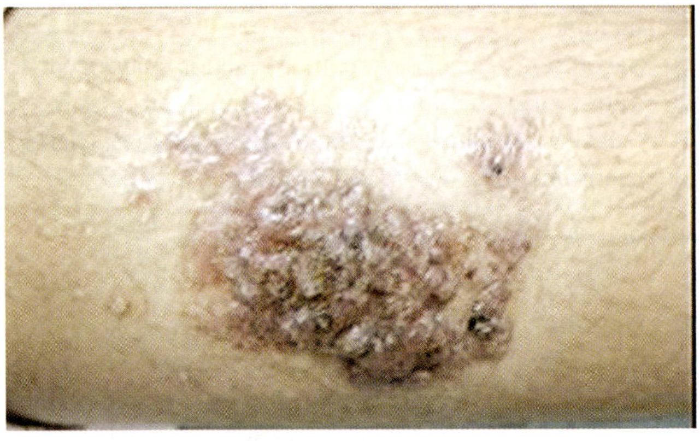

Fig. 16.16: Grouped, vesicles—skin colored to hemorrhagic—"Frog spawn appearance" (Lymphangioma)

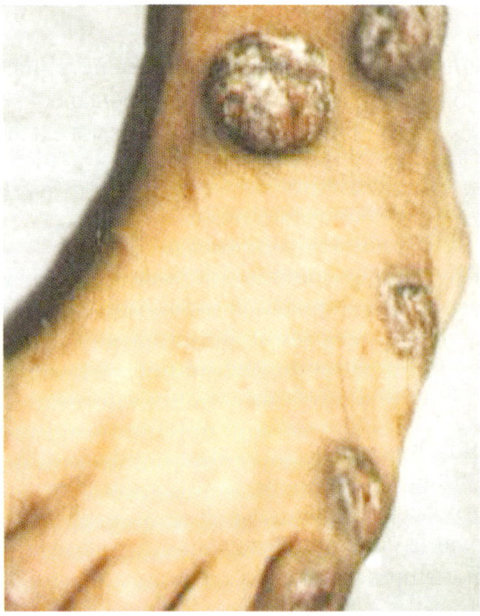

Fig. 16.17: Purplish nodules

NEVUS CELL TUMORS

Nevus cell tumors can be classified as melanocytic nevi or as malignant melanoma. Nevi, in turn are classified as (Fig. 16.18):

- Junctional or active nevus.
- Intradermal or resting nevus.
- Compound nevus.

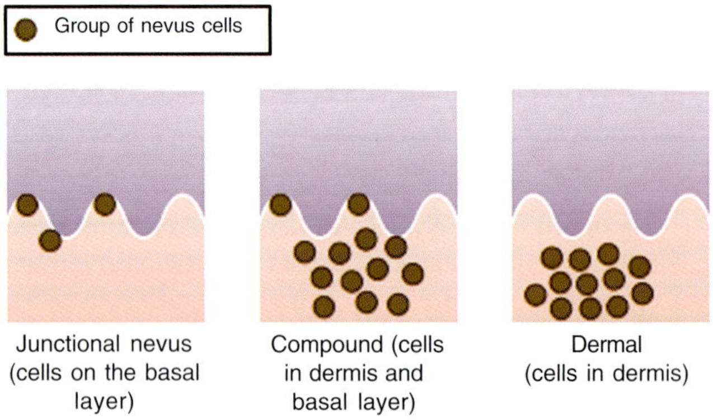

Fig. 16.18

MELANOCYTIC NEVI

Clinically, one never can be positive with which histopathologic type of nevus one is dealing, but certain criteria are helpful in establishing a differentiation between the forms.

Description

Clinically, nevi can be pigmented or nonpigmented, flat or

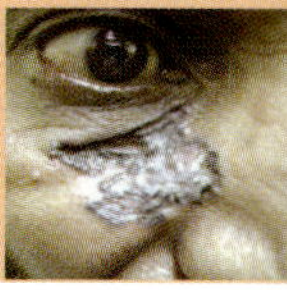

elevated, hairy or nonhairy, warty, papillomatous, or pedunculated. They can have a small or a wide base.

The brown or black-pigmented, flat or slightly elevated, nonhairy nevi are usually **junctional nevi.**

The nonpigmented or pigmented, elevated, hairy nevi are more likely to be the **intradermal nevi.**

A nevus with a depigmented area surrounding it is called a **halo nevus, Sutton's nevus or leukoderma acquisitum centrifugum** (Fig. 16.19). The nevus in the center of the halo that histologically has an inflammatory infiltrate around it usually involutes in several months in contradiction to the rarer noninflammatory halo nevus which may not involute. Excision of the halo nevus is usually not indicated unless the central nevus has the appearance of melanoma.

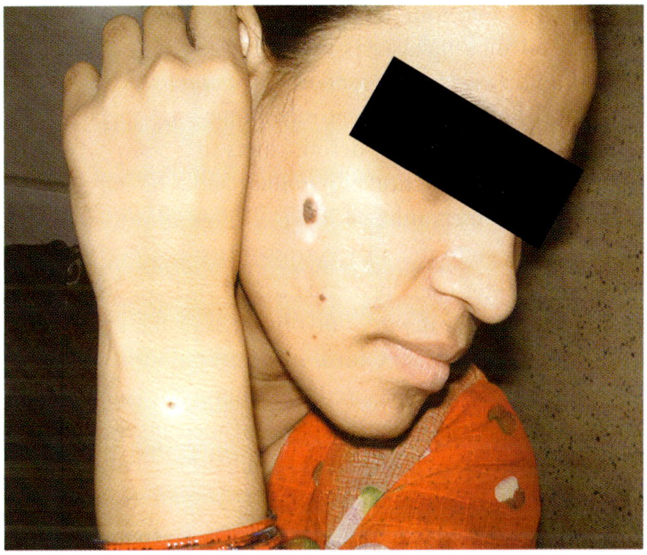

Fig. 16.19: Halo nevus

Course

A child is born with no, or relatively few, nevi, but with increasing age, particularly after puberty, nevi slowly become larger, can remain flat or become elevated, and may become hairy and darker. A change is also seen histologically with age. A junctional-type active nevus, although it may remain as such throughout the life of the person, more commonly changes slowly into an intradermal or resting nevus. Some nevi do not become evident until adult or later life, but the precursor cells for the nevus were present at birth. A malignant melanoma can originate from a junctional nevus, compound nevus, very rarely an intradermal nevus, and from dysplastic nevi, particularly in relationship to ultraviolet exposure. Most melanomas arise de novo. A benign junctional nevus in a child can histologically look like a malignant melanoma. Known as a Spitz nevus, this poses a difficult diagnostic and management problem. It is usually a dome-shaped reddish-brown tumor and rarely can occur in adults.

Treatment

- Surgical excision with tissue examination is the best method of removal. However, hairy, raised, pigmented nevi have been removed by shave excision with biopsy for years with no proof that this form of removal has caused a malignant melanoma.

First, following local anesthesia, perform a shave biopsy. Then electrosurgery can be done with the coagulating or cutting current or with cautery or applying aluminum chloride. The site should not be covered and will heal in 7 to 14 days, depending on the size. If the hairs regrow, they can be removed later by electrosurgical epilation.

Lentigines: These are to be differentiated from freckles (ephelides). A freckle histologically shows hyperpigmentation of the basal layer but no elongation of the rete pegs and no increase in the number of clear cells and dendritic cells. Juvenile lentigines (lentigo simplex) begin to appear in childhood and occur on all parts of the body.

Senile lentigines, (solar lentigo) also known as **"liver spots"**, occur in elderly persons on the dorsa of the hands, the forearms, and the face and are related to sun exposure. Solar ink-spot lentigo is commonly seen on sun-exposed areas and has a characteristic black, splotchy, reticulated pattern. **Lentigo maligna melanoma (Hutchinson's Freckle)** is a dark brown or black macular, malignant lesion, usually on the face or arms of elderly persons, that has a slow peripheral growth. Lentigines can be caused by ionizing radiation, a tanning bed, a sunlamp, PUVA therapy, and, most commonly, from sun exposure.

MALIGNANT MELANOMA

The incidence of malignant melanoma has increased considerably. Predisposing factors for the development of malignant melanoma include heredity, complexion (fair skin, red or blonde hair, blue eyes), ultraviolet exposure, and the presence of large bathing trunk congenital nevi (greater than 20 cm). The person with hereditary dysplastic nevi is more prone to develop a malignant melanoma. An appreciable percentage of melanomas arise from preexisting nevi. The incidence of malignant melanoma is increasing faster than any other cancer. The best chance for a cure lies in early diagnosis and prompt adequate treatment of the primary lesion.

Clinical Features

Sites: Skin, mucous membranes, eyes, CNS.

- Malignant characteristics of a mole include (ABCD).
  A - Asymmetry.
  B - Border (irregular).

C - Colour (varied).

D - Diameter (increasing or > 6 mm).

- Risk factors: Numerous moles, fair skin, red hair, positive family history, people who burn but do not tan, large congenital nevi, familial dysplastic nevus syndrome (100%).
- **Most common sites:** Back (M), calves (F).
- **Worse prognosis if:** Male, on scalp, hands, feet, late lesion.
- **Better prognosis if:** Pre-existing nevus present.

TYPES

There are four major types of malignant melanomas. They differ in terms of mode of onset, course, prognosis and incidence (Fig. 16.20).

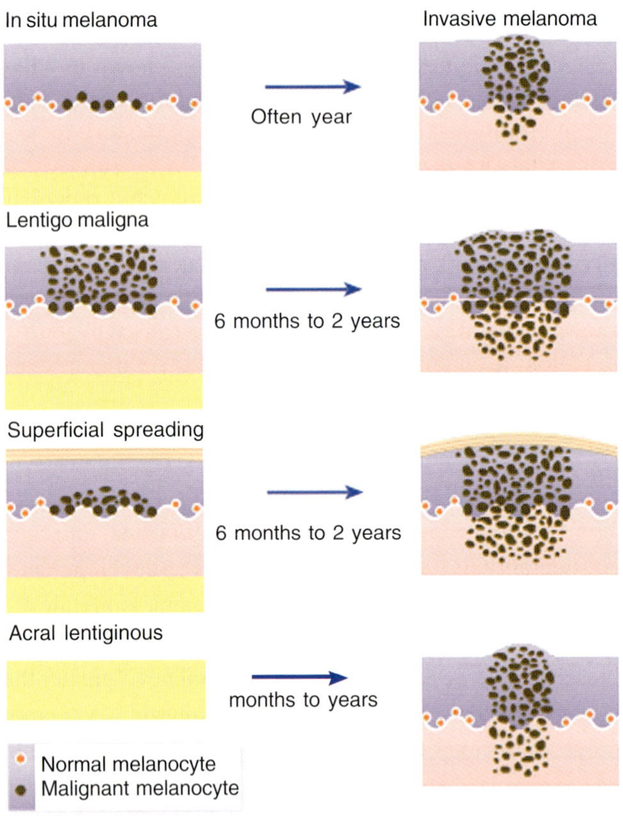

Fig. 16.20: Major types of malignant melanomas

- The most common melanoma is the **superficial spreading melanoma,** which develops from an in situ lesion. It grows slowly with a resulting good prognosis.
- **Nodular melanomas** grow quite rapidly and have a poorer prognosis.
- **Acral lentiginous melanoma**, the least frequent type, occurs, as the title signifies, on the palms, soles, and around the nails as well as perioral and perirectal; is the most common type seen in dark-skinned Caucasians; ulcerates; and metastasizes rapidly, so that it has a poor prognosis.
- **Lentigo maligna melanoma** develops from a lentigo maligna, occurs on the exposed areas of the body in the elderly, mainly on the forearms and face, grows slowly peripherally, and has a high survival rate.

Course

Classification of Invasion (Fig. 16.21): *See* Plastic Surgery Notes:

- *Breslow's Thickness of Invasion*
  1. <0.76 mm–metastasis in 0%.
  2. 0.76-1.5 mm–metastasis in 25%.
  3. 1.5-3.99 mm–metastasis in 50%.
  4. >4 mm–metastasis in 66%.
- *Clark's Levels of Cutaneous Invasion*

  Level I–above basement membrane–rare mets.

  Level II–in papillary dermis–mets in 2-5%.

  Level III–to junction of papillary and reticular dermis–mets in upto 20%.

  Level IV–into reticular dermis–mets in 40%.

  Level V–into subcutaneous tissue–mets in 70%.

The greater the depth of involvement of the growth, the worse the prognosis. **Clark** has defined five levels of invasion; **Breslow** measured the tumor thickness with a micrometer placed in the eyepiece of the microscope.

Risk groups have been defined using these measurements. For instance, a melanoma less than 0.76 mm thick and not invading the reticular dermis is in a low-risk group. Regional lymph node involvement or distant metastases gravely affect the prognosis. The most common sites of distant metastases to other organs are the *lung, liver, brain and bowel.*

Differential Diagnosis

- **Benign nevus:** No recent change in lesion, not black,

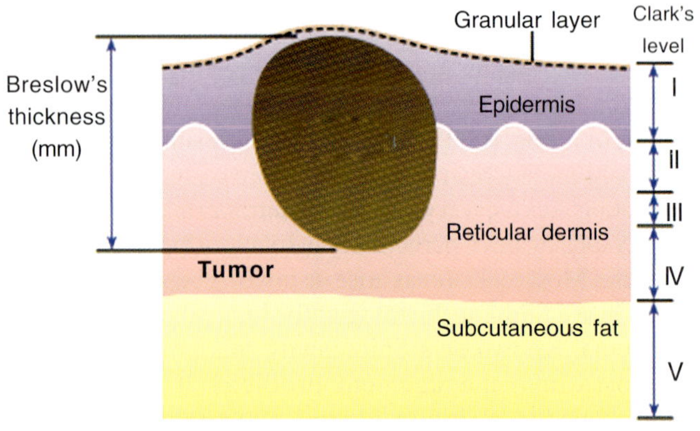

Fig. 16.21: Staging of melanoma

border smooth, single color, symmetrical, no bleeding; hairy nevi are most frequently benign, but if there is any question as to the diagnosis, a biopsy, preferably by complete excision, is indicated.

The other lesions to be thought of in the differential diagnosis are the same as under nevi (see earlier section), with the addition of a pigmented basal cell epithelioma (biopsy indicated for diagnosis) and a subungual hematoma (history of recent injury; if in doubt, perform a biopsy, especially in a light-skinned person).

Treatment

Rapid and adequate therapy is indicated after the diagnosis and staging are completed. The procedures include wide surgical excision, lymph node dissection (often involving sentinel lymph node biopsy involving gamma probe guidance as the initial step), chemotherapy and immunotherapy.

LYMPHOMAS (TABLE 16.2)

Table 16.2: Classification of lymphomas of skin

	T-cell lymphoma	*B-cell lymphoma*
Indolent	Mycosis fungoides Mycosis fungoides-associated follicular mucinosis Pagetoid reticulosis $CD30^+$ cutaneous large T-cell (anaplastic; immunoblastic; pleomorphic) Lymphomatoid papulosis	Follicle center cell lymphoma Immunocytoma (marginal zone B-cell lymphoma)
Intermediate	—	Large B-cell lymphoma of the leg
Aggressive	Sézary syndrome CD30-negative cutaneous large T-cell lymphoma (immunoblastic; pleomorphic)	—
Provisional	Granulomatous slack skin Cutaneous T-cell lymphoma, small/medium-sized Subcutaneous panniculitis-like T-cell lymphoma	Intravascular large B-cell lymphoma Plasmacytoma

Monomorphous Group

- The **non-Hodgkin's lymphomas** are referred to as monomorphous lymphomas because, in contrast to Hodgkin's disease, they lack a significant admixture of inflammatory cells and are composed almost entirely of lymphoma cells largely derived from B or T lymphocytes. A classification of cutaneous lymphomas follows.
- Lymphomas may have specific skin lesions containing the lymphomatous infiltrate, or nonspecific lesions may be seen. These latter consist of macules, papules, tumors, purpuric lesions, blisters, eczematous lesions, exfoliative dermatitis, and secondarily infected excoriations.

Polymorphous Group

- **Hodgkin's disease:** Specific lesions are very rare, but nonspecific dermatoses are commonly seen.
- **Mycosis fungoides**
  - **Sézary's syndrome:** This is a very rare form of exfoliative dermatitis that occurs at an early leukemic stage of a CTCL. It is diagnosed by finding unusually large monocytoid cells (socalled Sézary cells) in the blood and in the skin. This cell is indistinguishable from the mycosis cell, both of which are derived from the T-cell.

MYCOSIS FUNGOIDES (CUTANEOUS T-CELL LYMPHOMA)

This polymorphous lymphoma involves the skin only, except in some rare cases that terminally invade the lymph nodes and the visceral organs. As is true with most lymphomas, the histologic type may change gradually to another form of lymphoma, with progression of the disease. However, most cases of mycosis fungoides begin as such and terminate unchanged.

Mycosis fungoides is a thymus-derived (T)-helper cell lymphocyte malignancy. The name cutaneous T-cell lymphoma (CTCL) is preferred by many.

Monoclonal antibodies and gene rearrangement studies may help in the histologic diagnosis of this disease.

Associations with human T-cell lymphotrophic virus types I and II and Epstein-Barr virus are found in some patients with mycosis fungoides.

Most cases are CD_4 positive with clonal arrangements of the T-cell receptor. There is a rare, very aggressive subtype that is CD_3 positive that expresses a different T-cell receptor.

Description

The clinical picture of this disease is classic and is divided into three stages: the **erythematous stage, the plaque stage, and the tumor stage.** The course usually proceeds in order, but all stages may be evident at the same time, or the first two stages may be bypassed (the d'emblée type of mycosis fungoides).

- **Erythematous stage:** Commonly seen are scaly, red, rather sharply defined patches that resemble atopic eczema, psoriasis, or parapsoriasis. The eruption may become diffuse as an exfoliative dermatitis. Itching is usually quite severe.

- **Plaque stage:** The red scaly patches develop induration and some elevation, with central healing that result in ring-shaped lesions. This stage is to be differentiated from tertiary syphilis, psoriasis, erythema multiforme perstans, mycotic infections and other lymphomas.
- **Tumor stage:** This terminal stage is characterized by nodular and tumor growths of the plaques, often with ulceration and secondary bacterial infection. These tumors are to be differentiated from any of the granulomas, prognosis is poor.

Other Forms

1. Erythrodermic.
2. Follicular.
3. Icthyosiform.
4. Purpuric.

Course

The early stages may progress slowly, with exacerbations and remissions over many years, or the disease may be rapidly fulminating. Once the tumor stage is reached, the eventual fatal outcome is more imminent. Gene rearrangement studies may help make the diagnosis in skin lesions and may help predict the prognosis of positive lymphadenopathy.

Treatment

The combined services of a dermatologist, an oncologist, a radiologist, and a hematologist are required for the management of this sometimes fatal disease.

Topical

Locally, for early cases, a tar cream (LCD 5% in a water-washable base or in a corticosteroid cream) plus ultraviolet B therapy is quite beneficial. Local nitrogen mustard solution or ointment on the erythematous and plaque-stage lesions has proved to be effective for some cases. BCNU is also reported to be efficacious topically.

Phototherapy

PUVA therapy is also temporarily effective in resolving lesions. Narrow band UVB (311 nm) is considered to be safer by some authors and often as effective.

Systemic

Use of systemic therapy depends on the stage and extent of the disease. Most therapists believe that one should treat the symptoms and signs only as they appear.

Corticosteroids are quite helpful, especially for the first two stages.

Radiation therapy for the superficial type is effective for plaque and small tumor lesions; electron beam radiation therapy can be administered to the total body, either early or late in the disease.

Systemic chemotherapeutic agents enter into the therapy routine in the plaque and tumor stages of mycosis fungoides but are usually unsuccessful.

These include the alkylating agents cyclophosphamide, chlorambucil, and nitrogen mustard; the plant alkaloid vincristine the antimetabolite methotrexate; the antibiotic doxorubicin; and the antibiotic derivative bleomycin.

Monoclonal antibodies are also being used for therapy, as is interferon α2a.

Recent Advances

Extracorporeal photophoresis therapy and systemic retinoids are other recent therapeutic modalities. *Bexarotene* (it is an RXR receptor agonist) can be used topically and systemically. *Fludarabine* can be used systemically. Advanced recalcitrant disease can be treated with *allogenic and hematopoietic stem cell transplant*. A *recombinant fusion protein* (Ontak) can be beneficial in severe disease that is CD25 positive.

MYELOSIS

- **Leukemia:** Refers to circulating abnormal blood cells; may be seen along with lymphomas, but in skin almost always associated with myelosis, such as myeloid leukemia. Cutaneous lesions are quite uncommon but may be specific or nonspecific.

PSEUDOLYMPHOMA OF SPIEGLER-FENDT

- A benign, localized erythematous, nodular dermatosis usually on the face, with clinical and histologic features that make a distinction from lymphoma difficult. Some cases may eventually be diagnosed as a lymphoma.

HEMANGIOMAS AND MALFORMATIONS

In 1982, Mulliken and Glowacki proposed a classification system for vascular birthmarks that correlated natural history and physical examination with cellular features.

This scheme divided vascular lesions of infancy and childhood into two major types: hemangiomas, which exhibit endothelial hyperplasia malformations and malformations which have normal endothelial turnover.

Most hemangiomas of infancy are not present at birth but appear postnatally. They grow rapidly during the first year (proliferating phase), undergo slow, spontaneous regression during childhood (involuting phase), and remain stable thereafter (involuted phase). Histologically, the proliferating phase is characterized by increased mitotic activity, whereas the involuting phase is characterized by apoptosis, gradual fibrosis, and variable fatty infiltration.

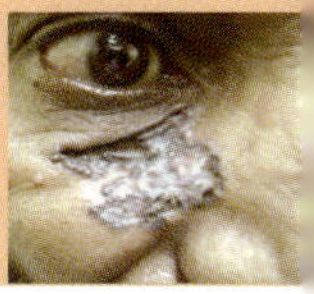

Vascular Tumors

- Hemangioma (infantile hemangioma)
  Superficial and/or deep components
  (Proliferative phase and involutional phase)
- Cherry angioma (senile angioma)
- Pyogenic granuloma
- Tufted angioma*
- Kaposiform hemangioendothelioma*
- Angiokeratoma
- Glomeruloid hemangioma
- Targetoid hemosiderotic hemangioma
- Spindle cell hemangioendothelioma
- Angiolymphoid hyperplasia with eosinophilla**
- Reactive angioendotheliomatosis†
- Bacillary angiomatosis
- Hemangiopericytoma

Vascular Malformations

Low flow
Capillary malformation (CM; portwine stain; nevus flammeus)
Venous malformation (VM)
Lymphatic malformation (LM)
Superfical/microcystic (lymphangioma circumsciptum)
Deep/macrocystic (cystic hygroma)
Combined (capillary-venous-lymphatic malformation; CVLM)
High flow
Arterial-venous fistula (AVF)
Arterial-venous malformation (AVM)
Arterial malformation (AM)

* Associated with Kasabach-Merritt syndrome.
** Associated with peripheral blood eosinophilia, enlargement of regional lymph nodes and salivary glands.
† Can be associated with paraproteinemia, cryoglobinemia, bacterial endocarditis, and atherosclerosis (diffuse dermal angiomatosis).

Malformations

Present at birth. Do not involute ('salmon' patch is exception):

1. Capillary ('salmon' patch and 'portwine' stain)
2. Arterial
3. Venous
4. Combined.

Vascular malformations are errors of morphogenesis that are presumed to occur between *the fourth and tenth weeks* of intrauterine life. Most vascular malformations are present at birth, although they may not be apparent; others do not appear until years later. Once manifest, they grow proportionately with the patient; however, rapid enlargement can occur as a result of trauma, hormonal changes (puberty, pregnancy, oral contraceptive), thrombosis, infection, or surgical intervention. Histologically, vascular malformations are characterized by dilated channels with abnormal walls lined by normal, quiescent endothelium.

Hemangiomas

Usually appear after birth. More common in females, 50-60% on head and neck. Involute by 5-9 years after initial proliferation.

1. Superficial (capillary)
2. Deep (cavernous)
3. Mixed.

This binary biologic classification has gained wide acceptance and has required only minor modifications to incorporate new information. Rather than specify all vascular birthmarks as either hemangioma or malformation, it is more appropriate to use the categorical terms vascular tumors and vascular malformations. Vascular malformations are subclassified according to the basic structural components into capillary, venous, lymphatic, arterial and combined forms. In addition, it is clinically useful to separate rheologically vascular anomalies into slow-flow (capillary, lymphatic, venous, combined) and fast-flow (arterial, combined) types. Abbreviated designations are formed by the first letter of the major anomalous channels.

MALFORMATIONS

'Salmon' Patches ('Stork bites')

These common malformations, present in about 50% of all babies, are caused by dilatated capillaries in the superficial dermis. They are dull red, often telangiectatic macules, most commonly on the nape of the neck ('erythema nuchae'), the forehead and the upper eyelids (Fig. 16.22). Nuchal lesions may remain unchanged, but patches in other areas usually disappear within a year.

'Portwine' Stains

These are also present at birth and are caused by dilatated dermal capillaries. They are pale, pink to purple macules, and vary from the barely noticeable to the grossly disfiguring. Most occur on the face or trunk . They persist, and in middle age may darken and become studded with angiomatous nodules. Occasionally a port-wine stain of the trigeminal area is associated with a vascular malformation of the leptomeninges on the same side, which may cause epilepsy or hemiparesis (**Sturge-Weber syndrome**), or with glaucoma.

Excellent results have been obtained with 585-nm flash lamp-pumped pulsed dye laser. Treatment sessions can begin in babies and anesthesia is not always necessary. If a trial patch is satisfactory, 40–50 pulses can be delivered

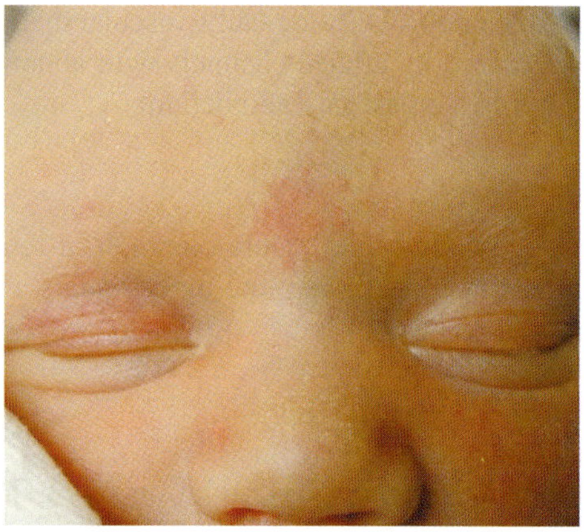

Fig. 16.22: Salmon patch on the forehead

in a session and the procedure can be repeated at 3-monthly intervals.

On the other hand, some adults become very adept at using cosmetic camouflage.

Combined Vascular Malformations of the Limbs

A large portwine stain of a limb may be associated with overgrowth of all the soft tissues of that limb with or without bony hypertrophy. There may be underlying venous malformations **(Klippel Trenaunay syndrome)**, arteriovenous fistulae **(Parkes Weber syndrome)** or mixed venous-lymphatic malformations.

Other rare syndromes are given below in Table 16.3.

Table 16.3

Syndrome/Association	*Features of vascular lesion(s)/Associated clinical features*
Kasabach-Merritt syndrome	Kaposiform hemangioendothelioma or tufted angioma; large, rapidly growing ecchymotic mass (cutaneous or retroperitoneal).
	Thrombocytopenia, microangiopathic hemolytic anemia, consumption coagulopathy (disseminated intravascular coagulation, DIC); occurs primarily in infants: 20-40% mortality.
Diffuse neonatal hemangiomatosis	Multiple small cutaneous hemangiomas+visceral hemangiomas (most often of the liver).
	Hepatomegaly, anemia, high-output cardiac failure.
Airway hemangiomas	Hemangiomas in 'beard' distribution. Large cervicofacial hemangiomas.
PHACES syndrome	Hoarseness, stridor, respiratory failure posterior fossa malformations; Hemangiomas; Arterial, Cardiac, and/or Eye anomalies; Sternal/abdominal clefting or ectopia **cordis.**
Spinal dysraphism, and/or urogenital anomalies	Hemangiomas in a lumbosacral distribution*. Cherry angiomas, glomeruloid hemangiomas.
POEMS syndrome	Polyneuropathy, Organomegaly, Endocrinopathy, M-protein (monoclonal gammopathy), skin changes; diffuse hyperpigmentation, edema, sclerodermoid changes.
Sturge-Weber syndrome (encephalotrigeminal angiomatosis)	Facial CM in V1 (+/-V2, V3) dermatomal distribution (un-> bilateral) + ipsilateral leptomeningeal vascular malformation +/- choroidal vascular malformation.
	Seizures, mental retardation, contralateral hemiplegia/hemiatrophy of the body, ipsilateral glaucoma, ipsilateral facial soft tissue/bony hypertrophy: pathognomonic radiographic feature of 'tram-track' cerebral gyral calcifications.
Bonnet-Dechaume-Blanc syndrome	Facial CM+ ipsilateral AVM of the retina and intracranial optic pathway.
Wyburn-Mason syndrome	Ipsilateral visual impairment, various contralateral neurologic manifestations.
von Hippel-Lindau syndrome	CM of head and neck.

Contd.

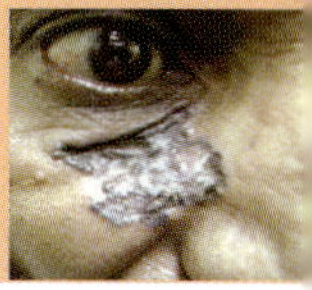

Contd.

	AD inheritance; skin findings in 5%; retinal and CNS (posterior fossa, spine) hemangioblastoma, renal cell carcinoma, pheochromocytoma, renal and pancreatic cysts, polycythemia.
Kippel-Trenaunay syndrome (angioosteohypertrophy syndrome)	CVM/CVLM of lower extremity (95%)>> upper extremity> trunk; 85% unilateral.
	Soft tissue/bony hypertrophy of affected limb(s) (occasionally atrophy), venous ulcers, lymphedema, phleboliths, occasionally gastrointestinal bleeding or hematuria.
Parkes Weber syndrome	Variant of Klippel-Trenaunay syndrome with clinically significant AVF.
	As above, but often with more progressive deformity over time.
Cutis marmorata telangiectasia congenita (CMTC)	Localized, segmental or generalized reticulated vascular network on extremities>trunk>face,+/- CM, +/- cutaneous atrophy.
	Atrophy or hypertrophy of affected limb/limb-length discrepancy, glaucoma, mental retardation; aplasia cutis+transverse limb defects (Adams-Oliver syndrome); macrocephaly + syndactyly+joint laxity+CM of philtrum (macrocephaly-CMTC).
Phakomatosis pigmentovascularis	CM.
	Epidermal nevus, dermal melanocytosis and/or speckled lentiginous nevus (nevus spilus) +/-nevus anemicus; may have systemic features of Sturge-Weber syndrome, Klippel-Trenaunay syndrome or nevus of Ota.
Blue rubber bleb nevus syndrome	Multiple VM of skin, gastrointestinal tract> other organ systems.
	Gastrointestinal bleeding, anemia.
Maffucci syndrome	Multiple VM/VLM, most often of distal extremities; spindle cell hemangioendothelioma.
	Multiple enchondromas of long bones (most often the metacarpals and phalanges of the hands), chondrosarcoma (15-30%), skeletal deformities, short stature.
Proteus syndrome	CM/LM/CVM/CLM, most often of extremities. Asymmetric soft tissue/body hypertrophy, macrodactyly, cerebriform hyperplasia of soles>palms, macrocephaly, lipomas/regional absence of fat, epidermal nevi.
Gorham syndrome	Multiple CVLM/LM of the skin, mediastinum and bones.
	Massive osteolysis/'disappearing bones', skeletal deformities, pathologic fractures, pulmonary and neurologic complications.
Bannayan-Riley-Ruvalcaba syndrome	Multiple CM/VM.
	AD inheritance, allelic with Cowden syndrome; macrocephaly, multiple lipomas, mental retardation, pigmented macules of the penis, intestinal hamartomatous polyps.
Cobb syndrome (cutaneomeningospinal angiomatosis)	CM/LM/angiokeratomas in a dermatomal distribution+vascular malformation in the corresponding segment of the spinal cord.
	Neurologic manifestations of spinal cord compression, kyphoscoliosis.
Fabry disease	Angiokeratoma corporis diffusum—small dark red papules symmetrically in a 'bathing trunk' distribution, +/-mucosal involvement.

Contd.

Contd.

	X-linked recessive lysosomal storage disease due to α-galactosidase A deficiency; acral paresthesias, painful crises, hypohidrosis, whorl-like corneal and lenticular opacities, progressive renal and coronary artery disease, cerebrovascular accidents.
Fucosidosis	Angiokeratoma coporis diffusum (as described above). AR lysosomal storage disease due to α-L-fucosidase deficiency; mental retardation, spastic paresis, seizures, recurrent sinus and pulmonary infections.

HEMANGIOMA OF INFANCY

Hemangioma is the **most common** tumor of infancy. Hemangiomas develop in premature infants weighing between 1500 and 2500 g at a frequency equal to that in full-term babies, whereas 23 percent of premature infants weighing less than 1000 g manifest a hemangioma. **Females** are affected more commonly than males in a 3:1 ratio. Approximately 30 percent of hemangiomas are nascent at birth; two-thirds become apparent during the first to fourth weeks of life (Fig. 16.23).

The hemangioma's initial **proliferative phase** (Fig. 16.23) of rapid postnatal growth lasts for 3 to 9 months; rarely beyond 18 months.

The phase of **involution** occurs gradually over 2 to 6 years and is complete by the age of 7 to 10 years.

The initial signs of a nascent hemangioma can be a hypopigmented blanched macule with or without telangiectasia (similar in appearance to a nevus anemicus) or an erythematous to ecchymotic patch that is superficial, often with an irregular surface and borders (Fig. 16.24). Several large draining veins typically radiate from the tumor.

Eighty percent of affected infants have a single lesion, most commonly located on the head and neck (60 percent), followed by the trunk (25 percent), and the extremities (15 percent). Multiple hemangiomas occur in 20 percent of affected infants. Often these cutaneous tumors are tiny, dome-shaped lesions associated with hemangiomas in visceral organs such as the liver.

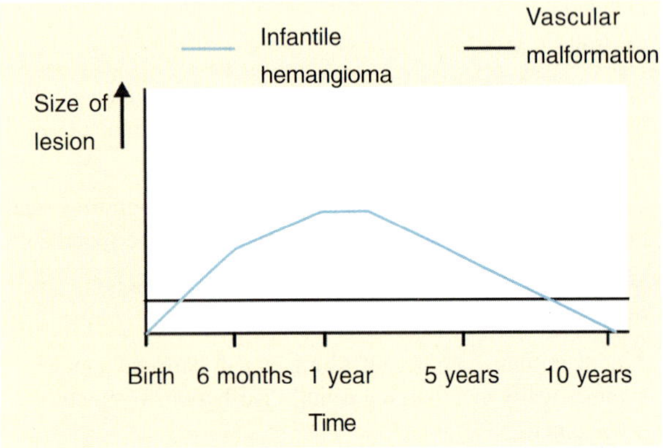

Fig. 16.23: Course and evolution of vascular tumor

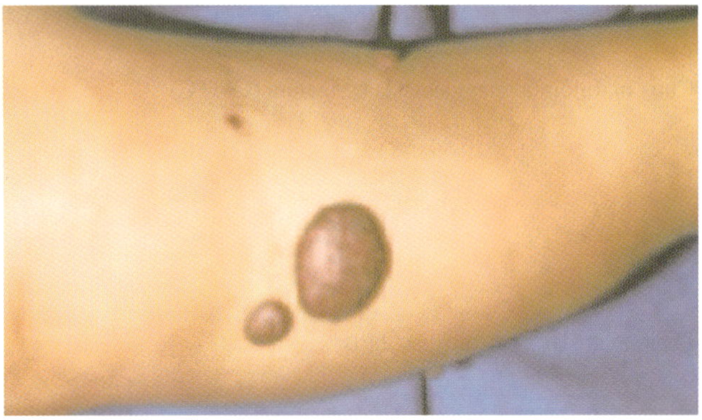

Fig. 16.24: Superficial hemangioma

Atypical Presentations

There are several unusual presentations, including deep (subcutaneous) hemangioma, telangiectatic hemangioma, arteriovenous malformation (AVM)-like hemangioma, multiple cutaneous hemangiomas, and congenital hemangioma.

Deep hemangioma (Fig. 16.25)**:** Deep hemangiomas (old term, cavernous hemangioma) proliferate in the lower dermis and subcutaneous tissue without penetration of the papillary dermis. They present as a localized, firm, rubbery subcutaneous mass that can be slightly raised with a bluish color or with telangiectasias involving the overlying skin, or they may be deep enough that the overlying skin is completely flat and of normal hue.

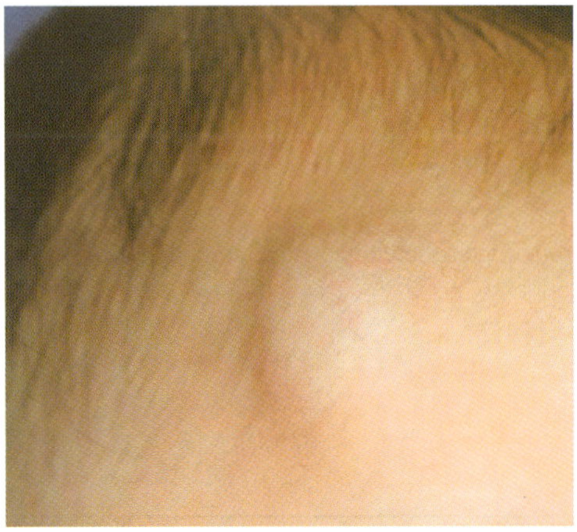

Fig. 16.25: Deep hemangioma

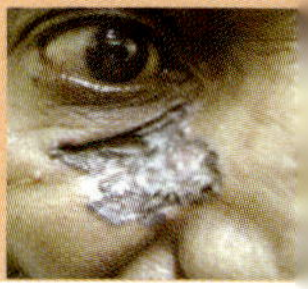

Associated Structural Anomalies

PHACE syndrome: Posterior fossa malformations, hemangioma (especially a segmental lesion), arterial abnormalities, coarctation of the aorta, and eye abnormalities. Lumbosacral hemangiomas may signal the presence of spinal dysraphism and should be evaluated by magnetic resonance imaging (MRI). These hemangiomas are often clinically distinctive, being telangiectatic, macular, or diffuse, sometimes with an acrochordon. Pelvic and perineal hemangiomas may be associated with urogenital and anorectal anomalies (e.g., anterior or vestibular anus, hemiclitoris, atrophy or absence of the labia minora and hypospadias).

Complications

- Bleeding.
- Ulceration.
- Infection.
- Airway obstruction.
- Feeding difficulty.

Treatment

The treatment of hemangiomas that are not of the obstructive type has been the subject of considerable discussion. To begin with, the size, depth, and location of the hemangiomas, and the pressure on the physician from parents and relatives, are factors that must be considered in every case.

There are those who favor treating almost every superficial or cavernous hemangioma, and there are others who believe that all hemangiomas should be left alone to involute spontaneously. It has been showed that around 85% of hemangiomas disappeared without any appreciable scar by the age of 7 years. They also found that the hemangiomas usually stopped growing by the age of 1 year.

To summarize, the advantages of **early treatment** of small superficial or cavernous hemangiomas are as follows:

1. The lesion is eliminated completely, or almost completely.
2. It is not left to chance the fact that it might or might not enlarge considerably.
3. Apprehension on the part of the parents and relatives regarding the course of the lesion is alleviated; and
4. With properly applied cryotherapy no mark is left, or only a slight one that would be no worse than that resulting from leaving the hemangioma alone.

The advantages of **not treating** one of these hemangiomas are as follows:

- The residuum after 5 to 7 years may be better cosmetically than if the lesion had been treated.
- The cost of therapy and trauma to the patient is saved.

Therapy

Treatment is probably indicated in about 25 percent of hemangiomas—the 5 percent that ulcerate; the 20 percent that compress, distort, or obstruct vital structures such as the eyes, nose, ears, or larynx; and the less than 1 percent of truly life-threatening tumors.

Intralesional glucocorticoids can be used for small hemangiomas (1 to 2 cm) localized to critical sites such as the lip, nasal tip, cheek, or ear. Triamcinolone is injected slowly (dose of 3 to 5 mg/kg every 4 to 6 weeks) for 1 to 5 total injections. Injection into an upper eyelid hemangioma carries a slight risk of retrobulbar hematoma, and there are two case reports of microvascular embolism causing blindness due to occlusion of the central retinal artery.

The high-potency topical steroid clobetasol propionate may be used to treat small superficial lesions.

Indications

1. Around eyelids.
2. Around larynx/Airway.
3. Other vital structures.
4. Ulceration.

Systemic glucocorticoids are the first-line pharmacologic treatment for deforming, endangering, or life-threatening hemangiomas. Prednisone or prednisolone is given at a dose of *2 to 3 mg/kg per day for 4 to 6 weeks*, after which time the dosage is tapered gradually for several months. If the drug dosage is lowered or stopped before the age of *8 to 10 months*, rebound growth often occurs. The response to oral glucocorticoids is excellent, with approximately 84 percent showing accelerated involution or cessation of growth (response rate) with a mean prednisone equivalent daily dose of 2.9 mg/kg given over 1.8 months. The optimal dosage is controversial. Response is 75 percent with a dosage of prednisone between 2 and 3 mg/kg per day, whereas a dosage higher than 3 mg/kg results in a response as high as 94 percent but greater adverse effects. Dosages lower than 2 mg/kg per day result in a 69 percent response rate, but the rebound rate (enlargement after tapering response occurred) is 70 percent. If there *is no response after 2 to 3 weeks* of therapy, the tumor is unlikely to respond to a higher dose, and the glucocorticoids should be discontinued.

Interferon-α2a and -2b are indicated in the treatment of endangering and life-threatening hemangiomas, specifically for tumors unresponsive to glucocorticoids. The drug is given subcutaneously at a dose of 3 million U/ml twice daily for 6 to 12 months. Side effects include transient fever, neutropenia, and minor elevations in liver enzymes.

Laser therapy: Treatment of hemangiomas with the flash-lamp pulsed-dye laser has been a subject of considerable controversy over the past decade. This laser uses a wavelength of 585 nm, specific for the absorption of oxyhemoglobin, the treatment target. In addition, the pulse duration is extremely short (400 ms), allowing for effective coagulation of vessels without extensive thermal diffusion to surrounding tissue that could result in scarring.

Surgical therapy: Surgical resection may be indicated at any time during the life cycle of a hemangioma. Excision is often necessary for fibrofatty tissue and abnormal skin after involution (when the child is 8 to 12 years old). Surgical intervention in early childhood should be considered for special situations.

ULCERATION (Fig. 16.26)

It is managed with gentle cleansing and application of topical antibiotics and barrier creams. Biocclusive dressings may be helpful, especially in the anogenital area, where the tumor is frequently contaminated. Systemic antibiotics are used for infection. Other modalities for treatment of ulcerated hemangioma include intralesional and systemic corticosteroids, excision, and interferon-α. Pain may be controlled with topical lidocaine ointment and oral acetominophen with or without codeine. Ulcerations generally heal within 2 to 3 weeks with topical care, leaving a scar.

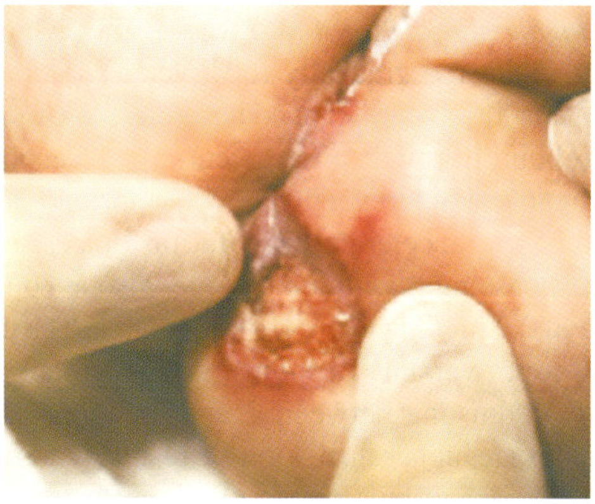

Fig. 16.26: Ulcerated hemangioma

MISCELLANEOUS

Cherry hemangiomas are also called senile hemangiomas. These pinhead-sized or slightly larger, bright red, flat or raised tumors are present in many young adults and in practically all elderly persons. They cause no disability except when they are injured and bleed. They tend to be inherited. Treatment is usually not desired, but if it is, light electrosurgery or laser is effective.

Venous Lake

Another vascular lesion that occurs in older persons is a venous lake. Clinically, it is a soft, compressible, flat or slightly elevated, bluish-red, 3 to 6 mm lesion, usually located on the lips or the ears. Lack of induration and rapid growth distinguish it from a melanoma. Lack of pulsation distinguishes a venous lake on the lower lip from a tortuous segment of the inferior labial artery.

Treatment is usually not desired, only reassurance concerning its nonmalignant nature.

Angiokeratomas

Three forms of angiokeratoma are known:

- Mibelli's form occurs on the dorsa of the fingers, the toes and the knees;
- Fabry's form occurs over the entire trunk in an extensive pattern; and
- The Fordyce form occurs on the scrotum.

The lesions are dark-red, pinhead-sized papules with a somewhat warty appearance. Treatment is not indicated for Mibelli form and the Fordyce form. The Fabry form (angiokeratoma corporis diffusum), however, is the cutaneous manifestation of a systemic phospholipid storage disease in which phospholipids are deposited in the skin, as well as in various internal organs. Death usually occurs in the fifth decade from the result of such deposits in the smooth muscles of the blood vessels, in the heart, and in the kidneys.

REFERENCES

- Barnhill RL: Color atlas and synopsis of pigmented lesions, New York, McGraw-Hill, 1995.
- Bernstein SC, Lim KK, Brodland DG, *et al.:* The many faces of squamous cell carcinoma, Dermatol Surg 1996;22:243.
- Bowers RE, Graham EA, Tomlinson KM: The natural history of the strawberry nevus, Arch Dermatol 1960;82:667.
- Dalton JA, *et al.:* Cutaneous T-cell lymphoma, Int J Dermatol 1997;36:801.
- Drake LA, Ceilley RI, *et al.:* Guidelines of care for actinic keratoses, J Am Acad Dermatol 1995;32:1.
- Drake LA, Salasche SJ, Ceilley RI, *et al.:* Guidelines of care for basal cell carcinoma, J Am Acad Dermatol 1992; 26:117.
- Drake LA, Ceilley RI, *et al.:* Guidelines of care for nevi: II. Nonmelanocytic nevi, hamartomas, neoplasms and potentially malignant lesions, J Am Acad Dermatol 1995;32:1.
- Drake LA, Chanco Turner ML, Ceilley RI, *et al.:* Guidelines of care for malignant melanoma. J Am Acad Dermatol 1993;28:638.
- Drake LA, Salasche S, Ceilley RI, *et al.*: Guidelines of care for cutaneous squamous cell carcinoma, J Am Acad Dermatol 1993;28:628.
- Lever WF, Schaumburg-Lever G: Histopathology of the skin, 8th edn., Philadelphia, JB Lippincott, 1997.
- Zackheim HS: Cutaneous T-cell lymphoma, mycosis fungoides and Sézary syndrome, Boca Raton, FL, CRC Press, 2005.

CHAPTER 17

DISORDERS OF THE MUCOSA (ORAL AND GENITAL)

DISEASES OF THE MUCOUS MEMBRANES

Mucous membranes are covered with a modified stratified squamous epithelium that lacks a stratum corneum. This makes them moist and susceptible to infection, and to conditions not seen elsewhere.

A brief overview of common conditions is given below:

Condition	*Cause*	*Treatment*
Black hairy tongue	Pigmentation and hypertrophy of filiform papillae caused due to bacterial overgrowth	Brush the tongue
Fissured tongue	Congenital, Down's syndrome, ageing changes	No treatment needed
Furred tongue	Hypertrophy of the filiform papillae	Brush the tongue
Geographic tongue	Familial, atopic, psoriasis, reiters	Topical steroids
Glossodynia	Trauma, candida, menopause, diabetes, nutritional, dry mouth	Treat the cause, use tricyclic antidepressants
Hairy leukoplakia	Epstein-Barr virus infection in patients with HIV/AIDS	Highly active anti retroviral therapy (HAART)
Herpetic glossitis	Painful fissures without vesicles	Acyclovir group
Macroglossia	Developmental, tumours, infections, amyloidosis, thyroid	Treat the cause
Median rhomboid glossitis	Developmental defect and candidiasis Smoking and dentures worsen	No treatment needed
Smooth tongue	Nutritional deficiency, sprue, malabsorption	Vitamins, nutrition
Varices	Blue compressible blebs of veins	No treatment needed

GEOGRAPHIC TONGUE

Geographic tongue is an extremely common condition of the tongue that usually occurs without symptoms. When these lesions are noticed for the first time by the individual, they may initiate fears of cancer.

Clinical Features (Fig. 17.1)

Irregularly shaped (map-like or geographic) pale-red patches are seen on the tongue. Close examination reveals that the filiform papillae are flatter or denuded in these areas. The patches slowly migrate over the tongue surface and heal without scarring.

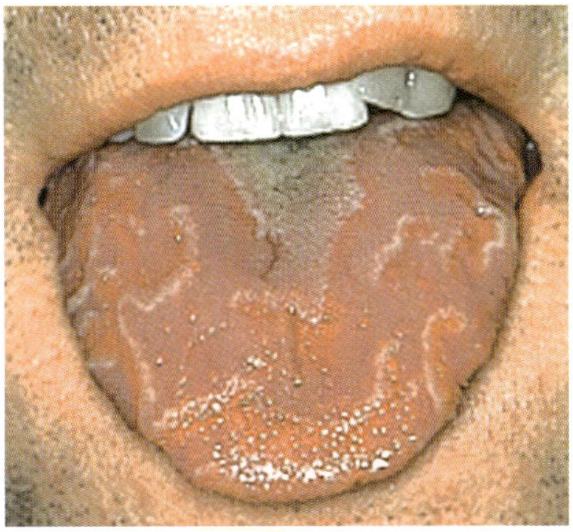

Fig. 17.1: Geographic tongue

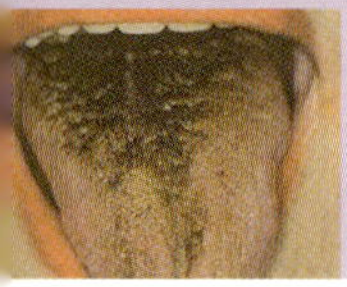

The cause is unknown, but the lesions seem to be more extensive during a systemic illness. It has been suggested by some authors that the geographic tongue is a form of psoriasis.

Treatment

- Reassure patient that these are not cancerous lesions.
- There is no effective or necessary therapy. However, if patient complains of burning and tenderness, prescribe Triamcinolone in Orabase.

FORDYCE'S SPOTS

This is a physiologic variant of oral sebaceous glands in which more than the normal number exist. When they are suddenly noticed, the person becomes concerned as to the diagnosis. The lesions are asymptomatic, yellowish-orange, 1- to 2-mm papules on the lips and labia minora and glans penis. No treatment is necessary; they are benign.

CONTACT STOMATITIS (Fig. 17.2)

This underdiagnosed problem usually causes a transient soreness, associated with a diffuse redness of the lips and buccal gingivae.

Mouthwashes, hard sweets (candies) and hot pizzas are common causes of the irritant type, whereas cinnamon, vanilla, peppermint, spearmint and dentifrices are the most common causes of allergic contact stomatitis.

When local stomatitis or ulcers occur near a gold tooth filling, gold allergy should be suspected, but patch testing is needed before recommending that the filling should be removed.

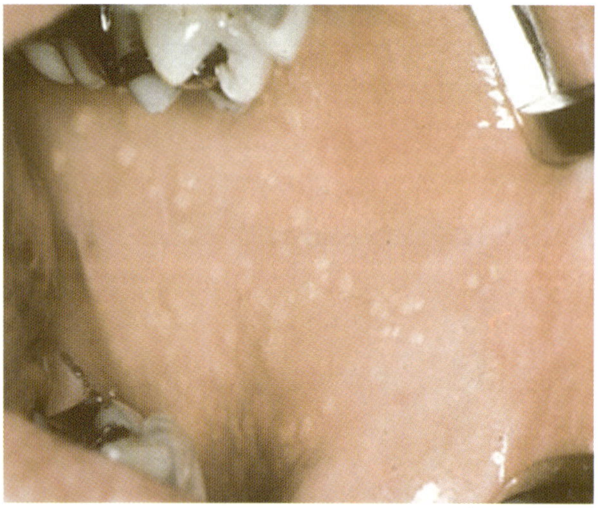

Fig. 17.2: Contact stomatitis

BULLOUS DISEASES

Pemphigus causes large painful long-lasting erosions. The whole mouth can be involved, but more often it affects just the lips and buccal mucosa.

Desquamative gingivitis can occur. The ulcers are large, appear without warning and last months. A biopsy may show an intraepithelial acantholysis and should not be taken from an ulcer, but from normal-appearing mucosa in an active area. Direct immunofluorescence (biopsy normal mucosa) shows antibody rimming each keratinocyte.

Cicatricial (scarring) pemphigoid affects the mucous membranes predominantly, but occasionally affects the skin too. The eyelid conjunctiva and other mucosae can also be affected; scarring often results. Cicatricial pemphigoid is also a cause of desquamative gingivitis. Biopsy shows a subepidermal bulla, and direct immunofluorescence a linear band of IgG and C3 at the dermal-mucosal junction.

APHTHOUS STOMATITIS

Factors associated with RAS (Recurrent Aphthous Stomatitis)
Local
Oral trauma (biting, tooth brushing)
Microbial
Various viruses
***Genetic**
Nutritional
Vitamin deficiencies (B vitamins, Fe, Zn) Food allergies
Tobacco Use (Inverse Relationship)
Stress
Endocrine
Hematological
*Most likely cause

Clinical Characteristics (Fig. 17.3)

The clinical characteristics of RAS are important since no specific diagnostic test is available. The major characteristics of RAS are a recurrence of one or more painful ulcers at intervals of days to months. Approximately 10% of patients record monthly recurrences, but most sufferers report three or four episodes of new lesions per year.

The ulcers are almost always located on the non-keratinized mucosa of the mouth, which may include the buccal mucosa, the floor of the mouth, and the bottom surface of the tongue.

Clinicians tend to divide RAS into three clinically distinct groups. The three groups consist of minor, major and herpetiform lesions. The clinical characteristics of each type of RAS lesion is summarized:

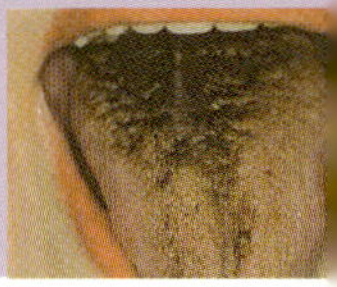

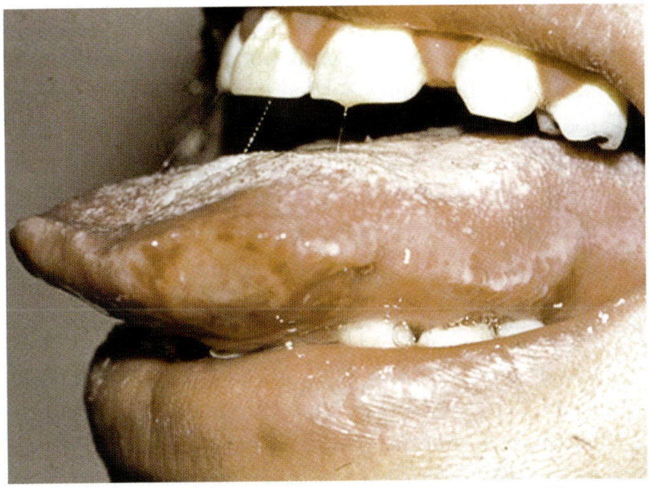

Fig. 17.3: Aphthous ulcer

RAS classification			
Characteristics	*Minor (Mikulicz)*	*Major (Sutton's)*	*Herpetiform*
Percentage of RAS case	70-87%	7-20%	7-10%
Total lesions per occurrence	1-5	1-10	< 150
Size (diameter) of lesions	<1cm	>1cm	1-2 mm
Lesion morphology	Shallow, with raised, oval border	Deeper may be irregular	Shallow, round, coalesce together
Time to heal completely	7-14 days	Upto 6 weeks	7-10 days
Scars upon healing	No	Yes	No

SPECIFIC INVESTIGATIONS

- Complete blood count.
- Vitamin B_1, B_2, B_6 and B_{12}, folate, zinc, and iron levels.
- Culture/polymerase chain reaction of aphthae to exclude herpes simplex virus (HSV).

Management

Because there is no definitive treatment, the emphasis is on measures that may afford symptomatic relief. These include application of *topical anaesthetics* such as *lidocaine, narcotics, sucralfate suspension,* 0.2% *chlorhexidine gluconate* mouthwash, *tetracycline* suspension 250 mg/5 ml.

Topical corticosteroids are the mainstay of therapy. For milder disease, intermediate strength corticosteroids such as *fluocinonide* are used. Potent corticosteroids such as *clobetasol* or *halobetasol* are appropriate for more severe episodes. Applications can be as frequent as five to ten times daily. Gel or ointment formulations are preferable. These can be applied in equal parts with an occlusive dressing such as Ora base for better adherence. *Intralesional triamcinolone acetonide* are helpful for major aphthae. Initial concentrations of 5-10 mg/mL are used which may be increased upto 40 mg/mL. Repeat injections over 2-4 week intervals are advised.

RAS that elicits severe pain may require intermittent *systemic corticosteroid therapy.* Prednisone can be given 40-60 mg daily with a 2-week taper or as 'burst therapy' for shorter periods.

Concomitant therapy with topical corticosteroids may be helpful.

Colchicine 0.6 mg two to three times daily and *thalidomide* 100-200 mg daily are the most effective steroid-sparing agents. *Dapsone* 100 mg daily, *pentoxiphyline* 400 mg three times daily, and *levamisole* 50 mg three times daily for 3 days every 2 weeks may also lead to suppression of aphthae.

Trigger avoidance is the key. Predisposing factors include food (nuts, chocolate, tomatoes and spices), trauma, menstruation or stress. A *food diary* may be of value in identification of an offending agent. *Hormonal therapy* may alleviate RAS associated with menstruation.

SUMMARY OF THERAPIES

First Line Therapies

- **Vitamin and mineral deficiency replacement**.
- **Topical corticosteroids.**
- Intralesional corticosteroids.
- Amlexanox *(Paste).*
- **Tetracycline.**
- Antimicrobial mouth rinses.

Commonly used Therapies

Use of tetracycline suspension 250 mg/5 mL four times daily in patients with RAS: The suspension is held in the mouth for 2 minutes then swallowed. It was found that tetracycline therapy significantly reduced ulcer duration, size and pain, but did not alter the recurrence rate.

0.2% chlorhexidine gluconate mouthwash three times daily for 6 weeks was also found to be useful.

Second Line Therapies

- **Oral corticosteroids.**

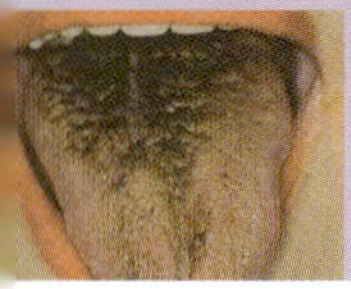

- **Colchicine.**
- Thalidomide.

Third Line Therapies

- **Dapsone**
- **Pentoxifylline**
- **Levamisole**
- Topical cyclosporine
- **Azathioprine**
- Topical 5-aminosalicylic acid
- Topical diclofenac in hyaluronate
- Triclosan
- Acyclovir
- Etretinate
- CO_2 laser
- Etanercept.

Commonly used Therapies

A study revealed that complete or partial clearing of aphthae was achieved in 11 of 19 patients with previously resistant oral aphthae, oral and genital aphthae, or Behcet's disease with dapsone 100 mg daily. The average duration of treatment was 19 days. Concomitant therapy consisted of zinc sulfate and co-trimoxazole.

Another drug found useful in patients with minor RAS was pentoxifylline 400 mg three times daily over a 6-month period, (50% did not experience a recurrence and 27% experienced a reduced number and duration of ulcers).

In recalcitrant cases azathioprine 50 mg twice daily with ibuprofen 600 mg four times daily and dexamethasone elixirr 0.5 mg/5 mL swish and rinse can be used.

HERPES SIMPLEX

Herpes simplex virus infection can occur as a group of umbilicated vesicles on the mucous membranes of the lips, the conjunctiva, the penis and the labia. Frequently recurring episodes of this disease can be quite disabling. Recurrent intraoral herpes simplex is uncommon but the primary outbreak can have extensive intraoral mucous membrane involvement.

OTHER MUCOSAL LESIONS AND CONDITIONS

Mucosal lesions can also be caused by the following:

- **Physical causes:** Sucking of lips, pressure sores, burns, actinic or sunlight cheilitis, factitial disorders, tobacco, and other chemicals.
- **Infectious diseases (from viruses, bacteria, spirochetes, fungi and animal parasites):** Gangrenous bacterial infections are called **noma. Ludwig's angina** is an acute cellulitis of the floor of the mouth caused by bacteria, abscesses, and sinuses and may be due to dental infection. **Trench mouth, or Plaut-Vincent's** disease, is an acute ulcerative infection of the mucous membranes caused by a combination of a spirochete and a fusiform bacillus.
- **Systemic diseases:** These include lesions seen with hematologic diseases (e.g., leukemia, agranulocytosis from drugs or other causes, thrombocytopenia, pernicious anemia, cyclic or periodic neutropenia), immunocompromised conditions (such as the acquired immunodeficiency syndrome, organ transplants, lymphomas), collagen diseases (lupus erythematosus and scleroderma), pigmentary diseases (e.g., Addison's disease, Peutz-Jeghers syndrome), and autoimmune diseases, which cross over in several categories but include pemphigus and benign mucosal pemphigoid.
- **Drugs:** Phenytoin sodium causes a hyperplastic gingivitis; bismuth orally and intramuscularly causes a bluish-black line at the edge of the dental gum; certain drugs cause hemorrhage and secondary infection of the mucous membranes.
- **Halitosis:** Halitosis, or fetor oris, is a disagreeable odor of the breath.
- **Periadenitis mucosa necrotica recurrens:** Also known as **Sutton's** disease, this is a painful, recurrent, ulcerating disease of the mucous membranes of the oral cavity. The single or multiple deep ulcers exceed 10 mm and heal with scarring. Systemic corticosteroids may be indicated. It is considered by some to be a very severe type of aphthous ulcer.
- **Hand-foot-mouth disease:** A common vesicular eruption of the hands, feet and mouth. Usually affecting children, it lasts upto 2 weeks. Most cases are caused by **coxsackievirus A16.**
- **Koplik's spots:** Bright red, pinpoint-sized lesions on the mucous membranes of the cheek are seen in patients before the appearance of the rash of **measles.**
- **Erythema multiforme:** Causes "bulls eye" lesions on the skin and erosions of the mucus membranes that may be severe. The most common causes are herpes simplex and drug allergies.
- **Burning tongue (glossodynia):** This rather common complaint, particularly among middle-aged women, is usually accompanied by no visible pathology. The cause is unknown, and therapy is of little value, but the many

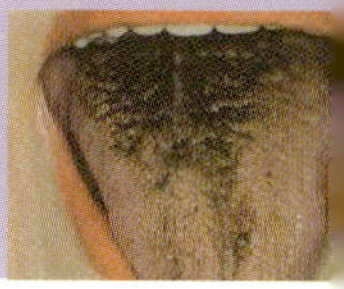

diseases and local factors that cause painful tongue must be ruled out from a diagnostic viewpoint. The entire mouth can also burn. Tricyclic antidepressants have been used with some success.

- **Black tongue (hairy tongue, lingua nigra) (Fig. 17.4):** Over-growth of the papillae of the tongue, apparently caused by an imbalance of bacterial flora, is due to the use of antibiotics and other agents. Black tongue without papillae hypertrophy can be seen with tobacco abuse, crack cocaine smoking, lansoprazole, chewing bismuth, methyldopa, minocycline, and hydroxychloroquine.

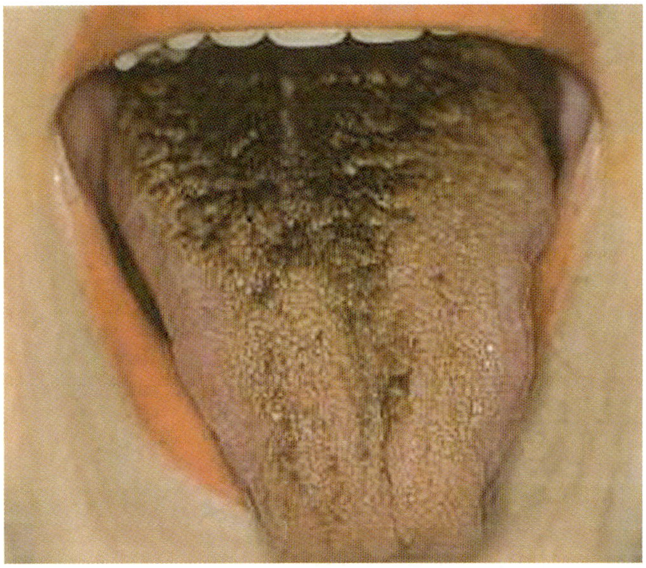

Fig. 17.4: Black hairy tongue

- **Hairy leukoplakia of the tongue:** A slightly raised, poorly demarcated lesion with a corrugated or "hairy" surface appears on the sides of the tongue. It is seen mainly in immunosuppressed homosexual men infected with human immunodeficiency virus. Human papillomavirus and Epstein-Barr virus have been identified in biopsy specimens. It is benign and no therapy is necessary.
- **Moeller's glossitis:** This painful, persistent, red eruption on the sides and the tip of the tongue persists for weeks or months, subsides, and then recurs. The cause is unknown.
- **Furrowed tongue (grooved tongue, scrotal tongue):** The tongue is usually larger than normal, containing deep longitudinal and lateral grooves of congenital origin, due to syphilis, or as part of **Melkersson-Rosenthal syndrome**.
- **Glossitis rhomboidea mediana:** This rare disorder, characterized by a smooth reddish lesion, usually occurs in the center of the tongue. This term is a misnomer because there is no inflammation and the reddish plaque may not always be in the center.
- **Sjögren's syndrome:** This rare entity is characterized by dryness of all of the mucous membranes and of the skin in middle-aged women. Keratoconjuntivitis sicca is used to describe the severe dryness of the eyes seen in this syndrome. The primary form of this syndrome is in many cases associated with a cutaneous vasculitis. The secondary type of Sjögren's syndrome is associated with rheumatic and collagen diseases.
- **Cheilitis glandularis:** This chronic disorder of the lips is manifested by swelling and secondary inflammation, caused by hypertrophy of the mucous glands and their ducts.

Some other oral lumps, bumps and colour changes

- **Mucocoeles** are collections of mucin following the rupture of a minor salivary gland duct. They are blue tinted soft translucent nodules, usually of the lips, and arise suddenly without pain.
- **Yellow patches** in the mouth may suggest pseudoxanthoma elasticum.
- **Brown macules** on the lips should trigger thoughts about the dominantly inherited Peutz-Jeghers syndrome and its bowel polyps and tumours.
- **Neurofibromas** may occur, especially in patients with widespread cutaneous neurofibromatosis.
- **Telangiectasia** may suggest hereditary haemorrhagic telangiectasia. These patients may also have telangiectases in their intestinal tract leading to gastrointestinal bleeding, and arteriovenous fistulae especially in the lungs that may lead to cerebral embolism.
- **Venous lakes** are blue or black papules on the lips. These melanoma-like lesions worry patients and doctors alike, but pressure with a diascope or glass slide causes them to blanch (Fig. 17.5).

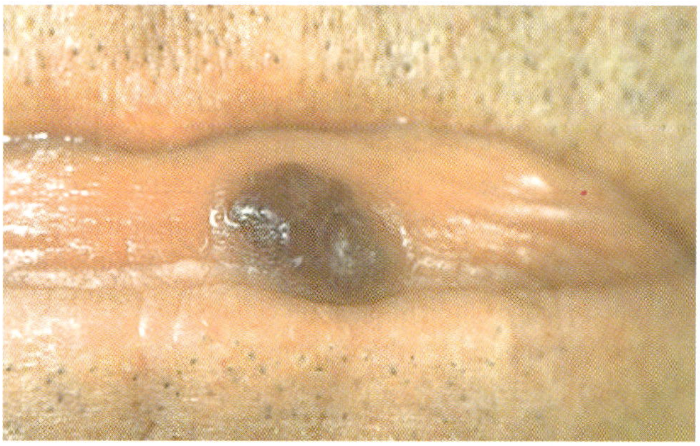

Fig. 17.5: Venous lakes

- Multiple, somewhat translucent, papules may suggest **Cowden's** syndrome. These are fibromas. Patients with Cowden's syndrome have facial papules and nodules (tricholemmomas and fibromas), fibrocystic disease of the breasts and a great propensity to develop malignant tumours of the breast, thyroid and other organs.
- Patients with the **multiple mucosal neuroma** syndrome have neuromas in their mouths, and 75% of those with this autosomal dominantly inherited disorder also have medullary carcinoma of the thyroid. Many also develop pheochromocytomas. Many small bumps appear along the lips, tongue and buccal mucosae.
- **Pyogenic granulomas** of the gingiva appear as quick growing red bleeding papules. They are reactive proliferations of blood vessels and often develop in pregnancy ('pregnancy tumours').
- **Fibromas** may result from dentures, or from resolving or indolent pyogenic granulomas, but can also appear without reason, usually on the gingiva of adults. Tooth bites may cause fibromas to appear on the tongue and on the buccal mucosae. Cowden's disease should be considered if multiple lesions are present.
- **Warts** in the mouth are not uncommon.

SQUAMOUS CELL CARCINOMA

Cause

Predisposing factors include smoking or chewing tobacco products, and the 'straight-shot' drinking of alcohol. Cancer can also occur in the plaques and ulcers of lichen planus. Lip cancers may be sun-induced.

Clinical Features

A thickening or nodule develops, usually on the lower lip, and often in a field of actinic chelitis (rough scaling mucosa from sun damage). Inside the mouth, the tongue is the most common site to be affected, often on its undersurface. The cancer itself appears either as an indurated ulcer with steep edges, or as a diffuse hardness or nodule. Red or white thickened plaques are common precursors, and the cancer may be surrounded by these changes. Plaques and hard areas may ulcerate.

THE GENITALIA

Common conditions are given below:

Pearly penile papules (Fig. 17.6)	Pinhead-sized angiofibromas of the glans penis
Fordyce spots	Ectopic sebaceous glands of the glans penis
Angiokeratomas	Black papules on scrotum
Balanitis	Many types, but poor hygiene is common
Warts (condyloma acuminata)	Cauliflower-like growths of moist genital skin
Fixed drug eruptions	Red plaques or ulcers can be localized to the penis
Lichen planus	Look for lesions in the mouth or on the skin to confirm the diagnosis
Psoriasis	Often favours the glans penis
Paget's disease	Intraepithelial adenocarcinoma appearing as a marginated red plaque
Infections	Syphilis, herpes simplex, chancroid, lymphogranuloma venereum

NORMAL ANATOMICAL VARIANTS

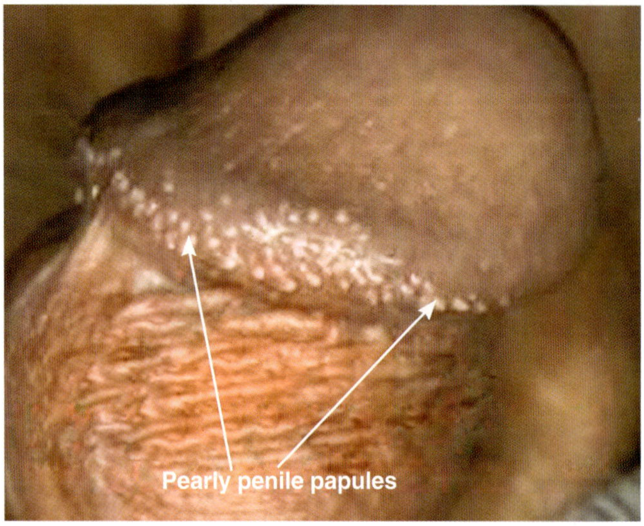

Fig. 17.6: Pearly penile papules

Lymphocele (Fig. 17.7)

This is a cord like swelling just below the head of the penis and can be quite alarming when it's first discovered.

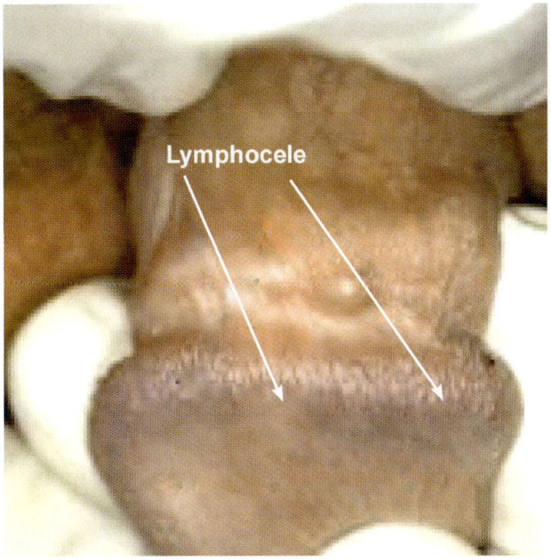

Fig. 17.7: Lymphocele

Lymphatics can become enlarged after vigorous sex or masturbation.

Vestibular Glands (Fig. 17.8)

Just at the entrance to the vagina there are two small symmetrical glands and in some women they can be quite large and can easily be mistaken for genital warts.

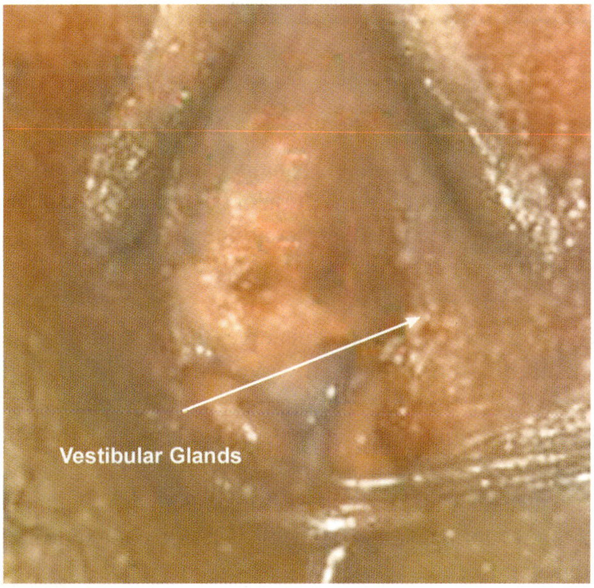

Fig. 17.8: Vestibular glands

The Fordyce Spots (Fig. 17.9)

These small white glands are just underneath the skin and appear in patches in both the male and female genital areas.

In males they are more often found around the prepuce or the skin that pulls back. They can be very prominent in some people and can be easily mistaken for genital warts (Fig. 17.9).

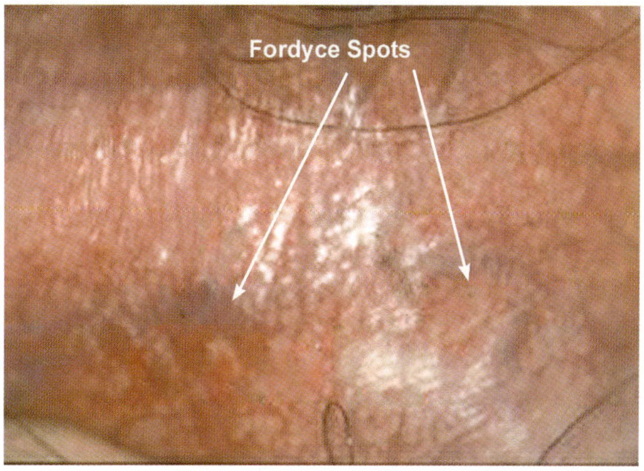

Fig. 17.9: Fordyce spots

Sebaceous Cysts (Fig. 17.10)

These are quite firm, yellow lumps, that collect just underneath the skin in both male and female, and can occur anywhere in the genital area.

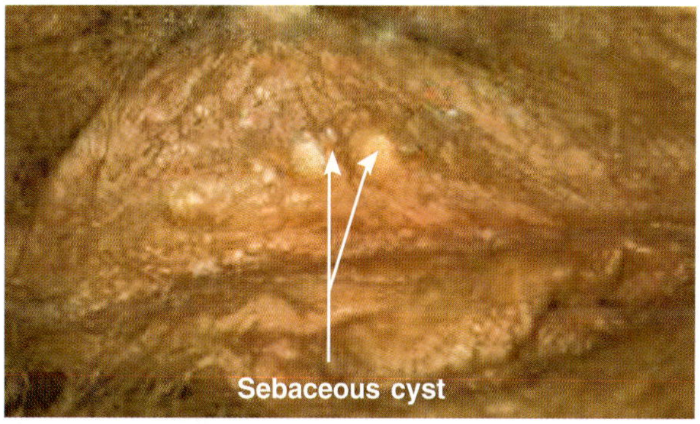

Fig. 17.10: Sebaceous cyst

BALANITIS AND BALANOPOSTHITIS

Balanitis is an inflammatory condition of the glans penis; posthitis is an inflammation of the foreskin; and balanoposthitis is an inflammation of the contiguous and opposing mucosa of the glans penis and prepuce. Balanoposthitis does not occur in an adequately circumcised male.

Characteristic findings include erythema, swelling, discharge, dysuria, bleeding, and ulceration of the glans. In most cases, no single infectious agent is the cause; bacterial cultures of the exudate in the space commonly produc*e a mixed growth, but, at times, Staphylococcus aureus* and group A (GAS) or group B *Streptococcus* (GBS) can be recovered alone. At times, perianal streptococcal cellulitis, cause by GAS, can be accompanied by acute balanoposthitis.

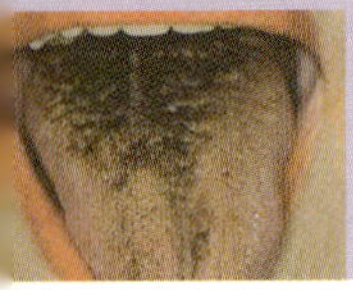

Diabetes mellitus with glucosuria is a common predisposing disease. Sexually transmissible agents that can cause balanoposthitis include *Candida albicans, Gonococcus, Gardnerella vaginalis* and *Trichomonas vaginalis*. Clinical findings include "rash", itching, burning sensation, erythema, erosion/ulceration, pseudomembrane, and/or subpreputial exudate. Invasive infection can complicate balanoposthitis (penile cellulitis), especially in the immunocompromised host.

Management of acute balanoposthitis is based on elimination of any predisposing factors in the pathogenesis, identification of a specific etiologic agent, and retraction of the foreskin, if possible, to eliminate the preputial sac, allowing the opposing epithelial surfaces to dry out. In some cases of recurrent balanoposthitis, the sexual partner also must be treated to prevent recolonization of the specific infectious agent; circumcision is indicated in some cases, especially if phimosis exists.

Vulvovaginitis

Inflammatory diseases of the vagina often also affect the vulva, but the vagina alone can be affected. Vaginitis causes discharge, odour, painful intercourse and itching or burning sensations. The differential diagnosis includes candidiasis, trichomoniasis, bacterial vaginosis, cytolytic vaginosis and atrophic vaginitis. The diagnosis can be made by the appearance of the discharge both grossly and under the microscope.

Lichen Sclerosus (Fig. 17.11)

The affected areas on the vulva, penis, perineum and/or perianal skin show well-marginated white thin fragile patches with a crinkled surface. Itching can be severe, especially in women. The fragility of the atrophic areas may lead to purpura and erosions. Scratching can cause lichenification, and diagnostic confusion. Women are more commonly afflicted than men, but pre-adolescent girls and boys also can develop this problem. In girls, the white patches circling the vulva and anus take on an hourglass shape around the orifices.

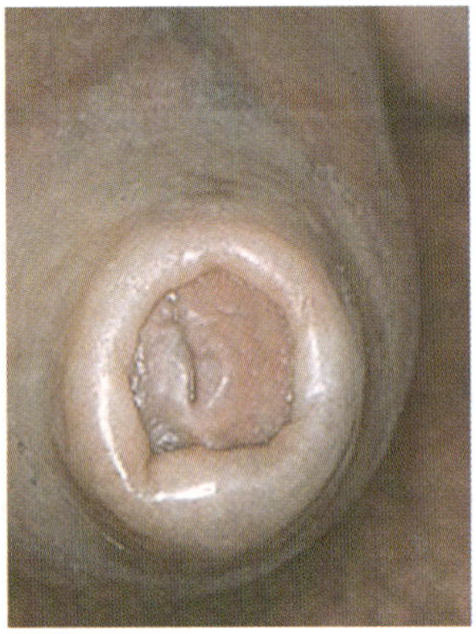

Fig. 17.11: Lichen sclerosus

Course

As time goes on, scarring occurs. In adult women, the clitoral prepuce may scar over the clitoris, and the vaginal introitus may narrow, preventing enjoyable sexual intercourse. Scarring is rare in girls and boys; treatment may prevent scarring in adults.

Differential Diagnosis

The sharply marginated white patches of vitiligo can afflict the vulva and penis but lack atrophy, and typical vitiligo may be found elsewhere on the body.

Neurodermatitis may be superimposed upon lichen sclerosus after incessant scratching.

Treatment

At first sight it might seem unwise to rub potent topical steroids onto atrophic thin occluded skin.

Yet, treatment with potent topical steroids not only reduces itch, pain and misery, but also reverses hypopigmentation and atrophy by shutting down its cause. However, atrophy, striae and other complications can develop on untreated adjacent skin, if the medication spreads there.

Ointments are preferable to creams. Only small amounts (15 g) should be dispensed. After a course of 8-12 weeks, weaker topical steroids can be used to maintain a remission.

VULVAL AND SCROTAL PRURITUS

Cause

Itching of the genital skin is usually caused by skin disease, or by rubbing, sweating, irritation or occlusion. Once started, genital itching seems able to continue on its own.

Presentation

The vulva and scrotum contain nerves that normally transmit pleasurable sensations. However, itching itself is not pleasurable, although scratching is. Itch may be present all day, but more frequently appears or worsens at night. Once scratching has started, it perpetuates itself. The history is of an incessant and embarrassing scratching. Examination may show normal skin, or the tell-tale signs of excoriations and lichenification.

Differential Diagnosis

Itch is part of many inflammatory skin diseases. In the groin its most common causes are tinea, candida, erythrasma, atopic dermatitis, psoriasis, pubic lice, intertrigo and irritant or allergic contact dermatitis.

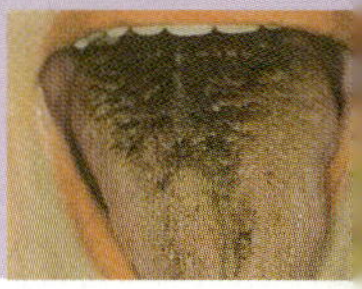

However, patients with 'essential' pruritus show no skin changes other than those elicited by scratching. Sometimes the cause is psychogenic.

Treatment

Low potency topical corticosteroids sometimes help by suppressing secondary inflammation; however, atrophy sometimes quickly occurs, and then the itch is replaced by a burning sensation. A better approach is to eliminate the trigger factors for itch such as hot baths, tight clothing, rough fabrics, sweating, cool air, the chronic wetness of vaginal secretions, menstrual pads and soaps. Antipruritic creams, such as pramoxine cream or menthol in a light emollient base, help to abort the itch-scratch-itch cycles.

Many patients benefit from systemic antihistamines or tricyclic drugs such as amitriptyline or doxepin.

DERMATOSES

Condition	*Clinical comments*
Tinea cruris	Involves the groin but seldom the scrotum
Candidiasis	Beefy red with satellite papules and pustules
Erythrasma	Brown patches of the upper thigh
Irritant contact dermatitis	Burning sensations may predominate
Allergic contact dermatitis	The scrotum may be oedematous
Inverse psoriasis	Beefy red marginated plaques extend up the gluteal fold
Seborrheic dermatitis	To confirm the diagnosis look at the scalp for disease.
Neurodermatitis	It feels wonderful to scratch an itchy groin
Intertrigo	Skin breaks down from maceration

SQUAMOUS CELL CARCINOMA

Cause

Human papilloma viruses, especially HPV types **6, 11, 16 and 18**, often play a part. These are sexually transmitted, so the risk of carcinoma of the vulva or penis is greatest in those who have had many sexual partners.

Squamous cell carcinoma of the glans penis is especially common in the *uncircumcised.* Smegma can incite inflammation leading to both phimosis and carcinoma. Exposure to tar also predisposes to scrotal carcinoma. Other predisposing factors are immunosuppression, lichen sclerosus and, possibly, lichen planus.

Cancer can also develop from **bowenoid papulosis** on the penis that resemble dark seborrheic keratoses clinically, and Bowen's disease histologically. The female equivalent is vulvar intraepithelial neoplasia.

Presentation

In men, a glistening irregular red moist patch; **Bowen's disease/erythroplasia of Queyrat)** (Fig. 17.12) develops on an uncircumcised penis, either on the glans or on the inner prepuce. Maceration may make it look white until evaporation reveals its true colour. It enlarges slowly, and invasion and tumour formation may not occur for years in immunocompetent men.

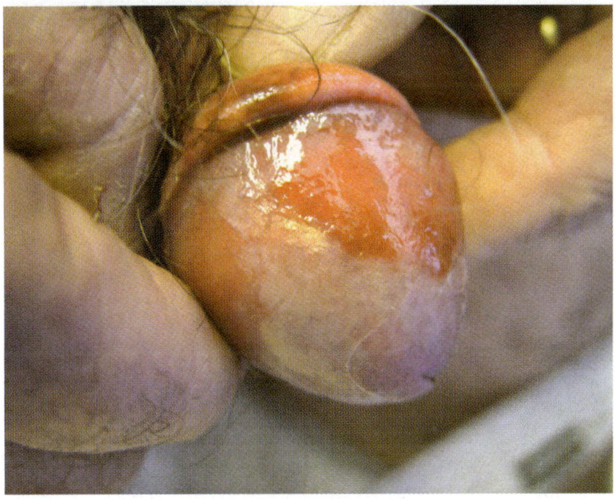

Fig. 17.12: Erythroplasia of queyrat

In women, the precursor lesion is often **Bowen's disease** presenting as a sharply marginated, very slowly growing, mildly hyperkeratotic or slightly scaling, oddly shaped red patch or plaque that is usually a single lesion on one labia or in the perineum. This may become huge (upto 10 cm diameter). Sometimes cancer of the penis or labia resembles a large wart destroying the underlying tissue, **or present as tumorous nodules.**

Treatment

Mohs' micrographic excision is probably the best treatment for small and minimally invasive carcinomas, but partial penectomy is indicated if the tumour is large. Precursor lesions such as warts, bowenoid papulosis, vulvar intraepithelial neoplasia and Bowen's disease can be destroyed with laser surgery or cryotherapy. In some patients, topical applications of the cytokine-inducer imiquimod cream or the chemotherapeutic 5-fluorouracil cream can be curative.

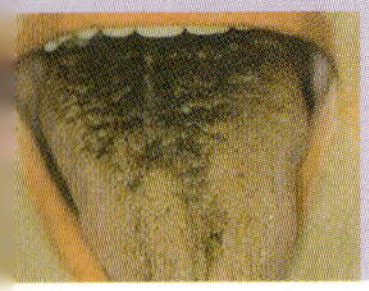

PLASMA CELL BALANITIS (BALANITIS CIRCUMSCRIPTA PLASMACELLULARIS OR ZOON'S BALANITIS) (Fig. 17.13)

This presents as a solitary, persistent plaque on the glans of uncircumcised, middle-aged to older men. The etiology and pathogenesis are unknown. The duration of the lesion prior to presentation ranges from several months to a decade or more. The clinical presentation is usually an *erythematous, shiny, moist, and glistening macular to slightly raised plaque on the glans penis* (Fig. 17.13). The color of the lesion is usually bright red, but it may be the color of **cayenne pepper** due to microhemorrhage and hemosiderin deposition.

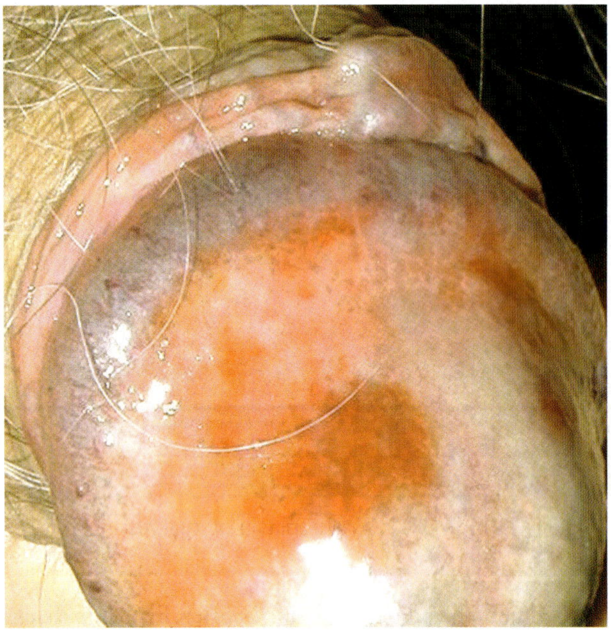

Fig. 17.13: Zoon's balanitis

Histologic features include a thinned epidermis showing "lozenge" keratinocytes (i.e., diamond-shaped acanthocytes), an occasional dyskeratotic keratinocyte, and mild spongiosis. Dermal findings include a dense bandlike or lichenoid mixed infiltrate with a predominance of plasma cells and vascular proliferation. There is poor response to all local modalities of therapy; circumcision is curative.

Rarer Conditions of Genital Mucous Membranes

- **Fusospirochetal balanitis:** This uncommon infection of the penis is characterized by superficial erosions. It must be differentiated from syphilis by a darkfield examination and blood serology.
- **Angiokeratomas:** Angiokeratomas of the scrotum and penis are common genital lesions characterized by ectasia of superficial dermal blood vessels and hyperkeratosis. Lesions occur on the scrotum or periurethral glans, may be solitary or multiple, and increase in number with age. Penile angiokeratomas are thin-walled and occasionally bleed spontaneously with trauma. Clinically, the lesions are soft and compressible, purple, 1- to 5-mm papules. Angiokeratomas are occasionally solitary but are more commonly multiple with up to 50 to 100 caviar-like scrotal papules. They may uncommonly afflict the female (Fig. 17.14).

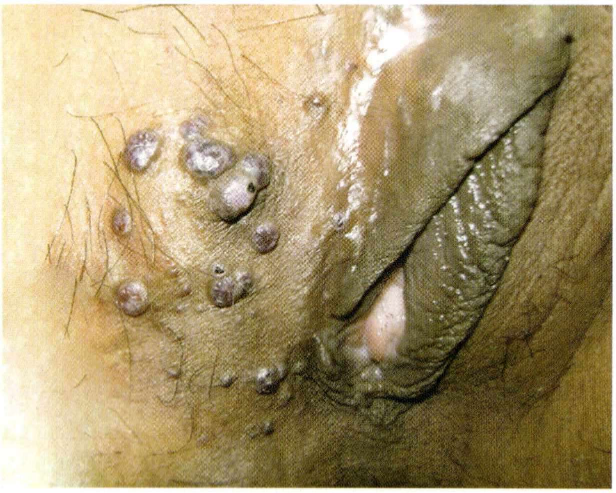

Fig. 17.14: Angiokeratomas

- **Allergic contact dermatitis (ACD):** This occurs on the penis and scrotum and often is more florid and symptomatic than on other sites. In nonsensitized individuals, a minimum of 5 to 7 days elapses from the time of contact to onset of symptoms. In a previously sensitized individual, however, the time varies with the quantity of allergen and the individual reactivity but can be as short as 4 to 6 hours. The extreme reactivity and tremendous vascularity of the penis maximize the intensity of the ACD.

REFERENCES

- Double-blind trial of tetracycline in recurrent aphthous ulceration Graykowski EA, Kingman A, J Oral Patho 11978; 7:376-82.
- Chlorhexidine gluconate mouthwash in the management of minor aphthous ulceration: A double-blind, placebo controlled cross-over trial, Hunter L, Addy M. Br Dent J 1987; 162:106-10.
- Prevention of recurrent aphthous stomatitis with colchicine: An open trial, Katz J, Langevitz P, Shemer J, *et al.* J Am Acad Dermato 11994; 31:459-61.
- Dapsone use with oral-genital ulcers, Handfield-Jones S, Allen BR, Littlewood SM, Br J Dermatol 1985; 113:501.
- Treatment of recurrent aphthous stomatitis with pentoxifylline, Pizarro A, Navarro A, Fonseca E, *et al.* Br J Dermatol 1995; 133:659-60.

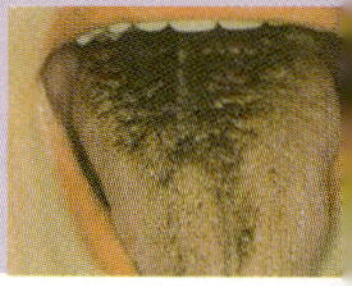

- Combination immunosuppressant and topical stem therapy for treatment of recurrent major aphthae Brown RS, Bottomley WK, Oral Surg Oral Med Oral Pat 1990; 69:42-44.
- Eisen D, Lynch DP: The mouth: Diagnosis and treatment, St Louis, Mosby, 1998.
- Eversole LR: Immunopathology of oral mucosal ulcerative, desquamative and bullous disease: Selected review of the literature, Oral Surg Oral Med Oral Pathol 1994; 77:555.
- Novick NL: Diseases of the mucous membrane, Clin Dermatol 1987; 5.
- Bork, K., Hoede, N., Korting, G.W., Burgdorf, W.H.C. and Young, S.H. (1996): Diseases of the Oral Mucosa and Lips, W.B. Saunders, Philadelphia, PA.
- Lynch, P.J. and Edwards, L. (1994) Genital Dermatology. Churchill Livingstone, Edinburgh.
- Ridley, C.M., Oriel, J.D. and Robinson, A. (2000): Vulval Disease, Arnold, London.

CHAPTER **18**

DISORDERS OF HAIR AND NAILS

Hair

HAIR PHYSIOLOGY

There are three types of hair:
- Lanugo.
- Vellus, and
- Terminal hair.

Lanugo

Lanugo hair are long, unmedullated hair seen in utero and are shed during the end of pregnancy and the first several months postpartum.

Vellus

Vellus (intermediate hair) are short, nonpigmented hair produced by follicles that penetrate only into the papillary dermis.

Terminal Hair

Terminal hair are produced by follicles that penetrate into the reticular dermis and are usually medullated (have a medulla) and are wider than the inner root sheath of the follicle that produces them. Hair on the scalp and beard area are examples of terminal hair. In the inherited types of balding, some terminal hair are lost and vellus hair are seen instead.

CYCLES

There is an **anagen** (growth) phase (about **85% to 95%** of scalp hair are in this phase), **catagen** (regressive) phase (about **1%** of scalp hair are in this phase), and a **telogen** (resting) phase (about **10% to 15%** of scalp hair are in this phase).

The length of the anagen phase determines the length of the hair. The **anagen** phase for human scalp hair is usually between **2 and 6** years and the hair on the scalp grows about 1 cm per month; therefore, some people can never have very long hair on the scalp even if they never cut their hair. Growth phases of hair on other body parts are much shorter than on the scalp. It is normal to lose **between 50 and 100 scalp** hair per day. Plucking the resting hair from follicles that have already entered anagen can advance the onset of the next anagen phase. Shaving the hair has no effect on the hair cycle. The telogen phase is the period between the completion of follicular regression (catagen) and the onset of the next anagen phase. On the human scalp, the telogen phase lasts about 2 to 4 months. The catagen phase on the human scalp lasts 2 to 4 weeks.

HIRSUTISM AND HYPERTRICHOSIS

Hirsutism is the excessive growth of terminal hair in an adult male sexual pattern in a female or child. Hypertrichosis is hair growth that is abnormal for the age, gender, or race of an individual or for a particular area of the body. Medications can cause either of these problems (Table 18.1).

Table 18.1: Drugs that can cause hirsutism and hypertrichosis

	Drugs
Hirsutism	Androgens
	Danazol
	Progesterone
Hypertrichosis	Acetazolamide
	Corticosteroids
	Cyclosporine
	Diazoxide
	Interferon
	Latanoprost
	Minoxidil
	Penicillamine
	Phenytoin
	Psoralens
	Streptomycin

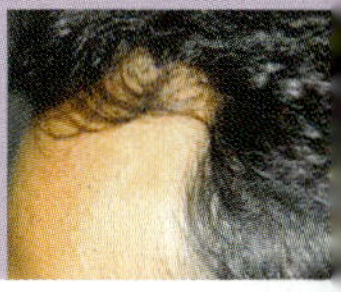

HIRSUTISM

Cause and Distribution

The prevalence of hirsutism in women overall is said to vary from 5% to 15%. The most common diagnosis associated with hirsutism is **polycystic ovary syndrome** (PCOS). About 5% to 15% of cases of hirsutism are idiopathic.

Laboratory Findings (Table 18.2)

Sometimes a serum **testosterone** and 17 α-hydroxyprogesterone may be sufficient, but women with irregular menses and hirsutism should be screened for thyroid dysfunction and prolactin disorders.

A **DHEAS** test is useful for screening for adrenal tumors, but is not reliable for screening late-onset congenital adrenal hyperplasia. The presence of striae, central obesity, and peripheral weakness make the diagnosis of **Cushing's syndrome** possible, in which case a 24-hour urine free cortisol test is indicated.

Normally, 78% of testosterone in women is bound to sex-hormone binding globulin **(SHBG)**, only 1% to 2% is free (which is the bioactive portion), and 20% is bound to albumin. SHBG may be reduced in amount by obesity, hypothyroidism, and hyperinsulinemia, thereby increasing free testosterone levels and therefore possibly leading to hirsutism.

An early morning follicular phase 17-α–OH progesterone level is one of the better tests to screen for congenital adrenal hyperplasia. There are some rare enzyme deficiencies that can lead to **congenital adrenal hyperplasia** that might be better done by an endocrinologist.

PCOS has a prevalence of 6% in all women and is the most common diagnosis associated with hirsutism. Stein and Leventhal were the first to describe this syndrome of amenorrhea, obesity, and hirsutism in association with sclerocystic ovaries. PCOS may be better described as chronic anovulation and hyperandrogenism with the exclusion of androgen-secreting tumors, nonclassic adrenal hyperplasia, and hyperprolactinemia. Insulin resistance with compensatory hyperinsulinemia is a prominent feature in many but not all cases of PCOS.

Commonly found laboratory abnormalities in PCOS include an elevated total testosterone (about twice normal), an elevated luteinizing hormone level (that is at least twice the value for follicle-stimulating hormone), a slight elevation in prolactin, and a slight elevation in DHEAS. The prostate-specific antigen test may or may not be helpful in distinguishing women with PCOS from those with idiopathic hirsutism.

Treatment

Treatment of hirsutism involves finding the cause and obtaining the help of an endocrinologist in some cases.

Oral spironolactone (Aldactone) may be helpful in PCOS and idiopathic hirsutism. Spironolactone interferes with androgen biosynthesis, blocks the action of androgens at the receptor level, and decreases the 5 α-reductase levels in the follicle. Six months of treatment with spironolactone at 100 to 200 mg per day is at least worth a trial. It is

Table 18.2: Causes of hirsutism, associated laboratory findings and recommended additional testing

Diagnosis	*Testosterone*	*17-OHP*	*LH/FSH*	*Prolactin*	*DHEAS*	*Cortisol*	*Additional testing*
Congenital adrenal hyperplasia	N to ↑	↑	N/N	N	N to ↑	N to ↓	ACTH stimulation may be necessary
Polycystic ovary syndrome	N to ↑	N	N to ↑	N to ↑	N to ↑	N	Primarily a clinical diagnosis consider laboratory testing and ultrasonography of ovaries to rule out other disoder/tumors. Consider screening lipids, glucose
Ovarian tumor	↑	N	N/N	N	N	N	Ultrasonography of CT to image tumors
Adrenal tumor	↑	N	N/N	N	↑	N to ↑	Ultrasonography or CT or image tumor
Pharmacologic agent (exogenous) (exogenous)	N	N	N/N	N	N	N	Withdrawal of offending agent recommended
Idiopathic	N	N	N/N	N	N	N	
Familial	N	N	N/N	N	N	N	

important that this not be given to women who are not using adequate contraception because it is teratogenic.

Oral contraceptives, flutamide (not approved by FDA), finasteride, **cyproterone acetate** are some other treatments that are available. The use of the antihyperglycemic **metformin** does reduce markers of insulin resistance in PCOS and this may help treat hirsutism. Removal of hair as discussed under treatment of hypertrichosis may be a helpful adjunct to treatments mentioned here.

HYPERTRICHOSIS

Hypertrichosis can result from the conversion of vellus hair to terminal hair, more hair being in a prolonged anagen (growth) phase (and therefore a decrease in the number of hair in the telogen phase), or an increase in hair follicle density.

Presentation and Characteristics

It is helpful to divide hypertrichosis into congenital or acquired and then into generalized and localized types.

Congenital generalized hypertrichosis and congenital hypertrichosis lanuginosa are both very rare inherited disorders, "Dog-faced" or "Monkey-faced" people in circus side shows may have had the former diagnosis. Congenital hypertrichosis may be a feature of numerous inherited syndromes such as mucopolysaccharidoses, leprechaunism, and Cornelia de Lange syndrome. Of particular note is fetuses exposed to hydantoin (Dilantin) during the first 9 weeks of gestation who may have hypertrichosis as part of the fetal hydantoin syndrome. Hypertrichosis may be seen in fetal alcohol syndrome.

Congenital localized hypertrichosis over the vertebral column ("faun tail") may be a marker of an underlying spinal abnormality. Magnetic resonance imaging is strongly recommended in such cases since the underlying problems may require early surgical intervention to prevent neurologic damage. Congenital hypertrichosis of the ears may be seen in the babies of diabetic mothers or in babies with XYY syndrome. Hairy elbows may be present at birth or acquired and may or may not be associated with other abnormalities.

Acquired hypertrichosis may be generalized or localized. Generalized acquired hypertrichosis may be seen as acquired hypertrichosis lanuginosa ("malignant down"), which is a rare, but striking marker of an internal malignancy (usually lung or colon cancer but a multiplicity of underlying tumors have been associated). Generalized acquired hypertrichosis may occur in diverse conditions including:

- Porphyrias.
- Dermatomyositis.
- Anorexia nervosa.
- Mercury intoxication (acrodynia).
- Insulin-resistant diabetes.
- Hypothyroidism.
- Postencephalitis.
- Multiple sclerosis.
- Head injuries, and
- POEMS syndrome (polyneuropathy, organomegaly, endocrinopathy, M protein and skin changes: hyperpigmentation, hypertrichosis, skin thickening, edema, digital clubbing, and cutaneous angiomas and others).

Multiple **drugs** can cause hypertrichosis. Which can be generalized or localized hypertrichosis. A newer drug in this latter category is one for treatment of glaucoma called latanoprost, a prostaglandin $F_{2\alpha}$ analog that causes hypertrichosis and hyperpigmentation of the eyelashes in most patients using it.

Localized acquired hypertrichosis on the pinnae may be an inherited trait (especially in men from India), or it may be seen with diabetes or with AIDS. Localized hypertrichosis may develop under orthopedic casts or in areas that are chronically traumatized such as lichen simplex chronicus (neurodermatitis), areas in which habitual self inflicted biting occurs, over thrombophlebitis, or over areas of osteomyelitis.

Treatment

Treatment of hypertrichosis may include shaving, depilatories, bleaching, plucking, waxing (a method of plucking of multiple hair simultaneously), laser, and electrolysis. Electrolysis may require more than one treatment and should be done by someone trained in the procedure who uses sterile patient exclusive needles so as to prevent transmission of blood-borne disease. Shaving, contrary to popular belief, does not increase the amount of hair that regrows. Chemical depilatories and bleaching agents are available over the counter and frequently prove effective but may irritate the skin of some users. Waxing and plucking have the advantage of removing the unwanted hair for longer periods without retreatment than does shaving or chemical removal. Electrolysis can cause scarring and is expensive. Laser may be helpful in selected cases especially dark hair in fair skinned patients. A newer topical cream for treatment of hypertrichosis is **eflornithine hydrochloride**, an irreversible inhibitor of ornithine decarboxylase that slows (but does not remove hair) hair growth. This drug is used systemically for treatment of African trypanosomiasis and its side effect of hair loss has been utilized in this cream. It is best not used in pregnant or nursing women and over vast surface areas.

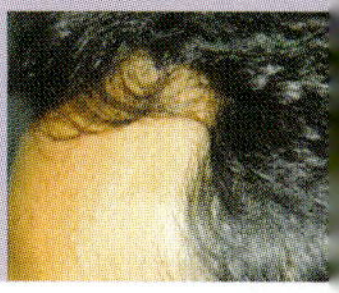

Classification of Alopecia

I. DIFFUSE

Non-Scarring

1. **Abnormality of hair production:**
   a. Congenital hypotrichosis or atrichia—Isolated abnormality or associated with syndromes.
2. **Hair shaft abnormalities associated with breakage:**
   a. Trichorrhexis nodosa
      - Congenital
      - Acquired
   b. Trichoschisis
   c. Pili torti
   d. Trichorrhexis invaginata (Netherton's syndrome)
   e. Monilethrix.
3. **Hair shaft abnormalities associated with unruly hair:**
   a. Uncombable hair syndrome
   b. Woolly hair
   c. Maria-Unna type of hereditary hypotrichosis.
4. **Abnormalities of cycling (shedding):**
   a. **Telogen effluvium**
   b. **Anagen effluvium**
      - Causes
        –Systemic chemotherapy
        –Radiotherapy to scalp
        –Thallium poisoning
        –Mercury intoxication
        –Boric acid intoxication
        –Severe protein malnutrition
   c. **Loose anagen syndrome**
   d. **Alopecia areata.**
5. **Androgenetic alopecia.**

II. FOCAL HAIR LOSS

A. Non-Scarring

1. **Abnormality of hair production**
   – Triangular alopecia
   – Androgenetic alopecia.
2. **Alopecia areata**
3. **Hair breakage**
   a. Trichotillomania
   b. Traction alopecia
   c. Tinea capitis
   d. Primary or acquired localized hair shaft abnormality
      - Trichorrhexis nodosa
      - Pili torti
      - Bubble hair.
4. **Unruly hair**
   a. Hair shaft abnormality—Woolly hair nevus
      - Acquired progressive kinking.
5. **Abnormality of cycling**
   a. Alopecia areata
   b. Syphilis.

B. Scarring

1. **Developmental/Hereditary**
   a. Aplasia cutis congenita
   b. Hair follicle hamartomas
   c. Epidermolysis bullosa dystrophica
   d. Incontinentia pigmenti
   e. Conradi syndrome (Follicular atrophoderma + punctate chondrodystrophy + lamellar icthyosis + acanthosis nigricans).
   f. Scarring follicular keratosis
      - Atrophoderma vermiculata
      - Keratosis pilaris atrophicans
      - Keratosis follicularis spinulosa decalvans.
   g. Porokeratosis of Mibelli
   h. Darier's disease
   i. Ichthyosis
   j. Polyostotic fibrous dysplasia.
2. **Physical injuries**
   a. Mechanical
   b. Chemical
   c. Thermal
   d. Scalp necrosis after embolization surgery
   e. Radiodermatitis.
3. **Follicular inflammation with pustules**
   a. Tinea capitis
   b. Bacterial folliculitis
   c. Folliculitis decalvans
   d. Dissecting cellulitis of scalp
   e. Acne necrotica varioliformis
   f. Acne keloidalis nuchae
   g. Tufted folliculitis.
4. **Follicular inflammation without pustules**
   a. Pseudopelade of Brocq
   b. Follicular lichen planus
   c. Graham-Little syndrome

d. D.L.E.
e. Lichen sclerosus et atrophicus
f. Follicular mucinoses.

5. **Neoplastic**
   a. Basal cell carcinoma
   b. Squamous cell carcinoma
   c. Metastasis
   d. Lymphoma.
6. **Dermal inflammation leading to secondary follicular damage:**
   a. Cicatricial
   b. Morphea
   c. Facial hemiatrophy
   d. Dermatomyositis
   e. Necrobiosis lipoidica
   f. Sarcoidosis
   g. Pyoderma gangrenosum
   h. Syphilis
   i. Tuberculosis
   j. Leishmaniasis
   k. Myiasis
   l. Herpes zoster
   m. Ecthyma and deep secondary pyodermas
   n. Temporal arteritis.

ALOPECIA AREATA (Fig. 18.1)

Presentation and Characteristics

Reversible, patchy, well circumscribed loss of hair without atrophy with **Exclamation mark hair.**

Alopecia areata has a 0.1% to 0.2% prevalence in the general population. It may account for 1% to 3% of new patient visits to a dermatologist.

It is a *non-scarring*, usually patchy, but sometimes diffuse, hair loss of unclear cause that probably is autoimmune. It has typically an abrupt, asymptomatic onset (Fig. 18.2). Usually the scalp is involved but any hair-bearing area of the body may be affected. At the margin of the bald spots there may be broken off hair that are thicker distally and thinner proximally near the scalp like the top part of an exclamation point (!) and are very characteristic of this problem. Regrowth may be with *white colored* hair. In adults regrowth is often in 6 to 12 months.

Factors that bode a **poor prognosis** are young age at onset, extensive early hair loss (especially if severe marginal hair loss called ophiasis), associated atopy, positive family history, autoimmune disorder and associated nail changes.

If all the scalp hair is lost, the term alopecia totalis is used and if all the body hair is lost, the term alopecia universalis is used.

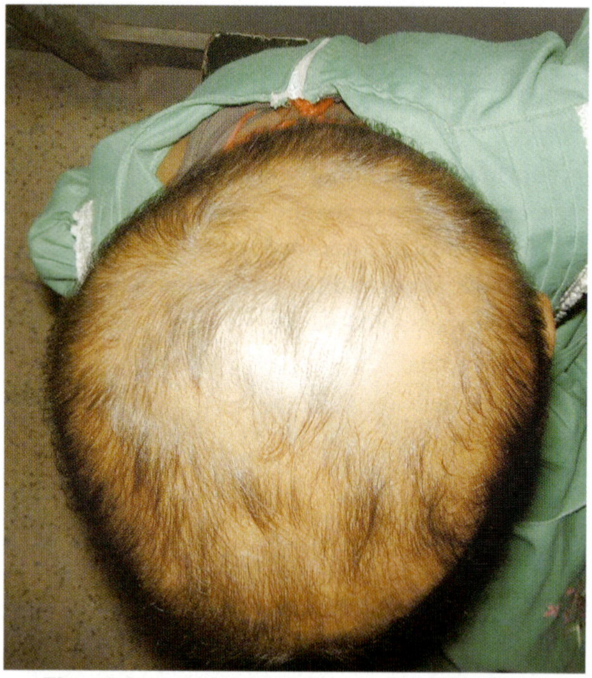

Fig. 18.1: Localised patches of alopecia areata

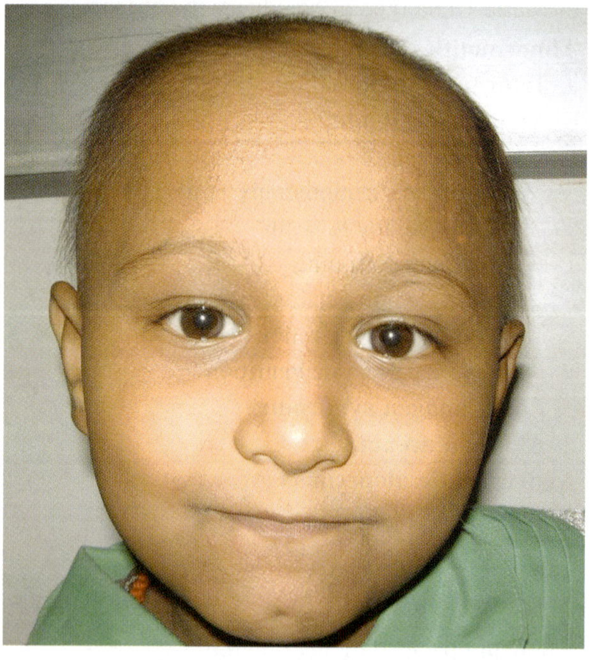

Fig. 18.2: Front view of the same patient

Nail

Nail pitting, longitudinal ridging, koilonychia, onycholysis, onychomadesis, and a host of other nail dystrophies may be associated in 10% to 66% of patients with alopecia areata and precede, accompany, or follow the hair disorder.

Association

An association of alopecia areata may be seen with multiple

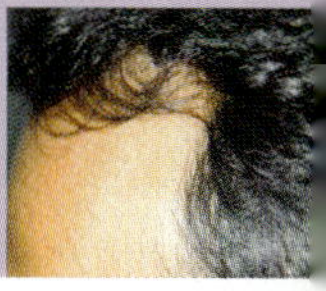

thyroid abnormalities including goiter, myxedema, and Hashimoto's thyroiditis. Patients are also more likely to have vitiligo, lupus, rheumatoid arthritis, pernicious anemia, inflammatory bowel disease, myasthenia gravis, lichen planus, or HIV infection. Patients with Down's syndrome, Turner's syndrome, and autoimmune polyglandular syndrome have an increased likelihood of developing alopecia areata.

Types

- Alopecia totalis.
- Alopecia universalis.
- Ophiasis.
- Sisaphio.
- Diffuse.

Ikeda's Classification

1. Common type.
2. Atopic type.
3. Prehypertensive type.
4. Combined type.

Aetiology

- Genetic.
- Autoimmunity.
- Infection.
- Emotional stress.

Histopathology

- Perivascular, peribulbar and outer root sheath infiltrate and follicular dystrophy (Swarm of bees appearance).
- Lymphocytic and eosinophilic inflammatory infiltrate.

Treatments for Alopecia Areata

Current Agents

- Corticosteroids
  – Topical
  – Intralesional
  – Systemic
- PUVA
- Minoxidil
- Topical sensitizers
- Anthralin
- Imiquimod.

Investigational Agents

- Cytokines
- Antibody
- Gene therapy
- Biologic therapy
- Adjunctive agents.

CORTICOSTEROID

Topical and Intralesional Corticosteroids

- Topical corticosteroids
  – Generally regarded as unhelpful.
  – Possibly helpful if clobestasol cream under occlusion is used.
- Intralesional corticosteroids
  – Treatment of choice for patchy disease <50% of scalp.
  – 64-97% response rate.
  – 10 mg/ml Maximum of 3 ml per visit.
  – Repeat every 4-6 weeks.

Systemic Corticosteroids

- Prednisolone (50-60 mg in tapering dose).
- 6 weeks to 3 months course.
- Allow no more than 2 courses per year.

Adjunctive Agents

- Minoxidil 5%: Used twice daily. Usually in combination with topical steroids under occlusion.
- Anthralin: Most useful in children and patients with less inflammatory disease.

Limited Hair Loss

1. The initial strategy may be no treatment as regrowth, particularly in paucilesional first episode alopecia areata, is common in 2-6 months.
2. Topical or intralesional corticosteroids (triamcinolone 2.5-10 mg per cc every 4-6 weeks).

Alternative Modalities:

1. Application of minoxidil 2%-5% every day or 2 times daily may be attempted.
2. Anthralin-induced irritant dermatitis is safe and may be beneficial. Application of anthralin 0.25%-1.0% in petrolatum or paste to the scalp for 20-30 minutes nightly at bedtime to induce an irritant dermatitis.
3. Contact allergen application like Diphencyprone or Squaric acid dibutyl ester may be efficacious.

A brief overview is presented below: (See Flowchart 18.1)

- The time duration may vary according to response.

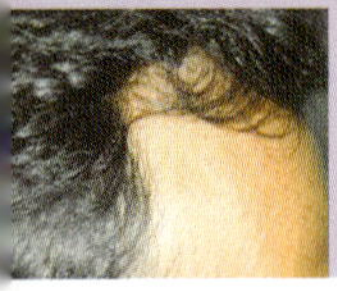

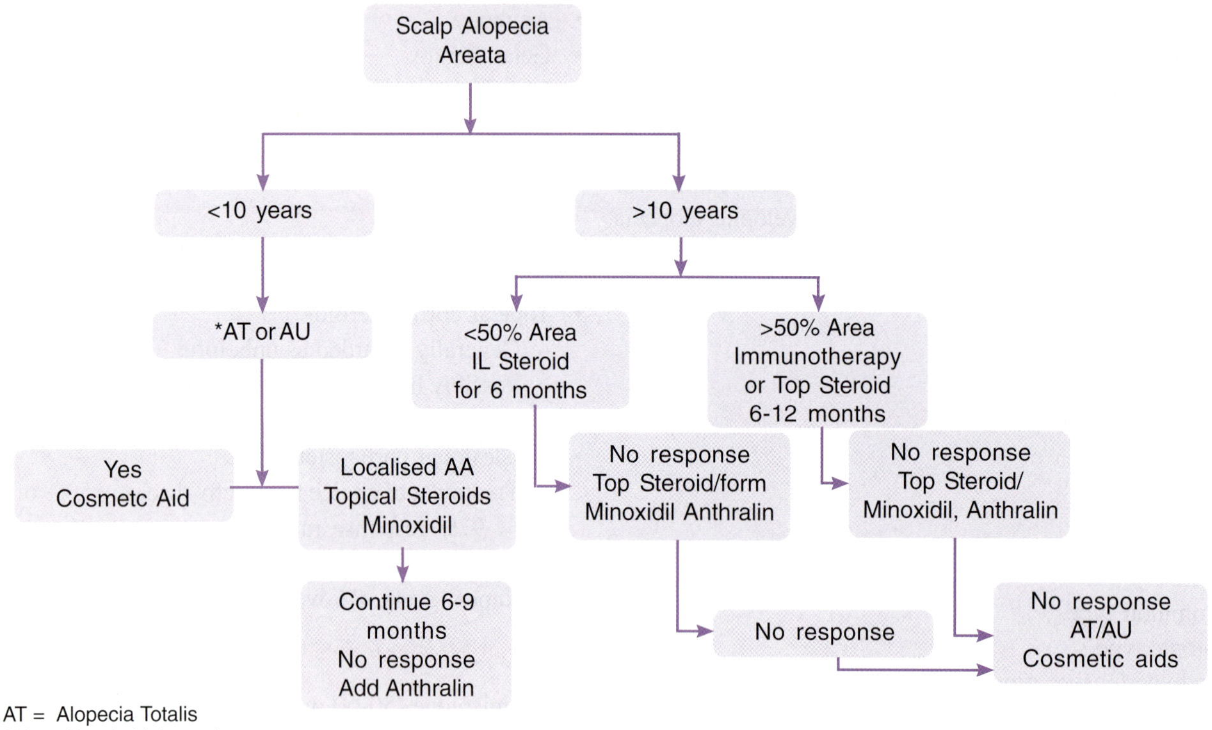

* AT = Alopecia Totalis
AU = Alpecia Universals

Flowchart 18.1

- In any case with extensive alopecia/non-responders consider wigs.
- Systemic steroids/PUVA are to be used with caution in limited cases and preferably not in children.

ANDROGENETIC ALOPECIA

Androgenetic (androgenic; pattern hair loss; female pattern hair loss; male pattern hair loss; diffuse hormonal alopecia; common baldness) is the most common cause of diffuse non-scarring hair loss in men and in women.

- Androgen dependent, genetically mediated.

A.D. Polygenic Variable penetrance

- Affects 50% of men and women.
- Usual onset—3rd to 4th decade.

Pathogenesis

Miniaturization of terminal hair follicle under the influence of androgens.

Testosterone—Dihydrotestosterone (DHT)
(5 times more potent).

- Enzyme responsible is 5α reductase.
- Type I (Skin and sebaceous glands).
- 5α reductase enzyme—Type II (Genitourinary tissue, papillae and ORS of hair follicles).

Diagnosis

a. **Increase in Telogen and Catagen hair and decrease in Anagen hair (Miniaturization of hair follicle)**
(Anagen: Telogen)
(12: 1) (N) → (5:1) (In Androgenetic Alopecia)
b. Mild- perifollicular histiocytic infiltrate depositing (Biopsy)
c. Perifollicular concentric collagen (Biopsy)
d. Decrease in size of hair follicle and wide variability in sizes

Normal		(MAGA)
(0.08 mm	Vs	0.04 mm and 0.06 mm)
Single peak		2 peaks

e. **Trichoscan**
f. **Hormonal studies** (FPHL): For androgen secreting tumor).
< 40% are hyper androgenic.
Indicated if:
Rapid progressive and sudden onset associated acne/ hirsutism/galactorrhoea/acanthosis.

1. **Free/total S. Testosterone and DHEAS.**

If > 2.5 x (N) Testosterone or > 200 ng/dl	or > 2 x (N) DHEAS or > 700 mg/dl (pre menstrual) or > 400 mg/dl (post menstrual)

SECTION - 8

Do radiographic search for tumor.
2. **S. prolactin if galactorrhoea.**
3. Screen for **congenital adrenal hyperplasia** if early morning 17-OH progesterone is elevated.

Clinical Features

It used to be thought that in women with female pattern hair loss, the frontal hair line was retained (unlike in men) and this could help distinguish it from telogen effluvium, in which there is often a temporal recession. Olsen has pointed out that many women with female pattern hair loss have a frontal accentuation of hair loss that may encroach on the frontal hair line in a "Christmas tree"–like pattern (with the base of the tree being the frontal hair line).

Severe female pattern hair loss in women may be a marker of insulin resistance and these women are perhaps more likely to have a paternal history of alopecia than women with a milder version of this problem. Female pattern hair loss is the preferred term and its onset may be early (3rd decade) or late (5th decade) with or without androgen excess. It is best to classify it in this way especially when reporting clinical trials of treatment. Most women with female pattern hair loss do not have androgen excess and androgen excess alone does not cause female pattern hair loss.

Male AGA - **Bitemporal recession + vertex predominance (Fig. 18.3).**
Hamilton - Norwood grading (8 grades).
Female AGA- Preservation of frontal hair line, progressive thinning on top of scalp **"Christmas tree pattern" (Fig. 18.4).**
Ludwig's classification (3 grades).

MEDICAL

- Medical: Male pattern hair loss (MPHL) (Flowchart 18.2).

Treatment

1. **Topical Minoxidil:** FDA approved for > 18 years
   - Enlarges miniaturized hair follicle (Vellus→Terminal in 30% pts).
     Best response in: Early stage.
   - Max diameter of **bald area < 10 cm.**
   - Pre **Rx hair density > 20 hair/cm^2.**
     Dose: 1 ml BD **life long**.
     Max. benefit: 4 months—1 year, thereafter marginal.

   Minoxidil is a vasodilator used in hypertension; it has a direct mitogenic and morphologic effect on follicular cells and does not have an antiandrogenic effect. Side effects of topical minoxidil include contact or irritant dermatitis (in less than 8%) and facial hypertrichosis in women using it (in at least 3% to 5% of those using the 2% concentration). The absorption of even the 5% concentration minoxidil is well below that necessary to change pulse rate, which is the most sensitive indicator of systemic minoxidil effects.
2. **Finasteride:** >18 years.
   Highly selective (inhibitor) of 5 alpha reductase enzyme Type 2.

5 α Reductase

Type 1–Ubiquitous, esp. sebaceous glands.
Type 2–Androgen dependent tissue—**Outer root sheath, dermal papillae.**

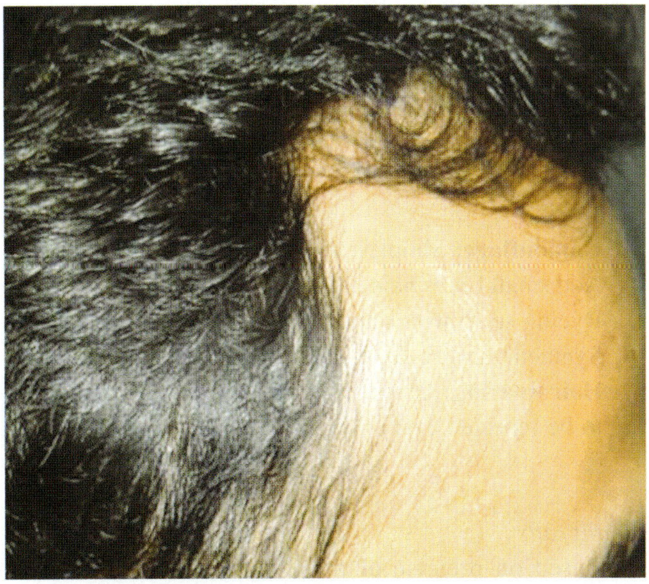

Fig. 18.3: Early stage of MPHL with recession of hair

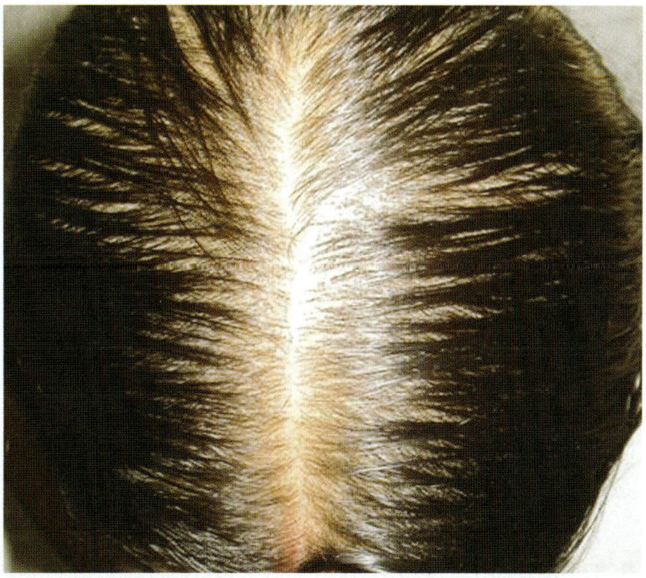

Fig. 18.4: FPHL—Christmas tree pattern

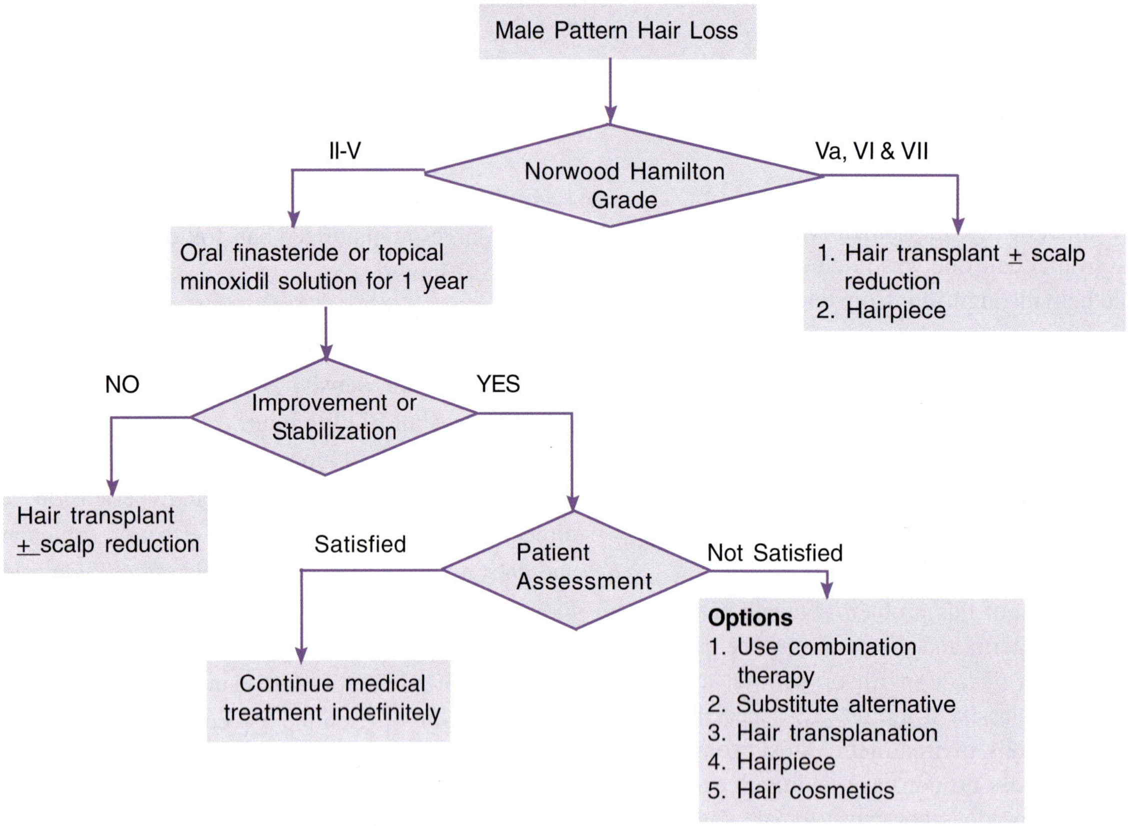

Flowchart 18.2

Effect:
- Increase hair weight.
- Increase anagen hair.
- Reverses miniaturization.

  Dose: 1 mg/day lifelong (decrease scalp DHT by 64% and serum DHT by 68%).

  Max Benefit: 1 year and continues till 2 years, thereafter marginal.

S/E:
- Loss of libido (1.8% while it is 1.3% with placebo).
- Erectile dysfunction (1.3% vs 0.7% with placebo).

  For young men, the use of finasteride 1 mg/d is an additional treatment option in male pattern alopecia. Finasteride is a 5-α-reductase inhibitor. The enzyme 5-α-reductase catalyzes conversion of testosterone to the more potent dihydrotestosterone. Women who are pregnant or nursing should not even handle finasteride pills (especially crushed or broken pills) to avoid teratogenic problems. Four percent of men aged 18 to 41 years of age taking finasteride may have decreased libido, erectile dysfunction, or a decreased volume of ejaculate. The drug must be taken indefinitely to maintain hair growth.

3. **Dutasteride:** 5 α R-type 1 and 2 nonselective inhibitor (0.5 mg/d – 53% decrease in scalp DHT).

Combined use of finasteride and topical minoxidil: Small-scale, variably controlled studies conducted on a primate model for androgenetic alopecia and on young men with mild to moderate MPHL suggest that combination therapy may be more effective than monotherapy, but further investigations are needed.

Non Approved Medications

2% ketoconazole shampoo (used 2 to 4 times weekly) + Finasteride, combined use of topical tretinoin and minoxidil.

Cosmetic (MPHL and FPHL)

1. **Camouflage:** Simplest easiest cheapest for mild AGA.
   Add small fibres held electrostatically.
   Dyeing scalp with same color as hair.
   Synthetic acrylic fibre—withstand wear and tear.
2. **Hair weaving:** Attached externally to existing hair—Need to be repeated every 4-6 weeks.

Surgical (MPHL and FPHL)

Autografts
- Based on premise of donor dominance (grafts from parietal and occipital areas) are less sensitive to androgens.

Grafts:

1. *Macrografts:* Cylindrical (frontal) Elliptical (occipital).
2. *Minigrafts:* 1.5-2.5 mm grafts with 3-4 hair/graft to mask doll hair look of macrografts.
3. *Micrografts:* 1-2 hair/graft, most natural frontal hairline.

FEMALE PATTERN HAIR LOSS (FPHL)

Medical (Flowchart 18.3)

1. **Topical Minoxidil** (2%)—FDA approved, 60% show improvement.
2. **Oral Anti Androgens**
   a. Spironolactone:
      Dose: 100-200 mg/d (usually 200 mg/d required).
      S/E: Premenstrual bleeding.
      - Breast enlargement.
      - Fatigue.
      - Feminization of fetus: use OCP's.

   b. Cyproterone acetate:
      MOA
      - Androgen receptor blocker
      - Potent progestin
      - Antigonadotrophic

   c. Flutamide.

TELOGEN EFFLUVIUM

Telogen effluvium is another important and the most common cause of diffuse non-scarring hair loss. It is the shedding of an abnormal number of hair in the telogen (resting) phase. Telogen effluvium may be triggered by:

- Childbirth.
- Major illness.
- High fever.
- Medications (Table 18.3).
- Rapid marked weight loss.

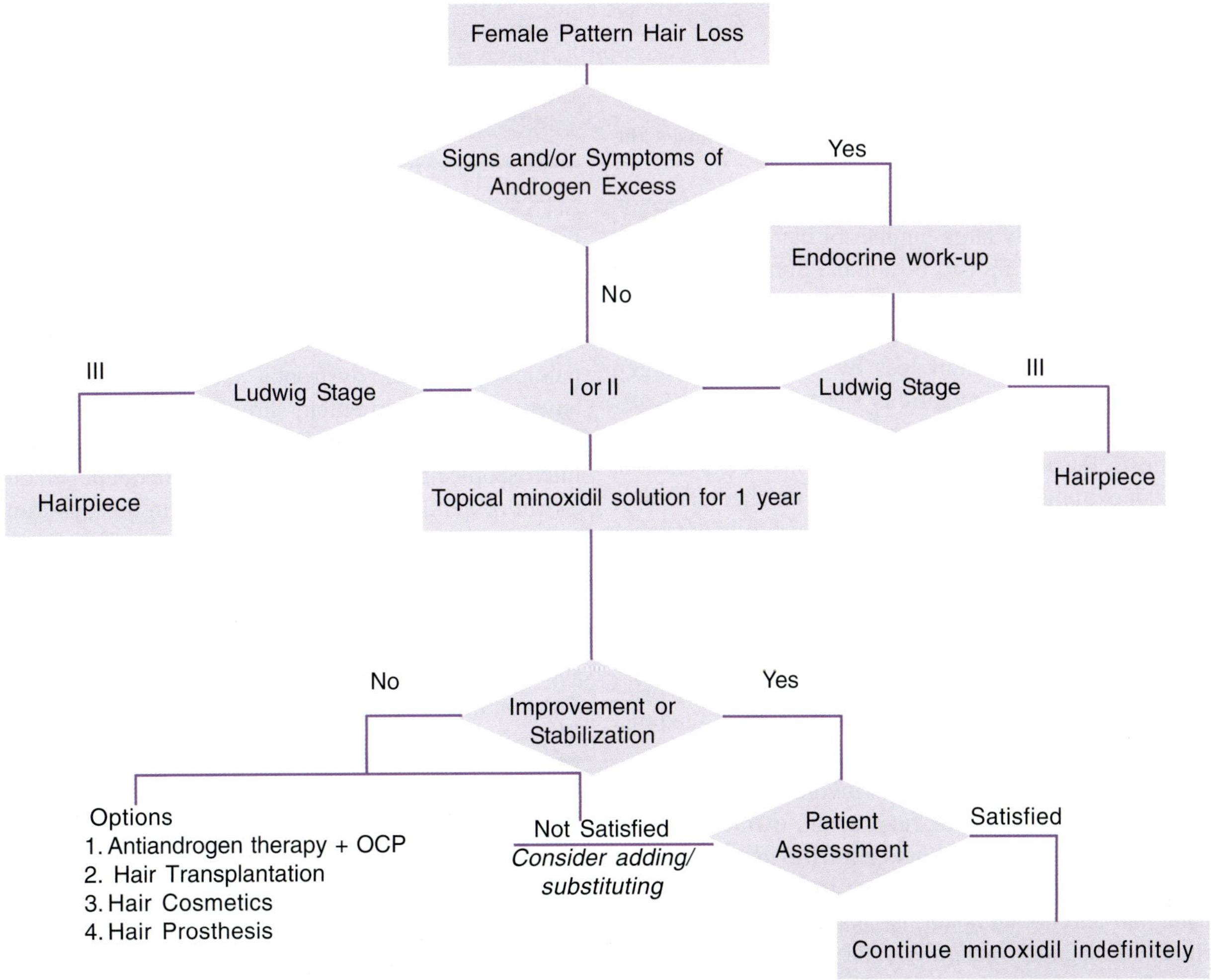

Flowchart 18.3

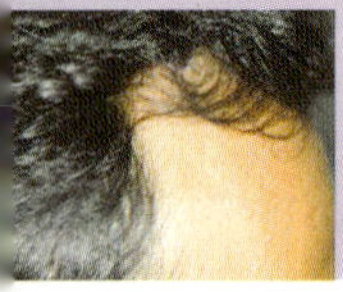

Table 18.3: Some drugs that can cause alopecia

Allopurinol	Interferon
Amiodarone	Isoniazid
Amphetamine	Itraconazole
Anabolic steroids	Levodopa
ACE inhibitors	Lithium
Anticoagulants	Minoxidil (temporary)
Anticonvulsants	MAOI
Antifungals (in high dose)	Nicotinic acid
Antimalarials	Nitrofurantoin
Antithyroid	NSAID
Benzimidazole	Oral contraceptive
β-Blockers	Progesterone
Bromocriptine	Retinoids
Captopril	Salicylates
Chemotherapeutic drugs	Sulfasalazine
Cholesterol-lowering agents	Tacrolimus
Cimetidine	Terfenadine
Colchicine	Testosterone
Corticosteroids	Tricyclic antidepressants
Gentamicin	
Gold	Vitamin A
Immunoglobulin	

Abbreviations: ACE, angiotensin-converting enzyme; MAOI, monamine oxidase inhibitors; NSAID, nonsteroidal anti-inflammatory drugs.

- Possibly smoking.
- Toxin exposure such as heavy metal intoxication; and
- Virtually any major insult to the body that causes the ratio of telogen to anagen hair to increase.

Within *2 or 3 months of the triggering event* the person notices an abnormally large number of hair coming out. It is usually reversible in 4 to 6 months. Some people with telogen effluvium may have a shortening of the anagen phase, which leads to shorter hair in addition. Multiple medications can cause hair loss by inducing a telogen effluvium but some medications such as *chemotherapy agents cause an anagen effluvium* because they interfere with mitosis. Because about 90% of scalp hair are in anagen, there is an extremely marked hair loss with chemotherapy. Both hypothyroidism and perhaps low ferritin may trigger a telogen effluvium.

There is a *chronic telogen effluvium* of unclear cause described primarily in middle aged women that affects the entire scalp, starts abruptly, often causes some temporal recession and fluctuates over a prolonged time. A brief overview of the investigations required is given below (Table 18.4).

Doing several hair pulls, which involves pulling firmly about 20 hair between your fingers and extracting more than 2 hair per pull, suggests a telogen effluvium. Inspecting the hair root under the microscope to make sure it is a telogen hair and not an abnormal anagen hair is important to clinch the diagnosis (and rule out loose anagen syndrome). Of course if a patient has vigorously shampooed and/or brushed their hair prior to seeing you the hair pull may not demonstrate an increased number of easily extractable telogen hair. On the other hand, if a patient only shampoos and or brushes their hair very infrequently, their hair pull test may be falsely elevated with excessively large numbers of telogen hair.

Treatment

Though various Oral vitamins have been travel unless the cause is nutritional the patients recover spontaneously.

Table 18.4: Laboratory studies to evaluate nonscarring alopecia

Baseline
Complete blood cell count
Ferritin
VDRL with dilutions
Thyroid screening
Microscopic examination of hair
Fungal culture
Other
Scalp biopsy
Antinuclear antibody
Hormones (*e.g.*, dehydroepiandrosterone sulfate, testosterone, androstenedione)
Borate and thallium levels
Heavy metal screens

LOOSE ANAGEN SYNDROME

Loose anagen syndrome is a disorder usually presenting in young blond girls (but can present in adults) that is sporadic or inherited (as autosomal dominant with variable expression and incomplete penetrance) characterized by easily (and painlessly) plucked dystrophic scalp hair. The plucked hair have misshapen, irregular, shrunken roots that may have a "mousetail"–like or "loose-sock"–like appearance microscopically. Normal anagen hair are not pulled out with a firm or gentle pull, but anagen hair in this syndrome are very easily extracted. In this condition there is a weak adhesion between the hair shaft cuticle and the inner root sheath cuticle. This may present clinically as a diffuse or as a patchy hair loss. It may be associated with other entities such as alopecia areata, Noonan's syndrome and AIDS. The condition may improve with age.

SCARRING ALOPECIA (CICATRICIAL ALOPECIA)

Lymphocytic (more common in women)

Central centrifugal cicatricial alopecia (CCCA)
Discoid lupus

Lichen planopilaris (LPP)
  Frontal fibrosing alopecia

Pseudopelade of Brocq

Neutrophilic (more common in men)
Folliculitis decalvans
Dissecting cellulitis
Mixed
Acne keloidalis
Acne necrotica
Erosive pustular dermatosis

Lymphocytic types are as common as *neutrophilic types* and more common in *middle-aged women* whereas neutrophilic types are more common in *middle-aged men*.

I. Lymphocytic Cicatricial Alopecia Includes

- **Central centrifugal cicatricial alopecia (CCCA)** (formerly called "hot comb alopecia" or more recently "follicular degeneration syndrome").
- **Discoid lupus erythematosus.**
- **LPP** (and its variant frontal fibrosing alopecia [FFA]), and
- **Pseudopelade of Brocq**

a. **CCCA** is usually seen in black women and begins in the crown early on and may be confused with female pattern alopecia (and perhaps it is a scarring variant). Typically it is thought that the inherited types of hair loss are nonscarring, but perhaps this is not entirely true. It is slowly progressive.

b. **LPP (Fig. 18.5)** presents typically in women as a patchy hair loss with perifollicular erythema, follicular spines and scarring. About half these patients develop other skin, mucous membrane, or nail changes of lichen planus. Treatments usually include (topical and intralesional) steroids and antimalarials. Sometimes retinoids, oral griseofulvin, cyclosporine, and methotrexate have been used. Some cases resolve spontaneously, others last for years; the average duration is 18 months.

- **FFA**, a variant of LPP, is usually seen in women in their 60s as a recession of the frontal and temporal hairline with perifollicular erythema within the marginal hairline that is asymptomatic. There may be loss of eyebrows as well.

c. **Pscudopclade of Brocq (Fig. 18.6)** usually in women and presents as a noninflammatory, intermittently progressive, scarring alopecia of unknown cause that starts on the crown and spreads in a pseudopod-like fashion at irregular intervals and has been described as resembling "**footprints in the snow**" on the affected scalp.

Slowly progressive cicatricial alopecia without clinically evident folliculitis and no marked inflammation.

Diagnostic Criteria

1. **Clinical:**
   a. Irregularly defined and confluent patches of alopecia
   b. Mild perifollicular erythema (early stage)
   c. Moderate atrophy (late stage)
   d. Female/Male = 3:1
   e. Long course (> 2 years)
   f. Slow progression with spontaneous termination.
2. **Direct immunofluorescence:** Negative or only IgM.
3. **Histological:**
   a. Absence of marked inflammation
   b. Absence of widespread scarring
   c. Absence of significant follicular plugging
   d. Absence or decrease of sebaceous glands
   e. Normal epidermis
   f. Fibrotic streams into subcutis.

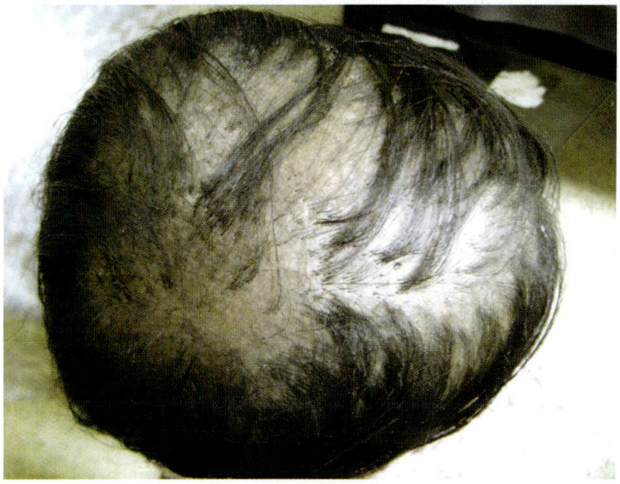

Fig. 18.5: Case of lichen plano pilaris—progressing to cicatricial alopecia

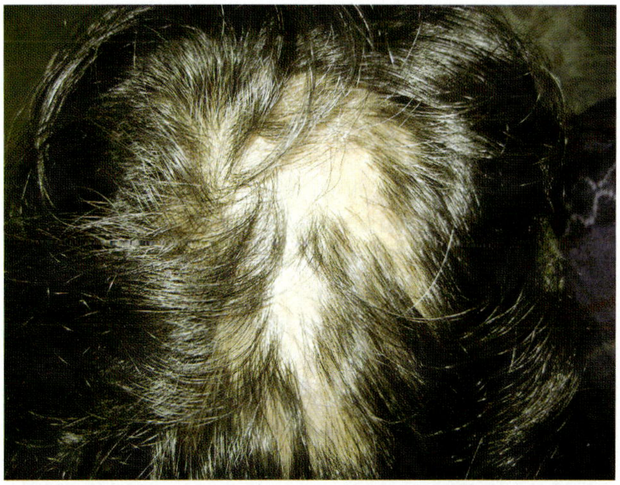

Fig. 18.6: Complete burnt out stage of cicatricial alopecia—pseudopelade

Treatment: I/L steroids not useful.

Surgical:

- Auto-grafting from unaffected to scarred scalp.
- Surgical expansion techniques.

A "**tufted folliculitis**" may result as the end stage of multiple types of scarring alopecias. It has the clinical appearance of "**doll's hair**"–numerous hair shafts exiting out of one aperture in multiple plugs. It is not diagnostic of any one disease, just as pseudopelade is not.

II. Neutrophilic Cicatricial Alopecias

Neutrophilic cicatricial alopecias include folliculitis decalvans and dissecting cellulitis/folliculitis (perifolliculitis capitis abscedens et suffodiens).

There is a cicatricial alopecia group in which the inflammatory infiltrate is mixed and this includes acne keloidalis (folliculitis keloidalis), acne (folliculitis) necrotica, and erosive pustular dermatosis.

- **Folliculitis decalvans** is a scarring folliculitis in which frequently staphylococcus aureus (and sometimes other bacteria) is cultured but response to antibiotics is not always that robust. In addition to giving the appropriate antibacterial agent based on culture and sensitivity, sometimes rifampin at 300 mg twice daily in combination is helpful. In addition to being a good medication to eradicate staphylococci it is effective for gram negative as well as gram positive organisms. It is capable of killing bacteria that are engulfed by phagocytic cells (may be one of the reasons it works so well in granulomatous diseases such as tuberculosis and leprosy). Rifampin does have numerous drug interactions and stains body fluids such as tears, saliva, perspiration, and urine a bright red color. Clindamycin at 300 mg/d can be used with rifampicin if other, safer antibiotics such as doxycycline are not effective but one should be aware of the risk of Clostridium difficile-induced diarrhea with clindamycin. Topical fusidic acid, oral zinc sulphate (400 mg/d), and steroids (topical and systemic), may be other considerations for therapy.
- **Dissecting cellulitis** is more common in young black men and begins as inflammatory, boggy nodules that drain with purulent drainage. Patients may be more likely to also have **hidradenitis suppurativa** and **acne conglobata** (often called the **follicular occlusion triad**). The cause is unknown and it tends to be a chronic problem. Usually it is not symptomatic but the disfiguring scarring and sometimes foul-smelling discharge are very problematic. Bacterial and fungal cultures should be performed. Treatment leaves a lot to be desired and has included various oral antibiotics (sometimes with the addition of rifampicin 600 mg/d to cephalexin or to ciprofloxacin), oral zinc sulphate 400 mg t.i.d. Oral isotretinoin is used in resistant cases for 4 to 5 months.

III. The Histologically Mixed Group of Cicatricial Alopecias includes Acne Keloidalis Primarily

This is more common in young black men and starts as smooth papules and pustules on the occipital scalp and posterior neck that evolve into keloid-like plaques. It may be asymptomatic or may have associated mild burning or itching. In mild cases a topical antibiotic may be helpful, but usually an oral antibiotic such as tetracycline (500 mg to 1 g total dose per day), doxycycline (100 to 200 m/d), minocycline (100 mg), or erythromycin (500 mg/d to 1 g/d) may prove helpful.

Acne necrotica presents usually as papules or necrotic pustules that are on the scalp and perhaps the face, neck, and chest that may lead to varioliform scars. It can be scarring or nonscarring. Oral antibiotics, intralesional or topical steroids, and even oral isotretinoin may be helpful for treatment.

Erosive pustular dermatosis is a pustular, necrotic, infundibular folliculitis with crusting that usually appears in older Caucasian women and later on has features of folliculitis decalvans.

MISCELLANEOUS HAIR DISORDERS

Traction Alopecia

Clinical features: Potentially reversible (early) hair loss: inadvertent process due to traction on scalp by physical force and certain hair styles/hairtyling devices.

Symmetrical along frontotemporal hair line:

• Afrocaribbeans (tight braids)	• Temporal hair loss
• Pony tails	• Frontotemporal hair loss
• Rollers	-do-
• **Sikh**	• Fronto parietal hair loss

Trichotillomania

- Greek – Hair pulling madness.
- Impulse control disorder.
- More common in females and children.
- Clinically, an ill-defined patch with twisted and broken hair at various distances from clinically normal scalp. Usually frontoparietal involvement.
- Histological, numerous empty canals; damaged follicles with intra epithelial and perifollicular haemorrhages and intrafollicular pigment casts.

Treatment

- Behaviour modification.
- Chlorpromazine.

Follicular Lichen Planus

Early lesion: Present as violaceous erythematous follicular papules with slight scaling. Later, follicular plugs and hair loss with scarring.

Well developed lesion: Smooth skin coloured patch of scarring alopecia with or without follicular plugging at periphery.

Graham-Little Syndrome

- Variant of L.P.
- Affects middle—aged or elderly women usually.
- Clinical findings.
- Progressive cicatricial alopecia of scalp with or without follicular plugging.
- Loss of axillary and pubic hair without clinically evident scarring.
- Widespread keratosis pilaris.

STRUCTURAL DEFECTS OF HAIR

A pictorial representation of the structural defects of hair disorders is elucidated in (Figs. 18.7 to 18.15).

a. *Trichoptilosis:* Hair are split and feathered (Fig. 18.7).
b. *Trichoclasis:* Transverse split in hair with retained cuticle.
c. *Trichoschisis*: Smooth transverse split in hair associated with trichothiodystrophy (Fig. 18.8).
d. *Trichorrhexis nodosa:* Localized longitudinal splitting of shaft, frayed ends are like two paint brush pushed into each other causing nodules along the shaft (Fig. 18.9).
e. *Trichonodosis:* Knots and loops in shaft.
f. *Trichorrhexis Invaginata:* Distal shaft pushed into bulbous receptacle on proximal shaft (bamboo hair) associated with Netherton Syndrome (Fig. 18.10-18.12).
g. *Pilus torti:* Twisting of hair along its long axis (Fig. 18.13).
h. *Monilethrix:* Shaft has alternate swellings and constrictions producing beaded effect (Fig. 18.14).
i. *Pseudomonilethrix:* Similar but only part of the shaft is involved.
j. *Loose anagen hair syndrome:* All pulled hair are anagen.
k. *Pilus annulatus:* Alternating band of dark and light hair (Fig. 18.15).

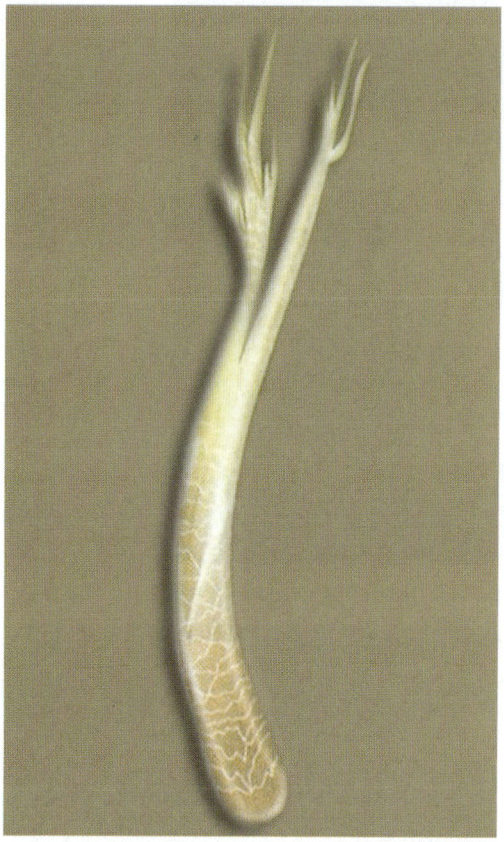

Fig. 18.7: Trichoptilosis

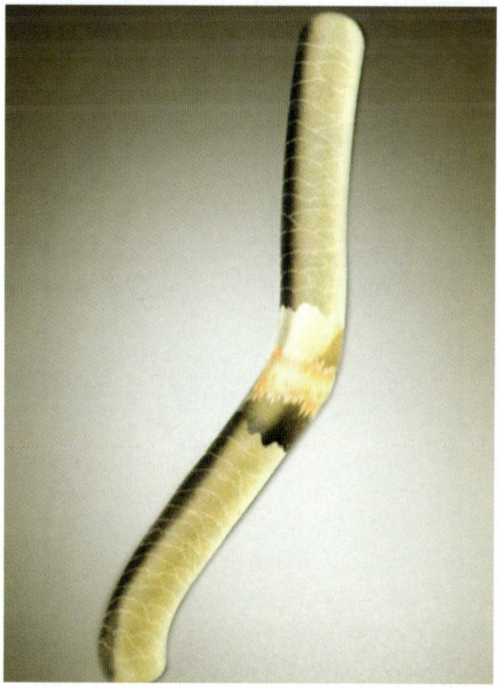

Fig. 18.8: Trichoschisis

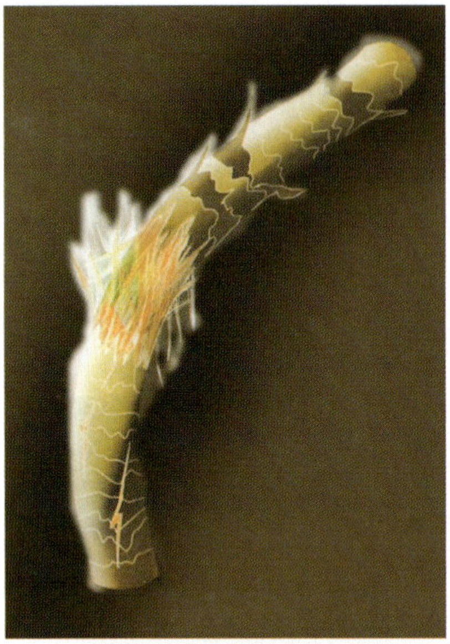

Fig. 18.9: Trichorrhexis nodosa

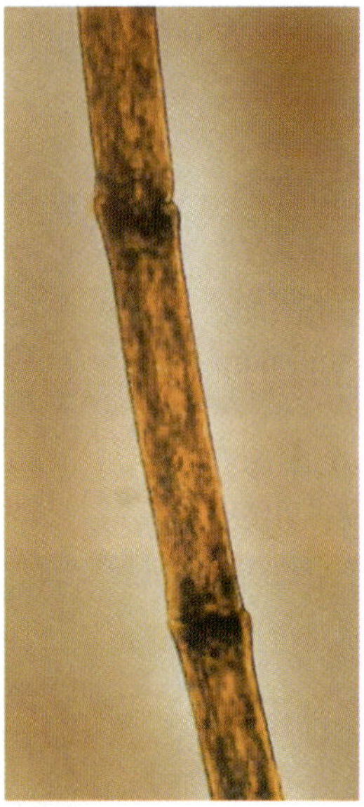

Fig. 18.10: Bamboo hair

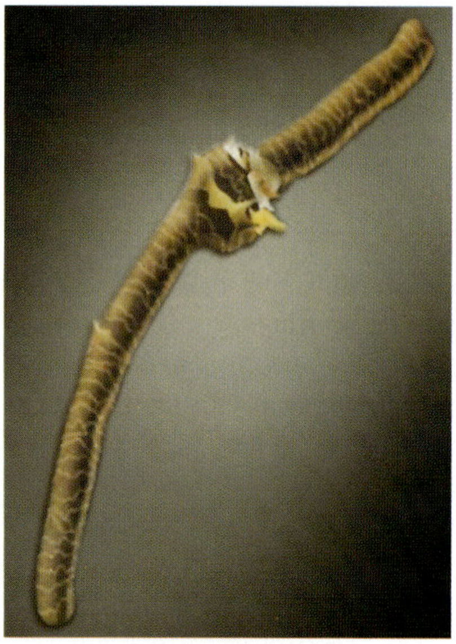

Fig. 18.11: Bamboo hair

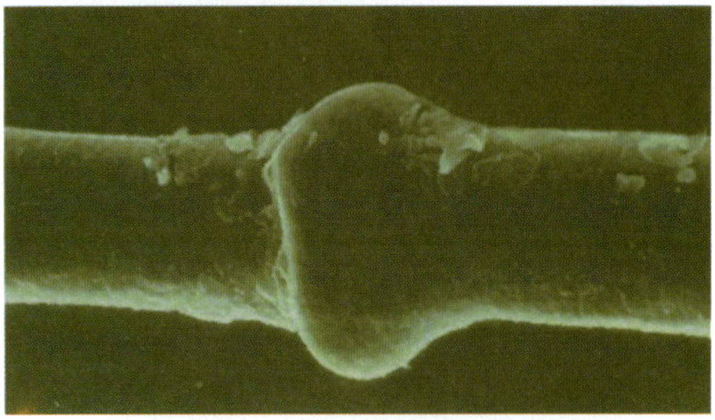

Fig. 18.12: Bamboo hair

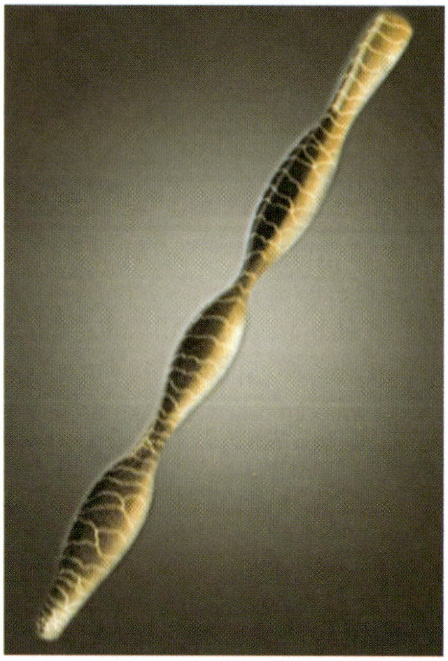

Fig. 18.14: Monilethrix

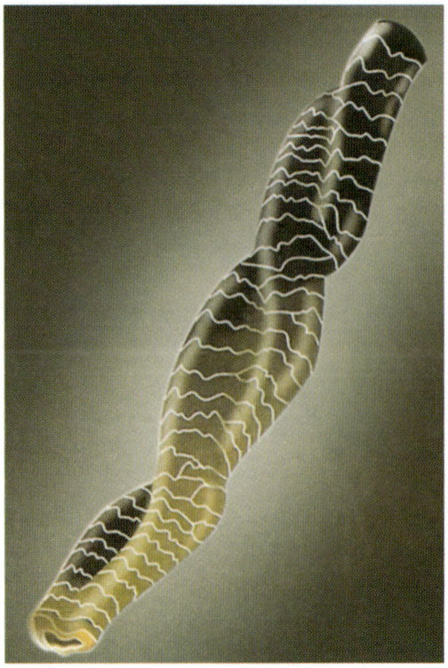

Fig. 18.13: Pilus torti

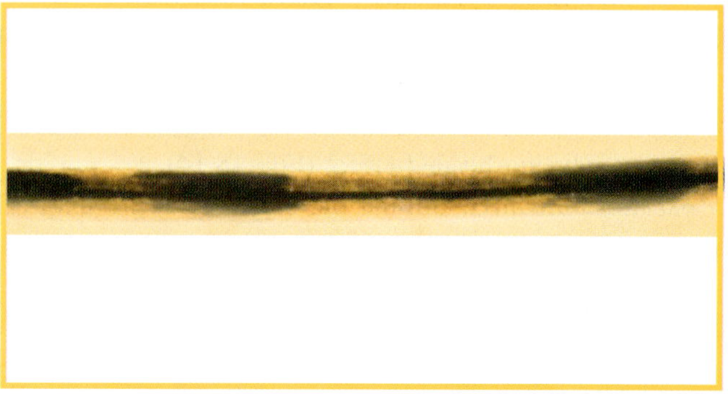

Fig. 18.15: Pilus annulatus

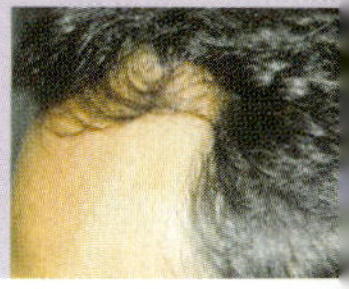

ALOPECIA DUE TO STRUCTURAL DEFECT

There are two types of disorders depending on the hair fragility:

A. Increased Hair Fragility

Monilethrix, Pseudomonilethrix, Pilus torti, Netherton Syndrome, Trichorrhexis nodosa,Trichiothiodystrophy.

B. No Hair Fragility

Pilus annulatus, wooly hair, uncombable hair syndrome.

- **Trichorrhexis nodosa** (Fig. 18.9) is the **most common hair** shaft disorder and most commonly is acquired secondary to damage from hair grooming procedures although it may be associated with hypothyroidism and with other rarer syndromes such as argininosuccinicaciduria or **Menkes' syndrome**. Severe scratching or other trauma as seen with lichen simplex chronicus or trichotillomania may lead to this hair shaft abnormality. Clinically, it presents as tiny white specks on the hair shaft that may superficially look like nits from head lice. When viewed microscopically these specks resemble the bristles of two broom ends interlocked and are the site of fractures. This condition is more likely to occur proximally in black hair and more distally in Caucasian or Asian hair. The resulting breakage may lead to the clinical complaint of the hair not growing very long.
- **Uncombable hair syndrome** ("spun glass hair") is an interesting hair shaft abnormality in which the hair shafts in cross-section are triangular and on electron microscopy there are longitudinal grooves. The onset is usually around 3 years of age when the hair seems particularly wild and unruly. Typically the hair is a silver-blond color and the problem may be generalized (usually) or localized. Spontaneous improvement may occur in childhood. Oral biotin may prove helpful. This same triangular hair-shaft abnormality has been described in loose anagen syndrome and after spironolactone therapy.
- **Acquired progressive kinking** of the hair is an odd entity that usually arises in the teens or early adult years in young white men. Gradually the hair becomes kinky, dry, and more unmanageable. The hair shaft is said to be elliptical with partial twists at irregular intervals. The anagen (growth) phase is said to be diminished. Oral retinoids or local radiation may induce a clinically similar problem. Interestingly, a seemingly converse clinical picture has been described in people of color with the acquired immunodeficiency syndrome who develop softer, silkier hair that replaces previously normal kinky hair. In addition, the color is said to become ashen and the hair becomes sparse.
- **Trichoptilosis ("split ends")** (Fig. 18.8) is the longitudinal splitting of the distal hair shaft as a result of weathering and is made more striking by overuse of various cosmetic hair styling and grooming procedures. Hair pulling and scratching may be causative. Various unusual inherited hair shaft defects are more prone to trichoptilosis.
- **Bubble hair** is the result of excessive heat from hair dryers (and perhaps other chemical treatments of the hair) leading to distinctive "bubbles" within the hair shaft. These hair may appear brittle and broken off. Interestingly with thallium intoxication a bubble-like inclusion can be seen within the hair shaft; typically thallium intoxication leads to massive hair loss.
- **Pseudofolliculitis barbae** is a problem typically seen in the beard area of black men caused by close shaving in curly or kinky hair that may cause the newly emerging hair shaft to grow back into the skin surface or pierce the follicular wall, causing inflammation. Clinically it presents as papulopustules that may lead to hyperpigmentation and scarring. Hair plucking and electrolysis can induce the same type of problem.

REFERENCES

- Camacho F, Montagna W: Trichology, diseases of the pilosebaceous follicle, Basel, S. Karger Publisher, 1998.
- Dawber R: Disease of Hair and Scalp, Oxford, Blackwell Science, 1997.
- Dawber R, Van Neste D: Hair and scalp disorders: Common presenting signs, differential diagnosis and treatment, Philadelphia, Lippincott, 1995.
- Olsen EA: Disorders of hair growth: Diagnosis and treatment. New York, McGraw-Hill, 2003.
- Whiting DA: Update on hair disorders, Dermatol Clin 1996;14(4).
- Whiting DA, Howsden FL: Color atlas of differential diagnosis of hair loss, Cedar Grove, NJ, Canfield Publishing, 1996.
- Management of Hair loss, Dermatological Therapy, Dermatology Clinics 2005; 23:2.

Nail

ANATOMY OF THE NAIL UNIT (Figs. 18.16 and 18.17)

The nail unit is a specialized appendage of the skin, composed of unique structures not found elsewhere in the body. The nail unit consists of the proximal and lateral nail folds, the nail matrix, the nail bed and the hyponychium.

The **nail plate** is the clear, firm section of the nail that is made of hard keratin. The nail plate is created by the nail matrix, a section of germative cells located proximal to the nail plate. The **nail matrix** contains a layer of actively dividing keratinocytes that mature and, after death, contribute to the formation of the nail plate. The nail plate is bordered by the proximal nail fold and two lateral nail folds. The **lunula** is the most distal portion of the matrix and is seen as a white, arched area under the nail plate and bordered by the proximal nail fold. The nail plate sits on top of the nail bed, which is highly vascular. The **hyponychium** is the section of skin located under the free edge of the nail plate between the nail bed and the distal nail groove.

Fingernails grow constantly at a rate of **0.1 mm per day or 3 mm per month**. At this rate, a fingernail can be totally replaced in 4 to 6 months. Toenails, however, grow at about half this rate. It can take *8 to 12 months for a toenail* to be totally replaced by a new nail.

1. DISEASES OF NAIL PLATE

Pits	Psoriasis, Fig. 18.18 alopecia areata, hand dermatitis, nail biting, lichen planus (very rare)
Horizontal ridges	Beau's lines, any inflammation affecting soft tissues around nails
Longitudinal ridges:	Pressure effect e.g. tumour in nail fold
• **Single**	Psoriasis, lichen planus, alopecia areata
• **Multiple**	Darier's disease
Thickening	Psoriasis, onychomycosis, pachyonychia congenita
Onycholysis (separation of nail plate from nail bed distally)	Idiopathic, psoriasis, onychomycosis, trauma, thyroid acropachy, drug induced photo-onycholysis e.g. tetracyclines
Subungual hyperkeratosis	Psoriasis, onychomycosis, trauma, ischaemia
Koilonychia	Iron deficiency, lichen planus, idiopathic
Colour changes	Infection: Pseudomonas (green) Fig. 18.19 Drugs: Tetracycline (yellow) Antimalarial (blue) Chlorpromazine (brown) Topical agents: Potassium permanganate Dyes: Systemic diseases: Cirrhosis hypoproteinaemia (white) Others: Cigarette smoking (brown) Subungual haematoma (reddish blue) Melanoma (black)
Leuconychia (whiteness of nail):	
True (affect nail plate)	Onychomycosis, trauma, congenital
Apparent (affect subungual tissues)	Anaemia, hypoproteinaemia
Pigmented streaks	Normal in pigmented skin, malignant melanoma, benign melanocytic naevi, Addison's disease

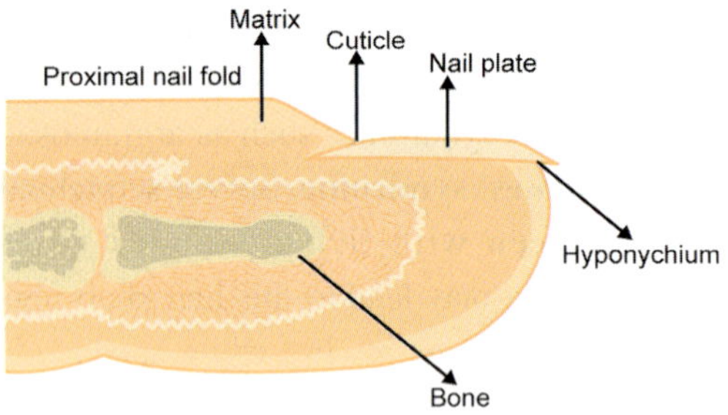

Fig. 18.16: Anatomy of the nail

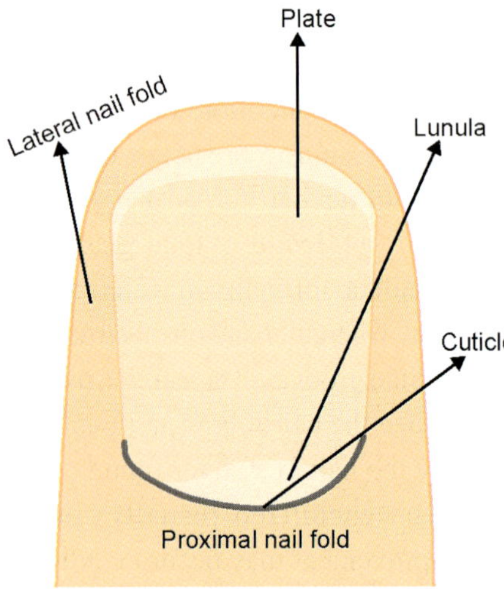

Fig. 18.17: Diagrammatic representation of nail

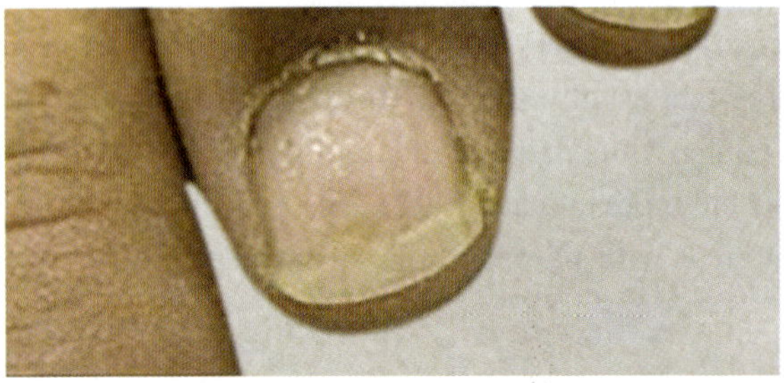

Fig. 18.18: Random, irregular, deep pits of psoriasis

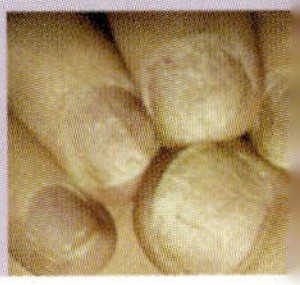

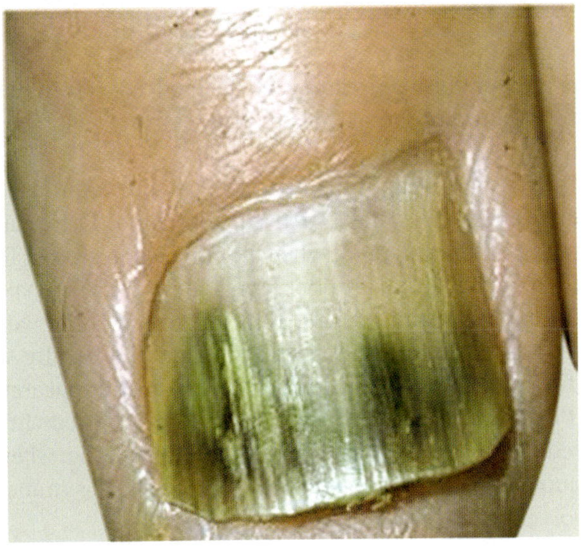

Fig. 18.19: Green discolouration due to pseudomonas

2. DISEASES OF NAIL FOLD

(i) Paronychia (inflammation of nail fold)	Acute Chronic
(ii) Trauma	Trauma, wet work, drugs e.g. etretinate
(iii) **Pterygium formation** (cuticle appears to grow out over the nail with loss of proximal nail fold)	Lichen planus, circulatory disorders, pemphigus
(iv) Palisading of dilated nail fold capillaries	Dermatomyositis, lupus erythematosus, scleroderma
(v) Infarcts at posterior or lateral folds	Vasculitis, e.g. rheumatoid diseases
(vi) Nailfold masses	Viral warts, myxoid cyst, periungual, fibromata, malignant melanoma.

3. DISEASES OF NAIL BED AND MATRIX

Tumor	Subungual exostosis
	Glomus tumor
	Naevus
	Malignant melanoma
Infection	Subungual wart

COMMON NAIL DISODERS

Effects of Trauma

Permanent ridges or splits in the nail plate can follow damage to the nail matrix. **Splinter haemorrhages** (Fig. 18.20), the linear nature of which is determined by longitudinal ridges and grooves in the nail bed, are most commonly seen under the nails of manual workers and are caused by minor trauma. They may also be a feature of *psoriasis* of the nail and of subacute *bacterial endocarditis.*

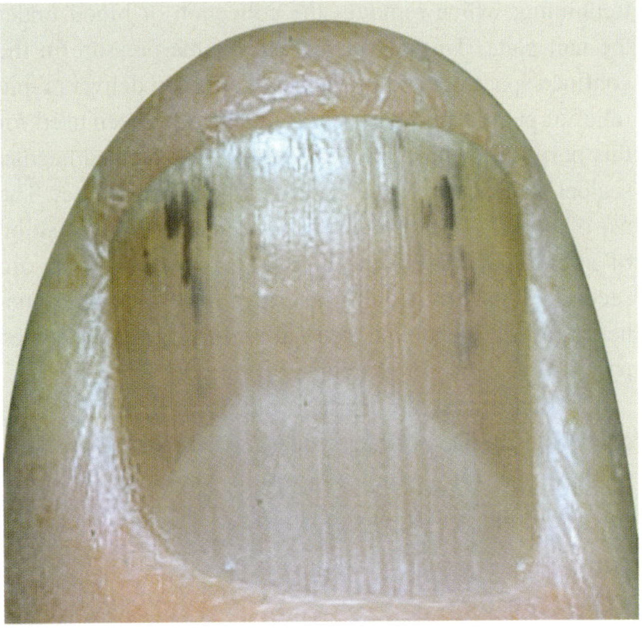

Fig. 18.20: Splinter hemorrhage

Subungual Hematoma (Fig. 18.21)

A common problem encountered by both dermatologists and primary care physicians is the **subungual hematoma**, a collection of blood beneath the nail plate. Clinically, it appears as a bluish or violaceous discoloration under the nail plate. The hematoma can produce a significant amount of pressure in the space between the nail bed and nail plate, causing intense pain. The most common cause of subungual hematoma is trauma to the nail: either a sudden, strong, external force, or repeated minor traumatic events occurring over time. Subungual hematomas form easily because the nail bed is a highly vascular structure, prone to bleeding if traumatized. Usually it is self limiting.

Treatment

The classic treatment for a subungual hematoma is nail

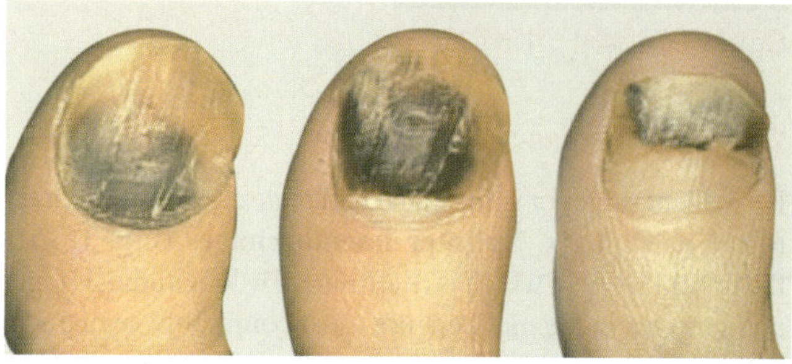

Fig. 18.21: Subungual hematoma

trephining, which removes the collection of blood under the nail plate. This maneuver relieves the pressure in the confined space created by the hematoma and delivers rapid relief of pain. A number of instruments have been used for this purpose, including a heated paper clip, heated needle, scalpel blade, cautery device, and carbon dioxide laser. The use of an extra-fine insulin syringe needle for the evacuation of subungual hematoma has been reported. To avoid secondary nail dystrophy resulting from the subungual hematoma, it is recommended that evacuation not be delayed past 6 to 12 hours after injury.

Chronic trauma from sport and from ill-fitting shoes contributes to haemorrhage under the nails of the big toes, to the gross thickening of toenails known as onychogryphosis and to ingrowing nails (Fig. 18.22).

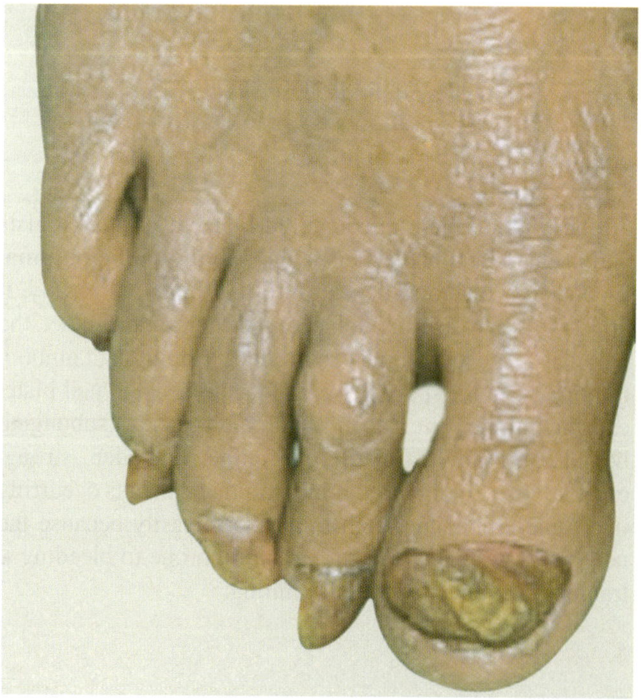

Fig. 18.22: Onychogryphosis

PINCER NAIL

The pincer nail deformity is defined as a transverse overcurvature of the nail plate, progressively pinching the nail bed.

The lateral edges of the nail plate can break through the skin, resulting in granulation tissue formation. There can be a trumpet-like appearance when the curvature increases from the proximal to distal portion. Involvement of the toenails is more common than the fingernails. A patient's life can be greatly affected by the pain, inflammation, difficulty with ill-fitting footwear, and an undesirable cosmetic appearance.

Pincer nails can be both familial and acquired. In the hereditary form, involvement is usually symmetric, whereas acquired pincer nails generally do not show symmetric involvement.

Diagnosis

There are a variety of causes of acquired pincer nails. The most common cause is deviation of the phalanges of the feet secondary to ill-fitting shoes. The most common skin disease causing an acquired pincer nail deformity is psoriasis. When tumors, such as an exostosis, implantation cyst, or myxoid cyst, are responsible for the pincer nail deformity, removal of the tumor may reverse the nail defect.

Pincer nails have also been reported in association with metastasis of colon carcinoma. Other causes of acquired pincer nail deformity include nail infection with the dermatophyte *T. rubrum*, placement of an arteriovenous fistula for hemodialysis, and use of beta blocker medications. Finger pincer nail deformity can be seen in association with osteoarthritis.

Treatment

Treatment of the pincer nail can be attempted without surgery by use of a brace placed on the nail plate and fixed on the lateral edges. This brace can be gradually adjusted and results in flattening of the nail plate.

Nail avulsion has not been shown to be a successful treatment, and in fact can aggravate the problem. Successful surgical treatments have corrected the pincer nail deformity by selective destruction of the lateral matrix horns. Further improvement can be obtained by surgically removing any possible bony defects contributing to the nail deformity. Permanent destruction of the nail matrix by phenol or surgical ablation may be required as a last resort.

ONYCHOCRYPTOSIS (INGROWN NAILS) (Fig. 18.23)

Onychocryptosis occurs most commonly when the distal lateral edge of the nail plate presses on the nail fold resulting

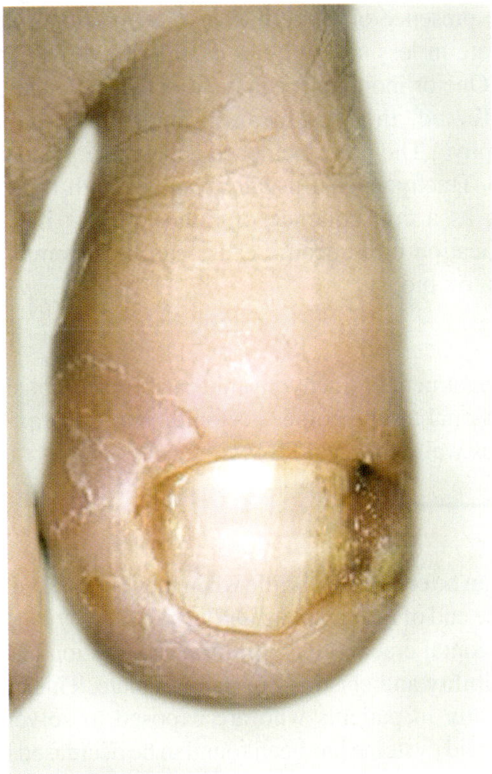

Fig. 18.23: Ingrowing toe nail with secondary infection

in inflammation and soft tissue hypertrophy, which can become secondarily infected. The great toenail is the most often affected site. This condition can be painful for patients and significantly restrict mobility.

Diagnosis

Onychocryptosis is often caused by, and is associated with, onychomycosis, resulting in a thickened and dystrophic nail. Incorrect technique in nail trimming can cause onychocryptosis. This occurs when the nail plate corners are cut in a curved manner and not allowed to grow over the toe. Other conditions predisposing patients to onychocryptosis include arthritis, circulatory disorders, hyperhidrosis and obesity. In younger patients, repetitive trauma, and poor foot hygiene are thought to contribute to this problem.

Treatment

Early disease can be treated with non-surgical therapy including the placement of a barrier (such as a wedge of fabric treated with an antiseptic solution) between the nail plate and nail fold that stays in place until the nail plate grows beyond the end of the toe. A separate option is excising the portion of the nail plate which is pressing on the nail fold. With the offending area removed, the inflamed nail fold can recover to its normal state while new nail forms.

RACKET NAIL

The racket nail is named after its similarity in shape to a tennis racket. The nail is short, broad and flat (Fig. 18.24). The cause is not because of the nail itself, but occurs rather in response to a deformity in the underlying soft tissue. The most common location is the thumb involved alone, but other digits may be involved as well. It is found more often in women, and affected patients are normal otherwise. Racket nails may be inherited in an autosomal dominant manner. One or both hands can be affected. This finding can be a source of embarrassment to patients, but does not otherwise affect functioning of the affected digit. Most cases of racket nail are congenital, but an acquired case of racket nails was reported in association with tertiary hyperparathyroidism.

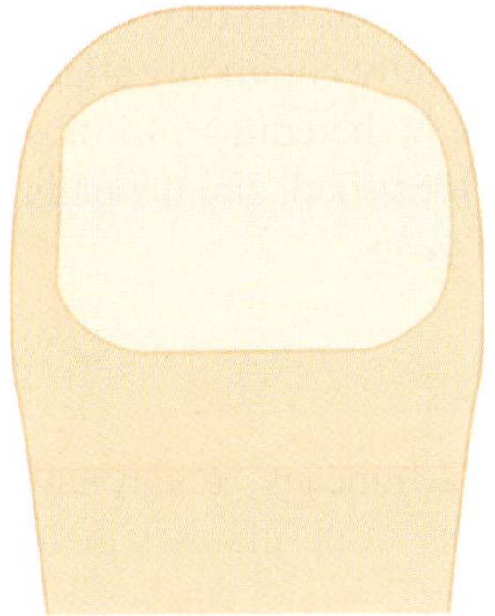

Fig. 18.24: Racket nail

HABIT-TIC DEFORMITY (Fig. 18.25)

The habit-tic deformity presents as evenly spaced, parallel transverse grooves with central depression in the nail plate.

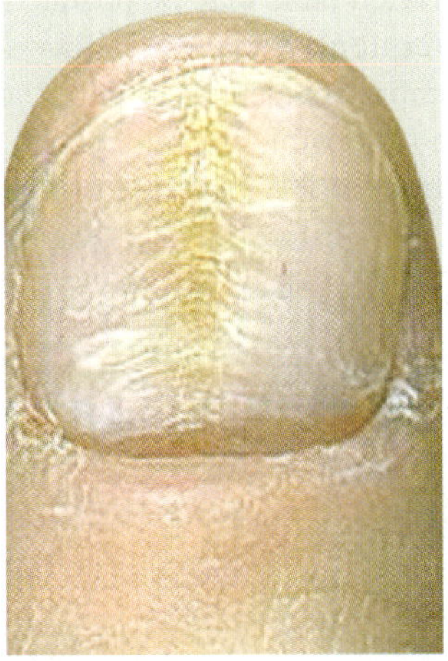

Fig. 18.25: Habit-tic deformity

The lunula is enlarged and the cuticle is often disrupted. The most commonly affected site is the thumb nail, but other nails can also be affected. This deformity is caused by repeated trauma to the nail matrix at the proximal nail fold secondary to picking. This can be a conscious or unconscious habit developed by the patient.

Body dysmorphic disorder, obsessive-compulsive disorder, and other psychiatric illnesses that involve a loss of impulse control can include ritualistic nail picking as part of the disease spectrum. The picking action can also be a nervous habit, unrelated to a specific psychiatric disorder. A case of the habit-tic deformity responding to treatment with fluoxetine has been reported.

MEDIAN CANALIFORM DYSTROPHY

Median canaliform dystrophy, also known as dystrophia unguium mediana canaliformis, is a nail plate defect in which a median (central) ridge develops, with short transverse ridges running from both sides of the central split. This has been described as an **"inverted fir tree configuration".** The thumb nails are the site most commonly affected. Median canaliform dystrophy can be hereditary. In most cases, an inciting cause cannot be identified, and the nails normalize in a period of months to years.

TRACHYONYCHIA

Trachyonychia (Fig. 18.26) means "rough nails" and can be associated with a variety of dermatoses including:

- Lichen planus.
- Psoriasis.
- Alopecia areata.
- Atopic dermatitis, and
- Ichthyosis vulgaris.

It has also been associated with immunoglobulin A deficiency. The affected nails may be opaque (sandpapered nails) or, less frequently, have a shiny appearance. Trachyonychia is more frequent in children, where it may be an isolated sign (idiopathic trachyonychia).

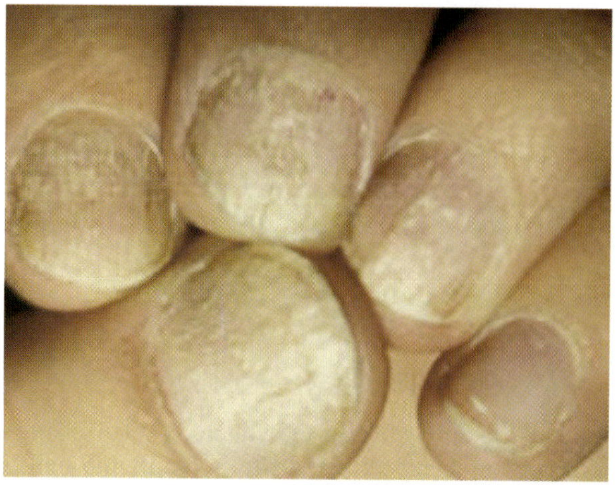

Fig. 18.26: Trachyonychia

The presence of numerous small, superficial pits in the nail plate in less severe cases can cause the nail to appear shiny. One or more nails can be affected. When all 20 nails are affected, this condition is known as "twenty nail dystrophy". The peak incidence is between 3 and 12 years of age. Trachyonychia usually resolves with time when it occurs as a consequence of lichen planus in children. Identification of a specific cause can be accomplished by nail matrix biopsy.

Treatment

Local treatment of trachyonychia can be accomplished with intralesional triamcinolone acetonide into the proximal nail folds, as well as topical PUVA.

BRITTLE NAILS

Nails can be considered brittle when they are easily damaged. The free end of the nail plate is often affected by longitudinal or horizontal cracking or splitting. Dehydration causes loss of flexibility and elasticity of the nail plate. This can occur commonly in patients who are exposed to solvents. The amino acid cysteine has been found to be decreased in brittle nails.

Brittle nails may be divided into three types, in isolation or combination:

1. Splitting, more often single than multiple, sometimes associated with shallow parallel furrows, called **onychorrhexis**, and running along the dorsum of the nail.
2. **Lamellar**, splitting involving either the free edge, following frequent water immersion, or the proximal surface of the nail associated with lichen planus, or oral retinoids therapy (Fig. 18.27).

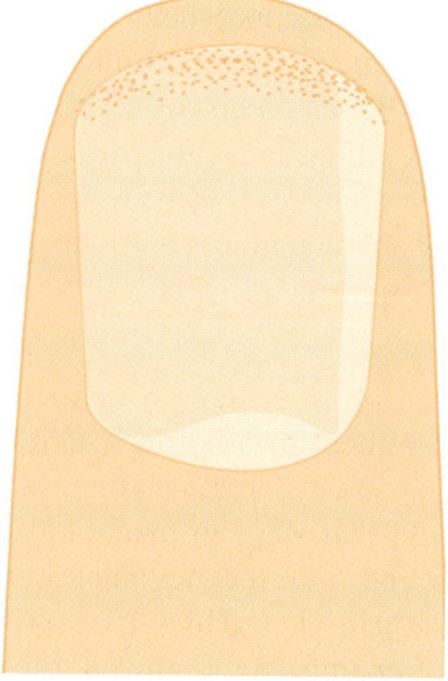

Fig. 18.27: Lamellar splits

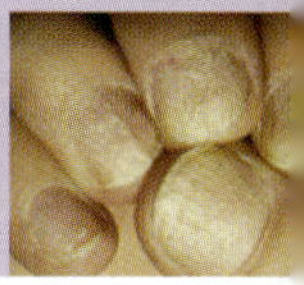

3. **Transverse** splitting and breaking of the lateral edge close to the free margin.

Causes

The dorsum of the nail may be friable in superficial onychomycosis as well as following nail enamel use. Friability may extend throughout the entire nail in advanced psoriasis and onychomycosis.

Dermatoses such as psoriasis, lichen planus, and alopecia areata can be associated with brittle nails.

Several systemic diseases are associated with brittle nails, including:

- Tuberculosis.
- Endocrinopathies.
- Iron deficiency anemia.
- Hemochromatosis.
- Glucagonoma; and
- Vitamin deficiencies.

Treatment

Treatment should first address any dermatologic or systemic disease that may be contributing to brittle nails. Cases of brittle nails can be divided into nails that are *hard and brittle* and nails that are *soft and brittle*.

Hard and brittle nails develop as a result of too little moisture, and the treatment goal is nail plate rehydration with the addition of a humidifier to the surrounding environment, daily emolliation, and nighttime nail soaks in water followed by urea or lactic acid creams. The nail plate can also be massaged with mineral oil after soaking to prevent drying.

Soft and brittle nails develop as a result of too much moisture. The treatment goal here is to avoid excess moisture by the use of cotton gloves or vinyl gloves for wet work, and avoidance of irritants.

Oral biotin, a B-complex vitamin, is considered the systemic treatment of choice for brittle nails. The recommended dose is 2.5 mg/d, taken for 3 to 6 months. The average time before clinical improvement is seen with biotin therapy is 2 months.

LONGITUDINAL MELANONYCHIA (MELANONYCHIA STRIATA)

Longitudinal melanonychia refers to a tan, brown, or black longitudinal band or streak affecting a nail. One or multiple nails can be involved. When multiple bands are present, the inciting cause is most likely non-neoplastic. Causes of multiple bands of longitudinal melanonychia include:

- Dermatologic disorders (Laugier-Hunziker syndrome, lichen planus, lichen striatus).
- Drugs (antimalarials, ketoconazole, minocycline, zidovudine, many chemotherapeutic agents).
- Bacterial and fungal infections.
- Racial variation.
- A variety of systemic diseases (Addison's disease, hyperbilirubinemia, hyperthyroidism, malnutrition, Peutz-Jeghers syndrome, porphyria and others).

The diagnosis of a nail unit melanoma is always in the differential diagnosis of longitudinal melanonychia, and can only be established or excluded by biopsy.

Presentation and Characteristics

A variety of other causes can be responsible for the clinical presentation of longitudinal melanonychia.

Pigment present from **exogenous** sources, such as dirt, tobacco, or tar, can usually be *scratched off* the nail plate. These sources usually do not present as a longitudinal streak. **Nail plate infection** with gram negative bacteria, such as Klebsiella and Proteus spp. can cause longitudinal melanonychia. When a greenish discoloration is present, infection with *pseudomonas aeruginosa is likely*. **Bacterial infection** causing a pigmented streak usually presents at the junction of the lateral and proximal nail folds. The border of this streak is usually variable. **Fungal infections** of the nail plate can also cause hyperpigmented streaks. These streaks are usually wider distally than proximally. **Subungual hematomas** caused by repeated minor trauma, usually from shoe friction, can cause an elliptical streak similar to longitudinal melanonychia. **Local irradiation** has also been reported to cause longitudinal melanonychia. A variety of **melanocytic lesions**, including acquired and congenital melanocytic nevi, benign and atypical melanocytic hyperplasias, and melanoma, can cause longitudinal melanonychia.

Situations in which **ungual melanoma** should be suspected in the presence of longitudinal melanonychia include longitudinal melanonychia, which:

- Begins in a single digit of a person during the fourth to sixth decade of life or later.
- Develops abruptly in a previously normal nail plate.
- Becomes suddenly darker or wider than 5 mm.
- Occurs in the thumb, index finger, or great toe.
- Occurs in a person with a history of digital trauma.
- Occurs singly in the digit of a dark-skinned patient.
- Demonstrates blurred lateral borders.
- Occurs in a person with a history or increased risk of melanoma; or
- Is accompanied by nail dystrophy.

COMMON INFECTIONS

Acute Paronychia

Bacterial infection (*Staph. Aureus, Strep. Pyogenes*) is the most common cause. There is acute swelling, tenderness and collection of pus in the nail fold. A swab should be taken if possible.

Give ampicillin 250 mg qid and cloxacillin 250 mg qid for 10 days. Analgesic should also be prescribed. Consider incision and drainage if swelling and pain does not improve quickly.

Chronic Paronychia

This is a multi-factorial condition:

1. Irritant dermatosis.
2. Infection: candidal; bacterial sometimes.
3. *Background eczema.*

All of the factors should be eliminated.

Treatment

Protection: Avoid water, detergent, soap if possible. Use rubber glove with inner cotton glove.

Emollient: Frequent application of bland emollient and use as a soap substitute.

Antibiotic: A course of systemic antibiotic should be considered in the first week.

Topical treatment: A combination of topical steroid and antifungal to the nail fold.

DERMATOSES

Psoriasis

Nail abnormalities are seen in 10 to 55 percent of adults with psoriasis. They are less common in children (7 to 13 percent). Psoriasis limited to the nails is quite frequent.

The following nail abnormalities are highly suggestive for a diagnosis of psoriasis: irregular pitting, salmon patches of the nail bed, and onycholysis. All these nail abnormalities are almost exclusively found in the fingernails (Fig. 18.28).

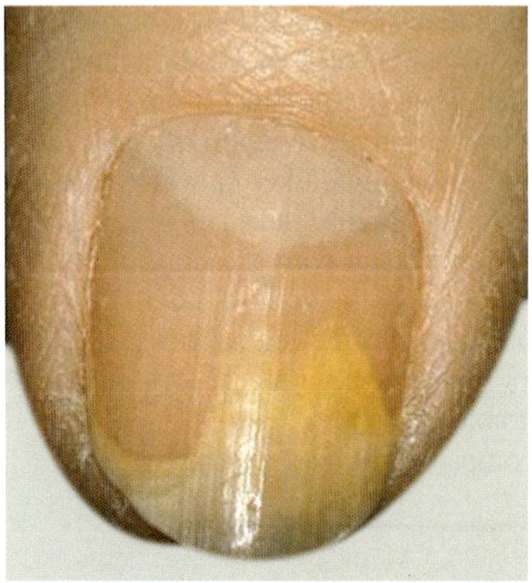

Fig. 18.28: Onycholysis, pitting and Salmon patch

Nail pitting results from the presence of easily detachable **parakeratotic** cells in the superficial layers of the nail plate. This nail abnormality indicates a disturbance in the maturation and keratinization of the proximal nail matrix. In psoriasis, pits are typically *deep, large, irregular in size and randomly distributed.*

Salmon patches appear as yellow or salmon-pink areas, irregular in size and shape, visible through the transparent nail plate. They result from a psoriatic involvement of the nail bed.

The term **onycholysis** describes the distal or lateral detachment of the nail plate from the nail bed.

In psoriasis, the onycholytic area is characteristically surrounded by an *erythematous* margin that marks its proximal border.

Other nail abnormalities that are not diagnostic, include splinter hemorrhages, nail bed hyperkeratosis, thickening and crumbling of the nail plate and chronic paronychia.

When psoriasis is limited to the toenails, differentiation from onychomycosis may be very difficult, because toenail psoriasis most commonly produces massive subungual hyperkeratosis and onycholysis clinically indistinguishable from those of onychomycosis. Psoriasis and onychomycosis are also frequently associated because psoriatic nails are more susceptible to fungal invasion than healthy nails.

Therapy

Nail psoriasis is difficult to treat.

When onycholysis is present, the detached nail plate should be removed. Systemic administration of methotrexate or cyclosporin A may improve the nail changes, but these drugs are not recommended in the absence of extensive skin psoriasis.

Intralesional steroid injections (10 mg/mL) are effective but very painful. Retinoids and PUVA are scarcely effective and may even worsen the nail changes. Topical application of creams containing steroids and salicylic acid, and/or topical application of calcipotriol ointment may be useful.

PUSTULAR PSORIASIS/HALLOPEAU'S ACRODERMATITIS CONTINUA

This condition frequently involves the nails and the periungual tissues. The disease, which is most frequently localized to one digit (usually a finger), typically shows a chronic course with periodic episodes of painful acute inflammation. In the acute phase, the affected digit shows severe inflammatory changes with pustular lesions of the nail bed and periungual skin. In the chronic phase, the nail bed and the periungual tissues show erythema and scaling. The nail plate is onycholytic or absent. The condition often improves with

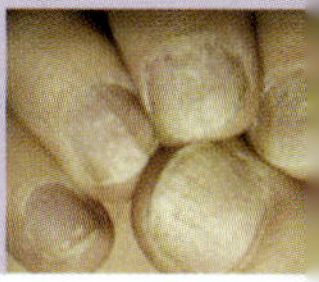

topical calcipotriol. Systemic retinoids may be useful in severe cases.

PARAKERATOSIS PUSTULOSA

This condition, which is exclusively seen in children, usually involves one finger, most commonly the thumb or the index finger. The affected nail shows subungual hyperkeratosis and onycholysis, which are usually more marked on one side of the nail.

LICHEN PLANUS

Nail involvement occurs in about 10 percent of patients with lichen planus. Nail abnormalities that are highly suggestive of lichen planus include dorsal pterygium and diffuse nail thinning and splitting (Fig. 18.29).

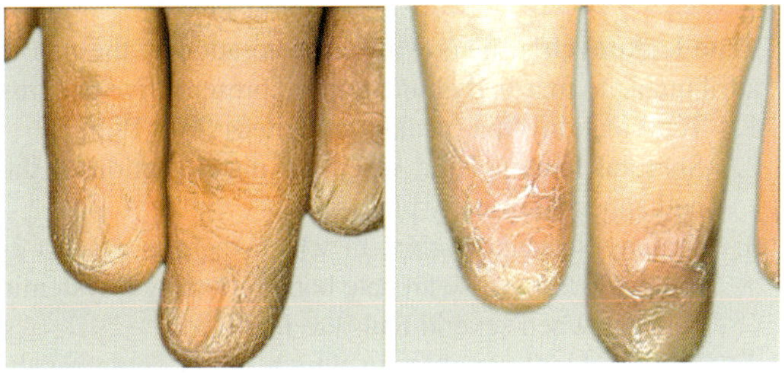

Fig. 18.29: Pterygium with anonychia and onychomadesis and scarring

Pterygium appears as an extension of the skin of the proximal nail fold that expands distally to adhere to the nail bed (Fig. 18.30).

Although lichen planus is the most common cause of nail pterygium, this lesion may be a consequence of nail matrix destruction by other conditions, including trauma, digital ischemia and bullous disorders.

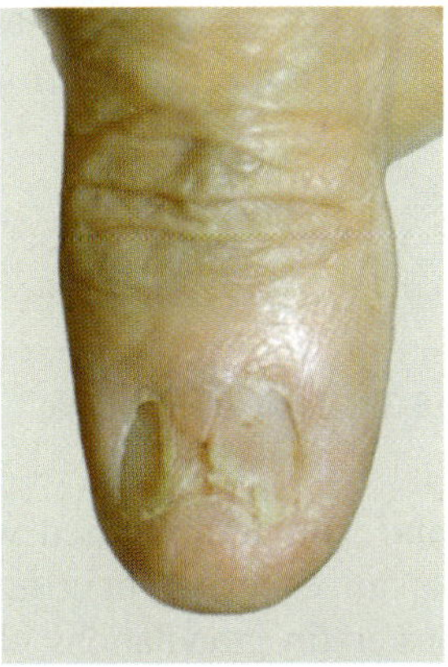

Fig. 18.30: Pterygium

Dorsal pterygium consists of a gradual shortening of the proximal nail groove, leading to progressive thinning of the nail plate and secondary fissuring caused by the fusion of the PNF to the matrix and subsequently to the nail bed. The portions of the divided nail plate progressively decrease in size as the pterygium widens. After several years, the pathologic process results in total loss of the nail, with permanent atrophy and sometimes scarring in the nail area. Pterygium is characteristic of lichen planus. It may also follow severe bullous dermatoses, radiotherapy, trauma, or digital ischemia. Rarely, it is congenital.

Ventral pterygium is a distal extension of the hyponychial tissue that is anchored to the undersurface of the nail, thereby obliterating the distal groove. Several conditions can cause ventral pterygium including: scleroderma associated with Raynaud's phenomenon, causalgia of the median nerve, trauma, and a reaction to a formaldehyde-containing nail cosmetic. Congenital forms exist (Fig. 18.31).

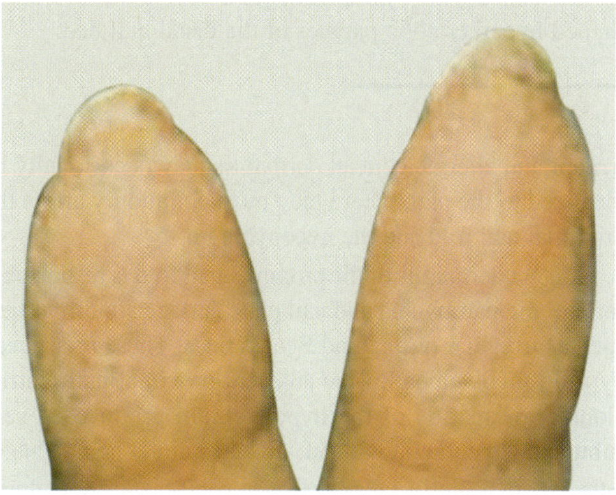

Fig. 18.31: Ventral pterygium

Nail thinning and splitting are consequences of diffuse and mild involvement of the nail matrix by lichen planus. The nail plate is diffusely or partially thinned and presents longitudinal ridging and splitting.

Nail bed lichen planus produces subungual hyperkeratosis and onycholysis.

Therapy

The definitive diagnosis of nail matrix lichen planus requires a nail biopsy. Except for trachyonychia, treatment of nail lichen planus is mandatory, because if left untreated, it may produce diffuse nail scarring. Systemic (triamcinolone 0.5 to 1 mg/kg IM every 30 days) or intralesional steroids are effective. Acitretin is also effective.

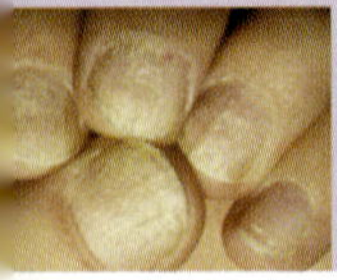

ALOPECIA AREATA

Nail abnormalities are frequent in patients with alopecia areata, particularly in children. They may precede or follow the onset of the disease and usually regress spontaneously. The changes include *geometric pitting, mottled erythema of the lunulae and trachyonychia.*

Pits are usually *small, superficial, and regularly* distributed in a **geometric pattern**.

Trachyonychia observed in 20-nail dystrophy describes nail roughness caused by excessive longitudinal striations. This nail sign is not exclusive to alopecia areata because it can also be a sign of other inflammatory disorders such as lichen planus, psoriasis, eczema, and pemphigus vulgaris.

DARIER'S DISEASE

The nail abnormalities are diagnostic and consist of longitudinal subungual white and red streaks. White streaks are associated with **V-shaped distal** notching due to wedge-shaped hyperkeratotic papules of the distal nail bed.

CONTACT DERMATITIS

Irritant and allergic contact dermatitis may occasionally be localized to the nail, where they most commonly affect the proximal nail fold and the hyponychium.

Contact dermatitis of the proximal nail fold is responsible for chronic paronychia and nail plate surface abnormalities, such as irregular pitting and Beau's lines. These are caused by mild involvement of the adjacent proximal nail matrix. Contact dermatitis of the hyponychium produces severe subungual hyperkeratosis and nail bed splinter hemorrhages Attempts to beautify nails can lead to contact allergy. Culprits include the acrylate adhesive used with artificial nails and formaldehyde in nail hardeners. In contrast, contact dermatitis caused by allergens in nail polish itself seldom affects the fingers but presents as small itchy eczematous areas where the nail plates rest against the skin during sleep. The eyelids, face and neck are favourite sites.

THE NAIL IN SYSTEMIC DISEASE

Clubbing is a bulbous enlargement of the terminal phalanx with an increase in the angle between the nail plate and the proximal fold to over 180°. Its association with chronic lung disease and with cyanotic heart disease is well known.

Rarely clubbing may be familial with no underlying cause. The mechanisms involved in its formation are still not known.

Koilonychia, a spooning and thinning of the nail plate, indicates iron deficiency (Fig. 18.32).

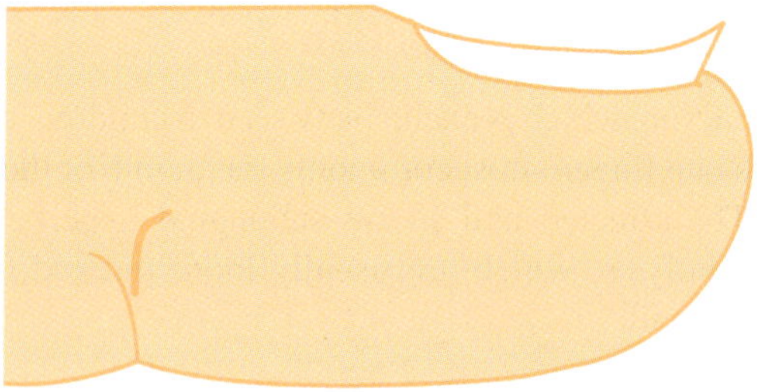

The concave, spoon-shaped nail of koilonychia (seen in iron deficiency)

Fig. 18.32: Koilonychia

COLOUR CHANGES

True leukonychia: This white discoloration of the nail is attributable to matrix dysfunction and presents five patterns

1. Total leukonychia (usually inherited) (Fig. 18.33).
2. Subtotal leukonychia, when the distal portion of the nail appears normally pink.
3. Transverse leukonychia, in which there is a 1- to 2-mm wide transverse arcuate band reflecting a systemic disorder when several nails are involved.
4. Punctate leukonychia, in which white spots result, usually from minor trauma (manicure); and
5. Longitudinal leukonychia, which may be associated with Darier's disease.

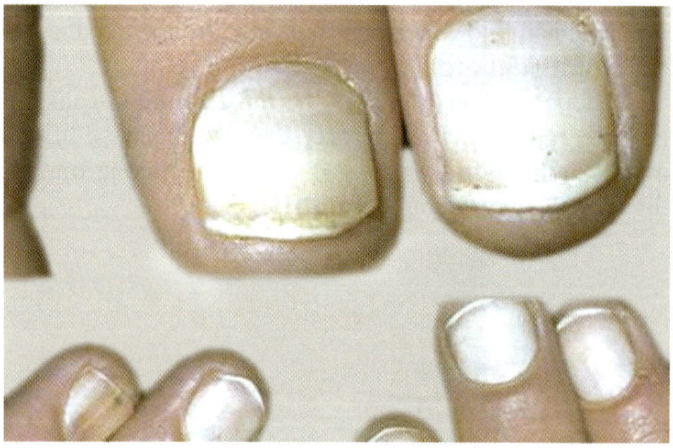

Fig. 18.33: Total leuconychia

Pseudoleukonychia: This term is used when the nail plate alteration has an external origin, such as in onychomycosis or in keratin granulations observed after nail enamel applications.

Apparent leukonychia: The white appearance of the nail is due to changes in the underlying tissue and may present as the following:

Terry's nail, in which the white discoloration stops suddenly 1 to 2 mm from the distal edge, leaving a pink-brown area 0.5 to 3.0 mm wide (Fig. 18.34). This condition, which involves all nails uniformly, is associated with cirrhosis of the liver, chronic congestive heart failure, or adult-onset diabetes mellitus.

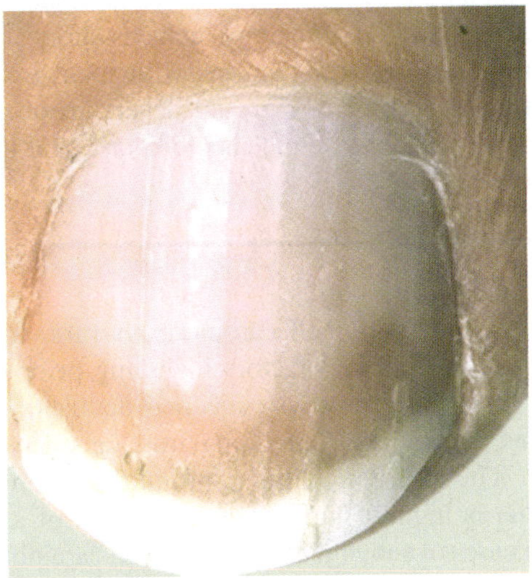

Fig. 18.34: Terry's nail

Half-and-half nail with the two parts showing a sharp demarcation. The proximal area is dull white, and the distal area (20 to 60 percent of the total length) is brownish. It has been reported in uremic patients (Fig. 18.35).

The 'half-and-half' nail, with a white proximal and red or brown distal half, is seen in a minority of patients with chronic renal failure.

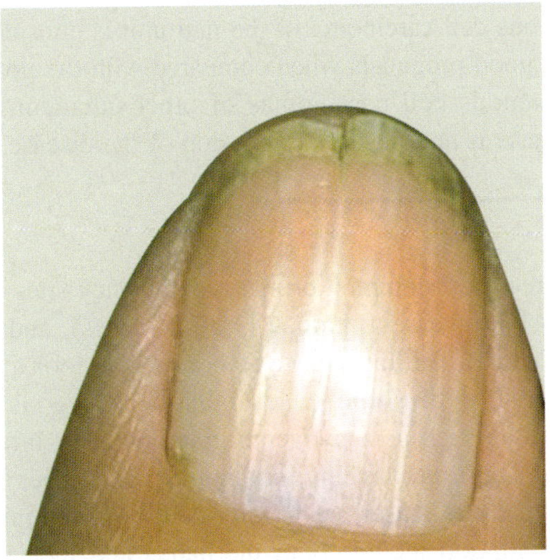

Fig. 18.35: Half-and-half nail

There are three causes for this one is vascular compromise, increased melanin deposition and in a minority of cases keratin defect.

Muehrcke's paired, narrow white bands parallel the lunula in the nail bed and are commonly associated with hypoalbuminemia or following chemotherapy.

NAIL DISCOLOURATION

Distinguish a discoloured nail bed from a discoloured nail plate.

Yellow Nail Syndrome: Yellow or green nails due to lymphatic obstruction in cardiopulmonary disease.

Green Nails: Pseudomonas/**candida** infection.

Yellow Nails: Due to **fungal nail infection**, Psoriasis.

Splinter Hemorrhages: These longitudinal hemorrhages in the distal nail bed conform to the pattern of subungual vessels. Emphasis has recently been given to their association with the antiphospholipid syndrome. Proximal splinter hemorrhages have been reported in bacterial endocarditis, trichinosis, and onychomatricoma. They may be seen following external trauma.

Beau's Lines (Fig. 18.36) are transverse grooves which appear synchronously on all nails a few weeks after an acute illness, and which grow steadily out to the free margin.

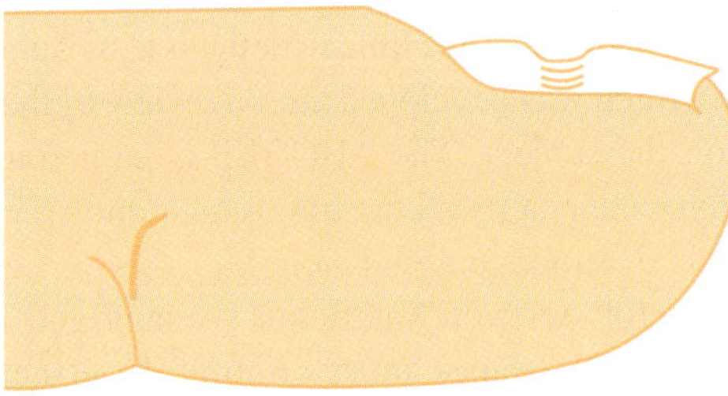

Fig. 18.36: Beau's line: A transverse furrow, across all nails, due to slow growth during a severe illness

Connective Tissue Disorders: Nail fold telangiectasia or erythema is a useful physical sign in dermatomyositis, systemic sclerosis and systemic lupus erythematosus. In dermatomyositis the cuticles become shaggy, and in systemic sclerosis loss of finger pulp leads to overcurvature of the nail plates. Thin nails, with longitudinal ridging and sometimes partial onycholysis, are seen when the peripheral circulation is impaired, as in Raynaud's phenomenon.

TUMORS OF THE NAIL UNIT

Subungual Melanoma

Subungual melanoma is an uncommon site for melanoma,

with an incidence of between 0.7% and 3.5% of all melanoma cases in the general population. The peak age of incidence of subungual melanoma is in the fifth to seventh decades. The two important signs of subungual melanoma are longitudinal melanonychia (discussed above) and **Hutchinson's sign**. Hutchinson's sign refers to the spread of pigment from the nail bed, matrix, and nail plate onto the adjacent cuticle and proximal and/or lateral nail folds.

Pseudo-Hutchinson's sign refers to periungual pigmentation unrelated to melanoma and can be found in the Laugier-Hunziker syndrome, use of certain medications, with the presence of infectious agents in the nail, secondary to ethnic variation, with a variety of systemic diseases, and other causes.

Diagnosis

There are four histologic subtypes of subungual melanoma, which includes lentigo maligna melanoma, superficial spreading melanoma, acral lentiginous melanoma, and nodular melanoma. It is also possible to develop a subungual melanoma without pigment, termed an amelanotic melanoma. The most important factors contributing to prognosis include the Breslow depth of invasion of the melanoma, presence of tumor ulceration, and presence of bone invasion.

The ABCDEF rule for clinical detection of subungual melanoma, which was developed after a review of the world literature on the subject. The ABCDEF is an acronym by which a physician can recall the important points regarding the diagnosis of subungual melanoma.

- A stands for African Americans, Asians and Native Americans, the races most commonly affected by subungual melanoma.
- B stands for the diagnostic sign of a brown to black pigmented nail band with blurred borders and a breadth of 3 mm or more.
- C stands for a recent, sudden, or rapid change in the size of the nail band or lack of change despite treatment.
- D stands for the digit most commonly affected by subungual melanoma, the thumb, followed by the hallux or index finger. A single digit affected by a pigmented band should raise the suspicion of subungual melanoma more than a situation where multiple digits are affected by pigmented bands.
- E stands for extension of pigment onto the proximal and/or lateral nail fold (Hutchinson's sign).
- F stands for family or personal history of the dysplastic nevus syndrome or previous melanoma, which would indicate an increased overall risk for subungual melanoma.

Final diagnosis of subungual melanoma requires a biopsy.

Treatment

Treatment of subungual melanoma depends on the extent of disease and the presence or absence of systemic metastasis. Evaluation of tumor burden can be accomplished with elective lymph node dissection or sentinel lymph node mapping and biopsy. However, such evaluation must be decided on a case-by-case basis, as lymph node dissection itself carries morbidity. Therapy includes surgical removal of the tumor with clear margins with local excision or amputation of the affected digit and, depending on the tumor burden, can include systemic chemotherapy and the use of interferon.

NAIL UNIT SQUAMOUS CELL CARCINOMA

Subungual squamous cell carcinoma is rare. It is often associated with inciting factors including prior radiation therapy (especially in physicians and dentists), nail unit infections with human papillomavirus, tar exposure, and trauma. The incidence of subungual squamous cell carcinoma is highest during 50 to 69 years of age. Most reported cases of subungual squamous cell carcinoma occur on the fingers, but cases have been described occurring on the toes as well. Usually only one digit is affected, the most common site being the thumb.

Diagnosis

Definitive diagnosis requires a biopsy. Delay in diagnosis is common as the presentation can resemble other common diseases of the nail unit including onychomycosis, verruca vulgaris, or a paronychia. Subungual squamous cell carcinoma involves the bone in between 20% and 55% of cases. Squamous cell carcinoma of the nail unit is considered to have a good prognosis when compared with the prognosis of squamous cell carcinomas of other cutaneous sites. Metastasis is an unusual progression of the disease.

SUBUNGUAL METASTASES

The three most common primary malignancy sites are the lung (41% of cases), kidney (11% of cases), and breast (9% of cases). The appearance of these lesions took a variety of forms, with some cases masquerading as other dermatoses such as a pyogenic granuloma, or infections such as acute paronychia, erysipelas and herpes zoster. Subungual metastases are usually painful. Anatomic sites of presentation include both the hands and feet. One or multiple digits can be affected.

An X-ray of the affected digit should be performed to evaluate bone involvement, a common complication of subungual metastases. A review of 39 patients with subungual metastases showed that in 44% of these cases the metastatic lesion was the initial expression of an undiagnosed malignancy or presented in the same month that the tumor was discovered.

DIGITAL MYXOID CYST

The digital myxoid cyst is also known as a digital mucoid cyst, digital mucous cyst, myxoid pseudocyst, and synovial cyst. The variety of terms for this disorder reflects the controversial origin of the cyst development. It usually presents as an asymptomatic, single, soft to rubbery nodule on the dorsal surface of a finger, located between the proximal nail fold and distal interphalangeal joint, lateral to the midline. The material encased in the cyst has been described as viscous or gelatinous. The surface of the cyst is usually smooth, but verrucous variants have also been reported. Most cases occur in patients between ages 40 and 70. Women are more commonly affected than men. The most commonly affected anatomic sites are the middle and index fingers, but are also sometimes found on the toes. Because of its location, the cyst can exert pressure on the nail matrix, resulting in a linear nail plate dystrophy and a groove in the nail. Occasionally, these cysts can have a connection with the nearby distal interphalangeal joint (Fig. 18.37).

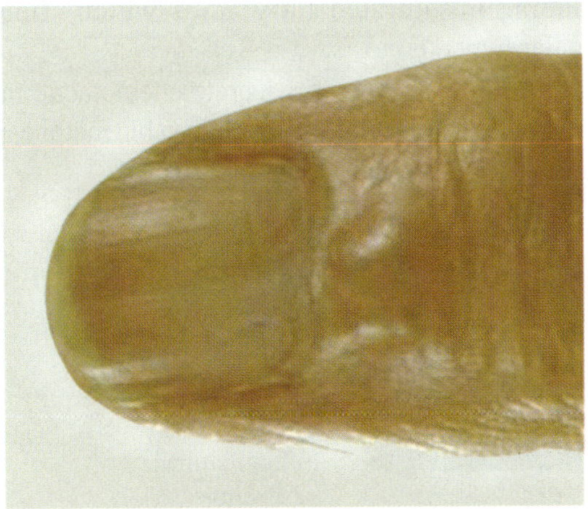

Fig. 18.37: Myxoid cyst

Treatment

When surgically excised, care must be taken to remove any communicating tracts between the cyst and joint, if present, to prevent recurrence. Other treatment options include cryotherapy, carbon dioxide laser vaporization, and injection of sclerosing solutions. Treatment with aspiration of the cyst contents and injection of intralesional steroids can have high recurrence rates.

GLOSSARY OF TERMS COMMONLY USED

Anonychia—The absence of a nail. This word comes from the Greek prefix "a-", meaning "without", and "onych-" meaning "nail".

Avulsion—The removal of the nail. May be done in a manner to allow the nail to grow back, or in a manner to prevent the regrowth of the nail.

Hangnail—A small loose flap of skin next to a nail plate.

Hapalonychia—Soft nails. Same as onychomalacia.

Ingrown Nails—Nails which are digging into the skin, thereby causing a break in the skin. Ingrown nails are characterized by inflammation and because of the break in the skin, they are frequently infected. We have a separate web page that discusses ingrown nails, and another web page that discusses nail surgery.

Onychalgia—Pain of the nail.

Onychogryphosis—Severe overgrowth of nails to the extent that the nails have the appearance of a ram's horn.

Onychoheterotopia—A nail in an abnormal location.

Onychitis— Inflammation of the nail bed.

Onychophagia—Chewing of the nails.

Onychophosis—Callus in the nail groove, common with incurvated nails.

Onychoptosis—Falling off of the nails. Often preceded by onycholysis.

Onychorrhexis—Abnormal brittleness of the nails.

Onychoschizia—Distal lamellar splitting/brittle nails due to water/detergent damage.

Onychosis—The condition of diseased nails. Synonymous with onychopathy.

Onychotillomania—Compulsive picking at a nail.

Platonychia—Increased curvature of the nail in the long axis (where the nail is growing around the tip of the toe).

REFERENCES

- Baran R, Dawber RPR: Baran and Dawber's diseases of the nails and their management, 3rd edn., Malden, MA, Blackwell Science, 2001.
- Hordinsky MK, Sawaya ME, Scher RK: Atlas of hair and nails, 1st edn., Philadelphia, Churchill Livingstone, 2000.
- Rich P, Scher RK: An atlas of diseases of the nail, 1st edn., New York, Parthenon Publishing Group, 2003.
- Uyttendaele H, Geyer A, Scher RK: Brittle nails: Pathogenesis and treatment, J Drugs Dermatol 2003; 2:48-49.

CHAPTER 19

DISORDERS OF APPENDAGEAL GLANDS

Sebaceous Glands

Acne Vulgaris

Acne is a self-limited disease affecting pilosebaceous unit, usually occurring in adolescents. Lesions are polymorphic consisting of comedones, papules, pustules. Pitted or hypertrophic scarring occurs. Acne affects both sexes. Exact cause is uncertain but multifactorial. The various factors affecting its occurrence are:

1. **Genetic:** Family history often positive especially in severe cases.
2. **Androgens:** Although high levels of testosterone and dihydrotestosterone do not directly corroborate with sebum secretion they are required for producing significant quantities of sebum. DHEA levels parallel sebum secretion through conversion to potent androgens.
3. **Diet:** Role of diet in the causation of acne is controversial and most studies have disapproved any correlation.

ETIOLOGY AND PATHOGENESIS (Fig. 19.1)

Interplay of 4 factors is important in the causation of acne:

1. **Follicular hyperkeratinization:** Normally keratinous material in follicle is loosely organized, with many lamellar granules. In acne, the primary lesion i.e. comedone is because of changes in follicular infundibulum. The keratinous material becomes more dense, keratohyalin granules increase and increased turnover of follicular cells. These effects occur under the influence of increased IL-1 of increased androgens.
2. **Colonization by *propionibacterium acnes:*** *P acnes* is anaerobic pleomorphic diptheroid. They are found in significantly high concentrations in individuals with acne. They act as source of follicular lipases and proteases and hyaluronidases which cause lipolysis of sebum producing unsaturated fatty acids which stimulate follicular hyperkeratosis.
3. **Inflammation:** *P acne* also secrete chemotactic factors which is a low molecular weight dialysable factor capable

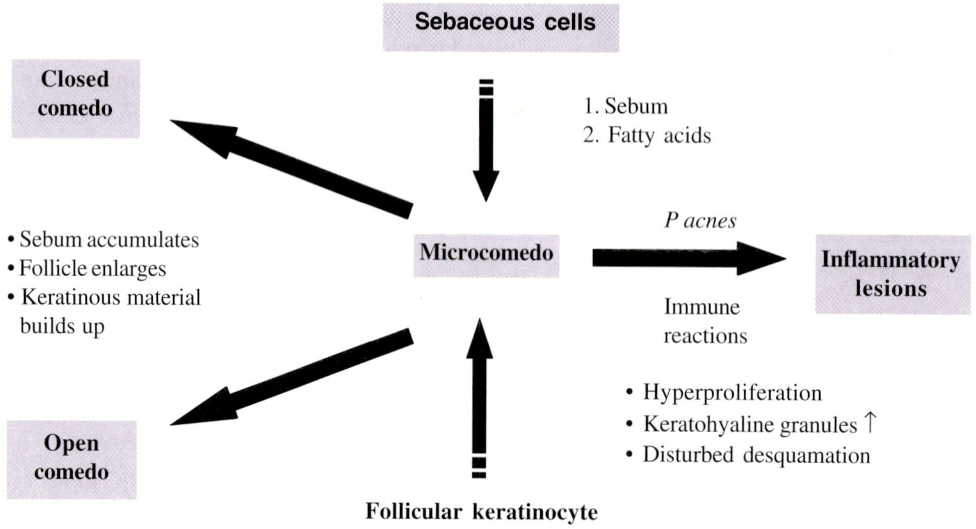

Fig. 19.1: Pathogenesis of acne vulgaris

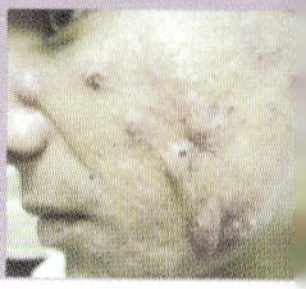

of attracting polymorphonuclear leucocytes which further cause release of hydrolytic enzymes and lead to follicular epithelial damage. Complement mediated damage also plays a significant role in its pathogenesis.

4. **Sebum production:** The triglyceride fraction of sebum which is unique to human beings is responsible for acne. There is increased sebum production but decreased linoleic acid concentration. Furthermore, agents which decrease sebum production reduce the severity of acne.

Clinical Manifestations

The primary lesions are COMEDONES—which are non-inflammatory papules produced by occlusion of pilosebaceous duct. They may be:

1. Closed (white) (Fig. 19.2).
2. Open (black) (Fig. 19.2).

Apart from the noninflammatory lesions, patients of acne have inflammatory lesions as well. These include:

1. Inflammatory papules.
2. Pustules.
3. Large tender fluctuant nodules (Fig. 19.3)
4. Cysts and sinuses.
5. Scars — Icepick (Fig. 19.4); Boxcar (19.4); Rolling (Fig. 19.5).

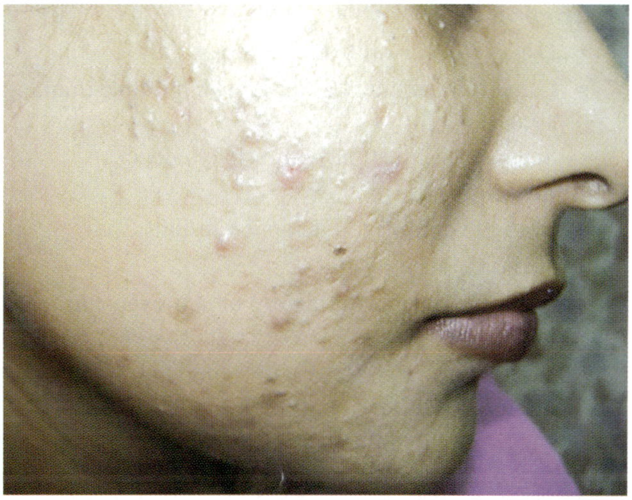

Fig. 19.2: Multiple closed and open comedones

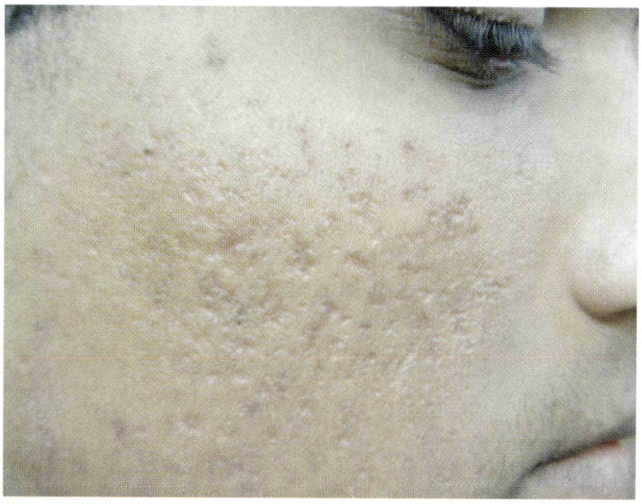

Fig. 19.4: Icepick and boxcar scars

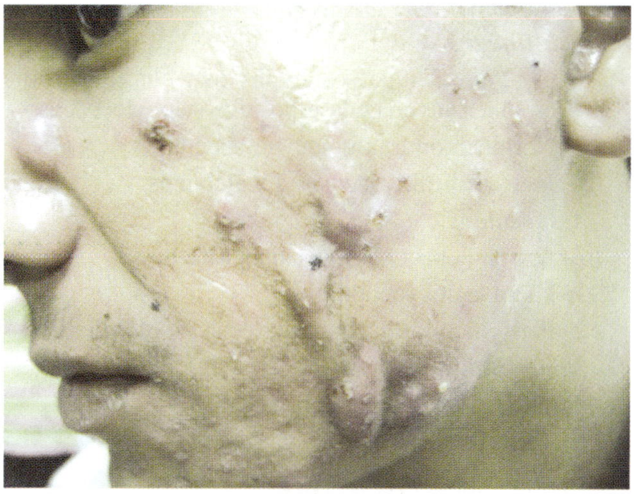

Fig. 19.3: Nodules and cyst

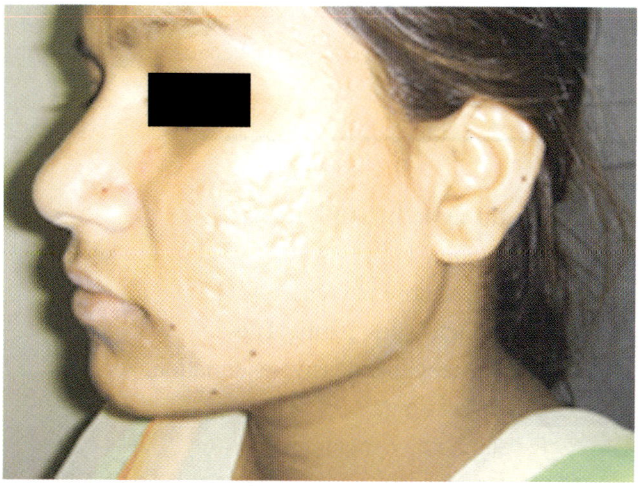

Fig. 19.5: Rolling scars

Most Common Sites

Primary site: Face (forehead, cheeks).
Others: Back, chest, shoulders.

Diagnosis and Differential Diagnosis

Diagnosis is mainly clinical based on the occurrence of polymorphic lesions on characteristic sites.

Differential Diagnosis

- Folliculitis.
- Rosacea.
- Acneiform disorders.
- Lupus millaris disseminatus faciei.

PATHOLOGY

The primary lesion is comedone which forms as an expanding mass of lipid-impregnated keratinous material in mid portion of follicles which leads to dilation of follicular wall. There is associated atrophy of sebaceous glands. On being traumatized inflammatory lesions develop in closed comedones leading to rupture of follicular wall and appear as pustule or nodule. Multichannelled tracts may form which may undergo fibrous contraction and contribute to scar formation.

LABORATORY FINDINGS

These can be done in recalcitrant/symptomatic patients.
- Elevated levels of serum androgens (>150 ng/ml) and DHEAS (>8000 ng/ml).
- In patients with associated PCOD→↑ LH: FSH ratio, serum progesterone, serum prolactin, fasting insulin.
- Increased levels of glucocorticoids and ACTH, gonadotrophins in acneiform eruptions because of exogenous cases.

MISCELLANEOUS TYPES/VARIANTS

1. **Neonatal acne/Infantile acne**
   - Self limiting.
   - Seen over nose and cheeks.
2. **Acne excoriee des jeunes files**
   - Mild acne with extensive excoriation.
   - Linear scarring.
   - Psychotherapy required.
3. **Steroid acne**
   - Appear 2 weeks after steroids are started.
   - Focal folliculitis with neutrophilic infiltrate, no hyperkeratinization.
   - Monomorphic lesions.
   - Trunk, shoulders and upper arms.
   - Comedones, cysts and scarring rare.
4. **Halogen acne**
   - Iodides and bromides are causative agents.
   - Inflammatory acne.
   - Associated with use of sedatives, expectorates, vitamins and drugs.
5. **Occupational acne**
   - Coal tar derivatives, cutting oils, chlorinated hydrocarbons.
   - Inflammatory acne (severe).
   - More on covered areas.
6. **Tropical acne**
   - Usually occur on trunk/buttocks.
   - Large inflammatory nodules with multiple draining areas.
   - Secondary infection with staphylococci.
7. **Acne aestivalis**
   - Multiple, uniform, red papular lesions.
   - Mallorce acne.
   - Young females with history of sun exposure.
8. **Acne conglobata**
   - Inflammatory disease with comedones, nodules, abscesses and draining sinus tracts.
   - Males usually affected (later age).
   - Chronic unremitting course.
   - Staphylococcus and streptococci recovered.
   - Back, buttocks, chest, abdomen, shoulders.
   - Comedones with multiple openings.
   - Multichannelled sinus tracts with foul smelling discharge.

   Lab findings
   - Coagulase negative staphylococcus, anaerobic diphtheroid, coagulase positive staphylococcus.
   - Normochromic normocytic anemia.
   - Increased ESR, increased γ globulins.

   Associations

   Acne conglobata often coexists with:
   1. Hidradenitis suppurativa.
   2. Perifolliculitis capitis abscedens et suffodiens.
9. **Acne fulminans**
   - Acute febrile ulcerative acne.
   - Teenage boys.
   - Face spared.
   - Polyarthralgia, myalgia, bony tenderness.
   - Explosive onset.
   - Ulcerative and crusted lesions common.

TREATMENT (Fig. 19.6)

Principle→Target the 4 steps of pathogenesis.

LOCAL THERAPY

1. **Cleansing:** For being effective the topical agent should be able to remove lipids and bacteria from within the follicle.
2. **Topical Agents:**
   a. *Retinoids:*
      - Mainly comedolytic.
      - May cause irritation/sun burns.
      - Bind to nuclear retinoic acid receptors which affects cell proliferation, cell differentiation and inflammation.
      - They reverse altered follicular keratinization.

   b. *Benzoyl peroxide:*
      - Antibacterial.
      - Decreased triglyceride hydrolysis.
      - Causes dryness, irritation and allergic contact dermatitis.

   c. *Topical antibiotics:*
      - Clindamycin, clarithromycin, erythromycin, nadifloxacin.
      - Combinations also preferred.
      - Decrease *P acne* concentration.

   d. *Azelaic acid:*
      - Useful in inflammatory and comedonal acne.
      - Also lightens the post-inflammatory hyperpigmentation.

SYSTEMIC THERAPY

A. **Antibiotics and Antibacterial Agents**
- Decrease sebum production.
- Decrease free fatty acid concentration.
- Decrease *P. acnes* concentration.
- Have anti-inflammatory activity.
- Gram negative folliculitis is a side effect.
  E.g. Tetracycline, minocycline, cotrimoxazole.

B. **Hormonal Therapy**
- Used in PCOD patients.
- Estrogens, antiandrogens, oral contraceptives, glucocorticoids, GnRH agonist.
- *Side effects:* Nausea, weight gain, amenorrhea, melasma, breast tenderness.
- Intralesional steroids are useful in nodulocystic acne.
- They inhibit sebum production and have anti-inflammatory properties.
- Physical therapy: Peels.
  Lasers.

Isotretinoin

- Affect all aspects of acne pathogenesis.
- Decrease sebum production, have indirect antibacterial activity, affect follicular hyperkeratinization.
- Dose = 0.5 to 1 mg/kg/d for 4-5 months and total dose should not exceed 120-180 mg/kg body weight.
- *Side effects:* Affect lipid profile, liver function, psychosis, hypertriglyceridemia, chelitis, xerosis, conjunctivitis, pruritis.

Diet

- No evidence supports that dietary elimination of foods e.g. shellfish, chocolates, sweets decreases acne.

REFERENCE

- Fitzpatrick's Dermatology in General Medicine, 6th edn 2003.

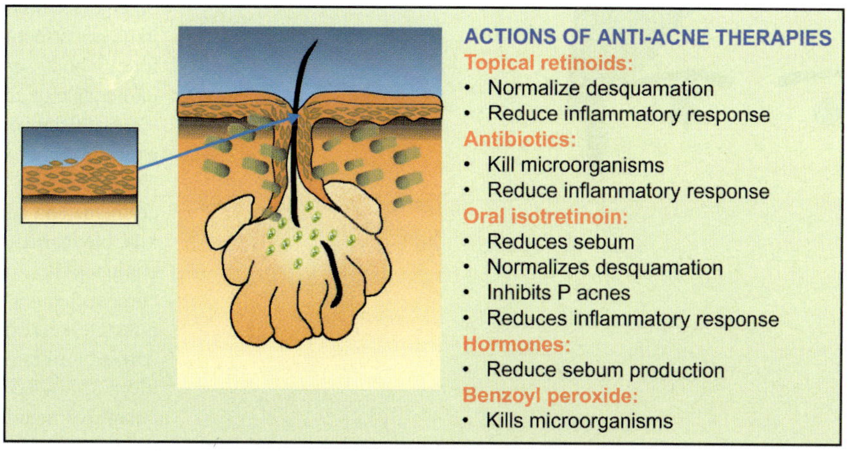

Fig. 19.6: Action and anti-acne therapies

Rosacea

Rosacea affects the face of adults, usually women.

Although its peak incidence is in the thirties and forties, it can also be seen in the young or old. It may coexist with acne but is distinct from it.

Cause and Histopathology

The cause is still unknown.

Those who flush easily in response to warmth, spicy food, alcohol or embarrassment.

Common Triggers of Rosacea Flares

Sunlight	Wind
Emotional stress	Humidity
(Laughter, embarrassment, anger, anxiety)	Skin care products, including:
Hot weather	• Astringents
Alcohol consumption	• Soaps
Spicy food	• Exfoliants
Exercise	• Make up perfumes
Hot baths, saunas, showers	• Sunscreens (especially those containing alcohol, witch hazel, fragrance and menthol)
Hot drinks	
Cold weather	
Menses, menopausal hot flash	

CLINICAL COURSE AND COMPLICATIONS

The cheeks, nose, centre of forehead, and chin are most commonly affected; the peri-orbital and peri-oral areas are spared (Fig. 19.7). Intermittent flushing is followed by a fixed erythema and telangiectasias.

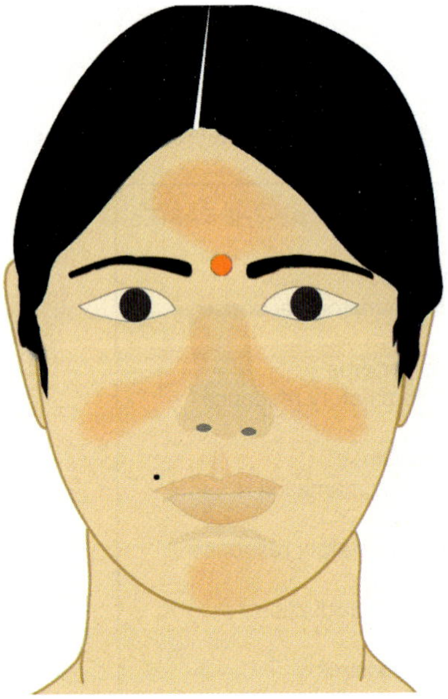

Fig. 19.7: Erythema, papule, pustule on centrofacial area

Discrete domed inflamed papules, papulopustules and rarely, nodules develop later. Rosacea, unlike acne, has no comedones or seborrhea.

Subtypes, Symptoms and Treatment of Rosacea

Subtype	*Symptoms*	*Treatment*
Erythematotelangiectatic	Facial erythema, flushing, burning, stinging, central facial edema, telangiectasias, roughness, scaling.	Avoid triggers Use Suncreen Green-tinted cosmetics Intense-pulsed light therapy.
Papulopustular	Persistent central facial erythema, transient papules and pustules, often in crops located on central face, perioral, perinasal, periocular regions. No comedones. May have symptoms of subtype 1.	Above, plus: Topical metronidazole, azelaic acid, sulfur. Oral tetracycline, or minocycline, or erythromycin. Isotretinoin if severse or resistant.
Phymatous (Fig. 19.8)	Patulous follicles, telangiectasias, fibrosis, thickened irregular skin surface, nodules, enlargement of tissue of nose (rhinophyma), chin, forehead, cheeks, ears. May have symptoms of subtypes 1 and 2.	Above, plus: debulking and reshaping surgery by electrocautery or CO_2 laser.
Ocular	Watery or dry eyes, burning, stinging, itching, sensitivity to light, gritty feeling, foreign body sensation, intolerance of contact lenses, telangiectasias along lid margin, chalazion, stye, erythema and edema of lids, blepharitis, conjunctivitis, possibly corneal changes such as punctate keratitis, corneal infiltrates or ulcers. May have cutaneous manifesta-tions.	Artificial tears Lid hygiene Possibly occular steroids.

Complications

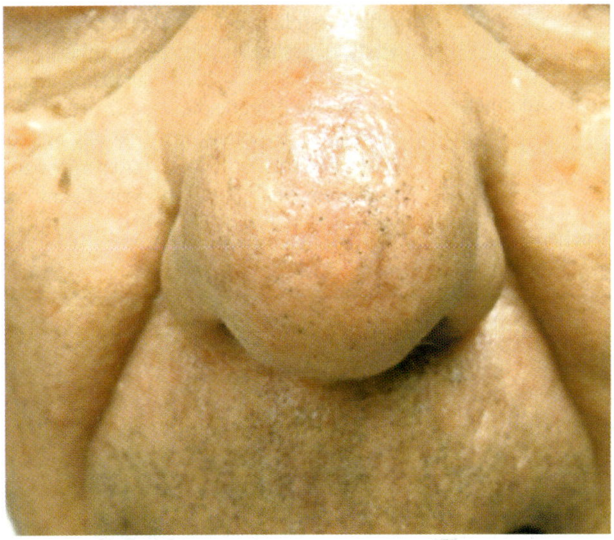

Fig. 19.8: Rhinophyma

Blepharitis, conjunctivitis and occasionally, keratitis. Rhinophyma, caused by hyperplasia of the sebaceous glands and connective tissue on the nose, is a striking complication that is more common in males. Lymphoedema, below the eyes and on the forehead, is a tiresome feature in a few cases. Some patients treated with potent topical steroids develop a rebound flare of pustules, worse than the original rosacea, when this treatment is stopped.

Treatment

Tetracyclines, prescribed as for acne, are the traditional treatment and are usually effective. Erythromycin is the antibiotic of second choice. Courses should last for at least 10 weeks and, after gaining control with 500-1000 mg daily, cut to 250 mg daily. The condition recurs in about half of the patients within 2 years, but repeated antibiotic courses, rather than prolonged maintenance ones, are generally recommended.

Topical 0.75% metronidazole gel, applied sparingly once daily, is nearly as effective as oral tetracycline and often prolongs remission. It can be tried before systemic treatment and is especially useful in treating 'stuttering' recurrent lesions that do not then need repeated systemic courses of antibiotics.

Rarely systemic metronidazole or isotretinoin is needed for stubborn rosacea.

Eccrine Sweat Glands

There are 2-3 million sweat glands distributed all over the body surface but they are most numerous on the palms, soles and axillae. Initially sweat is isotonic with plasma but, under normal conditions, it becomes hypotonic by the time it is discharged at the surface, after the tubular resorption of electrolytes and water under the influence of aldosterone and antidiuretic hormone.

In some ways the eccrine sweat duct is like a renal tubule. The pH of sweat is between 4.0 and 6.8; it contains sodium, potassium chloride, lactate, urea and ammonia.

The concentration of sodium chloride in sweat is increased in cystic fibrosis, and sweat can be analysed when this is suspected.

Sweat glands have an important role in temperature control, the skin surface being cooled by evaporation. Up to 10 L/day of sweat can be excreted.

Three stimuli induce sweating:

1. *Thermal sweating* is a reflex response to a raised environmental temperature and occurs all over the body, especially the chest, back, forehead, scalp and axillae.
2. *Emotional sweating* is provoked by fear or anxiety and is seen mainly on the palms, soles and axillae.
3. *Gustatory sweating* is provoked by hot spicy foods and affects the face.

The eccrine sweat glands are innervated by cholinergic fibres of the sympathetic nervous system. Sweating can therefore be induced by cholinergic, and blocked by anti-cholinergic drugs. Central control of sweating resides in the preoptic hypothalamic sweat centre.

THERMAL HYPERHIDROSIS

The 'thermostat' for sweating lies in the preoptic area of the hypothalamus. Sweating follows any rise in body temperature, whether this is caused by exercise, environmental heat or an illness. The sweating in acute infections, and in some chronic illnesses (e.g. Hodgkin's disease), may be a result of a lowering of the 'set' of this thermostat.

The classic sites are shown in Fig. 19.9.

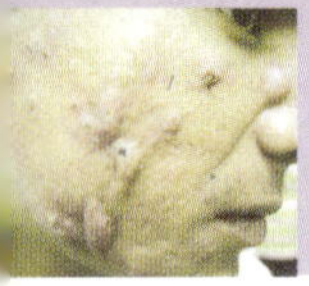

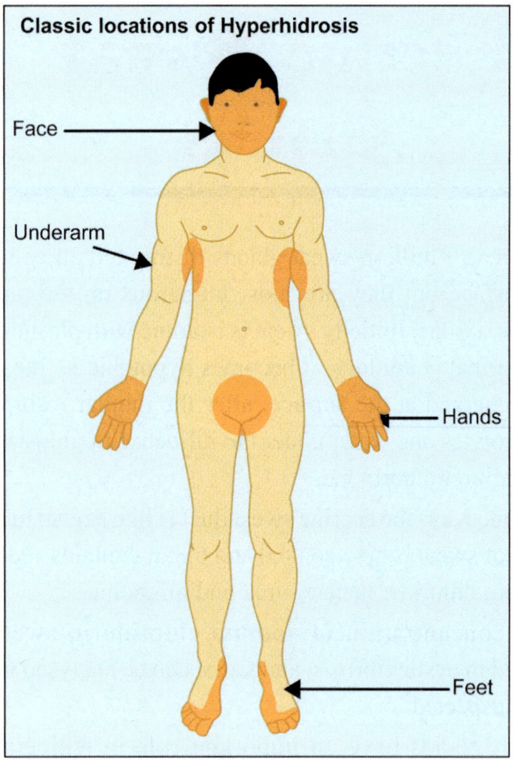

Fig. 19.9: Classic locations of hyperhidrosis

Causes of General Hyperhidrosis

Category	*Pathogenesis*	*Features*
Chronic infection	Tuberculosis, brucellosis	Night sweats
Neuroendocrine malignancy	Pheochromocytoma	Paroxysmal sweating, sudomotor cholinergic activation from excess catecholamines; responds to anticholinergics
Endocrinologic	Thyrotoxicosis, diabetes mellitus	Paroxysmal sweating, increased metabolism and increased sensitivity of nerve fibers to epinephrine; thyrotoxicosis responds to β blockade
Malignancy	Leukemia, lymphoma, renal cell carcinoma, Castleman disease	Night sweats, pruritus; may respond to plasmapheresis or histamine$_2$ receptor antagonists
Neurologic diseases	Acromegaly, carcinoid syndrome, diencephalic epilepsy, basilar artery occlusion–pontine ischemia	Paroxysmal sweating; pontine ischemia may damage descending inhibitory fibers
Biochemical agents	Acetylcholinesterase inhibitors, chemical warfare, pesticides	Responsive to removal of stimulus, anticholinergics
Spinal cord injury	Autonomic dysreflexia, orthostatic hypotension, posttraumatic syringomyelia	Can occur months to years after injury to spinal cord
Miscellaneous	Anxiety, hypoglycemia, menopause	

Contd.

Contd.

Local Hyperhidrosis

The most common areas to be affected are the palms, soles and axillae. Too much sweating is embarrassing, if not socially crippling.

Treatment

A simple treatment format is given below: (Fig. 19.10)

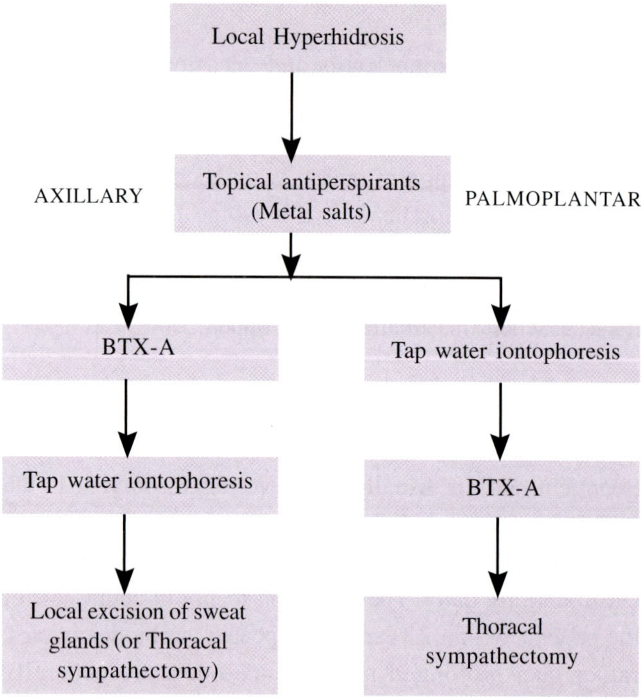

Fig. 19.10: Treatment of hyperhidrosis

Topical Applications

The most useful preparation for axillary hyperhidrosis is **20% aluminium chloride hexahydrate** in an alcohol base. At first it is applied to the dry axillae every night. Soon the interval can be increased, and many need the preparation only once or twice a week. The frequency may have to be cut down if the preparation irritates the skin, which is most likely if it is applied after shaving or when the skin is wet.

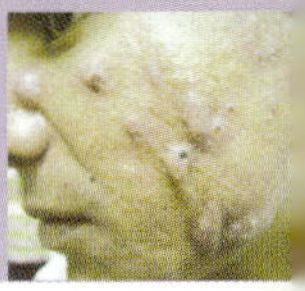

Iontophoresis

Iontophoresis with tap water or with the anticholinergic drug glycopyrronium bromide.

Botulinum toxin

This binds to presynaptic nerve membranes and then inhibits the release of acetylcholine. It is now the treatment of choice for severe axillary or plantar hyperhidrosis, unresponsive to medical measures. Subdermal aliquots of the toxin are injected into the hyperhidrotic area of the axilla or sole, one region at a single session. Sweating is abolished after a delay of 2-3 days. Repeat injections (about every eighth month) are necessary as the sweating returns when the toxin has gone. Antibodies may form against the toxin and diminish its long-term effectiveness. Botulinum toxin is used less often for palmar hyperhidrosis because of the risk of paralysing the intrinsic muscles of the hand.

Systemic Treatment

Oral anticholinergic agents such as pro-banthine and glycopyrronium bromide are sometimes tried but their side-effects limit their value.

Potassium permanganate soaks (1 : 10 000 aqueous solution) combat the bacterial superinfection of sweaty feet that is responsible for their foul smell. Patients should soak their feet for 15 min twice a day until the smell has improved and be warned that potassium permanganate stains the skin and everything else brown.

Occasionally **glutaraldehyde** solutions are used instead, but allergy and yellow-stained skin are potential complications. Topical clindamycin is also effective.

HYPOHIDROSIS AND ANHIDROSIS

Prematurity: The sweat glands function poorly in premature babies nursed in incubators and hot nurseries.

Anhidrosis Caused by Abnormality of the Sweat Glands (Heat Stroke)

Caused by sweat gland exhaustion, this is a medical emergency seen most often in elderly people moving to a hot climate. It can also occur in the young, during or after prolonged exercise, especially in hot climates. Patients present with hyperthermia, dry skin, weakness, headache, cramps and confusion, leading to vomiting, hypotension, oliguria, metabolic acidosis, hyperkalemia, delirium and death. They should be cooled down immediately with cold water, and fluids and electrolytes must be replaced.

Hypohidrotic Ectodermal Dysplasia

This rare disorder is inherited as an X-linked recessive trait, in which the sweat glands are either absent or decreased.

Affected boys have a characteristic facial appearance, with poor hair and teeth, and are intolerant of heat.

Anhidrosis Caused by Abnormalities of the Nervous System

Anhidrosis may follow abnormalities anywhere in the sympathetic system, from the hypothalamus to the peripheral nerves. It can therefore be a feature of multiple sclerosis, a cerebral tumour, trauma, Horner's syndrome or peripheral neuropathy (e.g. leprosy, alcoholic neuropathy and diabetes). Patients with widespread anhidrosis are heat-intolerant, developing nausea, dizziness, tachycardia and hyperthermia in hot surroundings.

Anhidrosis or Hypohidrosis Caused by Skin Disease

Local hypohidrosis has been reported in many skin diseases, especially those that scar (e.g. lupus erythematosus and morphoea). It may be a feature of Sjögren's syndrome, ichthyosis, psoriasis and miliaria profunda.

BROMHIDROSIS

Foul smelling sweat.

CHROMHIDROSIS

Chromhidrosis is production of colored sweat.

Types

Eccrine (very rare)—Generalised.

Apocrine—Axilla, anogenital skin, areola, face and scalp.

Pseudo Chromhidrosis

True Chromhidrosis

Corynebacterium species.

Chemicals/Paints/Dyes.

Color

Yellow, green, blue, brown or black (Fig. 19.11) due to concentration. or oxidation states of lipofuscin granules.

Higher states of oxidation of lipofuschin granules results in dark color and less fluorescence (at 360 nm).

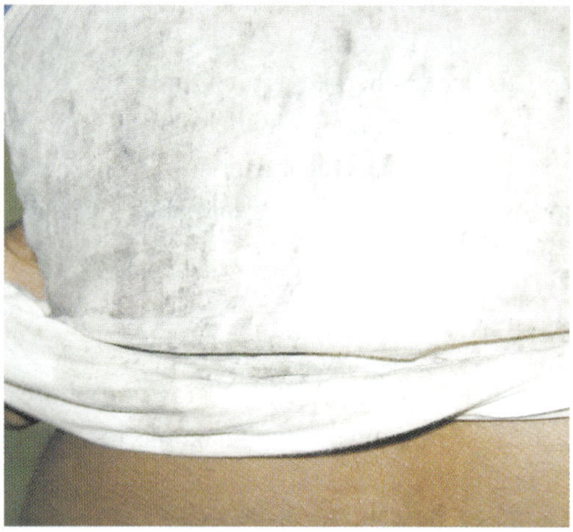

Fig. 19.11: Black sweat

Investigation

- Skin biopsy.
- H&E, PAS and Autofluorescence microscopy.
- Distilled water extraction from clothes.
- Ether extraction for sebum.
- Sweat harvested using pilocarpine hydrochloride.
- Early morning urine sample: Porphyrins and homogensitic acid.
- Skin scraping.
- Gram stain and cultures.

Treatment

Chromhidrosis

- Topical aluminum chloride.
- Topical Capsaicin (trans-8-methyl-*N*-vanillyl-6-nonenamide) 0.025% twice a day.
- Definitive treatment is surgical excision.

Pseudochromhidrosis

- Based on history and observation.
- Avoid exogenous dyes, paints or chemicals.
- Complete clearance with antibiotics both topical and systemic has been observed occasionally.

INTERFERENCE WITH SWEAT DELIVERY

Miliaria

This is the result of plugging or rupture of sweat ducts. It occurs in hot humid climates, at any age, and is common in over-clothed infants in hot nurseries. The physical signs depend on where the ducts are blocked (Fig. 19.12).

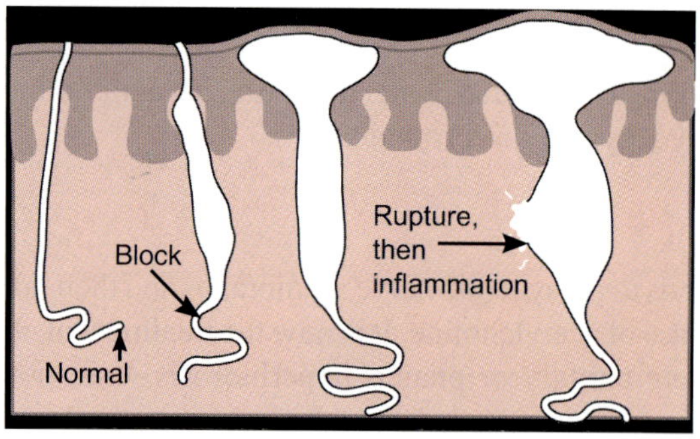

Fig. 19.12: Course of miliaria rubra

Miliaria crystallina: This presents as tiny clear non-inflamed vesicles that look like dew. This is the most superficial type, block within the S. corneum.

Miliaria rubra (prickly heat): Tiny erythematous and very itchy papules, block is in the epidermis.

Miliaria profunda: These consist of larger erythematous papules or pustules. This is the deepest type.

The block extends to the dermis.

Treatment

The best treatment is to move to a cooler climate or into air conditioning. Clothing that prevents the evaporation of sweat (e.g. nylon shirts) should be avoided; cotton is best.

Claims have been made for ascorbic acid by mouth. Topical steroids reduce irritation but should only be used briefiy. Calamine lotion cools and soothes the skin.

Apocrine Sweat Glands

Apocrine glands are limited to the axillae, nipples, periumbilical area and perineum. The action of bacteria on apocrine sweat is responsible for body odour. The glands are innervated by adrenergic fibres of the sympathetic nervous system.

Suppurative Hidradenitis (Apocrine Acne)

This is a severe chronic suppurative disorder of the apocrine glands. Many papules, pustules, cysts, sinuses and scars occur in the axillae, groin and perianal areas. The condition

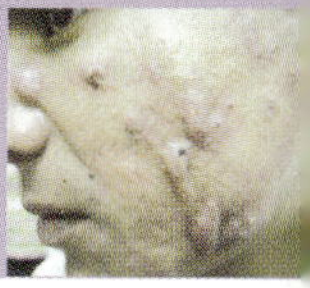

may coexist with conglobate acne. Its cause is unknown, but an underlying follicular abnormality seems likely. Slightly raised androgen levels are found in some affected females.

It is probably not an immunodeficiency or a primary infection of the apocrine glands, although staphylococcus aureus, anaerobic streptococci and bacterioides spp. are frequently present.

Treatment is unsatisfactory but should be as for acne vulgaris in the first instance. Systemic antibiotics help early lesions to resolve but are ineffective for chronic draining abscesses and sinuses. Incision and drainage of abscesses, and injections of intralesional triamcinolone (5-10 mg/mL) may reduce the incidence of deforming scars and sinus formation. Topical clindamycin has been shown to prevent new lesions from forming. Systemic antiandrogens help some women.

Severe cases need plastic surgery to remove large areas of affected skin.

Fox-Fordyce Disease

This rare disease of the apocrine ducts is comparable to miliaria rubra of the eccrine duct. It occurs in women after puberty. Itchy skin-coloured or light brown papules appear in the axillae and other areas where apocrine glands are found, such as the breasts and vulva. Treatment is not usually necessary but removal of the affected skin, or electrodessication of the most irritable lesions can be considered.

REFERENCES

- Collin, J. and Whatling, P. (2000): Treating hyperhidrosis. British Medical Journal 320, 1221-1222.
- Kreyden, O.P., Böni, R. and Burg, G. (2001): Hyper hidrosis and Botulinum Toxin in Dermatology.
- Karger, Basel Mortimer, P.S. and Lunniss, P.J. (2000) Hidradenitis suppurativa, Journal of The Royal Society of Medicine 93, 420-422.
- Plewig, G. and Kligman, A.M. (1992): Acne and Rosacea, Springer, Berlin.

CHAPTER **20**

DERMATOLOGICAL SIGNS OF INTERNAL DISEASE AND NUTRITIONAL DISORDERS

SKIN DISEASE AND CARDIOVASCULAR DISEASE

Multiple lentigines occur with **LEOPARD syndrome** (also known as **Moynahan's** syndrome), a mnemonic for *l*entigines, *e*lectrocardiographic changes, *o*cular telorism, *p*ulmonary stenosis, *a*bnormal genitalia, *r*etarded growth, and *d*eafness. Multiple lentigines also occur with **LAMB syndrome** (*l*entigines, *a*trial myxoma, *m*ucocutaneous myxomas, and *b*lue nevi) and **NAME syndrome** (*n*evi, *a*trial myxoma, *m*yxoid neurofibromas and *e*phelides).

Pseudoxanthoma elasticum (PXE) is an inherited (autosomal recessive) or acquired disease characterized by yellow papules over redundant skin folds on the neck, abdomen and groin. PXE represents a defect in elastic fibers, which become brittle and calcified. Skin biopsy reveals swollen, fragmented elastic fibers. Funduscopic examination reveals angioid streaks. PXE may include hypertension, peripheral vascular and coronary artery disease, retinal and gastrointestinal hemorrhage and strokes.

- *Differential diagnosis:* Cutis laxa, Ehlers-Danlos syndrome.
- *Treatment:* No definitive treatment is available.

Ehlers-Danlos Syndrome (EDS) is characterized by hyperextensibility, hypermobility, skin fragility, and "**fish-mouth**" scars, representing an abnormality in collagen biosynthesis. At least eleven types of EDS exist with varying associated features including mitral valve prolapse, blue sclerae, aneurysm, aortic dissection, hernias, angina, gastrointestinal bleeding (perforation), and peripheral vascular disease, depending on the type and severity of disease.

- *Differential diagnosis:* Cutis laxa.
- *Treatment:* Protection of the skin and treatment of **systemic** findings.

SKIN DISEASE AND PULMONARY DISEASE

Sarcoidosis is a multisystem, granulomatous disease of the lungs, bones, eyes and skin. Skin disease, affecting 15%-30% of patients, includes red to purple plaques of the nose (lupus pernio); midfacial papules; annular plaques; and plaques or nodules on the trunk and extremities. Erythema nodosum, the most common **cutaneous manifestation** of sarcoidosis, is an acute, painful panniculitis that usually affects the shins.

- *Differential diagnosis:* Trichoepitheliomas, rosacea, granuloma annulare.
- *Treatment:* **Systemic** corticosteroids, antimalarials.

SKIN DISEASE AND GASTROINTESTINAL DISEASE

Most patients with **dermatitis herpetiformis** have a gluten-sensitive enteropathy (see preceding section on this topic).

Hepatitis C infection may be associated with various skin **diseases**, namely leukocytoclastic vasculitis, **cutaneous** B-cell lymphoma, cryoglobulinemia, pruritus, porphyria cutanea tarda, urticaria, prurigo nodularis, and lichen planus.

Hereditary hemorrhagic telangiectasia (Osler-Weber-Rendu syndrome) is an autosomal dominant disorder characterized by numerous telangiectases on the skin and oral mucosa. Recurrent epistaxis is the most common presenting **manifestation** of the syndrome. Similar telangiectases may involve the lungs, liver, brain, eye, and gastrointestinal tract; hemorrhage may occur at any site. Pulmonary arteriovenous fistulas and CNS angioma may also occur.

- *Differential diagnosis:* Generalized essential telangiectasia.
- *Treatment:* Cauterization and iron supplementation in severe cases.

Peutz-Jeghers syndrome is an autosomal dominant disease characterized by lentigines on the skin and mucosa (lips, buccal mucosa, periorbital region, dorsal surfaces of the fingers and toes), and polyps of the small intestine. The polyps are usually benign hamartomas with low malignant potential.

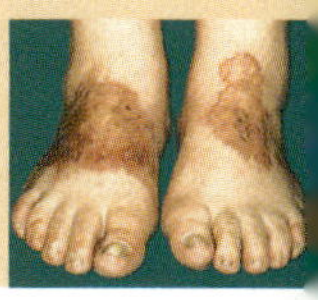

- *Differential diagnosis:* LEOPARD, NAME and LAMB syndromes.
- *Treatment*: Based on **systemic** symptoms.

Pyoderma gangrenosum (PG) is a neutrophilic dermatosis, characterized by painful ulcers with boggy, undermined edges and a border of gray or purple pigmentation. The ulcers usually occur on the legs and often follow trauma (**pathergy**). About 50% of affected patients have an underlying disorder, usually inflammatory bowel disease, rheumatoid arthritis, or a paraproteinemia, usually an IgA gammopathy.

- *Differential diagnosis:* Infection, vasculitis and factitious disorder.
- *Treatment:* **Systemic** corticosteroids, intralesional and topical corticosteroids, cyclosporine, other immunosuppressants.

SKIN DISEASE AND ENDOCRINE OR METABOLIC DISEASE

Diabetes Mellitus

The skin is affected in upto **one third** of patients with diabetes mellitus:

1. Associated with **microangiopathy** (e.g., necrobiosis lipoidica diabeticorum or diabetic dermopathy).
2. Related to a tendency to develop **infections** (e.g., furunculosis, extensive dermatophytosis, and refractory candidiasis).
3. Related to **vascular insufficiency** (e.g., peripheral gangrene).
4. Related to **neuropathy** (e.g., neurotropic ulcers).
5. Related to altered **metabolism** (e.g., eruptive xanthomas).
6. Related to complications of **treatment** (insulin lipoatrophy).

General Associations

Rubeosis

Characteristic chronic flushed appearance of the face and cheek, and even of the extremities, in patients with diabetes mellitus is termed rubeosis. There may be reduced vasoconstrictor tone in affected vessels, which allows for pooling of blood in the dermal venous plexus. The condition is improved by better diabetic control and may be worsened by vasodilators, including alcohol and caffeine.

Diabetic Dermopathy

Presence of atrophic hyperpigmented patches, primarily the lower legs. Although the condition occurs in a majority of elderly patients with diabetes mellitus, it is not specific to diabetes. Diabetic dermopathy may be a result of diabetic microangiopathy, and the presence of lesions appears to correlate with the presence of vasculopathy, neuropathy, and nephropathy.

Diabetic Bullae

The association of tense bullae, primarily on the lower extremities, and diabetes mellitus has long been recognized. Early studies describe an intraepidermal location. Electron microscopic studies of other patients strongly support a dermal-epidermal junction blister (i.e., lamina lucida) with the basal lamina on the floor of the blister. These blisters are nonscarring clinically.

Necrobiosis Lipoidica Diabeticorum

Necrobiosis lipoidica diabeticorum is clinically characterized by well-circumscribed, yellow-brown patches with pronounced epidermal atrophy (Fig. 20.1). The active border is raised and erythematous. These lesions may occur anywhere, but they favor the legs. Ulceration is not

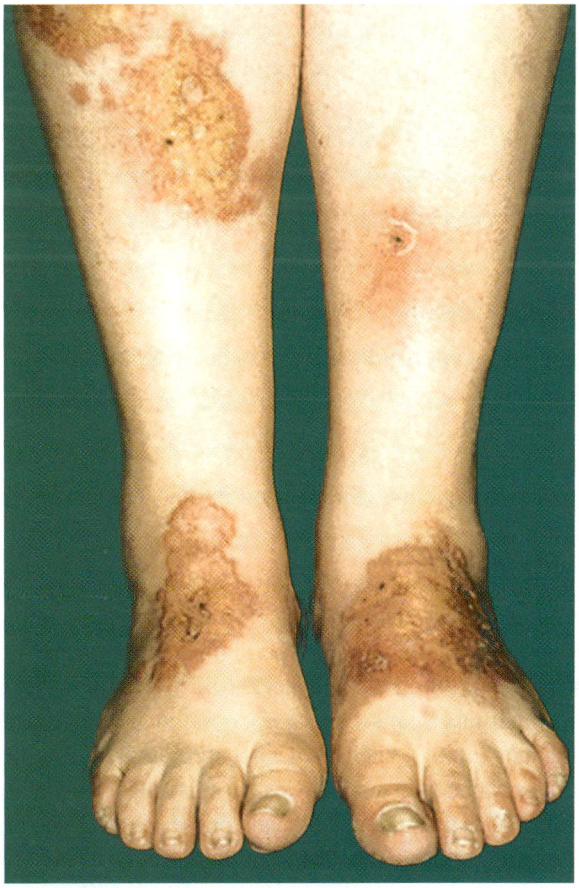

Fig. 20.1: Yellow-brown patches with pronounced epidermal atrophy

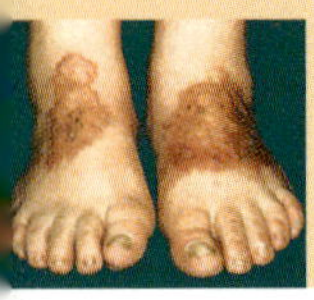

uncommon. Histopathologic examination of specimens shows a progression of neutrophilic vascular reaction to palisading granuloma formation with changes in collagen and with degeneration of adnexal structures.

About one third of patients with necrobiosis lipoidica diabeticorum have diabetes mellitus, about one third have only glucose intolerance and one third have normal glucose tolerance. Patients with necrobiosis lipoidica diabeticorum should be evaluated and followed for the possibility that they will develop diabetes mellitus at a later date. Excellent control of the diabetes, unfortunately, is not associated with improvement in necrobiosis lipoidica diabeticorum.

Intralesional corticosteroid therapy may be effective in preventing the expansion of lesions. Aspirin and dipyridamole may be effective in preventing the extension of lesions. Maintenance therapy with pentoxifylline, a vasodilator, has also been tried as a therapy for this condition.

Disseminated Granuloma Annulare

Granuloma annulare is clinically characterized by rings dermal papules that have histologic similarities to palisading granulomas of necrobiosis lipoidica diabeticorum.

Cutaneous Perforating Diseases

Kyrle's disease and perforating folliculitis are characterized by hyperkeratotic papules and nodules in which the histopathologic assessment confirms basophilic debris in the dermis with evidence of transepidermal elimination. Although these conditions are usually rare, their incidence in patients undergoing renal dialysis may be 5-10%.

Vitiligo

Vitiligo is an idiopathic disorder with a possible underlying autoimmune cause that is characterized by macular patches of total depigmentation. Melanocytes are absent from affected patches. Vitiligo occurs with greater frequency than expected in patients with adult-onset diabetes.

Acanthosis Nigricans and Lipodystrophy

Acanthosis nigricans is characterized by a typical velvety epidermal thickening with hyperpigmentation primarily in the axillary, inguinal, and neck folds. Although severe acanthosis nigricans can be associated with advanced malignant tumors, such as adenocarcinomas, it has been well associated with insulin resistance and diabetes mellitus.

It has been postulated that many obese patients who have what was previously labelled as pseudoacanthosis nigricans may actually have insulin resistance. **Insulin-like** growth factors have been postulated to account for the epidermal proliferation. Insulin resistance can occur in a number of clinical settings. **The type A** abnormality occurs in women with acanthosis nigricans and insulin resistance caused by insulin receptor abnormalities. These young, tall, hirsute women usually have polycystic ovaries. Patients with **the type B** abnormality have acanthosis nigricans and insulin resistance owing to antibodies to insulin receptors. These patients are usually older women with arthralgias, alopecia areata, proteinuria, and antinuclear and anti-DNA antibodies.

A host of generalized and partial lipodystrophies are associated with insulin resistance and acanthosis nigricans. These syndromes may be congenital or acquired, familial or sporadic, or generalized or complete. Localized lipodystrophy can occur at the sites used to inject insulin.

VASCULAR CHANGES

Diabetic microangiopathy is characterized histologically by endothelial cell proliferation and basement membrane thickening affecting the arterioles, venules and capillaries.

This small vessel vasculopathy may account for the **acral erysipelas-like erythema** described in elderly diabetic patients. This non-inflammatory, well-marginated erythema may evolve into superficial gangrene. **Dry gangrene** in diabetic patients, especially of the feet, may be the result of larger vessel obstruction. However, small vessel involvement usually plays an important adjunctive role. Gangrene of a foot that has strong peripheral pulses in a diabetic patient is an all-too-familiar consequence of small vessel involvement from diabetes mellitus.

The incidence of **large vessel atherosclerosis** of leg vessels is greatly increased in the diabetic patient population. This factor and the occurrence of small-vessel vasculopathy contribute to the incidence of difficult-to-control diabetic vascular ulcers, particularly on the lower legs and feet.

Large and small vessel peripheral vascular disease and the frequent peripheral gangrene and leg ulcers confirm that patients with diabetes mellitus require meticulous foot care.

Treatment of vascular ulcers requires aggressive use of topical and, at times, systemic antibiotics. Semipermeable membrane dressings are also helpful in treating these ulcers. Unfortunately, amputation of an extremity may be required when vascular flow is inadequate and cannot be surgically restored or when osteomyelitis and other infection cannot be controlled.

INFECTIONS

Bacterial

Erythrasma is an infection with *Corynebacterium*

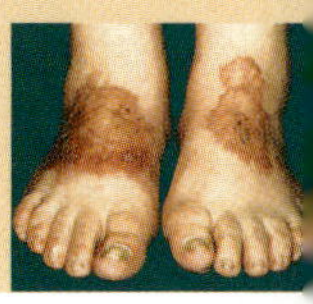

minutissimum, which is especially prevalent in the intertriginous areas of obese diabetic patients. A Wood's light examination confirms the diagnosis if a coral fluorescence (owing to a porphyrin produced by the organism) is seen. Topical therapy with erythromycin or clindamycin, in the formulation used to treat acne, is often adequate to eradicate the infection. Compresses, drying powders, meticulous local hygiene, and improved diabetic control reduce the risk of recurrence.

Impaired neutrophil function in patients with poorly controlled diabetes may account for the increased difficulty in eradicating infections caused by *Staphylococcus aureus* and with beta-hemolytic streptococci. **Impetigo, cellulitis, ecthyma and folliculitis, furuncles, and carbuncles** may occur. The diagnosis in each instance is confirmed by the clinical evaluation and by Gram stain and culture of the organism. In addition to local compresses, systemic antibiotic therapy to cover both organisms is usually indicated. Erythromycin or, for more aggressive infections, a penicillinase-resistant penicillin is often appropriate. Newer substitutes are available. Surgical incision and drainage are usually required to treat furuncles and carbuncles.

Superficial Fungal

The patient with poorly controlled diabetes is particularly at risk for the development of severe acute mucocutaneous **candidal** infections. Oral thrush, angular cheilitis, and candidal vaginitis and balanitis can become recurrent problems. These mucosal infections often respond to topical therapy with nystatin, the imidazoles, or other, newer topical antifungal agents and to better diabetic control. Refractory disease may necessitate therapy with systemic ketoconazole, fluconazole, or itraconazole. Candidal paronychia is characterized by chronic nail matrix dystrophy (as manifested by horizontal ridging of the entire nail plate) and loss of the cuticle. Secondary acute staphylococcal paronychia may occur as a complication.

There is controversy as to whether patients with diabetes mellitus have an increased incidence of dermatophytosis.

Tinea pedis must be aggressively treated. The diabetic patient may have macerated toe webs as a result of secondary bacterial infection of tinea pedis. A soft-tissue abscess followed by osteomyelitis and the need for amputation may be the result. The slightest cutaneous injury, especially when located acrally, must be treated aggressively to prevent a serious infection. Toenails must be trimmed straight across to prevent the development of ingrown toenails, which can become infected. Intermittent claudication, and particularly foot pain at rest, should be evaluated in conjunction with a consultation with a vascular surgeon.

Dermatophytosis, especially of the feet, can have devastating consequences in the diabetic patient, as discussed previously, and should be treated aggressively with topical imidazoles or other, newer topical antifungal agents whenever scaling of the toe webs recurs after an initially documented tinea pedis infection. Diabetes mellitus-associated dermatophyte onychomycosis is a good justification for oral antifungal therapy with agents such as terbinafine, itraconazole or fluconazolė. Maintenance prophylaxis with topical agents including nail laquers or lotions to the nails and/or antifungal powders to the feet and shoes is warranted.

Deep Fungal

Diabetes with ketosis that is debilitating puts the patient at risk for life-threatening mucormycosis. This occurs when various fungi of the phycomycetes group produce a necrotizing infection, especially in the nasopharyngeal area, that may lead to cerebral involvement and death. Prompt intensive supportive care and intravenous therapy with amphotericin B are required.

ASSOCIATIONS RELATED TO ALTERED METABOLISM

Eruptive Xanthomas

Patients with diabetes mellitus may occasionally develop a sudden eruption of yellow-red papules. Specimens from these lesions histologically show infiltration of the dermis with macrophages filled with lipid; these are called foam cells.

Yellow Skin

Many patients with diabetes mellitus have elevated serum carotene levels, and upto 10% of diabetic patients have a secondary yellowish discoloration of the skin. The elevation of carotene may relate to its impaired hepatic conversion. Treatment of this cosmetic problem involves a reduction of the dietary intake of foods rich in carotene, such as oranges, yellow fruits and vegetables, egg yolks and butter.

CUTANEOUS COMPLICATIONS OF ANTIDIABETIC THERAPY

Insulin allergy is more commonly seen with beef insulin than with pork insulin. Recombinant DNA-produced human insulins produce less allergy and lipodystrophy. Documented examples of insulin allergy include immediate hypersensitivity reactions that manifest cutaneously, such as urticaria; serum

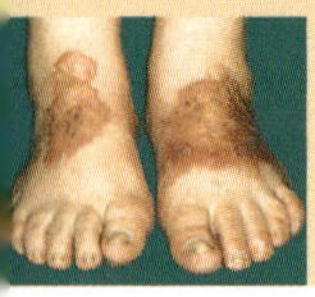

sickness-like reactions, which are often characterized by vasculitic or purpuric urticarial lesions; and delayed hypersensitivity reactions, which may present as localized nodules. Insulin lipodystrophy is less common than insulin allergy.

THYROID AND THE SKIN

Specific Lesions

Thyroglossal Duct Cysts

During embryonic life, the developing thyroid gland descends in the neck while maintaining its connection to the tongue by a narrow tube of undifferentiated epithelium, the thyroglossal duct. This structure may activate later in life, and the cells then differentiate into columnar, ciliated, or squamous epithelium or even into overt glandular tissue. Thyroglossal duct cysts account for 70% of the congenital cystic abnormalities of the neck. They usually present in the first decade of life.

Cutaneous Metastases

Papillary thyroid carcinoma accounts for the majority of thyroid malignancies in early life. It metastasizes to regional lymph nodes but only rarely distantly (including to the skin). By contrast, follicular carcinoma usually appears in middle-aged or elderly individuals, and distant metastases are more frequent. Anaplastic tumors, the giant or spindle cell subtypes, occur almost without exception in those older than age 60 years, grow rapidly, and possess a propensity for both nodal and distant metastases.

HYPERTHYROIDISM

Skin Fine, velvety, or smooth.
Warm and moist (increased sweating), rarely dry, hyperpigmentation (localized or generalized), vitiligo, urticaria or dermographism Pretibial myxedema and thyroid acropachy.

Hair Fine, thin alopecia (diffuse and mild; rarely severe), alopecia areata.

Nails Onycholysis, koilonychia, clubbing with thyroid acropachy.

The **most common** symptoms accompanying hyperthyroidism, regardless of the exact cause, are **systemic** rather than cutaneous. These include nervousness, emotional lability, weight loss despite an increased appetite, heat intolerance, hyperhidrosis, 'weakness', palpitations, and/or tremor. Patients often speak rapidly and complain bitterly about heat intolerance. Common clinical signs in thyrotoxic patients include sinus tachycardia; atrial fibrillation; increased systolic and lowered diastolic blood pressures; fine-to-coarse resting or intention tremors; proximal muscle weakness; and changes in the skin, hair and nails.

The skin is described as being **moist and warm**, the result of vasodilatation and increased cutaneous perfusion. Furthermore, the skin is characterized as **soft and velvety** in texture, comparable to that of an infant. The skin is usually less oily, and hyperthyroidism in adolescence is associated with a **decreased incidence of acne**. **Palmar erythema, episodic flushing** over the face and thorax, increased capillary fragility, and persistent erythema of the elbows may also occur. **Hyperhidrosis** may be either generalized or localized to the palms and soles.

Diffuse hair loss is present in 20-40% of hyperthyroid patients, although the severity of alopecia does not correlate with the severity of thyrotoxicosis. The hair itself is typically fine, soft, straight, and unable to retain a permanent wave.

Nail changes, present in about 5% of cases of hyperthyroidism, are often reversible following successful therapy. The nails are described as rapidly growing, soft and friable. Although not truly pathognomonic for thyrotoxicosis, the nails often assume a 'scoop shovel' configuration and/or onycholysis (**plummers nail**). Also seen are pigmentary changes.

GRAVES DISEASE

Pretibial myxedema—Bilateral raised, assymetrical, firm plaques and nodules on the legs.

Thyroid Acropachy—Clubbing, periosteal proliferation and swelling of soft tissue.

Exophthalmos.

HYPOTHYROIDISM

Skin Dry, rough, or coarse; cold and pale; puffy, boggy, or edematous **(myxedema). Yellow discoloration** as a result of carotenemia. **Ichthyosis and palmoplantar hyperkeratosis.** Easy bruising (capillary fragility). Eruptive bruising (capillary fragility). Eruptive and tuberous xanthomas (rare).

Hair Dull, coarse and brittle. Slow growth (increase in telogen or resting hairs). Alopecia (lateral third of eyebrows, rarely diffuse).

Nails Thin, brittle, striated. Slow growth. Onycholysis (rare).

The clinical manifestations of hypothyroidism, regardless of the exact cause, can be attributed to both a deceleration

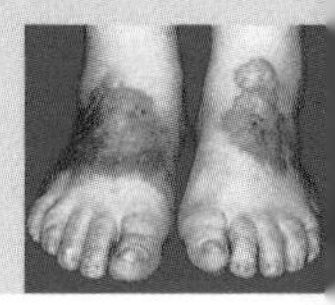

of cellular metabolic processes and to myxedema, the accumulation of acid mucopolysaccharides in various organs, such as the skin, vocal cords, and oropharynx. The exact pathogenesis of myxedema remains obscure, but most authorities have abandoned the hypothesis that it is the result of increased levels of TSH, which occurs in response to low thyroid hormone levels. The extracutaneous features of hypothyroidism include pleural and pericardial effusions, slow heart rate and reduced cardiac output, weight gain secondary to fluid retention, hoarseness, swollen lips and tongue, rheumatoid-like polyarthritis, and a wide variety of neurologic problems (such as slowed mentation). When hypothyroidism occurs in adolescence, delayed sexual maturation occurs; in adults, impotence, oligospermia, and amenorrhea are common. The symptoms often include weakness and fatigue, anorexia, cold intolerance, voice changes, muscle cramps, and the swelling of extremities. Such symptoms may easily be overlooked or ascribed merely to aging.

The most characteristic sign is generalized **myxedema,** which is caused by the dermal deposition of acid mucopolysaccharides (notably hyaluronic acid and chondroitin sulfate). The entire skin appears swollen, dry, waxy and pale. The **cutaneous pallor** is due both to vasoconstriction and to the increased water and mucopolysaccharide content in the dermis, which alters the refraction of incident light. The skin is also 'boggy' but nonpitting, especially around the eyes, lips, and acral portions. The skin is cool to the touch and may be so xerotic as to develop an **acquired ichthyosis**. The palms and sole are hypohydrotic and may demonstrate a **keratoderma**. **Carotenemia** may also be encountered on the volar and palmar surfaces as a result of decreased hepatic conversion of beta-carotene to vitamin A.

The hair in patients with hypothyroidism are dull, coarse and brittle. The growth rate is slowed, with an **increase in telogen (resting) hairs**. Although diffuse alopecia may be seen in patients with hypothyroidism, the classic pattern of hair loss is the loss of the lateral third of the eyebrows.

The nails are affected to some degree in 90% of all patients. They are typically thin, brittle, slow growing and striated (either in longitudinal or transverse fashion). Onycholysis, more commonly seen in hyperthyroid states, has also been reported to accompany myxedema. A list of skin findings in renal disorders is given below: (Table 20.1)

Table 20.1: Dermatologic manifestations

Systemic disorder	*Renal disorder*	*Dermatologic manifestations*
Diabetes mellitus	Diabetic nephropathy	Diabetic dermopathy Necrobiosis lipoidica Acanthosis nigricans Eruptive xanthomas Kyrle disease Scleredema
SLE	Glomerulonephritis Nephrotic syndrome	Purpura Chronic cutaneous lupus Subacute cutaneous lupus Photosensitivity Mucosal ulcers Vasculitis
Henoch-Schönlein purpura	Glomerulonephritis Vasculitis	Purpura
Wegener granulomatosis	Glomerulonephritis Vasculitis	Purpura Subcutaneous nodules Ulcers
Polyarteritis nodosa	Glomerulonephritis Vasculitis	Purpura Subcutaneous nodules Ulcers

Contd.

Contd.

Subacute bacterial endocarditis	Renal emboli Glomerulonephritis	Petechiae Purpura
Cholesterol emboli	Renal emboli	Petechiae Livedo reticularis Blue toes
HCV	Glomerulonephritis	Purpura Porphyria cutanea tarda Lichen planus Sclerodermatous plaques Cutaneous polyarteritis nodosa Necrolytic acral erythema
HIV	HIV-associated nephropathy	Eosinophilic folliculitis Oral hairy leukoplakia Bacillary angiomatosis Kaposi sarcoma
Systemic sclerosis	Malignant hypertension	Diffuse scleroderma
Amyloidosis	Nephrotic syndrome	Purpura Macroglossia
Fabry disease	Nephrotic syndrome	Angiokeratomas
Nail-patella syndrome	Renal tubular defects	Absent/displaced patella Absent/pitted nails
Tuberous sclerosis	Renal hamartomas Renal cell carcinoma	Adenoma sebaceum Ash-leaf macule Periungual fibromas Shagreen patch

SKIN SIGNS OF INTERNAL MALIGNANCY

Disorders that Strongly Associated with Cancer (Fitz Curth's Criteria)

- Acanthosis nigricans.
- The sign of Leser-Trelat.
- Bazex's syndrome.
- Cacinoid syndrome.
- Erythema gyratum repens.
- Hypertrichosis lanuginosa.
- Ectopic ACTH syndrome.
- Glucagonoma syndrome.
- Neutrophillic dermatoses.
- Paget's disease.
- Paraneoplastic pemphigus.

Disorders Associated Statistically with Cancer

- Bowen's disease.
- Dermatomyositis.
- Extramammary Paget's disease.
- Exfoliative dermatitis.
- Mycosis fungoides.
- Palmar keratoses.
- Generalized pruritus without a primary cutaneous eruption.
- Porphyria cutanea tarda.
- Pityriasis rotunda.

Dermatoses Possibly Associated with Cancer

- Arsenical keratoses.
- Erythema annulare centrifugum.
- Acquired ichthyosis.
- Multicentric reticulohistiocytosis.
- Necrobiotic xanthogranuloma.
- Classic pyoderma gangrenosum.
- Polymyositis.
- Tripe palms.

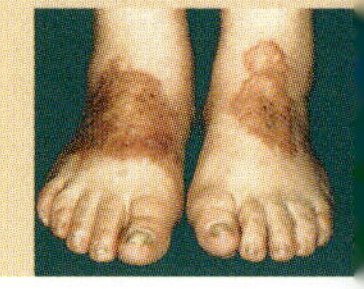

- Vasculitis.
- Vitiligo.
- **Cutaneous metastases.**
- Paraneoplastic syndromes.
- Heritable "cancer syndromes".

SISTER MARY JOSEPH NODULE

- Umbilical metastasis; poor prognosis.
- Precedes or follows diagnosis of CA.
- CA sites (decreasing order of frequency): **colon,** ovary, pancreas, endometrium, breast, small bowel.

PARANEOPLASTIC SYNDROMES

The skin often presents a clue that an internal malignancy is present. The combination of a malignancy and associated signs and symptoms that are seemingly unrelated to the actual tumor is called a "paraneoplastic" syndrome.

i. Erythema Gyratum Repens

- **"Wood-grain" pattern.**
- Wavy, erythematous, urticarial bands with scale.
- Slowly migrate.
- Breast, stomach, bladder, prostate, cervix; occasionally no CA.

ii. Glucagonoma Syndrome Necrolytic Migratory Erythema

- **Alpha cell tumor** of the pancreas; occasionally no neoplasm found.
- Abdomen, thighs and buttocks.
- Patchy erythema with flaccid vesicles and glossitis, angular cheilitis, normocytic anemia, low amino acid levels in serum.

iii. Sweet's Syndrome (Acute Febrile Neutrophilic Dermatosis)

- Bullae painful red plaques and papules—face, neck, upper chest, arms, legs.
- Usually females (4:1)—fever, leukocytosis prominent.
- Associations, benign—URIs, RA, Crohn's, sarcoidosis, Behcet's, pregnancy.
- Association, malignant—AML, myelodysplasia, lymphoma—may follow by months to years.
- **Treatment:** Prednisone.

iv. Trousseau's Sign

- Superficial migratory thrombophlebitis and neoplasia.
- 75% of CA in pancreas, stomach, lung, prostate, hematopoietic.
- Hypercoagulable state; thrombophlebitis resistant to therapy—sustained low grade DIC.

v. Pancreatic Panniculitis

- Fat necrosis, fever, eosinophilia, joint pain.
- Pancreatic CA; also acute or chronic pancreatitis.
- Circulating lipases and amylase.
- Tender red nodules stimulating erythema nodosum.

Heritable "Cancer Syndromes"

- Peutz-Jeghers.
- Torre.
- Cowden's.

Peutz-Jeghers Syndrome

- Multiple hamartomatous polyps in small bowel (most common), stomach and colon; low risk of bowel malignancy.
- Multiple lentigines (freckle-like) of lips, nose, oral mucosa, fingertips and nail beds.
- Non-intestinal malignancies increased: lung, ovary, endometrium, pancreas, myeloma.

Torre Syndrome

- Autosomal dominant; "cancer-family" syndrome.
- Multiple low-grade malignancies of the GI and GU tracts; occasionally breast, lymphoma; multiple GI polyps in 25%.
- Sebaceous neoplasms: Adenomas, carcinomas, sebaceous BCCs.

NUTRITION AND THE SKIN

Malabsorption

Nonspecific Cutaneous Symptoms

- Itching and acquired ichthyosis.
- Dry skin, elderly, cancer, liver and kidney disease and lymphoma.
- Melanosis
  - Symmetrical hyperpigmentation.
- Skin appendages
  - Brittle nails, hair loss.

Specific Cutaneous Effects

- Follicular hyperkeratosis (vit-A), ecchymosis and haematuria (vit-K), cheilitis, glossitis, neuritis and dermatitis (vit-B comp).

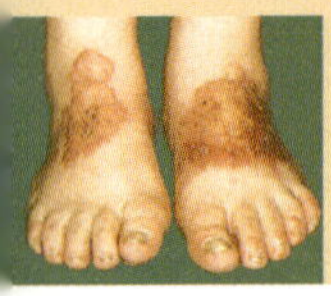

Investigation

- Analysis of serum calcium, zinc, folate and albumin level.
- Fecal fat excretion.
- X-ray of intestine.

Treatment

- Adequate intake of all nutrients
  - Wide variety of foods.

VITAMINS

- **Definition:** Biologically active organic compounds, have no direct function, acts as co-enzymes.
- Fat soluble
  - Vitamin A
  - Vitamin D
  - Vitamin E–Vitamin K.
- Water soluble
  - Vitamin B complex
  - Vitamin C.

1. Vitamin A

- Sources—liver, eggs, butter.
- Beta carotene is a provitamin A, which gets converted into vitamin A in the body.
- Sources of beta-carotene—fruits, carrots and green vegetable.
- Daily allowance is 5000 I.U. vitamin A equivalent to 6000-12000 I.U. of beta carotene.

Vitamin A Deficiency

- Mainly due to malabsorption.
- Often associated with deficiency of other fat soluble vitamins.

Clinical Features

- Xerophthalmia, follicular hyperkeratosis and generalized xerosis.
- **Phrynoderma**
  - Follicular papules seen mainly on dorsal and lateral aspect of extremities (Fig. 20.2).
- **Histology**
  - Lamellated hyperkeratosis around the hair follicle with keratinous plugs and atrophy of sebaceous gland.

Diagnosis and Treatment

- Low level vitamin A in blood is confirmatory.
- Supplementation of vitamin A and zinc.
  - Zinc acts on retinol binding protein.

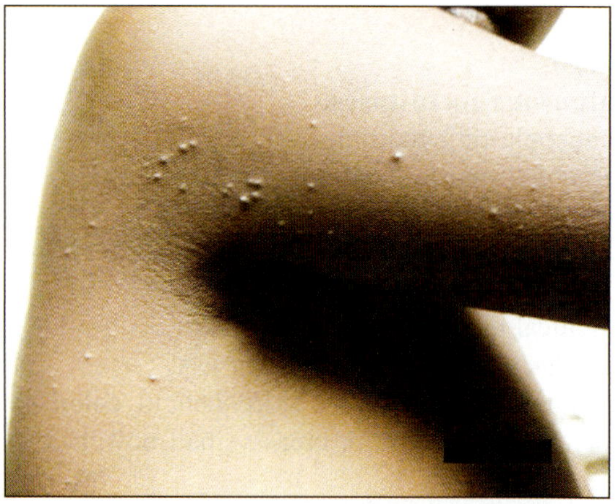

Fig. 20.2: Multiple follicular papules on the extensors of arm (Phrynoderma)

- Avoidance of alcohol.

2. Carotenoderma

- High intake of carrots.
- Orange discoloration due to deposition in S. corneum.
  - Palms, soles, sebaceous glands.
- Condition harmless and subsides gradually.

3. Vitamin B Complex

Thiamine (B_1).
Riboflavine (B_2).
Niacin (B_3).
Pyridoxine (B_6).
Cyanocobalamin (B_{12}).
Folic acid.
Pantothanic acid.
Biotin (vitamin H).

- **Sources**
  - Milk, yeast, cereals, liver, meat, eggs and vegetable.
- Cause of deficiency
  - Chronic illness, malnutrition.
- **Symptoms**
  - Associated with other deficiencies like pellagra, angular stomatitis (Fig. 20.3) and sore lips.
  - Tongue becomes purplish red and smooth.
  - Seborrheic dermatitis like eruption around orifices.
- **Treatment**
  - 5-15 mg riboflavine BD-TDS × 2 weeks.

a. Vitamin B_{12} (Cyanocobalamin)

- Involved in nucleic acid synthesis and erythrocyte production.
- Deficiency may occur in vegetarians.

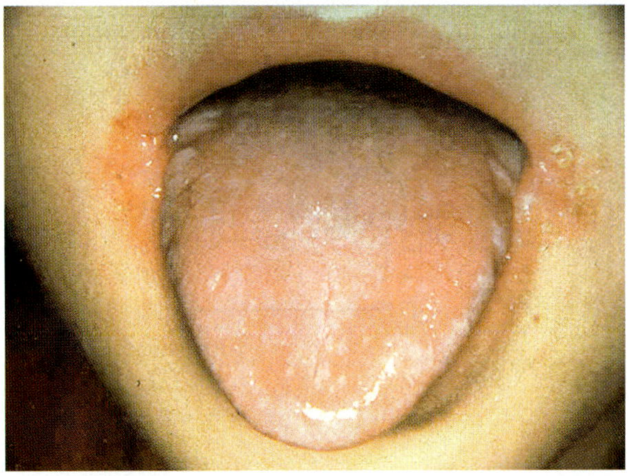

Fig. 20.3: Angular stomatitis and glossitis

Clinical Features

- **Hyperpigmentation** mainly in flexures.
- Pigmented streaks in nail.
- Enlarged and red tongue.

b. Folic Acid

- **Source**
  - Liver, meat, green leafy vegetables and milk.
- **Deficiency**
  - Pregnancy, drugs.

Clinical Features

- Cheilitis, glossitis and mucosal erosion.
- Pigmentation in flexures.
- Spotty pigmentation in palms and sole.

c. Biotin

- Involved in bacterial metabolism.
- **Deficiency**
  - Raw egg intake, short bowel syndrome, inborn error of biotin metabolism.

Clinical Features

- Alopecia, conjunctivitis, eczema around nose and mouth, hyperaesthesia, paraesthesia, depression and muscle pain.
- **Treatment**
  - Multivitamin preparation.

d. Niacin

- Essential component of two enzyme coenzyme I (NAD) and coenzyme II (NADP).
- **Deficiency**
  - Inadequate intake, chronic alcoholics, GI disease, psychiatric disturbance, INH.
- **Clinical Features—Pellagra**
  - **Triad–dermatitis, diarrhoea and dementia** (Fig. 20.4).

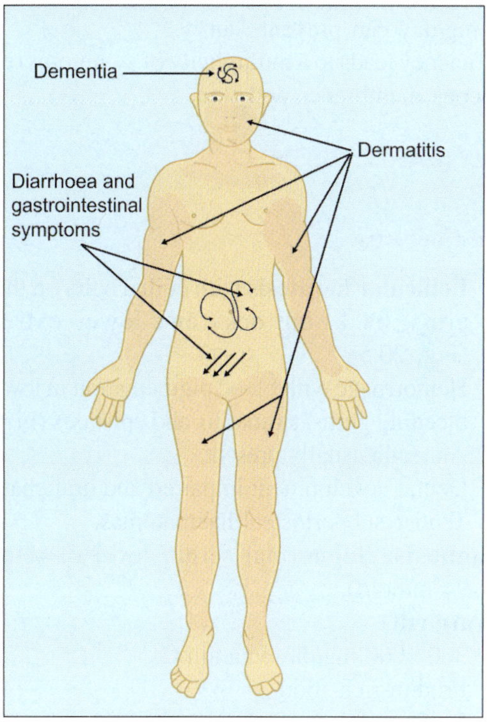

Fig. 20.4: Diagram depicting the features of pellagra

Dermatitis

- Redness and superficial scaling on **exposed** areas.
- Subside leaving dusky brown-red coloration.
- Exacerbation on re-exposure to sunlight.
- *Butterfly eruption* in face.
- Characteristic well marginated in front of neck—*Casal's necklace.*
- *Also on exposed part of limbs "glove and gauntlet sign".*

Diarrhoea

- Pain, diarrhoea and achlorhydria.
- **Histology**
  - Hyper and parakeratosis, acanthosis, and multiple melanin granules in epidermis.
- **Treatment**
  - Severe case—I/V 50-100 mg (Niacin) once or twice.
  - Orally 0.5 g/day in divided dose.

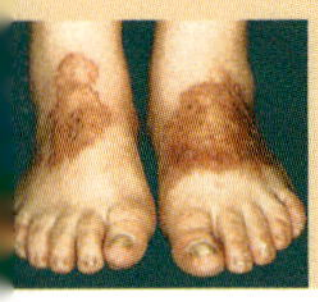

Vitamin C

- Cannot be synthesized in body.
- Plays central roles in collagen.
- Sources—cabbage, potatoes, green vegetables and fruits.
- Recommended daily dose 30-80 mg.
- 10 mg/day can prevent scurvy.
- Deficiency leads to a multiplicity of symptoms of bones, mucous membranes and skin.

SCURVY (BARLOW'S DISEASE)

Clinical Features

- **Follicular keratosis** with coiled hairs on the upper arms, back, buttocks and lower extremities (Fig. 20.5).
- Hemorrhage with blood pigmentation in lower legs, bleeding gums, stomatitis and epistaxis (Fig. 20.6).
- Anaemia usually present.
- Dental development impaired and oral changes.
- Tender subperiosteal haematomas.

- **Diagnosis:** Subnormal serum level of vitamin C (17-94 mmol/l).
- **Treatment**
  - 300-1000 mg/day vitamin C.
  - Protein-rich food.
  - Response is dramatic.

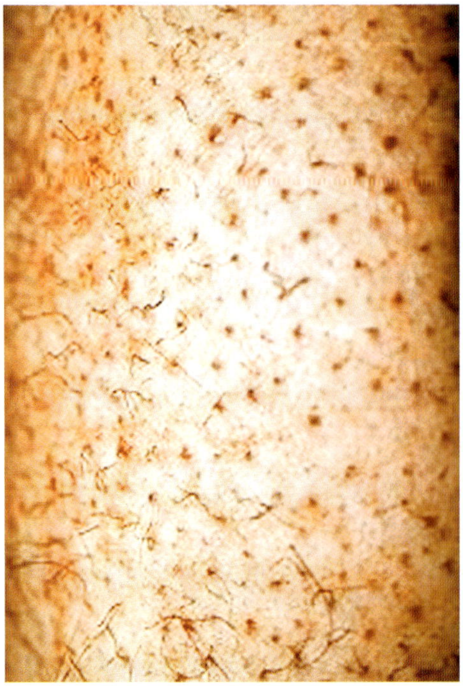

Fig. 20.5: Folliculär hemorrhagic papules with corkscrew hair (Scurvy)

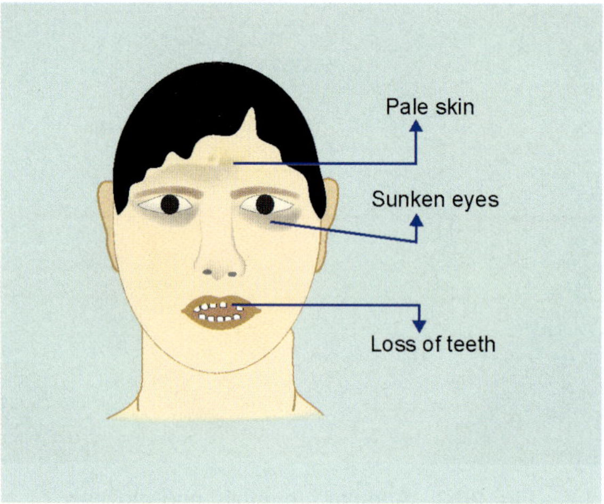

Fig. 20.6: Diagram depicting the features of scurvy

KWASHIORKOR

- *Most common and most widespread* nutritional disorder in developing countries.
- Common in children and in diet consisting corn, rice or beans.
- Onset during weaning and post weaning period.
- **Clinical Features (Fig. 20.7)**
  - Failure to thrive, mental development.

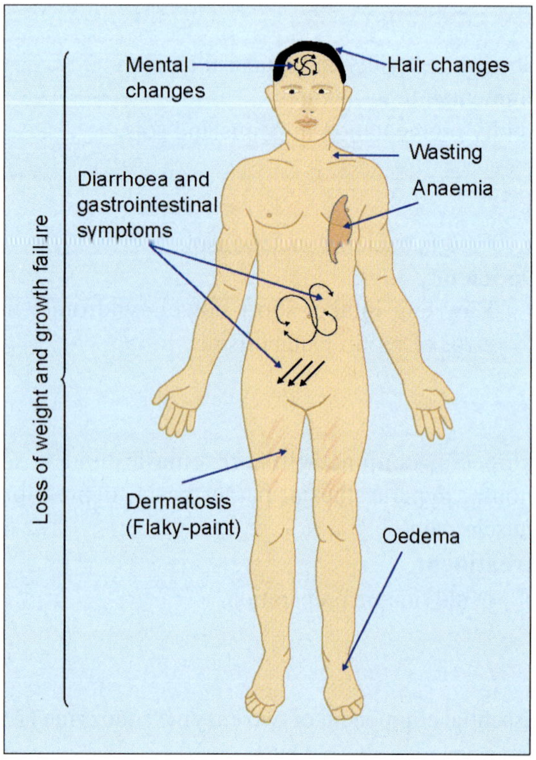

Fig. 20.7: Clinical features of kwashiorkor

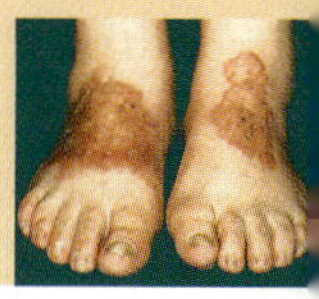

- Edema and muscle wasting (Figs. 20.8).

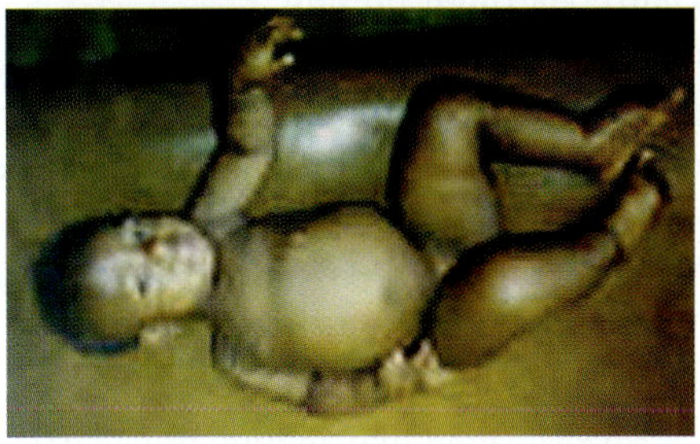

Fig. 20.8: Edema

Skin Lesion

- Edematous–purple or reddish brown–exfoliation.
- *Flaky paint or cracked skin* (Fig. 20.9).
- Hair are dry and lusterless or light brown, sparse and brittle.
- Hypopigmentation or patchy post inflammatory hyperpigmentation.
- Cheilitis, xerosis.

Diagnosis

- Dietary history, edema, skin changes.

- **Prevention and Treatment**
  - Increasing supply of animal proteins.
  - Education and social welfare in poor areas.

Differentiating Features between Kwashiorkor and Pellagra

Kwashiorkor

- Children > adult.
- Dermatitis with systemic signs of apathy and oedema.
- Eruption generalized, pale, ill-defined, cracked skin.

Pellagra

- Adult > children.
- Dermatitis precedes GI and neuropsychiatric symptoms.

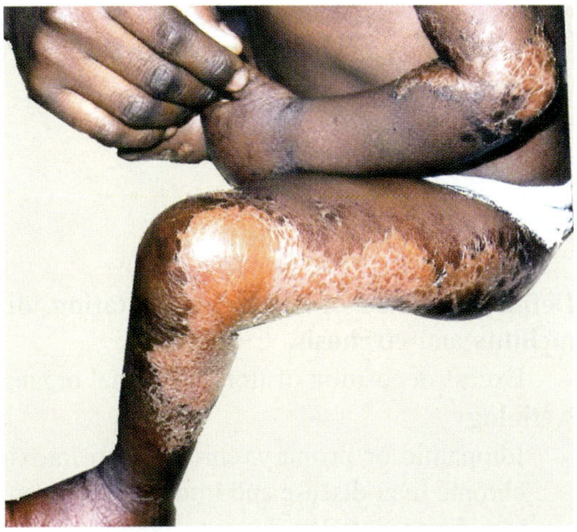

Fig. 20.9: Flaky paint dermatitis (Kwashiorkor)

- Exposed areas only; red thickened, well defined, later dry, branny scales.
- Normal.

MARASMUS

In marasmus the main deficiency is one of food in general, and therefore also of energy. It may occur at any age, most commonly upto about three and a half years.

Clinical Features of Nutritional Marasmus

The important features of kwashiorkor and nutritional marasmus are compared in Table 20.2.

Table 20.2: Comparison of the features of kwashiorkor and marasmus

Feature	*Kwashiorkor*	*Marasmus*
Growth failure	Present	Present
Wasting	Present	Present, marked
Oedema	Present (sometimes mild)	Absent
Hair changes	Common	Less common
Mental changes	Very common	Uncommon
Dermatosis, flaky-paint	Common	Does not occur
Appetite	Poor	Good
Anaemia	Severe (sometimes)	Present, less severe
Subcutaneous fat	Reduced but present	Absent
Face	May be oedematous	Drawn in, monkey-like
Fatty infiltration of liver	Present	Absent

The following are the main signs of marasmus (Fig. 20.10).

- ***Poor growth.***
- ***Wasting.***
- ***Alertness:*** Children with marasmus are quite often **not** disinterested like those with kwashiorkor. Instead the deep sunken eyes have a rather **wide-awake** appearance. Similarly, the child may be less miserable and less irritable.
- ***Appetite:*** The child often has a **good** appetite.
- ***Anaemia:*** Anaemia is usually present.
- ***Hair changes:*** Changes similar to those in kwashiorkor can occur. There is more frequently a change of texture than of colour.

Marasmic Kwashiorkor

Children with features of both nutritional marasmus and

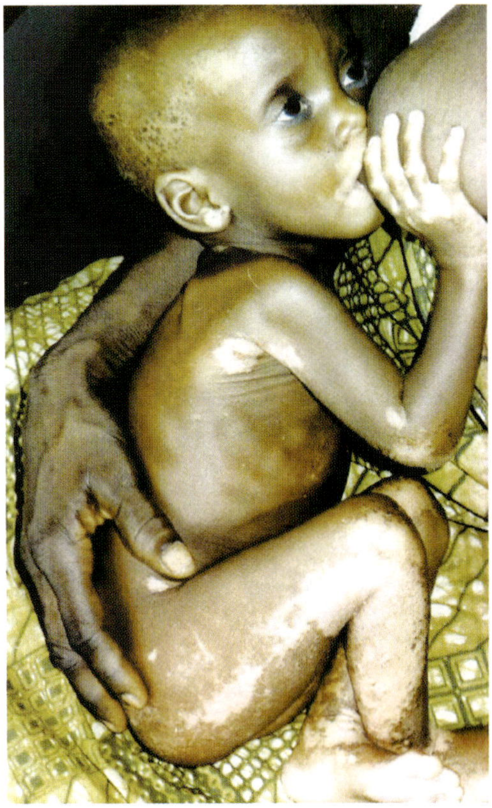

Fig. 20.10: Wasted appearance of a child of marasmus

kwashiorkor are diagnosed as having marasmic kwashiorkor. Children with marasmic kwashiorkor have all the features of nutritional marasmus including severe wasting, lack of subcutaneous fat and poor growth, and in addition to oedema, which is always present, they may also have any of the features of kwashiorkor described above. There may be skin changes including flaky-paint dermatosis, hair changes, mental changes and hepatomegaly. Many of these children have diarrhoea.

ACRODERMATITIS ENTEROPATHICA (AE)

- Essential trace element.
- Source: Shellfish, legumes, nuts, whole grains, green leafy vegetable.
- Supply mainly depends on protein content of food.
- Phytate and high fibre content food interfere the absorption.
- Zinc deficiency
  - Specific absorption defect—primary.
- Autosomal recessive
  - Disease of GI tract—secondary.
  - Zinc absorption is low in young patients with AE.
- **Clinical Features**
  - Starts at around 4-6 weeks of weaning.
  - Child turns peevish, withdrawn and photophobic.
  - Diarrhoea often present.
  - Growth is stunted.
  - Flat grayish,vesicobullous dermatitis surrounded by red brown erythema on hands, feet and periorificial areas.
  - Wound healing is poor and skin lesions do not heal.
  - The scalp hair is reduced.
- Growth retardation.
- Broken spearheaded like ending, transverse striation of the shaft, pseudomonilethrix, longitudinal split
  - Beau's line in nails.
- Prognosis
  - Without proper treatment—poor.
  - Lethal in 4-5 years.
- **Treatment**
  - Oral zinc 2 mg/kg/day.

Zinc Deficiency

- **Acute deficiency**
  - Cause— prolong total parenteral nutrition, chronic diarrhoea.
- Septicemia, photophobia, mental depression.
- Eczematous eruption on the hands, feet, in anogenital regions and periorificial areas.
- The finger flexural creases and the palms show characteristic flat, grayish, bullous lesions surrounded by red-brown erythema.
- Paronychial inflammation on finger and toes.
- **Chronic deficiency**
  - Listless and mentally depressed.
  - Skin lesions typically seen in trauma prone areas such as elbows, knees, knuckles and malleolar regions of ankles.
  - The lesions are well demarcated, thickened and brownish in colour.
  - Lichenification and the moderate scaling are often present.
  - Seborrhoeic dermatitis like changes.
  - Acne may flare up.

HAEMOCHROMATOSIS

- **Definition:** Triad of **hyper pigmentation**, **diabetes mellitus** and **cirrhosis.**
  - Excess deposition of iron in internal organs.
- **Aetiology**
  - Idiopathic or primary, chronic iron intoxication, chronic liver disease and iron overload, congenital transferrin deficiency.
  - Chronic alcoholism.

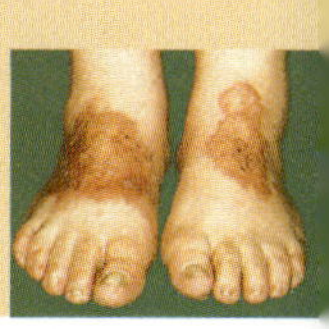

- **Clinical Features**
  - Gray-brown pigmentation especially in face, flexures and exposed areas.
  - Hair loss (75%).
  - Koilonychia.
  - Icthyosis.
  - Palmar edema, striae, leukonychia and spider angiomas.
- **Treatment**
  - Venesection – 500 ml weekly for 1-2 years.

REFERENCES

- Kahn LE, Russo G, Millikan LE: Genetic and acquired **cutaneous** disorders associated with internal malignancy, *Int. J Dermatol* 1995; 34: 749-758.
- Grattan C, Powell S, Humphreys F: Management and diagnostic guidelines for urticaria and angio-oedema. *Br J Dermatol* 2001; 144: 708-14.
- Scott JE, Ahmed AR: The blistering **diseases**, *Med Clin North Am* 1998; 82: 1239-1283.
- Von den Driesch P: Sweet's syndrome (acute febrile neutrophilic dermatosis), *J Am Acad Dermatol* 1994; 31:535.
- Poole S, Fenske NA: **Cutaneous** markers of internal malignancy I, II, *J Am Acad Dermatol* 1993; 28:1,147.
- Callen JP: Pyoderma gangrenosum, *Lancet* 1998; 351: 581-585.
- Perez MI, Kohn SR: **Cutaneous** manifestations of diabetes mellitus, *J Am Acad Dermatol* 1994; 30:519.
- Dermatological Signs of Internal Disease, 3rd edn., Vol 1, Callen and Lorizzo.
- Rook's Textbook of Dermatology, D. A. Burns , S. M. Breathnach, Neil Cox, Christopher E., Griffith's 7th edn 2004.
- Fitzpatrick's Dermatology in General Medicine, 6th edn 2003.
- Michael C. Latham: Human nutrition in the developing world *Food and Nutrition* Series - *No. 29,* Food and Agriculture Organization of the United Nations 1997.

CHAPTER **21**

PSYCHOCUTANEOUS DISORDERS

Most people accept that there are strong links between skin disease and the emotions, but only a few skin disorders, such as dermatitis artefacta, have emotional factors as their direct cause. The relationships between the mind and the skin are usually subtler and more complex than this. Nevertheless, patients with skin disorders do have a higher prevalence of psychiatric abnormalities than the general population.

CLASSIFICATION

Conditions that are **primarily psychiatric** but that commonly present to dermatologists:

1. **Delusions of parasitosis** (Ekbom's disease).
2. **Delusions of body image** (e.g. dysmorphophobia, body dysmorphic disorder, dermatological non-disease, atypical pain disorders).
3. (Glossodynia and essential vulvodynia).
4. **Phobic states** (e.g. syphilophobia, aids phobia, venereophobia, wart and mole phobia).
5. Compulsive hand washing.

DERMATOSES PRIMARILY FACTITIOUS IN ORIGIN

- Dermatitis artefacta.
- Artefact by proxy.
- Witchcraft syndrome.
- Dermatological pathomimicry.
- Malingering.
- Munchausen's syndrome.
- Munchausen's syndrome by proxy.
- Deliberate self-cutting.
- Self mutilation.
- Religious stigmata and psychogenic purpura.

DERMATOSES AGGRAVATED BY HARMFUL HABITS AND COMPULSIONS

- Lichen simplex chronicus.
- Neurotic excoriations.
- Prurigo nodularis.
- Acne excoriee.
- Hair plucking.
- Trichotillomania
- Trichophagia.
- Nail destruction.
- Onychotillomania.
- Lip-licking cheilitis.

Dermatoses due to Accentuated Physiological Responses

- Hyperhidrosis.
- Blushing.

Dermatoses in which Emotional Precipitating or Perpetuating Factors may be Important

- Vesicular eczema of the palms and soles.
- Atopic dermatitis in the adult.
- Seborrheic dermatitis.
- Psoriasis.
- Some cases of localized or generalized pruritus.
- Alopecia areata.
- Aphthosis.
- Rosacea.
- Chronic urticaria.

FIVE CATEGORIES OF PSYCHODERMATOLOGIC DISORDERS

1. **Psychophysiologic disorders**
   Atopic dermatitis, psoriasis, acne vulgaris, Lichen simplex chronicus, hyperhidrosis.
2. **Primary psychiatric disorders**
   Neurotic excoriations, delusions of parasitosis, factitial dermatitis, onychotillomania, trichotillomania.
3. **Secondary psychiatric disorders**
   Vitiligo, alopecia areata, nodulocystic acne.

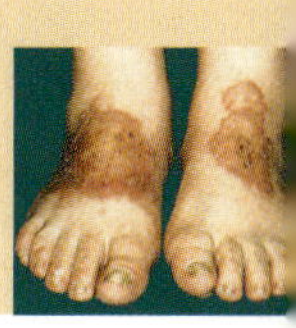

4. **Cutaneous sensory disorders**
   Post herpetic neuralgia.
5. The use of psychotropic medications for non-psychiatric indications.

DERMATOLOGICAL DELUSIONAL DISEASE

Delusions of Parasitosis

This term is better than 'parasitophobia', which implies a fear of becoming infested. Patients with delusions of parasitosis are unshakably convinced that they are already infested.

Underlying Defect

- Monosymptomatic hypochondriacal psychosis.
- Obsessional premorbid personality.
- Schizophrenia/depression.
- CVA in the non-dominant hemisphere.

Pimozide was once the most popular treatment for this condition but high doses carry cardiac risks. If pimozide is used, an electrocardiogram (ECG) should be performed before starting treatment and the drug should not be given to those with a prolonged Q-T interval or with a history of cardiac dysrhythmia. Patients on pimozide in excess of 16 mg daily need periodic ECG checks. Tardive dyskinesia may develop and persist despite withdrawal of the drug.

Risperidone, olanzapine and sulpiride are reasonable, and perhaps safer, alternatives.

Dermatological Non-Disease

This is a form of **dysmorphobia**. The clinician can find no skin abnormality, but the distress felt by the patient leads to anxiety, depression or even suicide. Such patients are not uncommon. They expect dermatological solutions for complaints such as hair loss, or burning, itching and redness of the face or genitals.

The dermatologist, who can see nothing wrong, cannot solve matters and no treatment seems to help. Such patients are reluctant to see a psychiatrist although some may suffer from a monosymptomatic hypochondriacal psychosis.

Areas Affected and Corresponding Complaints

- Face (Scarring, ↑ pores, ↑ greasiness).
- Scalp (Pruritus, burning, Pain).
- Genital area (increased scrotum and genital discomfort).
- **Vulvodynia** (vulval dermatosis, cyclic vulvitis, vulval Papillomatosis, essential vulvodynia.

PHOBIC STATES

Obsessive-Compulsive Disorder

Phobias about dirt and bacteria, warts, moles, anorexia nervosa, pseudojaundice, diffuse non-scarring alopecia, Sjögren-like syndrome, FDR, photosensitivity, severe perniösis, trichotillomania, onychotillomania, onychophagia, acne excoriee.

Mx.: SSRI, clomipramine, fluoxetine, psychotherapy.

SELF-INFLICTED AND SIMULATED DERMATOSES

Lichen Simplex and Neurodermatitis

Treatment: Doxepin
Behaviour therapy.

Neurotic Excoriations

- Psychosocial stresses (30-90%), compulsion, depression.
- Lesions in all stages of development at accessible sites. Patients with neurotic excoriations differ from those with other types of dermatitis artefacta in that they admit to picking and digging at their skin. This habit affects women more often than men and is most active at times of stress. The clinical picture is mixed, with crusted excoriations and pale scars, often with a hyperpigmented border, lying mainly on the face, neck, shoulders and arms. The condition may last for years and psychiatric treatment is seldom successful.
  Treatment: SSRI, clomipramine, doxepin.
- Empathic, supportive psychotherapy, cognitive behaviour therapy.

Acne Excoriée

Here the self-inflicted damage is based to some extent on the lesions of acne vulgaris, which may in themselves be mild, but become disfiguring when dug and squeezed to excess. The patients are usually young girls who may leave themselves with ugly scars. A psychiatric approach is often unhelpful and a daily ritual of attacking the lesions, helped by a magnifying mirror, may persist for years.

Trichotillomania

Irresistible urge to pull out hair.

Underlying Factors

Children—Anxiety, learning disability, Fe deficiency.

Adults—Depression, anxiety, OCD.

The diagnosis can usually be made on the history,but some parents do not know what is going on. The bald areas do not show the exclamation-mark hairs of alopecia areata, or the scaling and inflammation of scalp ringworm. The patches are irregular in outline and hair loss is never complete. Those hairs that remain are bent or broken, and of variable length.

The appearance of the scalp is called the '**Tonsure Pattern' or 'Friar Tuck**' pattern.

Treatment

Behaviour therapy, fluoxetine, low-dose pimozide.

Onychotillomania and Onychophabia

Similar disorder affecting nails.

Psychogenic Purpuras

a. Auto erythrocyte sensitization syndrome **(Gardner-Diamond syndrome).**
b. Psychogenic purpura without autoerythrocyte sensitization but without other abnormality.
c. With no measurable abnormality.
d. Purpura factitia.
e. Religious stigmata.

FACTITIOUS SKIN DISEASE

Dermatitis Artefacta

Here the skin lesions are caused and kept going by the patient's own actions, but parasites are not held to be to blame. Patients with dermatitis artefacta deny self trauma but, naturally, if treatment is left to them to carry out, their problems do not improve. Lesions will heal under occlusive dressings, but this does not alter the underlying psychiatric problems, and lesions may recur or crop up outside the bandaged areas.

Different types of dermatitis artefacta and the corresponding disorder are listed in Table 21.1.

Table 21.1

Type	*Personality*
Minor habits e.g. excoriated acne	Relatively normal
More obvious lesions	Hysterical or neurotic
Bizarre	Psychotic
Malingering	Criminal

The lesions favour accessible areas, and do not fit with known pathological processes. The diagnosis is often difficult to make, but an experienced clinician will suspect it because there are *no primary lesions* and because of the bizarre shape or grouping of the lesions, which may be rectilinear or oddly grouped.

Other Associated Features are:

1. 'Hollow history'.
2. Sudden appearance of complete lesions contrast with prolonged and elaborate descriptions of complications and failure to heal.
3. 'Mona Lisa' smile.
4. Exposed areas involved and the use of crude destructive processes.
5. Factitial cheilitis.
6. Chronic paronychia.
7. Hair artefact.
8. Artefact by proxy (witch craft syndrome).

Dermatological Pathomimicry

Intentional aggravation of existing dermatoses.

Dermatitis simulata: External disguise to simulate disease.

Self neglect: Diogenes syndrome.

Munchausen's Syndrome

Malingering

Produce false or grossly increased physical/psychological symptoms. Crude forms of dermatitis artefacta as cutaneous lesions. The psychological problems may be superficial and easily resolved, but sometimes psychiatric help is needed and the artefacts are part of a prolonged psychiatric illness. A few patients respond to banal treatments if given the chance to save face. Direct confrontation and accusations are usually best avoided.

COMMONLY USED DRUGS IN PSYCHOCUTANEOUS DISORDERS

Anxiety Disorder

- **Alprazolam**
  - Acute anxiety, additive antidepressant action.
  - Short t 1/2, duration of **Treatment:** 3-4 weeks, tapering required.

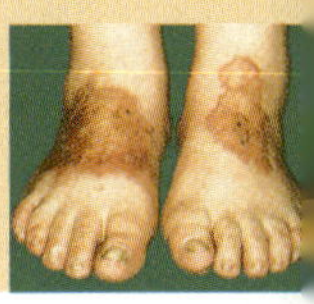

- **Buspirone**
  - Chronic anxiety
    Dose: 5-10 mg TDS/Q 1 D
  - No sedation/dependency.

ANTI DEPRESSANT DRUGS

SEROTONIN REUPTAKE INHIBITORS	Normal dose	Max Dose
Fluoxetine	10-20	10-60
Sertraline	50	50-200
Paroxetine	10-20	20-50
Fluvoxamine	50	100-200
Citalopram	20	20-60

Tricyclic Compounds

Clomipramine	25-50	100-200
Amitriptyline	50-75	100-150
Doxepin	25-75	100-150
Trimipramine	25-75	75-100
Imipramine	25-75	100-150

Doxepin: Tricyclic Antidepressant

- Depressed patient with Neurotic excoriations.
- Additional antipruritic (H^1) activity.
  Dose: 25 mg HS increase by 25 mg to a maximum of 100-300 mg dose.

NEWER DRUGS

Antidepressants

Bupropion	100	200-300
Nefazadone	100-150	200- 400
Venlafaxine	37.5-75	75-150

ANTI PSYCHOTIC DRUGS

- Pimozide 1 mg increased by **1 mg** till optimal clinical response (12 mg).
  Other Antipsychotic Agents:
  Risperidone, olanzapine.
- **RISPERIDONE** 1mg BD ↑ **every 05 - 07 d** →4-6 mg BD.
- **OLANZAPINE**: 5-10 mg → 10-15 mg/day.

HYPNOTHERAPY

Indication: Acne excoriee, alopecia areata, urticaria, vitiligo, psoriasis, pruritus, post herpetic neuralgia.

BIO FEEDBACK TECHNIQUE

Dyshidrotic eczema, hyperhidrosis.

BEHAVIOUR THERAPY

GROUP THERAPY

Psoriasis.

CHAPTER **22**

AGE SPECIFIC DERMATOSES

Pediatric Disorders

Skin conditions affecting children and adolescents often have special characteristics that differentiate them from their adult counterparts.

Between birth and maturity the surface area of the skin increases sevenfold. Infantile skin is similar to adult skin whereas skin during childhood shows some essential differences. This is in part a reflection of the hormonal milieu prevailing at that time.

Androgenic hormone levels, namely testosterone and dehydroepiandrosterone, are high during infancy and puberty. This correlates with the high levels of sebum secretion seen during these periods. These levels fall to the low levels of the rest of childhood by about the age of six months.

THE SKIN IN CHILDHOOD AND PUBERTY

- The skin, along with other organ systems, undergoes some degree of maturation during the hiatus of childhood, before the resumption of sexual development at puberty and the transition to adulthood.
- The skin disorders seen in children in part reflect these physiological changes, but many of the troublesome cutaneous problems result from intrinsic genetic abnormalities conditioned by environmental influences, e.g. atopic dermatitis.
- There is increased exposure to various infections, such as measles, chickenpox, impetigo, warts, molluscum contagiosum, scabies and infestation.
- There is also increased exposure to potential irritants, e.g. during sporting activities, rubber chemicals in footwear, wearing of jewellery and cosmetics, leading to allergic contact dermatitis.
- Some conditions have a predilection for pre-adolescents, e.g. atopic dermatitis, and lichen sclerosus et atrophicus. These two disorders tend to clear spontaneously with the onset of puberty.
- Atopic dermatitis is particularly important as it is maximally seen during childhood and may cause severe restrictions in day-to-day activity.
- Sexual abuse can cause dermatological complaints, e.g. vulval or perianal soreness and inflammation.
- Severe skin disease of any kind in childhood can have a considerable impact on the psyche and on general physical development, e.g. short stature in atopic children.
- Puberty brings on the development of secondary sexual characteristics, such as pubic and axillary hair, development of breasts etc. There is increased sebum secretion which may not be cosmetically desirable.

PHYSIOLOGICAL CHANGES

Minor Changes

1. **Rubor:** Transient erythema of newborn due to vasodilation.
2. **Cutis Marmorata (Fig. 22.1):** When a newborn infant is exposed to low environmental temperatures, an evanescent, *lacy, reticulated red and/or blue cutaneous* vascular pattern appears over most of the body surface. This vascular change represents an accentuated physiologic vasomotor response that disappears with increasing age.
3. **Physiological Exfoliation of Skin (Fig. 22.2):** This is most commonly seen in **postmature neonates**. The exact pathophysiology is not known. The baby at birth may present with a membrane like sheet around it like a colloidon baby. But soon sheds the membrane and there is scaling all over the body starting from head to toe.

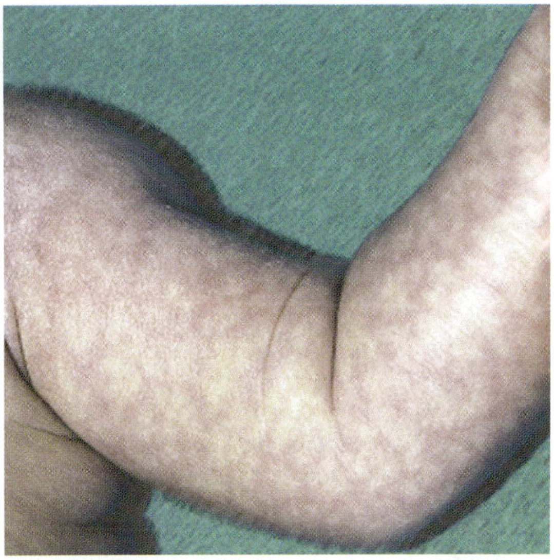

Fig. 22.1: Net like erythema (Cutis marmorata)

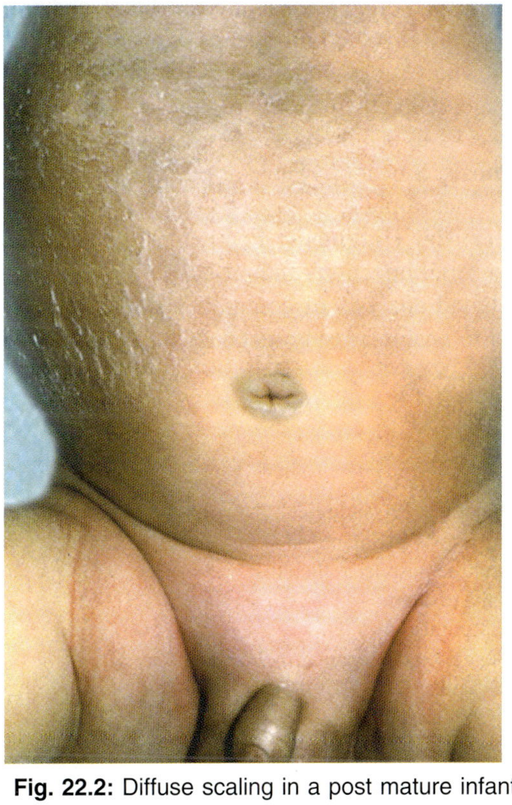

Fig. 22.2: Diffuse scaling in a post mature infant

The scaling gradually subsides over a period of 4-6 weeks.

4. **Harlequin Color Change:** Rare but dramatic vascular event occurs in the immediate newborn period and is most common in low birth weight infants. The immaturity of autonomic vasomotor control is felt to be responsible. When the infant is placed on the side, the body is bisected longitudinally into a pale upper half and a deep red dependent half. The color change lasts only for a few minutes and occasionally affects only a portion of the trunk or face. Changing the infant's position may reverse the pattern.
5. **Milia:** Milia are superficial epidermal inclusion cysts that contain laminated keratinized material. The lesion is a firm papule, 1-2 mm in diameter, pearly , opalescent white. In neonates they are scattered over face and gingivae and on the midline of the palate, where they are called *Epstein pearls*.
6. **Sebaceous Hyperplasia (Fig. 22.3):** Minute, profuse, yellow-white papules are frequently found on the forehead, nose, upper lip, and cheeks of the term infant; they represent hyperplastic sebaceous glands. Tiny papules gradually diminish in size and disappear entirely over first few weeks of life.
7. **Alopecia:** The hair loss occurs from the *front to back* and this is normal and is considered as a physiological telogen effluvium.
8. **Mongolian Spots:** Blue slate-gray macular lesions commonly occurring in the presacral area but may be found over posterior thighs, legs, back and shoulders. They may be solitary or numerous and often involve large areas. Mongolian spots usually fade during the first few years of life but occasionally persist.
9. **Sucking Blisters:** Sucking blisters are blisters apparent at birth as the result of intrauterine sucking; they are uncommon. They are usually solitary, intact oval blisters or erosions on non-inflamed skin of the newborn. They occur on the dorsal aspect of forearms, wrist or fingers or on the upper lip and resolve within a few days.

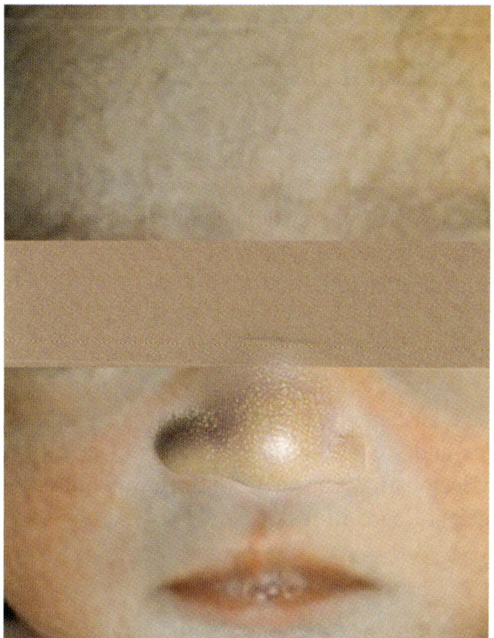

Fig. 22.3: Yellow-white papules on the nose

10. **Cradle Cap:** A very common misnomer, which is essentially a seborrheic dermatitis in infants. It is transient and is due to tarnsplacental migration of maternal hormones (Fig. 22.4).

Miscellaneous Changes

These include Neonatal mastitis, Neonatal acne/cephalic pustulosis (due to a combination of increased sebaceous gland activity and fungal infection).

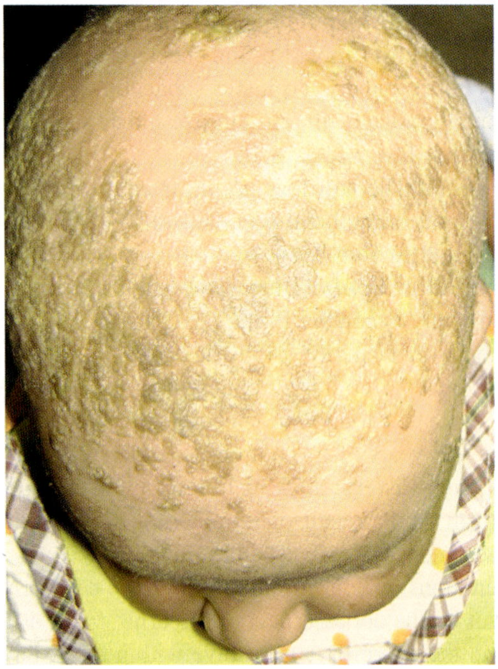

Fig. 22.4: Cradle cap

MAJOR CHANGES OF CLINICAL CONSEQUENCE

Erythema Toxicum (Fig. 22.5)

Erythema toxicum is transient, blotchy erythema seen in newborns. It occurs in 50% of term infants, and less commonly in premature infants. Cause is unknown. Blotchy erythematous macules 2-3 cm in diameter, with a tiny 1-4 mm central vesicle or pustule are seen in erythema toxicum. It usually begins at 24-48 hours of age. Lesions are seen on chest, back, face, genitalia and proximal extremities, sparing the palms and soles. Individual lesions clear in 4-5 days, and new lesions may occur from birth to tenth day of life. By 2 weeks of age, all lesions are resolved.

Transient Neonatal Pustular Melanosis (TNPM)

TNPM is a blotchy erythema of the newborn that heals with residual brown pigmentation. It is less common than erythema toxicum, and is more prevalent in the black

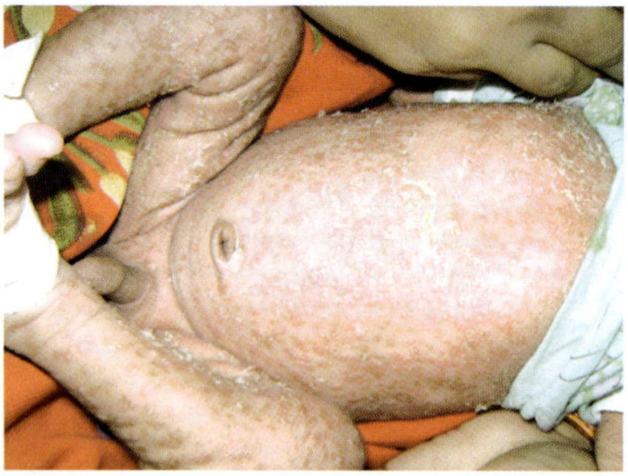

Fig. 22.5: Multiple, pustules, erythema with desquamation (Erythema toxicum)

population. Cause of this condition is not known. The lesions present at birth as vesicles, pustules or ruptured vesicles/ pustules with a collarette of surrounding scale. Pigmented macules are also often present at birth. Trunk and proximal extremities are involved, but palms and soles may also be involved. The vesicles and pustules usually disappear by 5 days of age, while the residual pigmented macules resolve over 3 weeks to 3 months.

Diagnosis: Smear of vesicle or pustular contents reveals numerous neutrophils.

Differential Diagnosis: Erythema toxicum, miliaria rubra, bacterial infections and pityrosporum folliculitis.

A detailed analysis of common pustular afflictions is provided to enable a ready reckoner for clinicians (Tables 22.1 and 22.2).

Table 22.1: Differential diagnosis of neonatal vesiculopustular diseases

Noninfectious: Physiological
Acropustulosis of infancy
Eosinophilic pustular folliculitis
Erythema toxicum
Miliaria putulsosa
Transient neonatal pustular melanosis
Noninfectious:
Acrodermatitis enteropathica
Epidermolysis bullosa
Herpes gestations – neonatal
Incontinentia pigmenti
Pemphigus vulgaris – neonatal
Infectious:
Impetigo neonatorum
BACTERIAL INFECTIONS
Chlamydia trachomatis
Eschericha coli
Hemophilus influenzae
Klebsiella pneumoniae
Listeria monocytogenes

Contd.

Contd.

Pseudomonas aeruginosa
Staphylococcus aureus
Streptococcus (group A beta-hemolytic)
Syphilis
FUNGAL
Candidiasis: Congenital
VIRAL INFECTIONS
CMV
Herpes
Varicella
INFESTATION
Scabies

Salmon Patch (Nevus Simplex) 'Stork Bite'

Small, pale pink, ill-defined, vascular macules that occur most commonly on glabella, eyelids, upper lip, and nuchal area of 30-40% of normal newborn infants. These lesions which represent localized vascular ectasia, persist for several months and may become more visible during crying or changes of environmental temperature. Most lesions on face disappear completely, but those on posterior neck and occipital areas often persist.

Differential Diagnosis: Portwine stain.

CUTANEOUS DEFECTS

Congenital and Early Onset Vascular Anomalies

Congenital vascular anomalies are divided into two broad categories:

- **Hemangiomas:** Proliferative lesions that grow and ultimately may involute (Fig. 22.6).
- **Vascular malformations:** Generally static lesions, although they may grow as the patient grows.

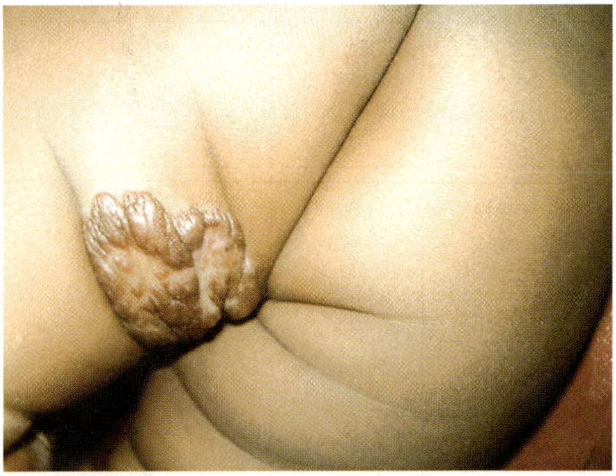

Fig. 22.6: Involuting hemangioma

Common infantile lesions such as nevus flammeus, 'stork bite', and 'salmon' patch are excluded from modern classifications of vascular anomalies. They occur mainly on the nape of the neck and forehead, and are viewed as dermal vascular ectasias that will fade. However:

- Facial lesions may be in the differential diagnosis of early lesions of portwine stain; and
- Nape of neck lesions may persist and become apparent again as hair thins in older patients.

Supernumerary Digit

A supernumerary digit is congenital and usually located at the ulnar side of the base of the fifth finger. It may range in size from a small papule to a large (sixth) digit. Surgery is appropriate if needed.

Accessory Tragus

A congenital, firm papule or multilobular nodule occurring in the preauricular area is characteristic. The lesion may consist of skin only, or skin and cartilage. It presumably develop from the auricular hillocks of the first branchial arch. These lesions may occasionally be bilateral or familial, or occur in association with other facial abnormalities. Congenital ear defects may be associated with kidney abnormalities, as both are formed at the same embryologic stage. The preauricular tag may be simply excised.

Accessory Nipple

Also known as polythelia, this lesion appears as a small, brown papule that may resemble a nipple, along the milk line that stretches from the axilla through the normal nipple to the groin. Accessory nipples may or may not have an areola and may be mistaken for congenital nevi. They may be excised for cosmetic reasons. Rarely, may undergo malignant change.

Wattle

Also known as cutaneous cervical tag, the wattle presents as a pedunculated, flesh-colored tag on the neck. Onset is usually by 3 years of age. A branchial sinus may be associated. The wattle probably represents either ectopic auricular cartilage or a remnant of the branchial arch system. Simple excision may be done if no sinus or fistula is associated.

Absent Dermatoglyphics

Rarely, a person may be born without dermatoglyphics.

Table 22.2: Comparison of the benign vesiculopustular diseases of the neonate and young infant

Disease	*General facts*	*Clinical features*	*Pathology*	*Stains*	*Treatment*
Acropustulosis of infancy	Hours after birth to 10 months 2-3 years	Red papules evolving into pustular and vesicular lesions in 1 day Seen on the hands and feet, both surfaces	Subcorneal pustules with neutrophils and occasionally eosinophils	Gram; neutrophils	Potent topical steroids, oral antihistamines; dapsone 2 mg/kg/day for severe cases
Candidiasis, congenital	Birth to 24 hours to 2 weeks	Pink red macules and papules evolving into pustules and vesicles Diffuse, generalized	Subcorneal pustules with pseudohyphae and spores	KOH: pseudohyphae and spores	Topical anticandidal agent (clotrimazole, or miconazole) preparation for 10 days: oral fluconazole if severe and for candida sepsis in premature infants
Candidiasis neonatal	**After** first week of life	Oral mucosa, diaper area	Same	Same	Same as above
Erythema toxicum neonatorum	Approximately 1/3 of full-term newborns 24-72 hours 1 week	Red macules and papules; white to pink pustules, vesicles Trunk, extremities, face	Subcorneal pustules with **eosinophils**	Gram: eosinophils	Self limiting
Eosinophilic pustular folliculitis	Very rare Birth to 1 year Years	Crops of papules, vesicles and pustules that crust **Primarily scalp** with some trunk and extremity lesions	Epidermal and dermal infiltrates of eosinophils associated with hair follicles	Gram: eosinophils	Topical and systemic steroids
Impetigo neonatorum	Second day to second week	Vesicles, pustules, plus bullae on an erythematous base Diaper area, neck, groin, axilla	Subcorneal pustules with Gram-positive cocci in clusters and neutrophils	Gram: Gram-positive cocci	Dicloxacillin, 12.5-25mg/kg/day; cephalexin, 40mg/kg/day; for 10-day course
Miliaria crystallina	First weeks of life, Lasts for Hours to days	Miliaria crystallina, clear vesicles Generalized	Subcorneal vesicles associated with sweat ducts	All stains negative	Cooling baths, air conditioning, removal of excess clothing
Miliaria rubra	First weeks of life, Hours to days	Miliaria rubra, grouped erythematous papules	Intraepidermal spongiosis and vesicles associated with sweat ducts	All stains negative	Same as above
Neonatal scabies	2-4 weeks	Vesicles and papules; rare burrows Hands, feet, trunk, genitalia	Subcorneal burrow with mite, eggs, scybala	Oil prep; mite, eggs, scybala	5% permethrin cream overnight
Transient neonatal pustular melanosis	At birth	Vesicles and pustules desquamate leaving brown macules Chin, neck, palms, soles	Macules: basilar hyperpigmentation; Pustula: intracorneal and subcorneal neutrophils and rare eosinophils	Gram Neutrophils	Self limiting

Midline Sacral Lesions (Fig. 22.7)

Lipomas, sinus tract, pigmented lesions, tufts of hair (e.g. faun tail nevus), and vascular patches are some of the congenital, sacral, cutaneous abnormalities that may be associated with an underlying spinal malformation also known as spinal dysraphism. Potential associations include tethered cord, spina bifida, and vertebral anomalies.

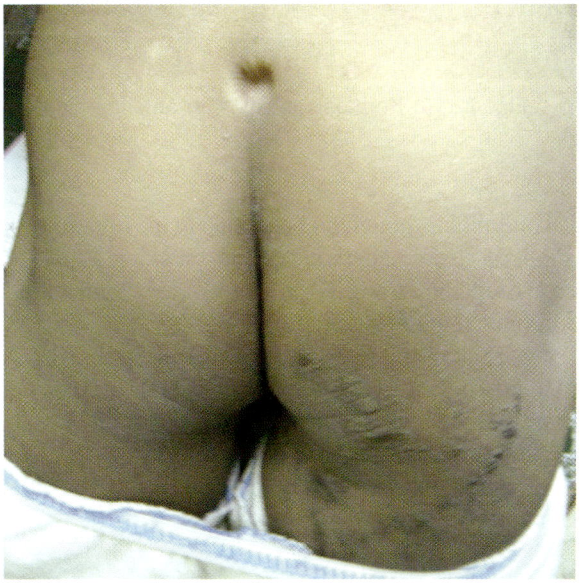

Fig. 22.7: Case of a sacral dimple with an associated epidermal nevus with an underlying spina bifida

Dermoid Cyst

The dermoid cyst is present at birth and is composed of epithelium and appendageal elements; it may contain bones, hair, or teeth. A round, subcutaneous, asymptomatic congenital nodule at the tail of the eyebrow, periorbitally, or on the nose or scalp is characteristic.

Preoperative MRI is recommended, although the yield for brow– frontotemporal lesions is low. An ophthalmologist should be consulted for orbital lesions.

Dermoids may be removed surgically. For isolated dermoids in the brow–frontotemporal region, simple excision may be done, although incision through the frontalis muscle is needed. After removal of lesions of the orbit, volume replacement may be needed for the larger lesions. Finally, those in the nasoglabellar region may show transcranial extension and craniotomy may be needed.

MISCELLANEOUS DERMATOSES

Blueberry Muffin Baby

The 'blueberry muffin' rash is defined as multiple, dark bluish skin nodules in the infant, which histologically represent dermal (extramedullary) hematopoiesis.

Infectious causes of this condition are conveniently summarized by the TORCH acronym for congenital infections: toxoplasmosis, other (syphilis, parvovirus, and other viral), rubella (the most common cause), cytomegalovirus and herpes simplex. Chronic prenatal anemia leading to blueberry muffin lesions in the neonate has been reported in association with severe hemolytic anemia such as congenital spherocytosis, rhesus hemolytic disease, and ABO incompatibility, or in anemia caused by twin-to-twin transfusion.

Clinically, one sees discrete, red to purple macules and papules, 3-8 mm in diameter, in a newborn. Leukemia cutis and metastatic rhabdomyosarcoma or neuroblastoma have been reported to cause similar lesions.

Treatment obviously depends on the cause.

Subcutaneous Fat Necrosis (Fig. 22.8)

Multiple, deep, subcutaneous nodules, or a panniculitis appearing within the first few weeks of life, are characteristic. The skin may be red-purple or flesh-colored. The lesions are not tender. The newborn is usually full term. The distribution of lesions may be in areas of trauma (e.g. from forceps). Hypercalcemia may be associated. Signs and symptoms of hypercalcemia include irritability, poor feeding and vomiting. Death has occurred from infection and cardiac arrest. Thrombocytopenia, hypoglycemia, and hyperlipidemia have also been associated. Usually, a history of obstetric trauma, meconium aspiration, neonatal asphyxia, hypothermia, or peripheral hypoxemia can be elicited.

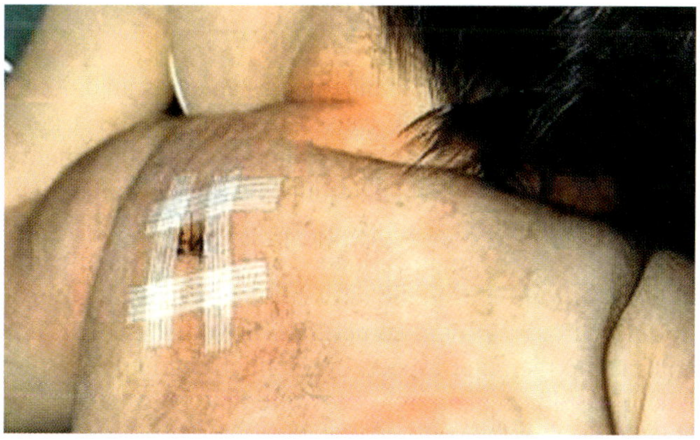

Fig. 22.8: Multiple, deep, subcutaneous nodules (Subcutaneous fat necriosis)

No treatment is needed, as the lesions remit spontaneously within weeks to months. The infant should be monitored for elevated calcium, especially if the disease is extensive. Treatment for hypercalcemia can include saline hydration, a low-calcium diet, furosemide, and glucocorticoid. For infants who fail to respond to standard measures, the use of oral biphosphonates, for example clodronate, has been reported to be very effective.

Sclerema Neonatorum (Fig. 22.9)

Sclerema is diffuse, fast spreading the thickening of skin in a sick **premature** newborn and is becoming rare as neonatal care improves worldwide. Premature newborns who suffer hypothermia are susceptible to the development of sclerema. Trunk is always involved. The onset is characteristically after 24 hours of age.

Careful monitoring of the skin temperature of ill-born newborns may prevent the development of sclerema. Supportive care in form of I/V Fluids, oxygen, control of infection may be required.

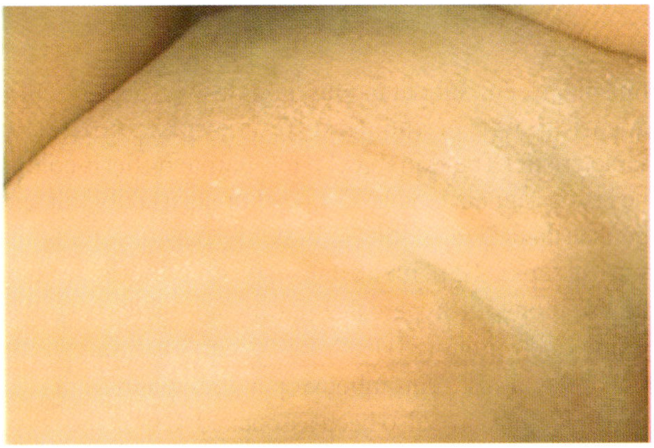

Fig. 22.9: Wax-like hardening of the back (Sclerema neonatorum)

Keratosis Pilaris

This common condition is inherited as an autosomal dominant trait, and is possibly caused by mutations in a gene lying on the short arm of chromosome 18. The abnormality lies in the keratinization of hair follicles,which become filled with horny plugs.

The changes begin in childhood and tend to become less obvious in adult life. In the most common type, the greyish horny follicular plugs, sometimes with red areolae, are confined to the outer aspects of the thighs and upper arms, where the skin feels rough. Less often the plugs affect the sides of the face; perifollicular erythema and loss of eyebrow hairs may then occur. The protruding kertain plug gives use to the **antenna sign** (Fig. 22.10).

Treatment

Treatment is not usually needed, although keratolytics such as salicylic acid or urea in a cream base may smooth the skin temporarily.

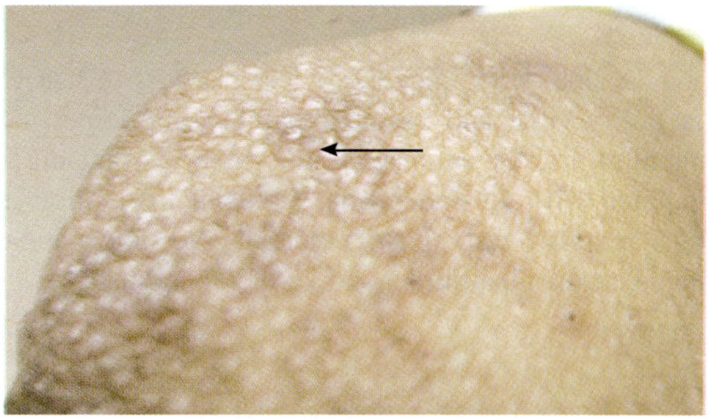

Fig. 22.10: Keratosis pilaris with antenna sign

Juvenile Plantar Dermatosis

This condition is thought to be related to the impermeability of modern socks and sweat gland blockage, and so has been called the 'toxic sock syndrome'. Some feel the condition is a manifestation of atopy.

The skin of the weight-bearing areas of the feet, particularly the forefeet and undersides of the toes, becomes dry and shiny with deep painful fissures that make walking difficult. The toe webs are spared. Onset can be at any time after shoes are first worn, and even if untreated the condition clears in the early teens.

Treatment

The child should use a commercially available cork insole in all shoes, and stick to cotton. An emollient such as emulsifying ointment or 1% ichthammol paste, or an emollient containing lactic acid, is as good as a topical steroid.

GROIN AND DIAPER AREA

Diaper Dermatitis

The term 'Diaper dermatitis' implies an inflammatory eruption of the diaper area. It can be regarded as prototype of irritant contact dermatitis. Hydration of the skin, friction between skin and the fabric of the napkin, urine and its degradation product, proteolytic and lipolytic enzymes and candida albicans level in the faeces are supposed to play etiologic role. Onset is from 3rd to the 12th week and the peak prevalence is seen between the 7th and 12th month. Both sexes and all races are equally affected.

It is manifested as confluent erythema and scaling on the convex surfaces in closest contact with the diaper i.e. the buttocks, the genitalia, the lower abdomen, pubic area and the upper thighs. The genitocrural folds are often spared (Fig. 22.11).

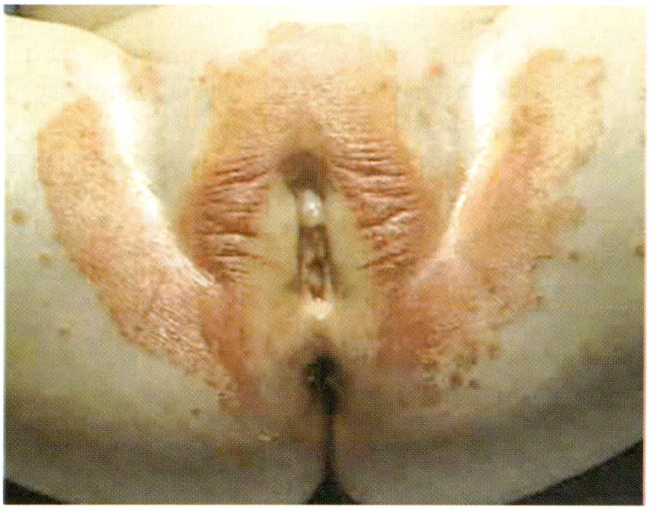

Fig. 22.11 : Diaper dermatitis

Management

The mother or caregiver should be advised regarding increasing the frequency of napkin changes and proper cleansing of the skin with either with a soft baby soap or a nonsoap nondetergent cleanser. Various barrier creams containing zinc oxide, titanium dioxide etc. can be used. Application of emollients help. In cases which do not respond to hygiene measures and application of emollients combinations of mild topical steroids with antifungals do help. Disposable diapers containing a superabsorbant material may help to maintain a dry environment.

Infantile Seborrheic Dermatitis

The term is used to describe an eruption having a predilection for the scalp and the proximal flexures and a favorable prognosis compared with atopic dermatitis. Eruption first appears between the 2nd week and the 6th month of life, most commonly between the 3rd and 8th week. It usually starts from the napkin area but may also appear on the face, scalp or trunk. The rash comprises erythema with greasy scaling with fine vesicles.

Granuloma Gluteale Infantum

Multiple, red-brown nodules in the diaper area of an infant occur in granuloma gluteale infantum. Most patients have been on topical fluorinated steroids for a diaper dermatitis. Stopping the topical steroid has led to slow resolution.

Jacquet Dermatitis

Jacquet dermatitis represents a primary irritant diaper dermatitis and may occur in the setting of urinary incontinence or infrequent diaper changes. Well-defined, punched-out ulcers or erosions with elevated borders occur on the penis, labia, or perianal area. The treatment is the same as for diaper dermatitis (discussed earlier).

EXANTHEM

- First disease (measles).
- Second disease (scarlet fever).
- Third disease (Rubella).
- Fourth—Dukes disease (enteroviral).
- Fifth disease—Erythema infectiosum.
- Sixth disease—Roseola infantum.

MEASLES (RUBEOLA)

This is one of the most common viral exanthem of childhood. Transmitted by direct contact with droplets from infected persons, rubeola is caused by measles virus (RNA virus of genus morbillivirus in the family paramyxoviridae).

Incubation period is 12-14 days to the first prodromal symptoms and another 2-4 days to the appearance of the rash.

Clinical Features

The prodromal phase usually lasts 3-5 days and is characterized by low grade fever, a dry cough, coryza and conjunctivitis (Fig. 22.12).

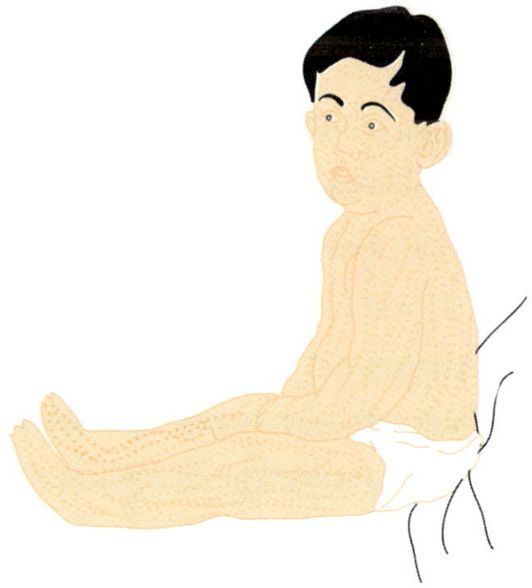

1. The virus is spread by breathing in virus-containing droplets or by touching contaminated surfaces.
2. The virus grows in cell in the back of the throat and lungs.
3. Infected person has a fever lasting two to four days, followed by a cough, runny nose and red, watery eyes.
4. A rash, lasting five to six days, appears about the face and head, spreading through the torso to the hands and feet.
5. The virus can be transmitted from four days prior to and four days after the appearance of the rash.

Fig. 22.12: Course of measles

These symptoms nearly always precede the appearance of **Koplik** spots, the pathognomonic sign of measles, by 2-3 days. **Koplik** spots are grayish white dots, usually as small as grains of sand, that have slight, reddish areolae; occasionally they are hemorrhagic. They tend to occur opposite the **lower molars** but may spread irregularly over the rest of the buccal mucosa. They appear and disappear rapidly, usually within 12-18 hours.

The temperature rises abruptly as the rash appears and often reaches 104 °F or higher. In uncomplicated cases, as the rash appears on the legs and feet, the symptoms subside rapidly within 2 days. The rash usually starts as faint macules on the lateral parts of the **neck, behind the ears,** along the hairline and the posterior parts of the cheek. The individual lesions become increasingly maculopapular as the rash spreads rapidly over the entire face, neck, upper arms, and upper parts of chest within the first 24 hours. During the succeeding 24 hours, the rash spreads over the back, abdomen, entire arm, and thighs. As it finally reaches the feet on the 2-3rd day. The rash fades downwards in the same sequence in which it appeared. *The severity of the disease is directly related to the extent and confluence of the rash.* The rash is often slightly hemorrhagic; in severe cases with a confluent rash, petechiae may be present in large numbers, and there may be extensive ecchymoses. Itching is generally slight. As the rash fades, branny desquamation and brownish discoloration occur and then disappear within 7-10 days.

Treatment

Entirely supportive: Antipyretics, maintain fluid intake, keep room comfortably warm.

Complications: Otitis media, pneumonia and encephalitis.

SCARLET FEVER

Scarlet fever is an infection caused by toxin-producing group A beta hemolytic **streptococci** (GABHS) found in secretions and discharge from the nose, ears, throat and skin. It may follow streptococcal wound infections or burns, as well as upper respiratory tract infections.

The cutaneous eruption of scarlet fever accompanies a streptococcal infection at another anatomic site, usually the tonsillopharynx. Abrupt onset of fever, headache, vomiting, malaise, chills and sore throat occurs. Rash appears 1-4 days after the onset.

Clinical Features

- The mucous membranes usually are bright red, and scattered petechiae and small **red papular lesions** on the soft palate are often present.
- During the first days of infection, the tongue is heavily coated with a white membrane through which edematous red papillae protrude (classic appearance of **white strawberry tongue).**
- By day 4 or 5, the white membrane sloughs off, revealing a shiny red tongue with prominent papillae **(red, strawberry tongue)**.
- Red, edematous, exudative tonsils are typically observed if the infection originates there.
- The characteristic exanthem consists of a fine erythematous punctate eruption that appears within 1-4 days following the onset of the illness. It first appears on the upper trunk and axillae and then becomes generalized, although it is usually more prominent in flexural areas, such as the axillae, popliteal fossae, and inguinal folds. It may also appear more intense at dependent sites and sites of pressure, such as the buttocks. The eruption imparts a dry rough texture to the skin that is reported to resemble the feel of **sandpaper.**
- Capillary fragility is increased, and often, transverse areas of hyperpigmentation with petechiae in the axillary, antecubital, and inguinal areas **(Pastia lines)** can be observed (Fig. 22.13).

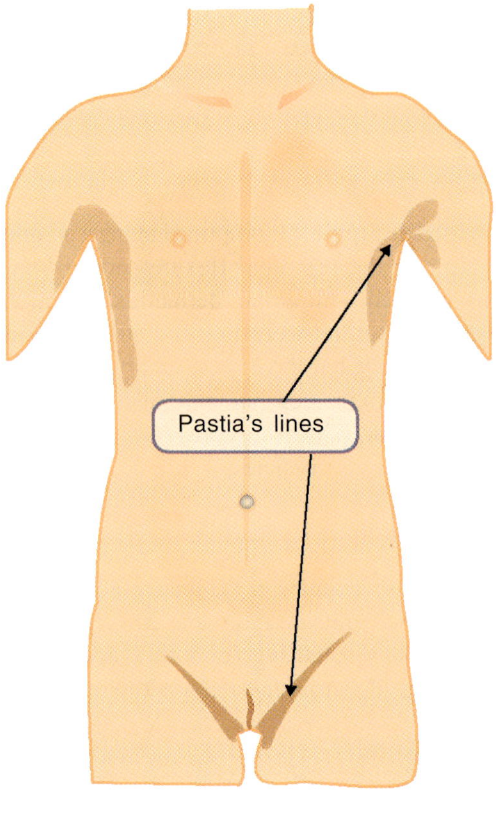

Fig. 22.13: Capillary fragility on the flexures (Pastia lines)

RUBELLA (GERMAN MEASLES OR THREE-DAY MEASLES)

Caused by Rubella virus, is an RNA virus of the genus Rubivirus in the family Togaviridae.

Spread either by droplet or transplacentally to the fetus, causing congenital infection. The peak incidence of rubella was among children 5-14 years of age but most cases now occur among susceptible teenagers and young adults. The incubation period is 14-21 days.

The prodromal symptoms are mild catarrhal symptoms. Approximately two thirds of infections are subclinical.

Clinical Features

The most characteristic sign is retroauricular, posterior cervical and postoccipital **lymphadenopathy**. Discrete rose-colored spots on the soft palate (**Forchheimer spots),** may appear in 20% of patients just before the onset of rash.

Lymphadenopathy is evident at least 24 hours before the rash appears and may remain for 1 week or more. The exanthem begins on face and spreads quickly. Its evolution is so rapid the rash may be fading on the face by the time it appears on the trunk. Discrete maculopapules are present in large numbers; there are also large areas of flushing that spread rapidly over the entire body, usually within 24 hours. The rash may be confluent, particularly on the face. During the *second day* the rash may assume a pinpoint appearance, especially over the trunk, resembling that of scarlet fever. Mild itching may occur. The eruption usually clears by the *third day.* Desquamation is minimal. Rubella without a rash has been described. In older children and adults, arthritis may affect around 30 percent of females and 5 percent of males. It characteristically involves the small joints of the hands and feet, occasionally the elbows, shoulders and spine.

Prophylaxis: Prophylactic recommendations include vaccination of all children with live attenuated vaccine either alone or in combination with measles and mumps vaccine, at the age of 15 months.

Treatment

There is no specific antiviral therapy; treatment is entirely supportive. Antipyretics are indicated for fever.

ENTEROVIRAL INFECTIONS

Herpangina

The principle cause is CVAs (serotypes 2-6, 8 and 10). Other viral etiologies include CVBs (serotypes 1-4), Es, adenoviruses and other EVs.

After an incubation period of approximately 4 days, the disease begins with acute onset of fever (temperature range, 38.5-40°C) accompanied by headache; sore throat; dysphagia; anorexia; and, occasionally, vomiting and abdominal pain.

The enanthem is characterized by the presence of gray-white minute papulovesicles about 1-2 mm in diameter. The lesions are surrounded by an erythematous halo, which progresses to a shallow ulcer. The lesions are self-limiting, resolving over 5-10 days. Lesions are most frequently found on tonsils, uvula; soft palate, and anterior pillars of the tonsillar fauces.

Hand-Foot-and-Mouth Disease (HFMD)

HFMD is most commonly associated with CVA16. HFMD is also associated with infection by CVA serotypes 4-7, 9 and 10; CVB serotypes 2 and 5; and EV71.

A brief prodromal period is characterized by low-grade fever, malaise, abdominal pain, and/or respiratory symptoms. Prominent historical features include oral pain and odynophagia.

Oral lesions begin as erythematous macules and papules that are 2-8 mm in diameter; these progress to form thin-walled vesicles (Fig. 22.14).

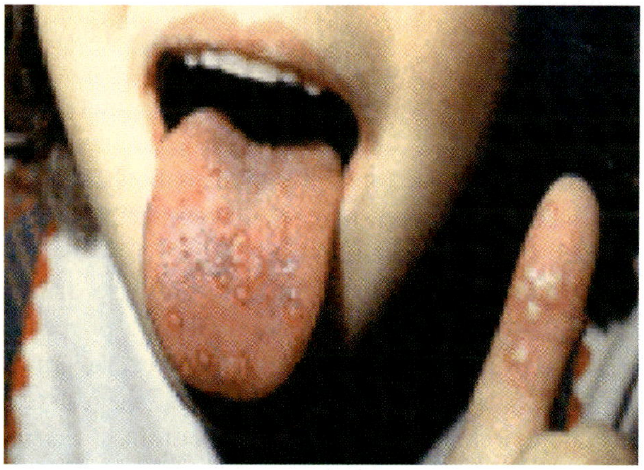

Fig. 22.14: Vesicular rash on the mouth and hand (Hand-foot-mouth disease)

Skin lesions are variably present, but they are characteristic when they occur.

They begin as erythematous macules or papules, which quickly become small (as large as 5 mm in diameter), gray, oval or linear vesicles surrounded by a red halo. The hands are more commonly involved than the feet. Lesions usually occur on the lateral aspects of the fingers and toes, especially around the nails, but they may be seen in the digital flexures and on the palms and soles. The lesions gradually disappear over 7-10 days without scarring.

Eruptive Pseudoangiomatosis

After the prodromal period, 2- to 4-mm blanchable, red papules resembling cherry angiomas appear.

The lesions usually number no more than 10, and they resolve spontaneously within 10 days.

They are distributed on the face, trunk and extremities.

Other Associations

- EV70 and CVA24—Acute hemorrhagic conjunctivitis.
- Coxsackie B5—Pustular stomatitis associated with erythema multiforme.
- Coxsackie A4—Widespread vesicular eruption.
- Coxsackie A16—Gianotti-Crosti–like eruption.
- Echovirus 2—Rubelliform eruption.
- Echoviruses 6, 11 and 25—Morbilliform eruption.
- Echovirus 9—Rubelliform or morbilliform eruptions.
- Echoviruses 11 and 19—Petechiae.
- Echovirus 19—Punctate macular eruption.
- Echovirus 11—Vesicular eruption.

ERYTHEMA INFECTIOSUM (FIFTH DISEASE)

Caused by *Parvovirus* B_{19}. It is a benign, self limited exanthematous illness of childhood. The incubation period for erythema infectiosum ranges from 4-28 days.The prodromal phase is mild and consists of low grade fever, headache, and symptoms of mild upper respiratory tract infection.

The hallmark of erythema infectiosum is the characteristic rash. The initial stage is an erythematous facial flushing, **"slapped cheek"** appearance (Fig. 22.15). The rash spreads to trunk and proximal extremities as diffuse macular erythema, in the 2nd stage. Central clearing of macular lesions occur promptly, giving the rash a **lacy, reticulated** appearance. Palms and soles are spared, and the rash tends to be more prominent over the extensor surfaces. Lesions are mildly itchy. The rash resolves without desquamation, but tends to wax and wane over 1-3 weeks.

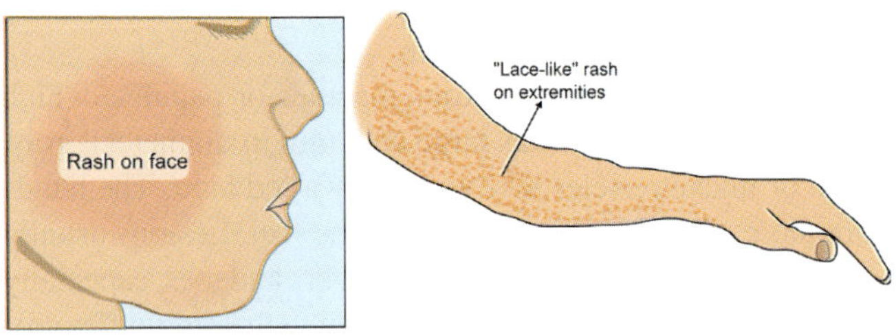

Fig. 22.15: Erythema infectiosum

ROSEOLA INFANTUM (EXANTHEM SUBITUM OR SIXTH DISEASE)

Common childhood viral infection caused by human herpes *virus 6 (HHV-6) mainly,* few cases also caused by HHV-7. Roseola is a mild febrile, exanthematous illness occurring almost exclusively during infancy. More than 95% cases occur in children younger than 3 years with a peak at 6-15 months of age.

The prodromal period is usually asymptomatic but may include mild upper respiratory tract signs. Mild cervical or occipital lymphadenopathy may be there.

Clinical illness is generally heralded by high temperature, usually ranging from 101-106°F, with an average 103°F. Some children may be irritable but most behave normally despite high temperatures. Febrile seizures may occur in upto 15% patients. In Asian countries, ulcers at the uvulopalatoglossal junction (***Nagayama spots***) are common in infants with roseola. Fever persists for 3-5 days and then typically resolves rather abruptly. Occasionally, the fever may gradually diminish over 24-36 hours. A rash appears within 12-24 hours of fever resolution. The rash is rose colored, and is distinctive. The rash begins as discrete, small (2-5mm), slightly raised pink lesions on trunk and usually spreads to the neck, face and proximal extremities. The rash is usually not pruritic, lesions are discrete but occasionally may become almost confluent. After 1-3 days rash fades. Supportive treatment is required.

KAWASAKI DISEASE (KD)

- The diagnostic criteria established by the Committee on Rheumatic Fever, Endocarditis and Kawasaki Disease; the Council on Cardiovascular Disease in the Young; and the American Heart Association include ***fever lasting longer than 5 days and 4 of the 5 main clinical features,*** *after diseases with similar findings have been excluded. The most recent guidelines suggest that if a patient presents with 4 or more of the principal criteria, KD can be diagnosed on day 4 of the fever.*
- The **5 major clinical findings** are as follows:
  - Change in the extremities, typically painful erythema and edema.
  - Polymorphous exanthem.
  - Changes in the lips and oropharyngeal mucosa.
  - Bilateral, nonexudative, bulbar conjunctival injection.
  - Unilateral nonsuppurative cervical lymphadenopathy.
- Patients who present with coronary artery disease can be diagnosed with KD if they have at least 3 of the 5 major diagnostic criteria.

– *Stage 1:* The acute stage begins with an onset of fever and lasts approximately 7-14 days. It is heralded by an abrupt febrile episode that is typically high-spiking and remittent, with peak temperatures typically ranging from 102-104ºF (39-40ºC). This fever is not responsive to antibiotics and antipyretics and can persist for up to 3-4 weeks if untreated. With appropriate therapy, high-dose aspirin, and IVIG, the fever typically remits within 48 hours. During the *acute* phase, the *mucocutaneous changes and lymphadenopathy* are most evident, and the diagnosis should be made in this phase.
– *Stage 2:* The subacute stage begins when the fevers have abated, and it continues until week 4-6. The hallmarks of this stage are desquamation of the digits, thrombocytosis, and the development of coronary aneurysms. This stage is when the patient is at highest risk for *sudden death.*
– *Stage 3:* The convalescent stage begins with the return of the acute phase reactants and other laboratory abnormalities to baseline. During this stage, most of the clinical findings resolve; however, deep transverse grooves across the nails (Beau lines) may become apparent 1-2 months after the onset of fever. During the convalescent stage, cardiac abnormalities may still be apparent, but in patients whose echocardiograms were previously normal, detection of new aneurysms is unusual after week 8 of the illness.

GIANNOTTI-CROSTI SYNDROME

Multifactorial, symmetrical, itchy, recurrent and bothersome eruption due to either viral causes or a hypersensitivity to insect bites (Fig. 22.16).

Other minor exanthems include papular-purpuric gloves and socks syndrome and unilateral exanthem.

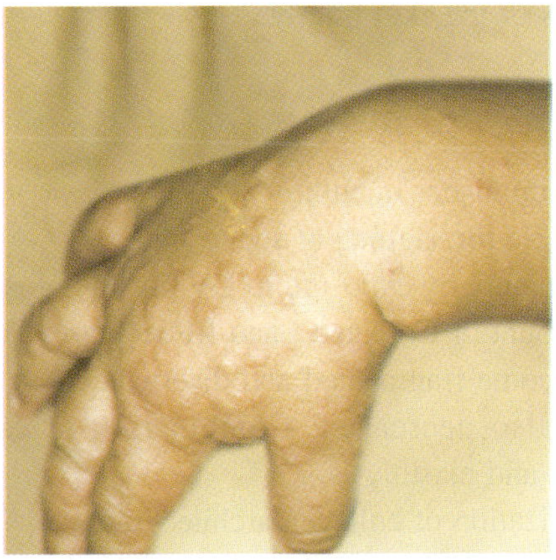

Fig. 22.16: Papulonodules on hands Giannotti-Crosti syndrome

DERMATOSES OF PUBERTY AND ADOLESCENCE

Acne Vulgaris

- Very common.
- Greater than 85-90% of boys and girls affected to some degree.
- Can cause severe psychological distress, both because of active lesions and post-acne scarring.

Acne Excoriée and Neurotic Excoriation

- A variant of acne vulgaris where minimal lesions are aggravated by self-inflicted trauma, e.g. repeated scratching of acne lesions.
- Chances of post-acne scarring higher.

Self-mutilation and Dermatitis Artefacta

- Psychosomatic.
- Mutilation varies from excoriated acne to severe habitual mutilation.
- Underlying mental state varied from mild anxiety to gross personality disorder, psychotic disturbance and instability.

Seborrheic Dermatitis

- Generally seen from adolescence onwards.
- Alterations in sebum that appear at puberty may be responsible.

Pityriasis Versicolor

- Caused by a yeast, malassezia furfur.
- Again alterations in sebum that appear at puberty may be responsible.

Hyperhidrosis

- Severe eccrine hyperhidrosis may occur at puberty.
- Responds well to medical treatment.

Axillary Bromhidrosis

- Bromhidrosis means bad odour.
- Can be very distressing.
- Again responds well to medical treatment.

Hidradenitis Suppurativa

- Inflammation and destructive changes in the apocrine glands.
- Leads to scarring and offensive odour.
- Generally seen in the axillary region.
- May be difficult to treat.

Fox-Fordyce Disease

- Fox-Fordyce disease is an infrequently occurring

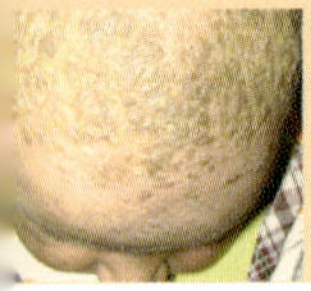

chronic pruritic papular eruption that localizes to areas where apocrine glands are found.

- The etiology is currently unknown.
- The observed pathophysiology is a keratin plug in the hair follicle infundibulum obstructing the apocrine acrosyringium and producing an apocrine anhidrosis.
- The primary lesion is a flesh-colored to reddish, smooth, dome-shaped, discrete, and follicular or perifollicular papule. Affected areas usually have many papules.
- Sweating is often absent in the affected area.

Polymorphic Light Eruption

- PMLE is an acquired disease and is the most common of the idiopathic photodermatoses, often beginning during adolescence.
- PMLE is characterized by recurrent, abnormal, delayed reactions to sunlight, ranging from erythematous papules, papulovesicles, and plaques to erythema multiforme-like lesions on sunlight-exposed surfaces.
- Within any one patient, only one clinical form is consistently manifested.

Epidermolysis Bullosa Simplex

- A genetic blistering disorder that may on occasion manifest during adolescence, the normal age of presentation being earlier.

Psoriasis

- 25% of patients of psoriasis have the onset of their disease during adolescence.
- Significant psychological morbidity is seen.

Atopic Dermatits

- Usually resolves with onset of puberty. However, disease may not abate in some patients.
- May rarely occur for the first time in puberty.

Other Relevant Pediatric Dermatoses that are covered in the book:

REFERENCES

- Pediatric Dermatology, 3rd edn. Edited by Lawrence, A Schachner and Ronald C Hansen 2003.
- Rook's Textbook of Dermatology, D. A. Burns, S. M. Breathnach, Neil Cox, Christopher E. Griffith's 7th edn 2004.
- Fitzpatrick's Dermatology in General Medicine, 6th edn 2003.

Dermatoses in Elderly

Ageing is the decline in the power of self-maintenance, the increase in susceptibility to disease and the growing probability of death as age advances. Ageing of the skin is a multifactorial process generating a lot of interest today because of the important social role that skin plays. The most obvious signs of an ageing skin are atrophy, laxity, wrinkling, sagging, dryness, yellowness, a multiplicity of pigmented and other blemishes and sparse grey hair.

Senescence in the skin involves:

- *Internal Factors*
  - Intrinsic genetically programmed changes in the skin.
  - Secondary skin changes due to senile changes in other organs.
- *External Factors*
  - Changes secondary to environmental factors.

Modern theories of ageing fall into two categories. The first views ageing as an ordered process finely programmed by the genes, similar to apoptosis. The second attributes ageing to progressive retention and amplification of errors in the replication of genetic information in the somatic cells. The following section will deal with the specific changes in different parts of the skin briefly.

DERMIS

- Dermis diminishes in bulk.
- Responsible for sagging of senile skin.
- Caused mainly by exposure to UV rays: Photoageing.
- Total amount of Collagen I and III decrease: Collagen fibers become fragmented and disoriented.
- Elastin also decreased: Combination of reduced synthesis and elastolysis.
- Disorganization of collagen architecture.
- Steady decrease in the number of mast cells and fibroblasts.

EPIDERMIS

Overall there is decreased thickness and disorganization of the epidermis. One notable exception is that the thickness of the stratum corneum remains relatively unchanged.

- Flattening of the dermal-epidermal junction.
- Cell turnover rate is halved between the third and seventh decades.
- Rate of epidermal repair and wound healing decrease.
- Stratum corneum function decreases: Increased permeability of skin, decreased water binding capacity, drying and flakiness of senile skin known as senile xerosis.

HAIR FOLLICLES

Changes in hair follicles are not uniform there being significant inter-site variations.

- *Scalp:* Decreased density of hair follicles, proliferative capacity of follicle unchanged, duration of anagen decreased resulting in decreased overall length of hair, hair shaft diameter decreases.
- *Beard:* As a result of decreased androgens the weight of the beard grown per day decreases after the fourth decade. The density here is maintained, the loss in beard thickness being explained by thinning of hair shafts.
- Axillary, pubic and chest hair follow a similar pattern.
- Some sites however show increased hair growth, viz. eyebrows and external auditory meatus in males.

GREYING OF HAIR

- Beyond 50 years of age about half the population has approximately 50% grey or white scalp/body hair.
- Bulbs of these hairs show various abnormalities including deficient or absent tyrosinase activity, the enzyme necessary for the first stages of melanin synthesis.
- Premature graying of hair may be associated with a number of disorders induced by organ specific antibodies.

GLANDS

As a rule of thumb the activities of most glands in the body decrease with age. The skin is no exception.

- *Sebaceous and apocrine glands:* Sebum secretion declines steadily through each decade by approximately 23% in men and 32% in women. The fatty acid composition also changes.
- *Eccrine glands:* There is a reduction in the number of glands and output per gland.

PIGMENTATION

Most pronounced in fair skinned races, irregularity of pigmentation is one of the most conspicuous changes associated with ageing. Individuals often seek treatment for the pigmentary changes.

- *Senile lentigines:* Also known as '*liver spots*' or '*age spots*', these are yellow or brown macules most often seen on the backs of the hands and exposed parts of the face in more than 50% of persons over 45 years of age. These are caused by a localized proliferation of melanocytes at the dermal-epidermal junction.

PRURITIS

'Senile pruritis' is a diagnosis of exclusion made after ruling out other causes of itching including xerosis. Most patients have an underlying cause. A rational approach to an elderly patient with itching is detailed under.

Itching in elderly person
↓
R/O primary cutaneous disorder
E.g. scabies, xerosis, candidiasis, early stage bullous pemphigoid, lichen sclerosus et atrophicus, eczema
↓
R/O systemic causes
E.g. renal or hepatic disease, anemia, thyroid disease
↓
R/O malignancy
E.g. lymphomas, leukemias, myelodysplastic disorders
↓
No cause found: Senile pruritis

SENILE XEROSIS AND ASTEATOTIC ECZEMA

- Elderly skin is often dry, although the exact cause for this is not known. The dryness is worse in the winter and may lead to considerable itching and distress. The changes are most pronounced over the lower limbs.
- If the surface texture of the skin assumes a cracked appearance the clinical picture resembles 'crazy paving'. This is known as asteatotic eczema *(eczema craquele).*
- The xerosis is exacerbated by frequent washing, soaps, central heating, low humidity etc.

ECZEMA

- Any type of eczema may occur in elderly patients.
- Seborrheic dermatitis, gravitational eczema are more common in the elderly.

- Atopic dermatitis, discoid eczema may continue into or present for the first time in old age.
- Allergic and irritant contact dermatitis are less common.
- Marked lichenification and chronic lichen simplex are also often seen.

LEG ULCERS

- Leg ulcers are a major problem.
- Most are caused by venous hypertension. Arterial disease is also important in causation.
- Poor wound healing leads to chronicity of lesions.

BULLOUS DISORDERS

- Bullous pemphigoid is much more common in elderly patients.

SKIN TUMOURS

- Skin tumours become commoner with age.
- *Benign:* Seborrheic keratoses, senile lentigines, skin tags.
- *Dysplastic:* Actinic keratoses.
- *Malignant:* Basal cell carcinoma, squamous cell carcinoma, malignant melanoma.

OTHERS

- Decubitus ulcers.
- *Psoriasis:* Flexural form particularly common.
- *Ectoparasite infestations:* Scabies, lice.
- *Herpes zoster:* Increased incidence, post herpetic neuralgia commoner.

Pregnancy Dermatoses

Pregnancy is a normal alternation and necessarily involves multiple physiologic and metabolic changes (Table 22.3). These changes have a profound effect on the skin. Most are minor and have no effect on the outcome of pregnancy. 'Dermatoses of pregnancy' are a group of dermatoses that are specifically related to pregnancy and the puerperium; distinct from physiological events, and not caused by exacerbation of pre-existing dermatoses (Table 22.4).

Table 22.3: Physiological changes in pregnancy

Condition	*Skin lesions*	*Trimester*	*Remarks*
Pigmentary and mechanical	Diffuse darkening, chloasma, darkening of linea alba, striae distensae	2nd-3rd trimester	Most cases resolve after childbirth, resolution may not be complete
Nails, hair	Hair remains in anagen, growth arrest of nails	Throughout	Telogen effluvium, beau's lines following delivery (3-6 months)
Eccrine activity	Increased, hyperhidrosis	Throughout	-
Sebaceous activity	Enlarged montgomery's glands on the areola	Throughout	-
Vascular changes	Spider angiomas, palmar erythema, varicose veins, haemorrhoids and DVT may occur rarely	Throughout	-
Tumour growth	Molluscum fibrosum gravidarum (skin tag), pyogenic granuloma, melanocytic nevi may increase in size	2nd-3rd trimester	Increased vascularity secondary to raised estrogen levels partly responsible. Malignant melanoma has a controversial relationship with pregnancy
Pruritis gravidarum	*No primary lesions* (some excoriations); 0.02 to 2.4% of pregnancies affected; mild variant of recurrent cholestasis of pregnancy	2nd-3rd trimester	Ursodeoxycholic acid effective if treatment needed, most cases resolve spontaneously soon after birth

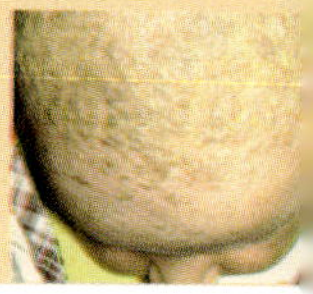

Table 22.4: Specific dermatoses of pregnancy

Condition	*Skin lesions*	*Trimester*	*Remarks*
PUPPP Pruritic urticarial papules and plaques of pregnancy also known as polymorphic eruption of pregnancy (1/200 pregnancies)	Papules, papulovesicles, urticarial lesions that begin on the abdomen, often around striae, typical sparing of the umbilicus, and spread peripherally; intense pruritis, EM like lesions may occur	3rd trimester	Mechanical cause suspected (stretching of skin), seen primarily in primigravidae, no effect on fetus, DIF negative: Differentiates it from prebullous pemphigoid gestationis
Pemphigoid gestationis also known as herpes gestationis (1/150 000 pregnancies)	Early papules and urticarial lesions, then grouped vesicles, abdomen a favoured site, may occur following delivery; intense pruritis	2nd-3rd trimester	Immunological cause; DIF shows linear deposition of C3 and IgG along BMZ; oral steroids needed; recurs with subsequent pregnancies; HLA association present; neonate may have blisters; premature delivery in 23% cases
Prurigo gestationis (1/300 pregnancies)	Prurigo nodularis like lesions: Excoriated papules scattered over the abdomen and extensor surface of extremities; *no urticarial lesions*	2nd-3rd trimester; occurs earlier than PUPPP	DIF negative, may recur with subsequent pregnancies, symptomatic management
Pruritic folliculitis of pregnancy	Similar papules but folliculocentric	2nd-3rd trimester	Symptomatic management
Impetigo herpetiformis (some authors have advised discarding the term and just considering the condition a psoriatic flare)	Widespread pustules on an erythematous base	3rd trimester	Basically a worsening of psoriasis by pregnancy; fetal death may occur; **oral corticosteroids** needed; recurs with subsequent pregnancies

CHAPTER **23**

MISCELLANEOUS INFILTRATIVE DISORDERS

EOSINOPHILIC TISSUE REACTIONS

A variety of eosinophilic syndromes may include skin involvement (Table 23.1).

Table 23.1: Dermatoses in which tissue eosinophilia is prominent

Eosinophilia usually the predominant component	*Eosinophilia often a significant feature*
Eosinophilic cellulitis (Wells' syndrome) Hypereosinophilic syndrome	1. Vasculitis associated with collagen vascular diseases
Scleroderma-like syndromes: Eosinophilic fasciitis, eosinophilia myalgia syndromes	2. Granuloma faciale (a vasculitis)
Eosinophilia with vasculitis: Churg-Strauss syndrome	3. **Drug eruptions**
Angiolymphoid hyperplasia with eosinophilia and Kimura Disease **Eosinophilic folliculitis** **Localized eosinophilic lesions:** Insect bites (early lesions), scabies	4. **Immunobullous disorders:** Bullous pemphigoid (dermal and epidermal), pemphigus (epidermal: eosinophilic spongiosis)
Edematous syndromes: Episodic angioedema with eosinophilia, solid facial edema with eosinophilia	5. Eosinophilic granuloma (a variant of Langerhans cell histiocytosis)

EOSINOPHILIC CELLULITIS (WELLS' SYNDROME)

Etiology and Pathogenesis

The etiology is uncertain, although some cases are felt to follow insect bites.

Clinical Features

Lesions usually affect distal limbs and resemble cellulitis. They are urticated or infiltrated, and may be annular or bullous. They gradually enlarge then resolve over a few weeks, but may recur at intervals. Tissue eosinophilia is very marked, and there may be a granulomatous reaction around large clumps of eosinophilic material known as flame figure (Fig. 23.1). Peripheral eosinophilia is less consistent.

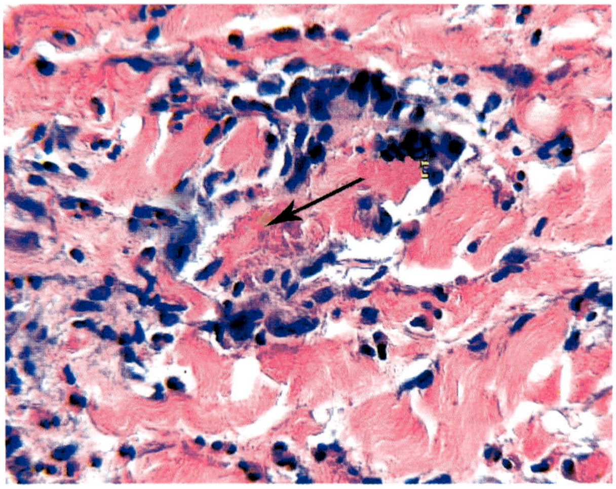

Fig. 23.1: Flame figure

Treatment

The condition usually responds well to systemic steroids (prednisolone, 40-60 mg daily, reduced over a few weeks).

Eosinophilic Fasciitis (Schulman Disease)

This condition presents as diffuse symmetric edema, usually most prominent on the lower leg, with peau d'orange appearance of the skin and symptoms of myalgia and tightness. It is sometimes apparently provoked by exercise. Dermal and fatty inflammation is minimal, but there is a predominantly lymphocytic fasciitis with a disproportionate eosinophilic infiltrate. The disorder is often quite steroid-

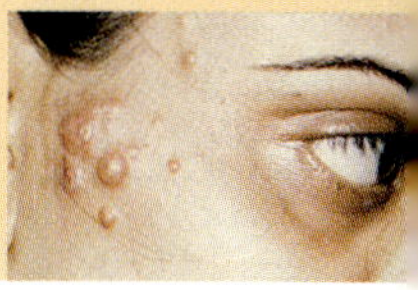

responsive, unlike acral scleroderma, but there may be progressive fibrotic changes and an association with morphea-like skin lesions. There is no specific serologic test, but typically there is an elevated eosinophil count, erythrocyte sedimentation rate, and gamma-globulin level.

Eosinophilia Myalgia Syndrome

This is a relatively recently described condition, which shares some features with eosinophilic fasciitis: Myalgia is prominent, and some patients have sclerodermoid skin lesions. Muscle spasm and weakness occur, and neuropathies are also associated with this disorder. Outbreaks have been associated with various toxins (contaminated batches of l-tryptophan, and toxic oil syndrome).

Hypereosinophilic Syndrome

This is a disorder of unknown etiology, which is probably reactive but in some cases behaves as an eosinophilic myeloproliferative state. It is defined by the presence of prolonged eosinophilia, for which other causes such as parasitic infections have been excluded, with internal organ involvement. Most patients are men, usually middle-aged or older.

Clinical Features

Persistent eosinophilia for which no other cause can be found is required to consider the diagnosis. Skin lesions include an itchy eczematous or papular eruption, which may become erythrodermic and occasionally develops blisters. Angioedema and dermographism may occur. Mucosal lesions affect the mouth and genitalia predominantly, and are usually erosive.

Internal organ involvement affects the heart (cardiomyopathy) and other organs (such as nephritis, pneumonitis and thromboses).

Treatment

Symptomatic treatment with topical steroids and oral antihistamines are of value. Systemic therapy includes prednisolone, azathioprine, dapsone, hydroxyurea, cyclophosphamide, interferon-alpha, vincristine, etoposide, and others.

ANGIOLYMPHOID HYPERPLASIA WITH EOSINOPHILIA AND KIMURA DISEASE

Angiolymphoid hyperplasia with eosinophilia (ALHE) is an uncommon condition in which there is a combination of angiomatous vessels, lymphoid infiltrate with germinal centers and eosinophilic infiltrate. The cause is unknown. Some parts of the spectrum behave as benign reactive processes, but others as invasive hemangiomatous processes.

Clinical Features

Lesions usually occur on the head and neck in elderly patients, and are reddish-colored nodules or cobblestoned plaques, which clinically may resemble malignant tumors such as basal cell carcinoma (Fig. 23.2).

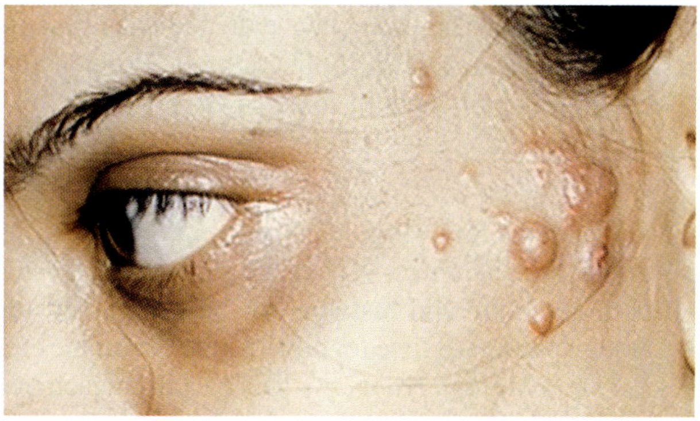

Fig. 23.2: Multiple papules and nodules on the preauricular area

Differential Diagnosis

This very much depends on the clinical pattern. Localized lesions may be confused with basal cell carcinoma or cysts. More extensive areas on the ear may resemble infective perichondritis, relapsing polychondritis, or pseudocyst of the auricle. Inflammatory conditions such as sarcoidosis or lymphocytomas may be considered, and even cutaneous lymphoma.

Treatment

Treatment is generally surgical excision or radiotherapy; local recurrences are common.

BENIGN LYMPHOCYTIC INFILTRATES

Several dermatologic disorders are characterized by a predominantly lymphocytic skin infiltrate.

1. Drug eruption.
2. Erythema annulare centrifugum.
3. Annular (figurate) erythemas.
4. Erythema multiforme.
5. Cutaneous lymphoma.
6. Lymphocytoma cutis.

Jessner Lymphocytic Infiltrate, Jessner-Kanof Disease

This is a benign lymphocytic infiltrate that most closely resembles lupus erythematosus (LE), and is considered by some to be a variant. Like LE, provocation by sunlight is a common feature.

Clinical Features

Lesions consist of (usually multiple) erythematous plaques and papules, which are most frequent on the head and upper trunk or upper arms in some instances, they may be markedly annular. They do not have the follicular plugging or atrophic changes seen in discoid LE. Premenstrual exacerbation is prominent in some cases.

Differential Diagnosis

This includes the following:

- *Lupus erythematosas*—The distinction from LE can be both clinically and histologically difficult, and may require passage of time for the situation to become clear.
- *Polymorphic light eruption*—This is usually much more obviously related to sunlight, although some patients with Jessner lymphocytic infiltrate do report photoaggravation.
- *Lymphocytoma cutis*—Usually a problem only if there are few and rather nodular lesions.
- *Other annular eruptions that may affect the face*—Such as sarcoidosis, and annular lesions in Sjögren syndrome; these are usually distinguished by histology or by other clinical or laboratory features.

Treatment

Response to treatment is unpredictable. Sunscreens may be useful prophylaxis. Topical steroids and systemic antimalarials or dapsone can be helpful.

Lymphocytoma Cutis (Spiegler-Fendt Sarcoid)

This term is used for a reactive B-lymphocyte proliferation that may resemble a cutaneous lymphoma but has benign behavior. Some cases may follow insect bites, scabies nodules and inoculations or tattoos.

Clinical Features

Lesions may be solitary or multiple, and consist of firm purplish colored dermal nodules. The face and upper trunk are common sites; lesions may affect the nipple.

Differential Diagnosis

The main differential diagnoses are insect bite reactions, cutaneous sarcoidosis and cutaneous lymphoma. On the face in particular, skin tumors such as basal cell carcinoma are in the differential. Cutaneous metastases occasionally need to be considered and, especially in the case of more widespread lesions, the other lymphocytic infiltrates discussed in this section.

Treatment

Some lesions regress spontaneously. Intralesional steroid injection is a useful therapy.

ERYTHEMA ANNULARE CENTRIFUGUM AND THE 'ANNULAR (FIGURATE) ERYTHEMAS'

Etiology and Pathogenesis

The annular or figurate erythemas are a poorly defined and poorly understood group of disorders, which are felt to be a reactive dermatosis. The most characteristic is **erythema annulare centrifugum** (EAC), which is usually idiopathic, although cases have occasionally been documented to be caused by a wide range of triggers, such as infections (dermatophytes and candida), drugs (chloroquine and penicillin), foods (blue cheese), and tumors (Hodgkin disease). It may also rarely occur as a familial disorder.

Erythema chronicum migrans due to borreliosis, **erythema marginatum** (a transient migratory rash in patients with rheumatic fever), and **erythema gyratum repens** due to gastrointestinal malignancy are usually included under the heading of annular erythemas. Neonatal LE is also often listed in this group but should probably be viewed as separate, as there is usually diagnostic serology.

Clinical Features

Erythema annulare centrifugum is an annular dermatosis with central clearing. It starts as a small macule with radial enlargement, occasionally over days but more typically over weeks or months. The edge is often urticated but with a trailing edge of scaling, and the central area clears, hence most lesions are erroneously diagnosed as ringworm dermatophyte infection.

GRANULOMATOUS REACTIONS

A granuloma is a focal chronic inflammatory response to tissue injury manifested by a histologic picture of an accumulation and proliferation of leukocytes, principally of the mononuclear type and its family of derivatives, the mononuclear phagocyte system. The immunologic components in granulomatous inflammation originate from cell-mediated or delayed hypersensitivity mechanisms controlled by thymus-dependent lymphocytes

(T lymphocytes). Five groups of granulomatous inflammations have been suggested:

- **Group 1 is the epithelioid granulomas**, which include sarcoidosis, tuberculosis in certain forms, tuberculoid leprosy, tertiary syphilis, zirconium granuloma, beryllium granuloma, mercurial granuloma and lichen nitidus.
- **Group 2, histiocytic granulomas,** include lepromatous leprosy, histoplasmosis and leishmaniasis.
- **Group 3 is the group of foreign-body granulomas**, including endogenous products (e.g., hair, fat, keratin), minerals (e.g., tattoos, silica, talc), plant and animal products (e.g., cactus, suture, oil, insect parts), and synthetic agents such as synthetic hair.
- **Group 4 is the necrobiotic/palisading granulomas,** such as granuloma annulare, necrobiosis lipoidica, rheumatoid nodule, rheumatic fever nodule, cat-scratch disease, and lymphogranuloma venereum.
- **Group 5 is the mixed inflammatory granulomas,** including many deep fungus infections such as blastomycosis and sporotrichosis, mycobacterial infections, granuloma inguinale, and chronic granulomatous disease.

Granuloma Annulare

Granuloma annulare (GA) is a relatively common disorder that has several morphologic variants. Some of these have an association with diabetes mellitus. Trauma may be involved in the pathogenesis, as lesions are often over bony prominences. Rarely, GA is recurrent on a seasonal basis (spring or summer). Pathologically, GA lesions occur in the mid-dermis and demonstrate necrobiosis (literally, death and life) of collagen, with mucin deposits between the damaged collagen and a surrounding infiltrate of lymphocytes and histiocytes.

Clinical Features

Lesions are most common over bony prominences such as knuckles, elbows, and the dorsum of fingers. The initial lesion is a firm, pink, yellowish, or skin-colored plaque, which gradually expands radially, and has the appearance of coalesced papules producing a cobblestoned morphology. (Fig. 23.3) About 50% of GA lesions resolve within 2 years, gradually flattening with some residual purplish staining. In the generalized form, the papules are usually much smaller, but more extensive sheets of superficial GA occur.

Clinical Variants

1. Localized
2. Generalized
3. Perforating
3. Subcutaneous

Treatment

Often, no treatment is required. During the early expanding phase, there may be erythema and itch, in which case topical corticosteroids can be useful. Photochemotherapy (PUVA) can be used, usually for those with more extensive lesions.

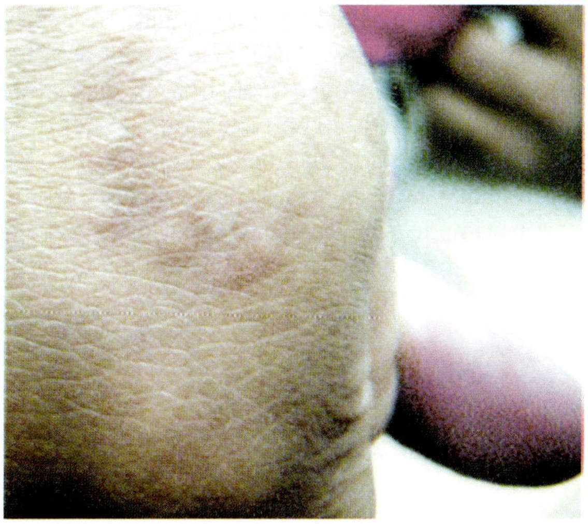

Fig. 23.3: Multiple, annular papules on the dorsum of the hand (Granuloma annulare)

Annular Elastolytic Giant Cell Granuloma

Annular elastolytic giant cell granuloma (AEGCG) may be a granulomatous reaction to damaged elastic fibers. It occurs in sun-damaged skin and, using appropriate histologic stains, fragments of elastic tissue can be seen within macrophages and giant cells. Like those of GA, lesions are typically annular, but often more serpiginous and without the cobblestoned character of GA. The two disorders are very similar histologically.

Sarcoidosis

The etiology is uncertain. Some evidence suggests an infective cause, combined with an abnormal degree of humoral and cell-mediated immune response. Polyclonal hypergammaglobulinemia is common in chronic sarcoidosis, and there is an association with a variety of autoimmune disorders and with Sjögren syndrome.

Clinical Features and Variants

Clinical Variants

1. Acute 2 Subacute 3. Chronic

Sarcoid skin lesions are extremely varied. They include erythematous or purplish plaques and nodules, papules (which may be widespread and very numerous in micropapular sarcoid), hypopigmented patches, atrophic lesions, and scar sarcoid. Lesions may mimic psoriasis or morphea, or may be subcutaneous. Atrophic, alopecic, pustular, and ulcerative lesions may occur. Massive

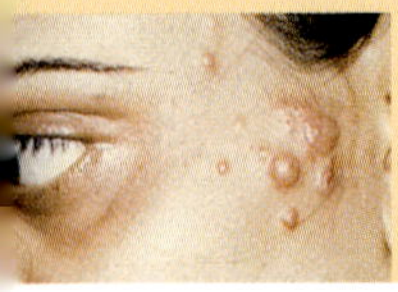

granulomatous nodules are uncommon but may resemble lymphedema if a limb is affected. Nails may be affected (usually with underlying osteolysis), as may mucous membranes. Diffuse erythrodermic or ichthyotic presentation causes particular diagnostic difficulty.

Additionally, non-specific lesions such as erythema nodosum occur in acute sarcoidosis, usually with hilar lymphadenopathy. The system involvement is varied (Table 23.2).

Table 23.2: Organ systems that may be involved in sarcoidosis

Organ system	*Comments*
Bones	Arthralgia in acute sarcoidosis, cysts (mainly digital)
Chest	Hilar lymphadenopathy in acute-onset sarcoidosis, pulmonary fibrosis in chronic disease
Eyes	Especially anterior uveitis
Heart	Commonly asymptomatic, but conduction defects and heart failure occur
Lymph nodes	Especially hilar, peripheral in about 25%
Neurologic	Especially facial palsy (may occur with uveitis and parotid enlargement)
Visceral organs	Splenomegaly, hepatomegaly

Lupus Pernio

This is a form of chronic cutaneous sarcoidosis that affects predominantly the central face and ears. It is typically purple, but the site on the face may lead to it being confused with LE. It is commonly associated with other features of chronic sarcoidosis, such as restrictive pulmonary disease or bone cysts.

Treatment

Treatment options for sarcoidosis include strong topical or intralesional corticosteroids, systemic steroids, antimalarials, and methotrexate, depending on the pattern and severity of both the skin disease and other organ involvement. In lupus pernio, physical modalities such as laser, electrocautery, or surgery may be useful. Methotrexate seems to be of particular benefit in verrucous lesions. Allopurinol appears to be beneficial, for uncertain reasons. PUVA may have a role, as does infliximab for severe disease.

FOREIGN BODY REACTION

Etiology and Pathogenesis

Foreign body granulomas (FBGs) may occur due to numerous agents, and the granulomas may be sarcoidal or necrobiotic in type. Examples include the following.

- Keratin from ruptured epidermoid cysts, folliculitis with disruption of hair shafts, and ingrowing hairs.
- *Plant materials*—Thorns, cactus spines, wood splinters, etc.
- *Animal derived*—Arthropod bites (e.g. tick mouth parts), sea urchin spines, and jellyfish stings.
- *Metabolic causes*—Calcinosis and gout.
- *Iatrogenic and other inoculations*—Suture material, talc, aluminium in vaccines, foreign collagen or silicone, paraffin (sclerosing lipogranuloma), and tattoo pigments.
- *Other essentially inert materials*—Silica, zirconium, and beryllium.

Clinical Features

Most foreign body reactions present either as a non-specific inflammatory nodule or in obvious relation to a preceding scar. The features may also vary according to the causative agent and type of injury; for example, granuloma formation due to illicit injection of paraffin for tissue augmentation may produce a broad area of abnormality, whereas a thorn injury is usually very localized. Pathologically, many foreign bodies will be visible by polarized light microscopy, thus confirming the diagnosis.

MULTICENTRIC RETICULOHISTIOCYTOSIS

Etiology and Pathogenesis

This is a granulomatous disorder, usually of unknown etiology but associated with internal malignancy in about 25% of cases.

Clinical Features

Lesions typically affect skin, bones, and joints, less commonly heart, lungs, eyes, and nervous system. Arthritis is usually manifest in the fingers and knees. The skin lesions usually consist of multiple reddish brown or purple nodules, usually affecting the dorsa of the hands and fingers, and the head and neck (especially around the ears).

MASTOCYTOSIS

Mastocytosis is divided on clinical grounds into the following types:

- *Type Ia:* Indolent mastocytosis, no systemic disease.
- *Type Ib:* Indolent mastocytosis, with systemic disease.
- *Type II:* Mastocytosis associated with a myeloproliferative (IIa) or myelodysplastic (IIb) disorder (skin lesions may or may not be present; urticaria, dermographism, or flushing usually occur).
- *Type III:* Lymphadenopathic mastocytosis with eosinophilia (also termed aggressive mastocytosis; rare, usually no skin lesions).

- *Type IV:* Mast cell leukemia (rare, usually no skin lesions).

Clinical Feature

Cutaneous mastocytosis presents with several different morphologies each of which has a different age group of predilection. Lesions in children contain many more mast cells than those in adults, hence the greater tendency for lesional urtication or blistering in the younger age group. Clinical features of the lesions include itch, urtication when rubbed (**Darier sign**), blistering in some cases, and pigmentation. Dermographism and urticarial lesions may occur more widely. Systemic symptoms include flushing, alcohol intolerance, headache (especially in adults), and peptic ulceration (Tables 23.3 and 23.4).

Table 23.3: Symptoms and organ-specific features that may occur in mastocytosis

Pattern	*Description*
Solitary mastocytoma	Yellow-brown plaque (may be macular or papular morphology). Urticates or blisters easily. Virtually always in children.
Urticaria pigmentosa: Childhood pattern	Variable number of yellow-brown macules, plaques; usually fewer if later age of onset. Usually urticate easily; especially if extensive and young age.
Urticaria pigmentosa: Adult pattern	Numerous red-brown macules or papules, usually each < 0.5 cm, mainly on trunk. May be difficult to urticate.
Diffuse cutaneous mastocytosis	Semiconfluent yellow–pale brown plaques, skin may be wrinkled and doughy.
Telangiectasia macularis eruptive perstans	Telangiectatic macules; may be discrete or semiconfluent. Urtication is often subtle. Usually adults.
Xanthelasmoid pattern	Yellowish plaques; may urticate. Rare.
No skin lesions	Systemic disease may occur without skin lesions.

- **Mastocytoma:** Usually presents as a solitary pink or brown itchy papule which wheals on rubbing. There are no systemic features.
- **Juvenile mastocytosis:** This is the most common type. Numerous pink or brown papules and macules develop over the trunk and limbs. There is no systemic involvement, and the condition is often mistaken for multiple melanocytic naevi.
- **Diffuse cutaneous mastocytosis:** This is rare and seen mostly in infants, being characterized by persistent dermographic wheals that appear after minor friction. The skin is diffusely infiltrated with mast cells, producing a thickened appearance like pigskin. The bone marrow, liver and spleen may be involved. Flushing is common. Death from massive histamine release is a real risk. Spontaneous improvement usually occurs.
- **Adult type:** Telangiectasia macularis eruptiva perstans (TMEP). Pink or pink-brown telangiectatic macules appear in early adult life and can spread to cover the whole body. The liver, spleen and bone are involved in up to 20% of cases but systemic features such as headaches, flushing and palpitations are unusual.

Table 23.4: Symptoms and organ-specific features that may occur in mastocytosis

Organ system	*Symptom or feature*
Skin	Itch (mediated by prostaglandin D2),wheals (leukotrienes), flushing (chymase), blisters (histamine)
General	General malaise or tiredness, fever
Cardiac	Palpitations, dizziness, fainting, chest pain
Respiratory	Dyspnea
Gastrointestinal and abdominal	Nausea or vomiting, diarrhea, cramps, dyspepsia; splenomegaly, hepatomegaly
Bone and bone marrow	Osteoporosis, bone pain
Neurologic	Headache

Investigations

About 20% of adults with urticaria pigmentosa will have some involvement of bone marrow or gastrointestinal tract, causing systemic features such as headache, **diarrhea**, or flushing. A small proportion, probably less than 2%, develop more aggressive disease associated with myeloproliferative features, lymphoma, neutropenia, lymphadenopathy and eosinophilia, or even mast cell leukemia. Such developments may bc accompanied by an apparently paradoxical improvement in skin symptoms, which presumably reflects development of a less well-differentiated mast cell population.

Measurement of mast cell tryptase or of urinary histamine or its metabolites (N-methyl histamine, 1,4-methylimidazole acetic acid, MeImAA) may be useful in assessment of systemic symptoms. A radiologic or isotope skeletal assessment is recommended in adults with mastocytosis, even in the absence of overt systemic disease, and a bone marrow biopsy is also recommended if there is either an abnormal complete blood count or evidence of bone lesions.

Treatment

This falls into three main categories for cutaneous disease.

Avoid triggers of mast cell degranulation

- This is especially important if there are significant systemic features due to widespread skin lesions. Friction is an important factor in causing urtication or blistering of lesions in children. More important is the potential for significant mediator release due to drugs such as opiates, aspirin, NSAIDs, alcohol, and many anesthetics (propofol, vecuronium, and fentanyl appear to be safe).

Local treatments

- These include topical corticosteroids, PUVA and UVA1 (the last is not widely available). If using topical corticosteroids, potent agents are required, so there is a risk of atrophy with prolonged use. Short-term use under occlusion may be worthwhile, or intralesional depot steroid (usually for localized mastocytomas). Rarely, troublesome mastocytomas may be treated by excision.

Systemic treatments

- In patients with more widespread urticaria pigmentosa, or with systemic symptoms, symptomatic treatment with oral H_1 antihistamines is usually required. H_2 antagonists are also useful, especially if there is associated peptic ulcer disease. Mast cell stabilizing agents, such as ketotifen and sodium cromoglycate, are also useful in some cases, as is doxepin (which has powerful antihistaminic activity).

LANGERHANS CELL HISTIOCYTOSIS AND OTHER HISTIOCYTOSES

Langerhans Cell Histiocytosis (Histiocytosis X)

This histiocytic disorder is most frequent in children. It causes a rash that resembles a severe **seborrheic rash**, with crusted papular lesions, erosions, granulomatous areas, and **purpuric areas** (Fig. 23.4). The rash may present on the nappy area, trunk or scalp. Internal involvement may occur, especially diabetes insipidus (in 25-50% with systemic disease), and treatment is usually with radiotherapy or chemotherapy or both.

Occasionally, solitary nodular skin lesions known as eosinophilic granuloma of the skin may occur as a rare variant of Langerhans cell histiocytosis (LCH), which may be cured by excision, radiotherapy, or intralesional steroid injection.

Juvenile Xanthogranuloma

Juvenile xanthogranuloma (JXG) is the most common of the histiocytic disorders. It occurs in children, usually as one or a few yellowish orange papules or nodules, most commonly on the scalp or face. However, involvement of

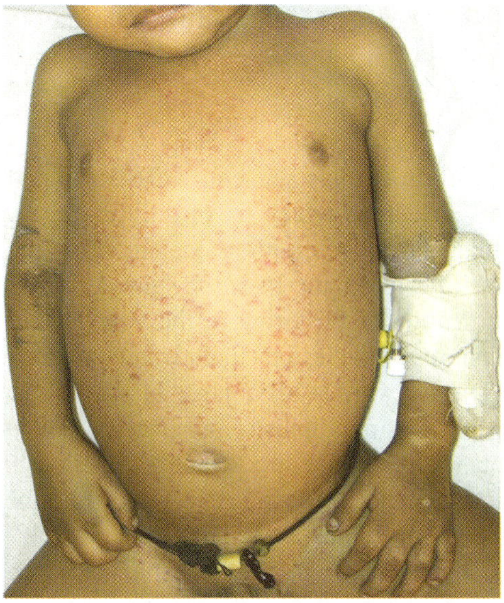

Fig. 23.4: Purpuric papules on the trunk and scalp with enlarged liver and spleen

the eyes may occur, and there is a rare association between JXG, neurofibromatosis type 1 (NF1), and juvenile myelomonocytic leukemia (although JXG and NF1 can coexist without leukemia also).

Other Histiocytoses

Most other histiocytoses are rare. They include the following types:

- *Familial:* Familial sky blue histiocytosis and hereditary progressive mucinous histiocytosis.
- *Eruptive or disseminated:* Benign cephalic histiocytosis (usually in children), generalized eruptive histiocytosis (mainly in adults), and xanthoma disseminatum.
- *Paraneoplastic*: Diffuse plane xanthomatosis and necrobiotic xanthogranuloma (with paraproteinemia).
- *Usually systemic but occasionally confined to skin*: Massive sinus histiocytosis (Rosai-Dorfman disease).

OTHER METABOLIC INFILTRATES AND DEPOSITS

Perforating Disorders

This is a group of disorders in which dermal tissue is extruded through the epidermis or into the follicles (perforating folliculitis), a process known as transepidermal elimination. This is an important group of disorders, as they are associated with systemic disease, notably diabetes and chronic renal failure. However, the same process of transepidermal elimination may occur sporadically and also occurs as isolated lesions in several other situations, which are usually more obvious. For example, subcutaneous suture material ('spitting' sutures), fragmented hair shafts (e.g. after simple folliculitis), or insect mouth parts may all be eliminated through the skin surface.

Types

1. Primary

- Reactive perforating collagenoses.
- Perforating folliculitis.
- Kurle's disease.
- Elastosis perforans serpiginosa.

2. Acquired

- Chronic renal failure with/without hemodialysis.
- Diabetes mellitus.

Calcinosis

Cutaneous calcinosis (Fig. 23.5) occurs by various mechanisms, the clinical features being very varied and depending on the disease entity (Table 23.5).

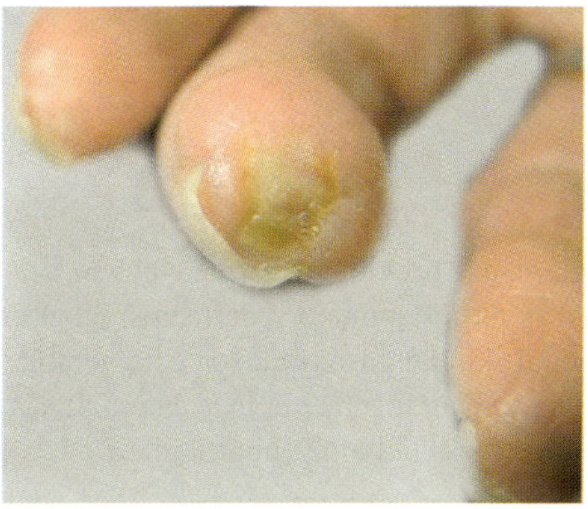

Fig. 23.5: Cutaneous calcinosis

Types of Calcinosis Cutis

- Circumscripta.
- Universalis.
- Pinnal.
- Scrotal/Vulval.
- Solitary.

- **Dystrophic calcification:** In this mechanism, calcium is deposited in previously abnormal tissue or is related to specific local factors. This occurs, for example, in some connective tissue disorders (widespread in juvenile dermatomyositis, locally in CREST [calcinosis, Raynaud phenomenon, esophageal dysfunction, sclerodactyly, and telangiectasia] syndrome); occasionally in longstanding venous stasis or Ehlers-Danlos syndrome, and after various injuries. Calcification of the ear occurs most commonly after cold injury but also in some endocrine disorders. There are also some specific entities in which calcification occurs, such as pilomatricoma (a benign tumor of hair follicle origin.
- **Metastatic calcification:** This occurs due to either *elevated calcium or phosphate levels,* or both. Most cases occur in renal failure with secondary hyperparathyroidism. Rarely, this may cause deposits of calcium in the skin; the more significant disorder that occurs is calcific uremic arteriolopathy.
- **Idiopathic calcification:** At least some examples of apparent idiopathic calcification are probably due to unrecognized injury and are really dystrophic in type.

Table 23.5: Some examples of cutaneous calcinosis

Mechanism of calcinosis	*Examples*
Dystrophic calcification. In this mechanism, calcium is deposited in previously abnormal tissue or is related to specific local factors	**Localized lesions:** Cysts, angiomas, lipomas **Post-traumatic:** Scars, hematomas, fat injury **Inflammatory diseases:** Sclerodermas, dermatomyositis, acne **Other skin conditions:** Venous stasis disease, pseudoxanthoma elasticum, Ehlers-Danlos syndrome
Metastatic calcification. This occurs due to either elevated calcium or phosphate levels, or both. Most cases occur in renal failure with secondary hyperparathyroidism	Hyperparathyroidism, pseudohypoparathyroidism, chronic renal failure, milk-alkali syndrome Sarcoidosis
Idiopathic calcification. At least some examples of apparent idiopathic calcification are probably due to unrecognized injury and are really dystrophic in type.	Calcinosis universalis, calcinosis circumscripta Solitary nodular calcinosis (cutaneous calculus) Idiopathic calcinosis of the scrotum

REFERENCES

- Braverman IM: Skin Signs of Systemic Disease, 3rd edn. Philadelphia: Saunders, 1998.
- Breathnach SM: Amyloid and amyloidoses, J Am Acad Dermatol 1988; 18: 1-16.
- Caputo R: Text Atlas of Histiocytic Syndromes, London: Martin Dunitz, 1998.
- Hartmann K, Henz BM: Mastocytosis: Recent advances in defining the disease, Br J Dermatol 2001; 144: 682-95.
- Rongioletti F, Rebora A: Updated classification of papular mucinosis, lichen myxedematosus, and scleromyxedema, J Am Acad Dermatol 2001; 44: 273-81.
- Stephens CJM, McKee PH, Black MM: The dermal mucinoses. Adv Dermatol 1993; 8: 201-26.
- Touart DM, Sau P: Cutaneous deposition diseases, Part 1, J Am Acad Dermatol 1998; 39: 149-71.
- Touart DM, Sau P: Cutaneous deposition diseases, Part 2, J Am Acad Dermatol 1998; 39: 527-44.

Disorders of Epidermis, Dermis and Subcutaneous Tissues

EPIDERMAL DISORDERS

Atrophy

Atrophy (thinning) of the epidermis occurs in numerous situations, but rarely in isolation. Causes include the following.

- *Aging*—Both chronologic and solar (in which it is associated with elastosis of the upper dermis).
- *Lichen sclerosus.*
- *Necrobiosis lipoidica.*
- *Lupus erythematosus.*
- *Poikilodermas.*
- *Iatrogenic*—Due to use of topical steroids and following radiotherapy.
- *Localized lesions*—Porokeratosis.

Epidermal Thickening

- *Local thickening in dermatoses*—for example psoriasis, keratodermas, acanthosis nigricans, diabetic finger pebbling, and any disorder where chronic rubbing or scratching of the skin is a feature.
- *Acanthosis in localized lesions*—For example prurigo nodularis, dermatofibroma, corns, and callosities.

Callosities, Corns and Similar Disorders

These arise due to pressure or other forms of chronic, low-grade damage. The most common types of corn are on the sole of the foot, where they may mimic plantar warts although they also occur between the toes.

Callosities occur at other sites of chronic friction, such as those related to sitting posture on the dorsum of the foot, or 'pickers' nodules', which are most commonly seen on the hands. Knuckle pads are a variation of this habit pattern.

DERMAL ATROPHY

Table 23.6: Some causes of dermal atrophy

Abnormal tissue	*Examples*
Collagen	Scars and striae Lichen sclerosus Ehlers-Danlos syndrome Atrophodermas Discoid lupus erythematosus Focal dermal hypoplasia (Goltz syndrome)
Elastic tissue	Cutis laxa Blepharochalasis Anetoderma
Mixed	Aging: Chronologic and solar, cigarette smoke

Lichen Sclerosus

Etiology and Pathogenesis

Lichen sclerosus (previously termed lichen sclerosus et atrophicus) is an inflammatory dermatosis that especially affects genital skin but also occurs at extragenital sites; the two forms may occur together or in isolation. It has a female predominance, especially in genital skin.

Clinical Features

The affected areas on the vulva, penis, perineum and/or perianal skin show well-marginated white thin fragile patches with a crinkled surface. Itching can be severe, especially in women. The fragility of the atrophic areas may lead to purpura and erosions. Scratching can cause lichenification, and diagnostic confusion. Women are more commonly afflicted than men, but pre-adolescent girls and boys also can develop this problem. In girls, the white patches circling the vulva and anus take on an **hourglass** shape around the orifices.

Course

As time goes on, scarring occurs. In adult women, the clitoral prepuce may scar over the clitoris, and the vaginal introitus may narrow, preventing enjoyable sexual intercourse. Scarring is rare in girls and boys:

- *Male genital (also known as **balanitis xerotica obliterans**):* Usually presents due to color change or functional impairment, such as difficulty with erection or micturition.

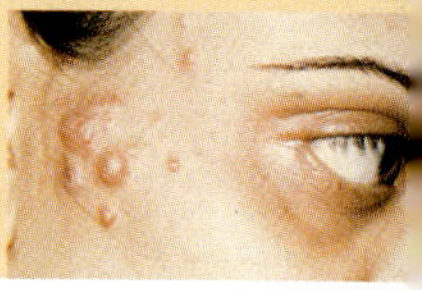

- *Female genital:* May be asymptomatic or present with itch or dyspareunia; in children, it may be felt to represent abuse, as the poor dermal support for blood vessels may lead to episodic bruising.
- *Extragenital:* Usually in women who also have genital lichen sclerosus; may be asymptomatic or present with itch.

Treatment

Treatment with potent topical steroids not only reduces itch, pain and misery, but also reverses hypopigmentation and atrophy by shutting down its cause. However, atrophy, striae and other complications can develop on untreated adjacent skin, if the medication spreads there. Ointments are preferable to creams. Only small amounts (15 g) should be dispensed. After a course of 8-12 weeks, weaker topical steroids can be used to maintain a remission.

Other modalities include topical estrogen, tacrolimus, systemic retinoids, chloroquine and systemic retinoids.

Ehlers-Danlos Syndrome (Cutis Hyperelastica)

Etiology and Pathogenesis

This is a group of inherited disorders characterized by hyperextensible skin, together with varying degrees of hyperextensibility of joints and abnormality of blood vessels.

- *Classic (mostly autosomal dominant)*—Includes types previously termed type I (gravis: hyperextensible skin with fragility, easy bruising, and atrophic scarring;) and type II (mitis: milder hyperextensibility and joint laxity of hands and feet).
- *Hypermobility (autosomal dominant)*—Type III or benign hypermobile syndrome: Generalized joint hypermobility, mild cutaneous features and floppy mitral valve.
- *Kyphoscoliosis (autosomal recessive)*—Type VI or ocular: patients have hyperextensible and dislocating joints, and ocular problems (blue sclerae, retinal detachment, and bleeding); skin features are usually less apparent.
- *Arthrochalasia (autosomal dominant)*—Types VIIa and VIIb: Mainly affects joints, but the skin is soft and velvety, and stretches easily, and there may be bruising and atrophic scars.
- *Dermatosparaxis (autosomal recessive)*—Type VIIc: The skin is very hyperelastic and fragile, with easy bruising.
- *Others*—Includes previous types V, VIII, X and XI.

Anetoderma

Etiology and Pathogenesis

Anetoderma is a localized area of lax skin, often with herniation of the underlying tissues, although lesions may be depressed:

- *Primary (idiopathic)*—Divided into forms with preceding inflammation **(Jadassohn-Pellizzari)** or without **(Schweninger-Buzzi)**, although these can coexist and the distinction is probably not very useful.
- *Postinflammatory or postinfective*—Usually after acne, chicken pox, borrelial acrodermatitis chronica atrophicans; also occurs in systemic lupus erythematosus and sarcoidosis.
- *Follicular*—This pattern is probably a variant of the postinfective group, infection causing perifollicular elastolysis, but is usefully considered as a distinct group, as follicular lesions may occur in isolation.

Striae and Scars

Striae (stretch marks) are primarily due to changes in dermal collagen, but the shearing of the dermis that occurs causes the overlying epidermis to be thinned, especially when there is already damage to the epidermis (e.g. in cases due to overuse of topical steroids).

Cutis Laxa

This is a defect of elastic tissue that may occur as dominant, recessive, X-linked recessive, and acquired forms. The acquired forms may be apparently idiopathic, paraneoplastic and some occur following inflammation of the skin. Similar changes can occur due to long-term penicillamine therapy. The striking clinical feature is laxity, with wrinkling and sagging of the skin, producing a prematurely aged facies. As well as the skin defect, there may be internal features such as hernias, emphysema and gastrointestinal diverticula.

Blepharochalasis

This disorder is rather like a localized form of cutis laxa confined to the upper eyelids, although it is sporadic in nature. It causes drooping of the upper eyelid, in some cases sufficiently obvious that a surgical correction is required.

Atrophodermas

These are a group of rather varied disorders in which there is a depression in the skin surface. Recognized patterns include the following:

- **Atrophoderma of Pasini and Pierini** (progressive idiopathic atrophoderma)—Variant of morphea although the inflammatory border and sclerotic component that occur in morphea are not features of this type of atrophoderma.
  Borrelia infection has been implicated in some cases.
  Lesions, solitary or multiple, usually occur on the lower part of the back, and consist of a brown-colored, depressed area of skin. There is a well-demarcated and palpable junction with the normal skin, and some lesions have follicular prominence. It usually presents in older children or young adults, mainly in females. There is no routinely useful treatment.
- **Atrophoderma vermiculatum** (honeycomb atrophy)—This usually affects the cheeks most noticeably, usually in children or young adults. It may occur in isolation on a sporadic basis, as an inherited condition, or with keratosis pilaris atrophicans and related disorders.
- **Follicular atrophoderma**—This may occur after inflammation such as that caused by acne or an infective folliculitis. It also occurs, with basal cell carcinomas, in a rare disorder termed Bazex syndrome.

DERMAL THICKENING

Table 23.7: Some causes of dermal thickening with the morphological presentation

Appearance	*Cause*	*Examples*
Discrete lesions with scaling or other surface change	Cellular infiltrate	Numerous inflammatory dermatoses, for example psoriasis, early discoid lupus
Smooth localized swelling	Fluid	Urticaria, localized edema
	Cellular infiltrate	Jessner lymphocytic infiltrate
	Other infiltrate	Some xanthomas, nodular mucinosis, discrete areas of calcinosis
	Altered connective tissue	Keloid scar, dermatofibroma, localized fibromas
Papular or cobblestoned appearance	Altered connective tissue	Granuloma annulare, pretibial myxedema
	Cellular infiltrate	Scleromyxedema, solar elastosis, connective tissue nevi, pseudoxanthoma elasticum
	Other infiltrates	Sarcoidosis, some psoriasis or eczema (especially lichenified) Some xanthomas, lichen amyloidosis
Smooth plaque lesions	Sclerotic disorders	Scleroderma, morphea, diabetic stiff skin
Peau d'orange appearance	Cellular infiltrate	Neoplastic infiltration
	Fluid altered connective tissue	Early pretibial myxedema, scleredema, some connective tissue nevi Some dependent edema

KELOIDS

Keloids are a persistent, proliferative type of scar tissue. They may arise after surgical procedures, the risk being greatest on the neck and upper trunk or upper arm in young adults. Inflamed lesions such as acne, tuberculosis inoculation sites, and ingrowing hairs may also cause keloids; some are apparently spontaneous. Hypertrophic scars appear similar but are confined to wound sites, do not proliferate laterally, and tend to gradually flatten with time.

Keloids are difficult to treat. Therapy is usually with topical or intralesional steroids. Silastic gel in various formulations may be helpful in some cases, and laser treatments (especially to early keloids with a vascular component) can be useful. Cryotherapy may reduce some of the bulk of a keloid scar. Surgical excision has the risk of further keloid, but may be successful if the wound is subsequently treated with steroid, silastic gel sheets, pressure bandaging, or radiotherapy. UVA1 may be proved useful; various intralesional cytotoxics and interferon have also been tried, with variable benefit.

Fibromatoses, Pachydermoperiostosis and Other Collagen Proliferations

Scleroderma (hard skin) is a feature of several skin disorders. This is discussed with a differential diagnosis in the context of collagen vascular disease the most common cause of a diffuse sclerodermatous process. Note that some cases may have a thickened dermis but are depressed below the normal skin surface contour (therefore appearing atrophic) due to deeper tethering.

Fibromatoses are uncommon. They may affect fibrous tissue at different levels in the skin, although some are confined to the dermis or to the deeper fascia (see later). They may present a diagnostic challenge, as deep, diffuse types may be difficult to distinguish with certainty from soft tissue sarcomas or other lesions, and are also difficult to remove surgically without risk of interfering with function.

Pachydermoperiostosis describes a thickening of tissues including the skin and deeper structures, including periosteum, as implied from its name. Finger clubbing is a type of pachydermoperiostosis that occurs in conjunction with internal malignancy, especially bronchial carcinoma. A more extreme version occurs as an autosomal dominant condition, which is particularly prominent in males. There is marked coarsening of facial features, with greasy skin and palmoplantar hyperhidrosis.

Periungual fibromas may occur as sporadic (usually solitary) lesions, at least some of which appear to be traumatic in origin. Multiple periungual fibromas are a feature of tuberous sclerosis.

Connective tissue nevi usually present in early childhood as yellowish white plaques with a cobblestoned surface. They may occur in tuberous sclerosis (collagen) and in Buschke-Ollendorff syndrome (elastic, nevi).

DISORDERS OF ELASTIC TISSUE

Pseudoxanthoma Elasticum

Etiology and Pathogenesis

Pseudoxanthoma elasticum (PXE) is a recessively inherited disorder, most individuals having a mutation in the gene MRP6. Some apparent dominantly inherited cases have also been reported.

Clinical

Skin and blood vessels are affected. The characteristic cutaneous lesions are grouped yellowish papules that predominantly affect the neck and axillae but also other flexural areas. There is also some sagging of the skin, giving rise to the description of a **plucked chicken** appearance. Internal organs may be affected, with papules on various mucosal surfaces; the elastic deficiency also affects the **Bruch** membrane in the eye, which develops ragged brown linear tears that resemble vessels and are known **as angioid streaks**.

The importance of the condition is the involvement of blood vessels internally, mid-sized arteries being predominantly affected. This is most commonly apparent as gastrointestinal bleeding, especially in pregnancy. Bleeding from the uterus or urogenital tract may occur, and retinal hemorrhage is a frequent complication. Hypertension, angina, peripheral vascular disease, and cerebrovascular bleeds are all potential causes of serious morbidity or death.

Elastosis Perforans Serpiginosa

This is a perforating dermatosis in which abnormal elastic fibers are extruded through the skin surface. Patients are usually older children or young adults. It is common in patients with trisomy 21 (Down syndrome), and also occurs due to prolonged high-dose penicillamine therapy (e.g. in Wilson disease) and in conjunction with other defects of connective tissue such as Marfan syndrome, Ehlers-Danlos syndrome and PXE.

The lesions are grouped papules, often with an annular or a serpiginous pattern, which typically occur on the neck and arms). They usually appear umbilicated or centrally crusted due to the elimination of altered elastic tissue through the skin.

Other Types of Elastosis and Related Disorders

- Solar elastosis.
- Hypermobility (autosomal dominant)—was termed type III or benign hypermobile syndrome: Generalized joint hypermobility, mild cutaneous features, and floppy mitral valve.
- Elastosis of striae (linear focal elastosis).
- Localized elastoma.
- Acquired digital cutis laxa (tree frog fingers), which may be associated with myeloma.
- Perifollicular elastolysis due to bacterial elastase.
- Mid-dermal elastolysis.
- Buschke-Ollendorff syndrome (dermatofibrosis lenticularis disseminata)—increased elastic tissue in skin lesions, associated with osteopoikilosis.
- Acrokeratoelastoidosis.
- Granulomatous disorders—notably annular elastolytic giant cell granuloma.

DISORDERS OF THE FAT AND SUBCUTANEOUS TISSUES

This section will discuss three groups of disorders, namely:
- Atrophy of the fat (lipoatrophy and lipodystrophy).
- Hypertrophy of fat (lipohypertrophy), and
- Inflammation of the fat (panniculitis).

Lipoatrophy and Lipodystrophy

Lipoatrophy

Localized areas of lipoatrophy may occur in the following situations:
- *Injection sites*—Insulin lipoatrophy and intralesional or depot steroid injections.
- *Postinflammatory*—Following panniculitis.
- *Idiopathic*—Thighs (**lipoatrophia semicircularis**, abdomen (**centrifugal lipodystrophy**).
- *Pressure*—Prolonged pressure may cause some fat atrophy, such as that seen on the shoulder of some women and due to bra straps. Pressure related to hard seats or leaning against a desk or bench may be the cause of lipoatrophia semicircularis.

Lipodystrophy

The most frequent of these uncommon disorders is partial lipodystrophy. This is poorly understood but may have an autoimmune basis. It may be familial. Most patients have a gradual loss of fat from the face and upper trunk, causing a cadaverous facies and easily visible musculature in women, in whom it is most frequent, it may be mistaken for a hyperandrogenic state. In some cases, there is a compensatory lipohypertrophy of the lower limbs.

The importance of this disorder is an association with **mesangiocapillary glomerulonephritis**, which occurs in the majority of affected individuals and which may be accompanied by **complement C3 deficiency** and **diabetes**. This may present during pregnancy or oral contraceptive use.

Total lipoatrophy is a much less common, autosomal recessive disease in which hyperlipidemia and insulin-resistant diabetes occur; hypertrichosis and complete loss of fat occur in infancy, diabetes occurring later. An acquired form, sometimes triggered by a febrile illness, also occurs.

Lipohypertrophy and Lipedema

Lipohypertrophy

Lipohypertrophy may occur as a localized phenomenon, multiple discrete lesions, or more diffusely. The most frequent type of localized lipohypertrophy is a lipoma, a benign tumor of adipose tissue. These may be solitary or multiple, the multiple lesions often being familial. Multiple discrete or more extensive areas of painful adiposity occur in *Dercum disease* (adiposis dolorosa), and isolated angiolipomas are also painful. Localized lipohypertrophy was also related to insulin injections, but it is now rare since the introduction of synthetic human insulins.

More extensive areas of lipohypertrophy occur in multiple symmetric lipomatosis (*Madelung disease*). Lipohypertrophy may occur as a compensatory feature in partial lipodystrophy (discussed earlier), and centripetal adiposity occurs in Cushing's syndrome. In cellulite, the dimpled appearance is due to fibrous tethering within the fat, rather than simply due to increased fatty tissue. A lipodystrophic disorder with central lipohypertrophy (*buffalo hump*, increased abdominal fat and breast hypertrophy) has been reported in patients with AIDS, the majority of cases being related to treatment with protease inhibitors.

Lipedema

Lipedema is a condition in which there is soft fatty swelling of the lower leg. It can be distinguished from simple edema or lymphedema by the fact that it is sharply limited at the ankle, the foot being unaffected. It also fails to respond to diuretics or compression.

Panniculitis

Etiology and Pathogenesis

Panniculitis is an inflammation of fat. Methods of

classification may be based on the causative mechanisms, the type of cellular infiltrate, the structures that are affected within the fat, and the presence of vasculitis. The most helpful approach is to divide panniculitis on histologic grounds according to the part of its structure that is predominantly affected by the inflammatory process.

Fat has two components, namely lobules made up of fat cells and septa between these (in which the vascular supply traverses the fat). Assessment of the pathologic site of the inflammation, i.e., mainly septal or mainly lobular, can be used to create a likely list of causative disorders; these can then be subdivided according to the presence or absence of vasculitis, and by the type of inflammatory infiltrate that is present.

Table 23.8: Some causes of panniculitis

Histologic pattern	*Examples and comments*
Septal, *with vasculitis*	Vasculitis (Polyarteritis nodosa, vasculitis in lupus erythematosus) **Thrombophlebitis**
Septal, *no vasculitis*	**Erythema nodosum, erythema nodosum migrans** **Granulomatous disorders** (Deep granuloma annulare, sclerodermas)
Lobular, *with vasculitis*	**Nodular vasculitis** (Eythema induratum (Bazin disease)) **Neutrophilic dermatoses** Behçet syndrome, neutrophilic panniculitis of rheumatoid disease **Leprosy** Erythema nodosum leprosum
Lobular, *no vasculitis*	**Cold and other injuries collagen vascular disorders** Lupus panniculitis (lupus erythematosus profundus), dermatomyositis **Pancreatic panniculitis** Pancreatic carcinoma or pancreatitis **Metabolic** Calciphylaxis, oxalosis, 1-antitrypsin deficiency (may be mainly septal or mixed) **Malignancies** Lymphoma, cytophagic histiocytic panniculitis, other malignant infiltration of the fat **Iatrogenic** **Idiopathic (Weber-Christian disease)**

Clinical

Most panniculitis lesions present as one or several deeply situated tender nodules. Inflammation is prominent in some causes, such as erythema nodosum. Lesions are typically on the lower legs or over fatty areas in the most common variants. A particular variant that can often be suspected clinically is lupus panniculitis (lupus erythematosus profundus, this typically affects the upper trunk or upper arms in young women, who usually have other features of lupus erythematosus. Panniculitis due to cold injury is also often clinically distinctive, occurring over lateral thighs or upper arms and with markedly cold lesions.

The clinical features of panniculitis lesions themselves may be characteristic of a specific diagnosis in some cases, such as most examples of erythema nodosum or cold injury. However, most causes of panniculitis are diagnosed from associated clinical features, biopsy features, or other tests; note also that diagnosing an eruption as erythema nodosum does not identify the triggering cause.

Treatment

The treatment of panniculitis depends on the cause; for example, lupus panniculitis is often responsive to oral antimalarials, and pancreatic panniculitis due to a carcinoma requires treatment of the tumor.

DISORDERS OF FASCIA

Fascial Defects and Piezogenic Pedal Papules

Herniation through fascial defects is a similar process to anetoderma in some respects, but without skin atrophy, as the overlying dermis is normal. This may occur over the anterior tibia, but is often not brought to medical attention or may be diagnosed as a protruberant vein. Piezogenic pedal papules are clinically characteristic lesions that are usually most apparent at the medial border of the heel. They represent small fatty herniations through fascial defects, producing pale or skin colored compressible nodules. They may be asymptomatic, but some patients complain of pain. They are often confused with warts, even though they have no epidermal component. The simplest treatment, if required, is support hosiery.

REFERENCES

- Rook's Textbook of Dermatology: D. A. Burns, S. M. Breathnach, Neil Cox, Christopher E., Griffith's 7th edn 2004.
- Fitzpatrick's Dermatology in General Medicine, 6th edn 2003.

Xerosis and Pruritus

Xerosis is a term used to describe a skin condition where there is a rough, dry textural feel to the skin, accompanied by fine scaling and sometimes fine fissuring. Increasing xerosis is usually accompanied by increasing itch. It is a description, not a diagnosis—it may result from a combination of environmental conditions (low humidity, degreasing of the skin by excessive bathing soap or detergent use), genetic disorders of keratinization (ichthyoses), Down syndrome, atopic eczema, endocrine disease states (hypothyroidism), and a host of underlying disease states such as chronic renal failure, liver disease, malnutrition, anorexia nervosa, essential fatty acid deficiency, Sjögren's syndrome, HIV infection, lymphoma, and carcinomatosis. It is more common in the elderly.

SPECIFIC INVESTIGATIONS

- Thyroid function tests.
- Renal function tests.
- Consider tests for Sjögren's syndrome, HIV infection, malignancy and malabsorption, if clinically indicated.
- Drug history.

Treatment

The anchors of therapy for xerosis after any underlying disorders (if possible) are corrected are *improvement of the humidity* in the patient's environment, *avoidance of exacerbating factors* such as soap and detergents, and the use of *emollients.*

Low environmental humidity both at home and work will exacerbate xerosis of any cause. Arid air is a problem in air conditioned homes, offices and vehicles. Hot dry air directed to the lower legs during the winter in the front of automobiles is a common cause of lower leg xerosis. In the home or workplace, humidifiers can be fitted over radiators; alternatively placing wet towels over them will increase air humidity.

Soaps and detergents degrease the skin, reduce epidermal thickness, and increase scale and itch, so are best avoided, and light emollient cleansers are suggested in their place. Bathing in tepid water is often preferred by patients, and patting the skin dry will produce less scale and dryness than vigorous toweling.

Emollients (that simply produce an impervious film over the epidermis and prevent 'transpiration') and humectants (such as lactic acid, urea, or glycerine that hold water in the epidermis osmotically) are the mainstays of therapy. They should be used liberally and as frequently as possible; emollients are particularly valuable after bathing or showering to hold water in the epidermis. Light emollients for use in the shower or bath may be preferred to *bath oils* by some. Choice of emollient is entirely personal to the patient.

Agents containing *a-hydroxy acids (AHAs)* may offer some advantages over conventional paraffin-based emollients, but this may be at the expense of irritation in some people. Low-concentration *salicylic acid* may help reduce scale in more severe xerosis, but it is essential to remember that systemic absorption and salicylism can occur. *Topical retinoids* have only been used in the more severe ichthyoses and are too irritating for use in xerosis. Systemic therapies have little part to play in most patients.

First Line Therapies

- Soap avoidance.
- Humidification.
- Emollients.
- Bath oils.

Second Line Therapies

Urea-containing creams

A comparison of 3% and 10% urea cream showed that both were effective at reducing scale, dryness, and laboratory parameters (transepidermal water loss and colorimetric changes). The 10% cream was better at restoring the skin's water barrier function.

Lactic acid-containing creams.

Ammonium lactate creams

Lactate 12% lotion was significantly more effective than a petrolatum-based cream in reducing the severity of xerosis during treatment and post-treatment phases.

AHA creams.

PRURITUS

Itch can be defined as the urge to scratch. It is a characteristic feature of many diseases of the skin and an unusual sign of some systemic diseases. Generalized itch in the absence of a diagnosable rash can pose both a diagnostic and therapeutic dilemma to even the most seasoned dermatologist. Although there is no magic bullet for pruritus, new understanding of the neurophysiology of itch may lead to specific therapies targeting particular pathways in the central nervous system.

Itching in Pathologic States

Pruritus associated with underlying internal disease is often multifactorial, involving both systemic and external factors,

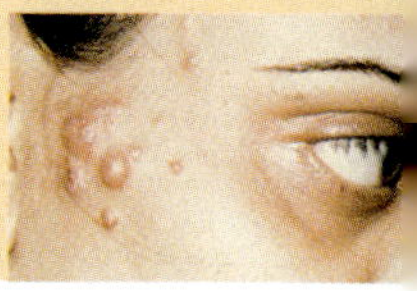

including ambient temperature and humidity. Itching associated with skin disease may also include central (neurogenic) and pruritogenic components.

Pruritus of Chronic Renal Disease

Pruritus is one of the most distressing symptoms of chronic renal failure. It affects 20 to 50 percent of patients, especially those on dialysis, although it is recently becoming less prevalent, probably due to more efficient dialysis techniques. Patients being dialyzed with membranes that are less permeable and biocompatible are more likely to suffer pruritus than those patients who are using more permeable polysulphone membranes. Patients with uremic pruritus often have a dry skin, but correction of this by emollients usually provides only mild relief. The expanding number of alleged pathogenetic factors bears testimony to the elusiveness of the causes. These include secondary hyperparathyroidism, increased numbers of dermal mast cells, elevated plasma histamine levels, abnormal levels of divalent cations, proliferation of sensory nerve endings in skin, release of pruritogenic cytokines during hemodialysis, and elevated levels of vitamin A.

Pruritus of Cholestasis

The pruritus of cholestasis is not completely understood, but may be a consequence of increased levels of endogenous opioids which was first demonstrated by Thornton and Losowsky in 1988.

The highly distressing and persistent pruritus of biliary obstruction often begins with an acral distribution, but later becomes more generalized. Both peripheral and central mechanisms are important. Cholestatic pruritus is associated with high plasma levels of bile salts, but there is little or no evidence of a correlation between concentrations of bile salts and itching, whether the bile salts are measured in the blood or skin itself.

Pruritus of Endocrine Disease

Generalized intractable itching is a recognized feature of thyrotoxicosis and may be a presenting symptom. This is usually due to increased blood flow, which raises the skin temperature, which, in turn, reduces the threshold to itching.

The skin is warm, moist and flushed. However, itching in thyrotoxicosis may be localized to the anogenital area, in which case, it is usually due to mucocutaneous candidosis. Hypothyroidism may also present with widespread pruritus, in this case, due to excessive skin dryness. The skin is cool, dry, slightly scaly, and may be thickened and sallow (myxedema).

Generalized itching is not a feature of diabetes mellitus. Although there was a suggestion in the early literature that widespread pruritus could be a presenting feature, this is not substantiated by more recent studies. However, anogenital itching is common, is often a presenting feature, and is due to mucocutaneous candidosis. Localized itching of the scalp can also be a manifestation of diabetic neuropathy, which may respond to topical capsaicin treatment.

Postmenopausal pruritus may be generalized or localized, and, in the latter case, it is usually anogenital and due to candidosis. Generalized pruritus is less common, often episodic, and associated with postmenopausal hot flushes. The presence of elevated plasma levels of pituitary luteinizing hormone and follicular stimulating hormone should support the diagnosis.

Iron Deficiency

The role of iron deficiency in the causation of pruritus is controversial. Several reports have implicated iron deficiency as a cause of pruritus in otherwise normal-looking skin. Pruritus and iron deficiency are sometimes associated in patients with polycythemia vera, the cause of the deficiency usually being venesection. In these patients, correction of iron deficiency is associated with clinical improvement. Although patients with iron deficiency may complain of pruritus, it is unlikely that iron deficiency is responsible and other causes should be sought.

Pruritus in Hematologic Disease

Itch is common in hematologic disorders. In Sézary syndrome (T cell leukemia) it is invariable, intense, and generalized. In polycythemia vera, it occurs in about 50 percent of patients, is often precipitated by contact with water ("bath itch") and is associated with raised blood histamine levels.

In Hodgkin's disease, it may be a presenting symptom, and may persist after remission. In cutaneous mastocytosis, itching occurs locally following rubbing the skin, although it can be widespread in severely affected patients, when it is usually associated with systemic symptoms. Itching may occur in patients with myeloid and lymphatic leukemia and myelodysplasia.

Pruritus as a Manifestation of Solid Malignant Tumors

Traditionally, the onset of pruritus in a middle-aged or elderly patient with an otherwise normal-looking skin prompts a thorough investigation for underlying systemic causes including internal neoplasia, although the latter is an uncommon cause. Although pruritus may occasionally be present years before the tumor becomes clinically detectable, even if resources are available, full investigation for a causative solid tumour is probably not worthwhile.

Pruritus of HIV-1 Infection

Itch is an early symptom of HIV disease and may be associated with skin disease (scabies, pediculosis, seborrheic eczema, xerosis) or a result of systemic causes (hepatic disease, renal disease, lymphoma, adverse drug reaction, systemic and skin infection including *Staphylococcus aureus* and Pityrosporum). However, it may occur as a primary symptom of HIV. Eosinophilic folliculitis is an intensely pruritic eruption characteristically occurring in HIV-positive individuals with a CD_4 count less than 300/μL. Clinically, it presents with follicular and non-follicular urticarial papules and plaques, which may or may not be pustular on the upper trunk, extremities and face.

Itching in Senescence

At least 50 percent of persons aged 70 years or older will suffer from prolonged bouts of troublesome pruritus. Pruritic skin diseases such as scabies, lichen planus, prebullous pemphigoid, pemphigoid nodularis, or low-grade eczema should be considered, as well as underlying systemic disease, especially cholestasis and renal failure. However, in many instances, no cause is found. In many of these cases, the cause is desiccation of the skin due to a combination of decline in natural moisturizing factors in ageing skin and low atmospheric humidity, as in a heated institutional environment. Occasionally, the pruritus may be provoked by water contact, mimicking aquagenic pruritus (discussed below). However, unlike true aquagenic pruritus, water-evoked itching in senescent skin responds well to emollient treatment.

Itching as a Manifestation of Psychiatric Disease

Localized pruritus, especially anogenital pruritus, is a common manifestation of chronic anxiety, although candidiasis with or without accompanying diabetes mellitus, pinworms, and dermatitis medicamentosa must always be excluded. In cases in which these have been excluded, sympathetic explanation of the cause of the itch, advice regarding local hygiene, change in lifestyle, and prescription of a mild anxiolytic drug such as a beta blocker may be all that is required. If the localized area is persistently rubbed, lichenification may develop (lichen simplex, neurodermatitis). Parasitophobia is a much more serious problem, the patient persisting in claiming skin infestation, although careful inspection reveals no evidence of parasites. The patient will often bring "evidence" in the form of collected fragments, although on examination the material proves to be nonspecific debris. Such patients have a delusional psychosis and a psychiatric referral is wise.

MISCELLANEOUS

Aquagenic Pruritus

Characteristically, local itching is provoked by contact with water at any temperature, provoking a bout of itching lasting for 30 to 60 min, with no visible signs in the skin. During attacks patients are usually considerably distressed, but there are no other systemic manifestations. Laboratory investigations are negative, but occasionally patients with aquagenic pruritus and normal blood indices can progress to polycythemia vera. The condition must be distinguished from water-induced itching of the elderly (unlike true aquagenic pruritus, this condition is relieved by emollients) and from the "bath itch" of polycythemia vera.

Nostalgia Paraesthetica

This is a common, chronic localized itch, affecting mainly the interscapular area especially the T2-T6 dermatomes, but occasionally with a more widespread distribution, involving the shoulders, back, and upper chest. The sensation perceived by the patient is part itch, part paraesthesia. There are no specific cutaneous signs, apart from those attributed to scratching and rubbing. Amyloid deposition may be found in skin biopsies, but this is a secondary event. The current view on etiology is that it is a neuropathic itch due to entrapment of spinal nerves as they emerge through the epaxial muscles of the back. It may respond to topical capsaicin treatment.

Brachioradial Pruritus

This localized pruritus is becoming increasingly common. Patients develop persistent pruritus of the outer surface of the upper arm, elbow and forearm, associated with clinical evidence of chronic sun damage and xerosis in the pruritic skin. The itch may gradually become more widespread. Results of phototesting are negative and the problem seems consequent upon straightforward chronic ultraviolet overexposure. It may respond to capsaicin cream.

Itching in Atopic Eczema

This remains a controversial area and the molecular basis of pruritus in atopic eczema remains largely unexplained. Whether the itch precedes the eczema, or the other way round is also an unresolved issue. What is certain is that an itch-scratch vicious cycle exists in atopic patients, in which scratch damage enhances itch. Itching is particularly acute in response to punctate stimuli such as wool fibers; rubbing

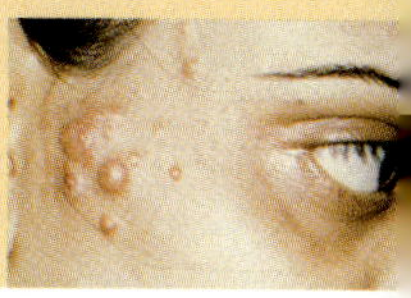

or scratching elicits surround inhibition. Allokinesis is a prominent feature of the itch of atopic eczema and explains the bouts of intense itching associated with sweating, sudden changes in temperature, dressing, and undressing. That there is a central (neurogenic) component to the itch of atopic eczema is suggested by the poor response to low sedation H 1 antihistamines. This also suggests that histamine is not a major mediator of atopic eczema; alternative candidates include cytokines. Opioid peptides may serve as central mediators because opioid antagonists are effective in some patients. Nocturnal scratching is a major problem in atopic eczema, occurs during sleep stages 1 and 2 (superficial sleep), and occupies 10 to 20 percent of the total sleeping time, leading to tiredness and irritability. Treatment should be directed first at managing dryness and infection—two important and remediable causes of itch. Sedative antihistamines may be useful. Topical steroids **allay** itching where this is a result of inflamed skin, using the lowest effective concentration. Phototherapy (UVB, photochemotherapy) may be effective in some patients. For selected, severely handicapped, treatment-resistant patients, recourse may be made to oral azathioprine or to cyclosporin. Tacrolimus, a topically applied macrolide immunosuppressive with an action resembling that of oral cyclosporin, has been shown to be effective in relieving the pruritus of atopic eczema.

SPECIFIC INVESTIGATIONS IN CASE OF PRURITUS

- Careful medication history.
- Complete physical examination.
- Complete blood count with differential.
- Thyroid function testing.
- Blood urea nitrogen, creatinine .
- Hepatic function testing .
- Fasting glucose.
- Chest radiograph (posteroanterior and lateral).
- Age-appropriate cancer screening.

Additional Testing to Consider

- HIV testing.
- Erythrocyte sedimentation rate.
- Serum iron and ferritin.
- Serum protein electrophoresis, urine protein electrophoresis.
- Stool for ova and parasites.

MANAGEMENT

The management of pruritus depends upon the cause, which may not be apparent. Presence of a rash and localization are two clues that can provide important information. Many dermatoses cause itch and it is beyond the scope of this chapter to discuss them all. In the search for a primary dermatosis, one must look for xerosis and scabies, because both can have subtle findings. Generalized pruritus (GP) can be defined as widespread itch without an identifiable primary rash, though nonspecific secondary changes may be present. In GP, the possibility of systemic disease should be considered and evaluation undertaken. A complete history and physical examination is mandatory. Interval re-evaluation should be undertaken because pruritus may precede the diagnosis of systemic disease by months to years.

In patients with generalized itching, with or without a rash, one of the more common and embarrassing errors is to miss the diagnosis of scabies; the most serious error is to miss the diagnosis of an underlying systemic disease such as Hodgkin's disease or hyperthyroidism. When it happens, failure to diagnose an underlying systemic illness tends to occur in the setting of a non-diagnostic dermatitis that has been created by rubbing and scratching, but is mistaken for a primary skin disease.

Other causes of GP to consider are psychogenic pruritus and, after all other causes have been excluded, idiopathic pruritus. Idiopathic pruritus is common in the elderly and may be a result of age-related changes of central and/or peripheral neural pathways. It is also important to consider localized forms of pruritus that can go undiagnosed for quite some time. By the time patients fail to respond to various treatments and obtain a dermatology referral, the itch has often been going on for months. The patients can hardly recall where the itch began and secondary changes hide the primary dermatosis. Aggressive treatment of the rash and pruritus may be effective and then reveal a previously localized itch.

TREATMENT

First Line Therapies

Localized pruritus

- Topical capsaicin.
- Lidocaine patch.
- Topical doxepin.

Generalized pruritus (also useful in hepatic or uremic pruritus)

- Emollients.
- Patient education regarding skin care regimen.
- Antihistamines (for their sedative effect).
- Doxepin.

Cholestatic pruritus

- Cholestyramine.
- Naltrexone.

Uremic pruritus

- UVB phototherapy.
- Erythropoietin.

Second Line Therapies

Generalized pruritus

- UVB phototherapy.
- PUVA.
- Gabapentin.
- Naltrexone.
- Mirtazapine.

Cholestatic pruritus

- Rifampin.
- Ursodeoxycholic acid.
- SSRIs.

Uremic pruritus

- Activated charcoal.
- Cholestyramine.
- Naltrexone.

Third Line Therapies

- Thalidomide.

In the case of most eczematous dermatoses, topical *corticosteroids* or *calcineurin inhibitors* are effective in treating the rash and relieving itch. In the case of xerosis, which may be difficult to recognize, an adequate skin care regimen and *emollients* are indispensable. A good skin care regimen involves the use of unscented bath oils, a humidifier, and the liberal use of emollients, especially after bathing. Irritating soaps, friction from washcloths, and prolonged hot showers should be avoided. In systemic disease, *treating the underying cause is essential*, but symptomatic treatment is often required (e.g. UVB phototherapy for hemodialysis patients with GP). In the management of pruritus that does not respond to simple measures, treatment should be stepwise and individualized based on severity.

Topical corticosteroid treatment may be tried if there is clinical evidence of inflammation. *Cooling agents* such as menthol may be applied liberally and can provide immediate relief in some cases. *Capsaicin* may be a good option for areas of localized itch, but is not practical for total body application. *UVB phototherapy* has been reported to relieve itch in patients with idiopathic GP, cholestasis and renal itch.

Sedating antihistamines are often employed in therapy for patients with itch; it is important to remember that their benefit derives from their soporific side effect. Nonsedating antihistamines may be of benefit, but are not reliably effective unless the disorder is mediated by histamine. The tricyclic antidepressant *doxepin* is a very potent antihistamine; it is unknown if any aspect of its antipruritic effect is independent of sedation. *Amitriptyline* and *mirtazapine* have been effective in brachioradial pruritus and lymphoma associated pruritus, respectively. *Selective serotonin reuptake inhibitors (SSRIs) paroxetine* and *fluoxetine* have improved pruritus in patients with polycythemia vera. *Gabapentin* has been effective in brachioradial pruritus, but its effect on GP has not yet been reported. Opioid antagonists, *Naltrexone,* have proven effective in randomized and open trials in a number of pruritic conditions.

Cholestatic Pruritus

Treatments for the itch of cholestasis may be targeted at decreasing levels of bile acid or blocking opioid action. *Cholestyramine* and *ursodeoxycholic* acid bind to bile acids in the intestinal tract and interrupt enterohepatic circulation. *Rifampin* and *phenobarbital* are hepatic enzyme inducers that may be effective in suppressing pruritus of cholestasis. *Naltrexone,* and *naloxone* were effective in randomized controlled trials. Opioid antagonists may precipitate a withdrawal syndrome in cholestatic patients due to high levels of endogenous opioids. Paroxetine and mirtazapine have been reported to improve itch in small series of patients with cholestasis. *Ondansetron,* a 5-HT3 receptor antagonist, has shown conflicting results in randomized, controlled trials.

Uremic Pruritus

Uremic pruritus is a misnomer because blood urea levels do not correlate with itch. UVB phototherapy is a mainstay of treatment and both narrowband and broadband are effective. Emollients improve xerosis and a good skin care regimen can help relieve itch. In patients with elevated calcium and phosphorus, *Parathyroidectomy* may lead to improvement of pruritus. *Erythropoietin* was found to improve pruritus and should be considered in any patients not already on this drug. Activated charcoal and thalidomide have been effective in clinical trials. Opioid antagonists were effective in one randomized controlled trial, but subsequent studies have not duplicated these results.

REFERENCES

- Treatment of Skin Disease, 2nd edn., Mark G Lebwohl, WR Heymann 2006.
- Evaluation of the patient with generalized pruritus, Kantor GR, In: Bernhard, JD edn. Itch: Mechanisms and management of pruritus. New York: McGraw-Hill; 1994:337-46.

- The diagnostic and therapeutic approach to idiopathic generalized pruritus. Yosipovitch G, David M. Int J Dermatol 1999; 38: 881-87.
- Pruritus in chronic liver disease: Mechanisms and treatment. Bergasa NY, Curr Gastroenterol Rep 2004; 6:10-16.
- Clinical evaluation of 40% urea and 12% ammonium lactate in the treatment of xerosis, Ademola J, Frazier C, Kim SJ, *et al.* Am J Clin Dermatol 2002; 3:217-22.
- Comparative efficacy of 12% ammonium lactate lotion and 5% lactic acid lotion in the treatment of moderate to severe xerosis, Rogers RS III, Callen J, Wehr R, Krochmal L.J. Am Acad Dermatol 1989; 21:714-16.

CHAPTER 24

THERAPY

Medical

BASIC PRINCIPLES

Treatment of most of the common skin conditions is simpler to understand when the physician is aware of three **basic principles:**

- The type of skin lesion, more than the cause, influences the kind of local medication used. The old **adage, "If it's wet, dry it with a wet dressing, and if it's dry, wet it with an ointment",** is true in most cases. For example, to treat a patient with an acute, oozing, crusting dermatitis of the dorsum of the hand, the physician should prescribe wet soaks. For a chronic-looking, dry, scaly patch of psoriasis on the elbow, an ointment is indicated because it holds moisture in the skin; an aqueous lotion or a wet dressing is more drying. Bear in mind, however, that the type of skin lesion can change rapidly under treatment. The patient must be followed closely after beginning therapy. An acute oozing dermatitis treated with water soaks can change, in 2 or 3 days, to a dry, scaly lesion that requires an ointment. Conversely, a chronic dry patch may become irritated with greasy ointment and begin to ooze.
- The **second basic principle** in treatment is first *do no harm and never overtreat*. It is important for the physician to know which of the chemicals prescribed for local use on the skin are the greatest irritants and sensitizers. It is no exaggeration to say that a commonly seen dermatitis is overtreatment contact dermatitis. The overtreatment is often performed by the patient, who has gone to the neighborhood chemist, or to a friend, and used any, and many, of the medications available for the treatment of skin diseases.
- **The third principle is to instruct the patient adequately** regarding the application of the medicine prescribed. The patient does not have to be told how to swallow a pill, but does have to be told how to put on a wet dressing. Most patients with skin disorders are ambulatory, so there is no nurse to help them; they are their own nurses. The success or the failure of therapy rests on adequate instruction of the patient or person responsible for the care. Even in hospitals, particularly when wet dressings or aqueous lotions are prescribed, it is wise for the physician to instruct the nurse regarding the procedure.
- Carefully instruct the patient or nurse regarding the local application of salves, lotions, wet dressings and baths. Thin coats of topical medications save money and are equally as effective as thick coats. Number of applications are more important than how thick the medication is put on. Also, applying medications *after hydration* such as bath, showers, and hand washing increases penetration and makes topical therapy more effective. Effectiveness can also be increased by occlusion.
- Change the therapy as the response indicates. If a new prescription is indicated and the patient has some of the first prescription left, instruct the patient to alternate using the old and new prescriptions.
- If a prescription is going to be relatively expensive, explain this fact to the patient.
- For many diseases, "therapy plus" is indicated. Advise the patient to continue to treat the skin problem for a specified period after the dermatosis has apparently cleared. This may prevent or slow down recurrences.
- Instruct the patient to telephone you if there are any questions or if the medicine appears to irritate the dermatosis.

TOPICAL THERAPY

Topical therapy is the most important aspect of dermatologic therapy. To be a good dermatologist, the basic knowledge of what vehicle to choose, how much to give, how often to apply it is very important. **Vehicle** includes all the constituents of formulation apart from active ingredients.

Factors determining choice of ideal vehicle: Ideal vehicle should be non toxic, non allergic, non irritant, stable, chemically inert, cosmetically acceptable and should not inactivate the drug. Vehicles include ointment, cream, gel, lotion, paste, powder.

Frequency of Application

- Frequent and liberal application of emollient.
- Even once daily application of corticosteroid is sufficient.
  - Frequency of application is not proportionate to the efficacy. On the other hand excessive topical application can result in irritation, systemic exposure to drug and unwanted side effects.

Quantity to be Applied

Rule of thumb for calculating BSA is that the surface area of one palm is about 0.5% of the total BSA. Rule of nines, as used in burns treatment, can be applied to estimate larger areas (each arm, each lower leg or foot, each thigh, anterior trunk, posterior trunk, and head and neck each account for 9% of BSA).

Quantity of Cream or Ointment to Prescribe (Fig. 24.1)

Several factors influence any general statements about dosage: the severity of the dermatosis, whether it is acute or chronic dermatosis, the base of the product (a petrolatum-based ointment spreads over the skin farther than a cream and is more moisturizing), whether it is dispensed in a tube or jar (patients use less from tubes), and the intelligence of the patient.

- 15 g of a cream used b.i.d. treats a mild hand dermatosis for 10 to 14 days.

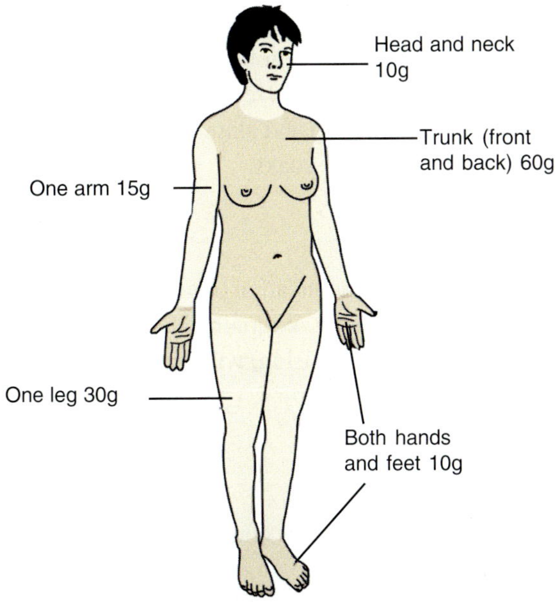

Fig. 24.1: Amount of cream required for different body parts

- 30 g of a cream used b.i.d. treats an arm for 14 days.
- 60 g of a cream used b.i.d. treats a leg for 14 days.
- 480 to 960 g or 1 to 2 lb of a cream used b.i.d. treats the entire body for 14 days. This is seldom a practical prescription, but unmedicated white petrolatum or a cream base is economical to use over a large surface area. Other therapeutic agents should be used to make the dermatoses less extensive (i.e., internal corticosteroids).

FTU (Finger tip unit)—Weight of a strip of cream or ointment squeezed from a tube and extending from the tip of the finger to the crease at the distal interphalangeal joint in an adult is 0.5 g. It is particularly useful for topical corticosteroid measurement.

Rule of Hand: Adult flat hand = 2 FTU = 1 gm ointment.

Time of Application

The best time to apply most medications is soon after bath when skin is hydrated (Increased penetration and efficacy) and clean. If both topical steroid and an emollient are to be used, the *steroid should be applied first followed by an emollient.*

Occlusion

Leads to increased penetration and efficacy. This can be done with plastic wrap, gloves, vinyl suit or shower cap for the scalp. Caution must be exercised with occlusion, as it can make the ultrapotent steroids too strong.

COMMON EXTRANEOUS FORMULATIONS

Creams are semisolid preparation containing both water and alcohol.

Two Types

- **Oil in water emulsion:** Also called aqueous cream or vanishing cream.
- **Water in oil emulsion:** Also called cold cream or oily cream.

Ointments

- Semisolid preparation that spread easily. Occlusive, hydrating, lubricating action. They are greasy, stain clothes, do not require preservative.

Gels

- Liquify on coming in contact with skin.
- **Sites:** Hair bearing areas, face.
- Nongreasy water washable, transparent, easy to apply and remove.
- **Disadvantages:** Require preservative, removed by perspirations.

Foams

Foams are pressurized dosage form containing active ingredient that upon valve actuation, emits fine dispersion of solid or liquid material in gaseous medium.

Used in psoriasis, eczema, seborrheic dermatitis.

Powders

Powders are the solid vehicles that absorb moisture and decrease friction, maceration along with antiseptic antifungal action.

- They also have cooling, soothing, protective and covering properties.

Lotions

- **Sites:** Scalp and other hairy areas, intertriginous areas.
- **Advantages:** Easy to apply, allow uniform coating and are preferred in children.
- **Disadvantages:** Require shaking, require preservatives, more drying than ointment.

Pastes

- Paste are much more stiffer and drying than ointments. They are less occlusive and less greasy.

Tincture

- It is an alcoholic solution or extract of non volatile substance.
- Solution of volatile substance is called spirit.

Baths and Soaks

- Used in treating widespread disease.
- Soothing, antipruritic, anti inflammatory action.

Emollients

The use of emollients is widespread. They are oily substances which form occlusive film over skin surface, prevent evaporation thus restore skin hydration. They sooth and soften the skin. Emollients are critically important in treating certain diseases, most notably the eczemas. In eczema, the barrier function of the skin is damaged and the water content reduced. Hydrating the skin with a shower or bath followed immediately by the application of a cream or ointment (no lotions) locks in the moisture and helps repair the barrier. Emollients help to reduce scaling in numerous other dermatoses, such as psoriasis.

In acute but non-infected exacerbations of eczema, application of emollients under damp tubular dressings (wet wraps) can be effective in some children. Particularly aimed at atopic dermatitis, in which staphylococcal infection is common, some emollients for direct application or for use in the bath are manufactured in plain versions or in versions with added antiseptic agents.

Wet Compresses

Used in the treatment of wet, exudative skin disease.They have anti inflammatory action and anti bacterial action.

Condy's Compresses

- Potassium permanganate is the agent used.
- It is used for wet dressing in concentration of 1:4000 – 1: 16000 dilution.
- It has astringent, antiseptic, fungicidal activity against candida. It also has oxidizing properties.
- **Disadvantages:** It stains and burns the skin. It gets rapidly inactivated.

Soaps

Occasionally, antibacterial soaps or skin-cleansing agents (sometimes as a bath additive) are recommended for patients with chronic *S. aureus* infection of the skin.

Soaks and Astringents

Soaks are often prescribed for exudative skin disease. The benefits are multiple and include a soothing effect on the skin, debridement, and potentially delivery of medication.

Potassium permanganate solution is useful as a soak for exudative pompholyx or venous eczema, having both astringent and antibacterial effects. Silver nitrate 0.5% (which also causes staining) and aluminum acetate solution are also used as astringent soaks.

Wraps

Wrapping the skin after application of topical agents can be very soothing to atopic skin. Wrapping after the application of a topical steroid (i.e. occlusion) will augment the potency of the steroid.

TOPICAL STEROIDS

As steroids constitute a major component of dermatology practice it is pertinent to begin with them. Below is an overview of the classification of the strength of steroids. (Tables 24.1 and 24.2).

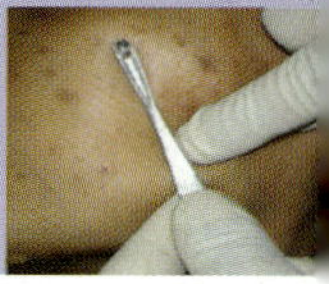

Table 24.1: Potency ranking of some commonly used topical corticosteroids*

Group I Clobetasol propionate cream/oint 0.05% Betamethasone diproprionate cream/oint 0.05% Halobetasone cream 0.05% Halobetasone ointment 0.05%	**Group IV** Mometasone furoate cream 0.1% Fluocinonide ointment 0.025% Fluocininide cream 0.2% Triamcinolone acetonide oint 0.1%
Group II Fluocinonide cream/oint 0.05% Mometasone furoate 0.1% Triamcinolone acetonide oint 0.5%	**Group V** Betamethasone valerate cream 0.1% Betamethasone valerate lotion 0.1% Fluticasone cream 0.1% Hydrocortisone butyrate cream 0.1% Prednicarbate cream 0.1 %
Group III Betamethasone valerate ointment 0.1% Fluticasone ointment 0.005% Triamcinolone acetonide cream 0.5%	**Group VI** Betamethasone valerate 0.1% Desonide cream 0.05% ointment 0.05% Fluocinolone cream 0.01% Fluocinolone solution 0.01%
	Group VII Methyprednisolone cream 1% Hydrocortisone cream 1.0%, 2.5% Hydrocortisone lotion 1.0%, 2.5%

* Group I is the superpotency category. Potency descends with each group, to group VII, which is the least potent (groups II and III are potent corticosteroids; IV and V are midstrength corticosteroids; VI and VII are mild corticosteroids). There is no significant difference between agents within groups II through VII. The compounds are arranged alphabetically within the groups.

Table 24.2: Topical steroids

Actions	**Anti-inflammatory** 1. Vasoconstriction 2. Decrease premeability of dermal vessels 3. Decrease phagocytic migration and activity 4. Depress fibroblastic activity 5. Decrease kinin formation 6. Inhibit phospholipase A2 activity and decrease products of arachidonic acid metabolism 7. Decrease fibrin formation 8. Stabilize lysosomal membranes **Immunosuppressive** Antigen—antibody interaction unaffected but inflammatory consequences lessened by above mechanisms and by inhibiting cytokines (e.g. IFN-α GM-CSF, IL-1,2,3 and TNF-α) Lympholytic Decrease epidermal proliferation
Side-effects	1. Thinning of epidermis 2. Thinning of dermis 3. Telangiectasia and striae 4. Bruising 5. Hirsutism 6. Folliculitis and acneiform eruptions 7. May worsen or disguise infections (bacterial, viral and fungal) 8. Systemic absorption (rare but may be important in infants, when applied in large quantities under polyethylene pants) 9. Tachyphylaxis—lessening of clinical effect with the same preparation 10. Rebound—worsening, sometimes dramatic on withdrawing treatment
Use	Eczema, proriasis in some instances (facial, flexural, and palms/soles) Many non-infective, inflammatory dermatoses.

GM-CSF, granulocyte macrophage colony-stimulating factor; IFN interferon; IL, interleukin; TNF, tumour necrosis factor.

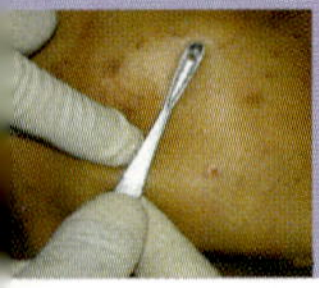

Guidelines for the Use of Topical Corticosteroids (TCS)

- Use TCS only when indicated.
- Avoid the use if high potency steroid i.e. group1 and 2 in children particularly in prepubertal age because on systemic absorption they cause growth retardation and premature closure of epiphysis.
- Moderate potency steroid should be used on trunk and extremities.
- Low potency steroid should be used on face, axillae groin, neck and diaper area.
- Limit use to once or twice daily application.
- Limit duration of therapy to 7-14 days.
- Group1-2 TCS should not be used under occlusion.
- Diaper dermatitis should be treated with group 4,5,6 TCS because diapers act as an occlusive and increase absorption.
- Steroid holidays should be given either by completely stopping the drug or by substituting bland emollients.
- Clinician must be vigilant to observe the side effect of TCS in children.

Highly Steroid Responsive Dermatosis

- Psoriasis.
- Atopic dermatitis.
- Seborrheic dermatitis.
- Nummular dermatitis.
- Irritant dermatitis.
- Lichen simplex chronicus.

Contraindication of Topical Corticosteroid

Absolute– Hypersensitivity to TCS or other component.
Relative– Infection at site of application, infestation, ulceration or chronic wound.

Important Adverse Effect of TCS

Local

- Epidermal atrophy, shiny, lax, wrinkled skin.
- Striae, telangiectasia.
- Perioral dermatitis.
- Glaucoma.
- Hirsutism, folliculitis, miliaria.
- Granuloma gluteale infantum.
- Systemic absorption.

TOPICAL RETINOIDS

Topical retinoids (.025%,.05%,0.1%) are comedolytic and anti-inflammatory.

- They cause epidermal differentiation and, thus, normalize follicular hyperproliferation and hyperkeratinization.
- Topical retinoids reduce the numbers of microcomedones, comedones and inflammatory lesions.
- They may be used alone or in combination with other acne medications.
- The most commonly prescribed topical retinoids include **adapalene** (0.1%) gel, **tazarotene (0.05-0.01%),** and tretinoin (0.025%, 0.05%, 0.1%).
- These retinoids should be applied once daily to clean, dry skin, but they may need to be applied less frequently if irritation occurs.
- Skin irritation with peeling and redness may be associated with the use of topical retinoids.

Tretinoin

It was initially used in acne for its comedolytic effect, but later it was found to decrease wrinkles and improve the signs of aging. As with other topical retinoids, it is usually prescribed in combination with an antimicrobial agent. Tretinoin helps open the pore, whereas the antimicrobial agent reduces the number of **P. acnes**.

Adapalene

It is both chemically and photochemically stable. It is applied once a day and is equivalent to tretinoin in terms of efficacy for acne.

Isotretinoin

Topical isotretinoin is used in treatment of acne.

Tazarotene

It is used for both acne and psoriasis. It has maximum efficacy in the treatment of acne as compared to adapalene and retinoic acid. For maximum benefit, it should be combined with antimicrobials. Tazarotene may also be used in psoriasis, usually with once daily application. Irritation is the most frequent side effect and can be minimized with the concomitant use of a topical steroid. An added benefit of this combination is that topical retinoids can reduce or prevent the atrophogenic effects of steroids. Tazarotene 0.1% cream was found effective against photoaging, with benefit similar to that of tretinoin 0.05%.

Tazarotene is contraindicated in pregnant women.

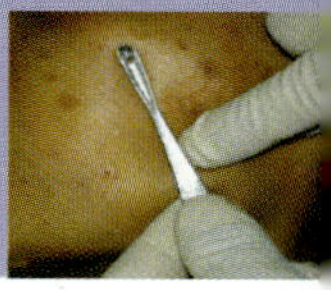

Bexarotene

Topical treatment for early stages of mycosis fungoides.

TOPICAL AGENTS FOR ACNE

Benzoyl peroxide: Benzoyl peroxide remains an excellent agent in the treatment of acne. Its has excellent ability to kill **P. acnes.**

Furthermore, bacterial resistance does not occur. Washes are less effective compared with the usually recommended water-based gels.

Azelaic acid: It has antimicrobial and anti comedonal actions. However, it is also used as a depigmenting agent, particularly for disorders such as melasma.

Topical antibiotics are not comedolytic, and bacterial resistance may develop to any of these agents.

- Commonly prescribed topical antibiotics include erythromycin and clindamycin alone or in combination with benzoyl peroxide (Combination should decrease the potential problem of resistance).

Sulphur-2-10%: Messy but safe.

Metronidazole

Topical metronidazole is used in treatment of rosacea.

AGENTS FOR SKIN INFECTIONS (Table 24.3)

Bacterial Infection

Antiseptics destroy or inhibit bacteria, fungi and viruses.

Table 24.3: A summary of common topical antibiotics/ antiseptics

Alcohol 70%	Gram +bacteria
Aluminium Hexahydrate 20%	Gram +, yeasts, Dermatophytes
Bacitracin	Gram +, anaerobes, tetanus, diphtheria
Chlorhexidine	Gram +/-, Pseudomonas, yeasts,
Gentamicin	Gram-/+, Pseudomonas, proteus,
Iodine	Bacteria, fungi, yeast, protozoa
Mupironic acid	Gram +, MRSA

Several antibiotics are available topically, including the following:

Aminoglycosides and polymyxins (e.g. neomycin)—Often used for otitis and some wounds, but contact sensitivity is relatively frequent.

Mupirocin—Mainly used for staphylococcal infection, but increasingly being reserved for infections due to *methicillin-resistant staphylococcus aureus (MRSA).*

Silver sulfadiazine—Especially used for burns.

Fusidic acid—Used for staphylococcal infection, and available as a combination product with steroids for infected eczema, but increasing bacterial resistance problems mean that use should be limited to short courses. An oral antibiotic is preferred for widespread impetigo or infected eczema.

Metronidazole—Mainly used for malodorous wounds, ulcers, or ulcerated tumors.

Antiseptics—These have a wider spectrum of activity than that of antibiotics; many are used topically, such as povidone–iodine, chlorhexidine, etc.

PREPARATIONS FOR PSORIASIS

Tar preparations—Tars may be derived from coal, wood (Cade oil), or fish (ichthammol and ichthyol) sources. They are anti-inflammatory and antiproliferative, and are helpful in psoriasis and in some eczemas.

Tars (coal tar solution, 3% to 10%; crude coal tar, 1% to 5%).

Coal tar (3-6%)—Keratoplastic and anti-inflammatory. Also available in combination-6% coal tar with 3% salicylic acid.

Consider for use in cases of:

- Atopic eczema.
- Psoriasis.
- Seborrheic dermatitis.
- Lichen simplex chronicus.
- Avoid in intertriginous areas (can cause a folliculitis and irritation).

Dithranol (anthralin) (0.02-2%)—Synthetic derivative of a tree bark extract. One of the most effective antipsoriatic agents available.

It reduces epidermal mitotic activity. Use alone or in combination with salicylic acid.

Disadvantage—Stain normal skin and clothing and is an irritant.

Calcipotriene is a synthetic vitamin D3 analog that regulates skin cell production and development. Inhibits epidermal proliferation, promotes keratinocyte differentiation, and has immunosuppressive effects on lymphoid cells.

Used in the treatment of moderate plaque psoriasis.

Tazarotene (0.05%, 0.1%)—Keratolytic and keratoplastic. Has irritant potential.

TOPICAL ANTI FUNGAL INFECTION

Agents available to treat fungal infections include the following:

Imidazoles—Several are available (e.g., ketoconazole, clotrimazole, miconazole etc.); they can treat yeasts or dermatophytes.

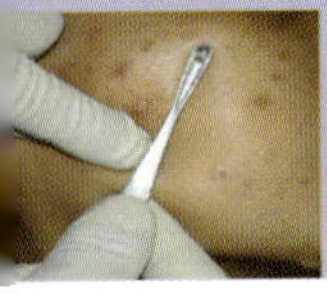

Allylamines (e.g. terbinafine)—They can treat yeasts or dermatophytes when used topically, and are fungicidal. It has the advantage of a fungicidal activity, whereas the imidazoles are fungistatic and usually less rapid in achieving benefit.

Nystatin (a polyene)—Usually reserved for the treatment of candida infection.

Amorolfine (a morpholine)—Used topically for nail dermatophyte infection, but benefit is usually limited to distal infection of relatively non-thickened nails; it is useful for superficial white onychomycosis and has activity against some moulds.

Ciclopirox olamine has a broad spectrum of action.

Undecylenic acid—It has notably lower potency.

ANTI VIRAL AGENTS

Topical aciclovir and related agents such as penciclovir are available for herpes simplex infection.

CALCINEURIN INHIBITORS

These are topical agents primarily used for treatment of eczema (mainly atopic dermatitis), psoriasis, vitiligo, discoid lupus erythematosus, and oral lichen planus.

Tacrolimus is a calcineurin inhibitor that is effective in treating atopic dermatitis in both adults and children. Applied twice daily. It is particularly effective for the face and neck but, unlike with topical steroids, there is no risk of skin atrophy. Patients using it for the first time should be told to expect itching and/or burning. Tacrolimus can be combined with phototherapy to improve vitiligo.

Pimecrolimus: Used for atopic dermatitis. As with tacrolimus, its great advantage over steroids is its lack of atrophic side effects.

OTHER TOPICAL AGENTS

Hydroquinone and Related Hypopigmenting Agents

Hydroquinone is a topical bleaching agent used primarily in melasma at concentrations of 2-5%. At higher concentrations, it can paradoxically cause increased pigmentation in the form of exogenous ochronosis. The combination of fluocinolone acetonide 0.01%, hydroquinone 4%, and tretinoin 0.05% is more efficacious at reducing pigmentation than any of these agents alone.

Azelaic acid also has a depigmenting activity.

Antiperspirants

The most commonly used antiperspirants agents contain aluminum chloride hexahydrate. They should ideally be applied at night, when sweating is at its least.

Use of glycopyrronium bromide, an anticholinergic agent, for its antiperspirant effect is most commonly as an additive to enhance the effect of iontophoresis but it can also be obtained in a cream base for application to the skin. Formaldehyde also has an antiperspirant effect and is sometimes used as a treatment for plantar hyperhidrosis.

5-Fluorouracil

5-Fluorouracil is a topical agent that selectively kills photodamaged keratinocytes. It is effective at reducing actinic keratoses and in treatment of Bowen disease, actinic cheilitis. It usually causes significant inflammation, crusting, and even erosion.

Imiquimod

Imiquimod is an immune modifier with antiviral and antineoplastic activities.

Mechanism of Action

Stimulation of production of proinflammatory cytokines through Toll-like receptor on the surface of dendritic cells of monocyte-macrophage lineage. This activation stimulates the patient's own immune system to attack both virally infected and tumor cells. Imiquimod is proved effective against genital warts as well as in treatment of superficial malignancies and their precursors, for example actinic keratoses, Bowen disease, superficial basal cell carcinoma, and lentigo maligna. It may have some benefit in the treatment of common warts and molluscum contagiosum.

Antipruritic Agents

They relieve itching in various ways. Commonly used chemicals include menthol (0.25%), phenol (0.5%), camphor (2%), pramoxine hydrochloride (1%), and coal tar solution.

These chemicals are added to various bases for the desired effect. Numerous safe and unsafe proprietary preparations for relief of itching are also available. The unsafe preparations are those that contain sensitizing antihistamines, benzocaine, and related-caine derivatives.

Keratoplastic Agents

Tend to increase the thickness of the horny layer. Salicylic acid (1% to 2%) is an example of a keratoplastic agent.

Keratolytics

Eemove or soften the horny layer. Commonly used agents of this type include salicylic acid (4% to 10%), resorcinol (2% to 4%), urea (20% to 50%) and sulfur (4% to 10%).

Urea in 5% to 10% concentration is moisturizing, whereas in 20% to 50% concentration, it is keratolytic.

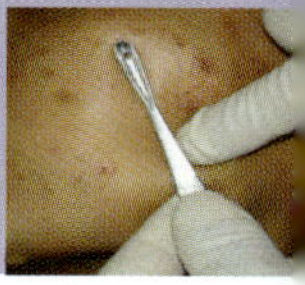

Alpha hydroxy acids, glycolic acid in 5% to 12% concentrations are moisturizers, whereas in higher concentrations upto 80%, they are keratolytic and can be used in the office for facial peeling, with caution.

Antiparasitic Agents

Destroy or inhibit living infestations. Examples include 5% permethrin cream for scabies, γ-benzene hexachloride cream and lotion for scabies and 1% for pediculosis, crotamiton for scabies, and permethrin 1% for pediculosis.

For scabies and lice, *10% sulfur* can be mixed in petrolatum and is effective and very safe, even in **infants and pregnant women,** but is malodorous and stains.

Minoxidil

Used for androgenic alopecias in either sex.

Eflornithine

Used for treatment of hirsutism. It inhibits ornithine decarboxylase. Benefits vary and are not usually apparent before 1 - 2 months. Relapse occurs when it is discontinued.

Sulfur (Sulfur Precipitated 3% to 10%)

Consider for use in cases of:

- Tinea of any area of body.
- Acne vulgaris and rosacea.
- Seborrheic dermatitis.

SUNSCREENS

Sunscreens are primarily used for photosensitive skin disease (Table 24.4).

Table 24.4: Classification and action spectrum of photosensitive skin disease

Photosensitive skin disease	*UVB*	*UVA*	*Visible*
Idiopathic			
Polymorphous light eruption	+	++	—
Hydroa vacciniforme	+	++	—
Solar urticaria	+	++	++
Chronic actinic dermatitis	+++	++	—
Exogenous chemical			
Photoallergic contact dermatitis	—	+++	—
Photoirritant contact dermatitis	—	+++	+
Photodrug reactions	+	+++	+
Genetic and metabolic			
Porphyria	+++	—	+++
Xeroderma pigmentosa	+++	—	—
Cockayne's syndrome	—	+++	—
Smith-Lemli-Opitz	—	—	—
Photoaggravated			
Lupus erythematosus	+++	++	—

Types of Sunscreens

- **Chemical sunscreens** (Table 24.5)
  – E.g. PABA esters, cinnamates, benzophenones.
- **Physical sunscreens**
  – E.g. zinc oxide, titanium dioxide, calamine.
- **Systemic sunscreens**
  – E.g. chloroquin, beta carotene.
- **Others**
  – Dihydroxyacetone, tannic acid.

Table 24.5: Classification of sunscreens (chemical)

Organic sunscreen	*Protection*	*UVB*	*UVAII*	*UVAI*
Anthranilates				
Menthyl anthranilate	260-380	complete	complete	partial
Benzophenones				
Dioxybenzone	250-390	complete	complete	partial
Oxybenzone	270-350	complete	complete	partial
Sulisobenzone (Eusolex 4360)	260-375	complete	complete	partial
Cinnamates				
Octocrylene	250-360	complete	complete	partial
Octyl methoxycinnamate (Parsol MCX)	290-320	complete	—	—
Dibenzoylmethanes				
Avobenzone (Parsol 1789)	320-400	—	complete	complete

EFFECT OF UV ON SKIN

UVA

- UVA (range 320-400 nm).
- UVA1 (340-400 nm) and UVA II (320 to 340 nm).
- Midday UVR is 10% UVB, 90% UVA.
- Erythremogenic activity weak but penetrates dermis.
- Induces development of slow natural tan, drug induced photosensitivity reactions.
- UVA may augment the effects of UVB in causing sunburn, photo-aging and skin carcinogenesis.

UVB

- UVB (Range 290-320 nm).
- Highest erythemogenic activity.
- Produces sunburn, hyperpigmentation, Vitamin D synthesis.
- Chronic exposure – Photoaging and skin cancer.

GENERAL PRINCIPLES OF SUNSCREEN

- Sunscreens that absorb both ultraviolet (UVA) and UVB

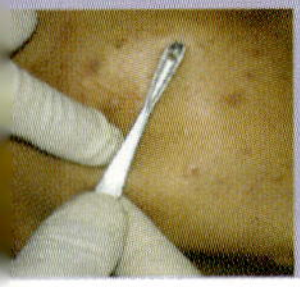

should be recommended, as drug-induced photosensitivity reactions are frequently caused by wavelengths within the UVA range.

- The ideal sunscreen should have a sun protection factor (SPF) of at least 15, and should be water resistant.
- Sunscreens should be applied daily to all sun-exposed areas *at least 30 min before* exposure to sunlight, and reapplied after swimming, washing, or perspiring heavily.
- Because 50% of ambient UV light is received in the shade, sitting in the shade does not protect against UV exposure.
- Patients should wear sun-protective clothing: tightly woven fabric, a broad-brimmed hat and sunglasses.
- Because *90% of UV light penetrates clouds,* patients should wear sunscreen and protective clothing even on cloudy days.
- Sun-blocking cosmetics can enhance appearance and self-esteem while shielding the skin from sunlight. In addition to using sunscreens, patients should also avoid sun exposure, particularly during the summer from 10 am-3 pm, even through window glass.
- Sun protection should include sunscreens if they do not contribute to the photosensitivity reaction.
- *Avoid sunscreens* that contain p-aminobenzoic acid (PABA) and/or benzophenones, which can sometimes cause photosensitivity or allergic contact dermatitis.
- *Fluorescent lights* should be covered *with plastic shields* to avoid leakage of UV radiation.
- If a patient notices that the sun can induce LE lesions through glass windows, film that blocks UV radiation should be applied to home, office, and automobile windows.
- Although some sunscreens can promote skin cancer, and sunlight avoidance can decrease Vitamin D levels, for photosensitive patients the benefits of sunlight protection greatly outweigh the risks. Vitamin D can be obtained in the diet or with supplements.

Sun Protection Factor

- SPF – The dose of UVR required to produce 1 minimal erythema dose (MED) on protected skin after application of $2mg/cm^2$ of product divided by the UVR to produce 1 MED on unprotected skin.
- Most available sunscreens provide good UVB protection.
- SPF is based on UVB exposure.

Physical Sunscreens

- Broad spectrum UVA and UVB radiation.
- Most common physical sunscreens—ZnO,Titanium dioxide.
- Near ideal sunscreens – chemically most, safe, photostable.
- Microsized particles reduce whitening appearance.
- Microfine ZnO has better absorption than Ti O2 at longer wavelength of UVA.

Sunscreen for Routine Use for Normal Skin in the Indian Context

- SPF protection does not actually increased proportionately with a designated SPF number.
- While SPF 2 equals 50% absorption, SPF 15 indicates 93% absorption and SPF 30 97% absorption.
- SPF 15- Adequate for routine use and cosmetically more acceptable.
- SPF **15+-** Compensates for inadequate use and for photodermatoses and persons *who stay mainly outdoors*.

Risks/Benefits

Although some sunscreens can promote skin cancer, and sunlight avoidance can decrease Vitamin D levels, for photosensitive patients the benefits of sunlight protection greatly outweigh the risks.

ANTIFUNGAL AGENTS (Table 24.6)

1. Allylamines (e.g. Terbinafine)

Inhibit squalene epoxidase to reduce ergosterol synthesis.

Topical treatment of choice for **tinea pedis**, tinea unguium and tinea coporis and tinea manuum.

For hyperkeratotic tinea pedis, oral therapy is preferred because it provides better skin penetration.

Good alternative (although more expensive) for **tinea barbae and tinea capitis.**

- **Adult oral:** 250 mg once daily.
- **Treatment course:** 2 weeks; 6 weeks for fingernail infections; 12 weeks for toenail infections.

Risk with Oral Therapy

- Safety and efficacy in pediatric patients under 12 years have not been established.
- Pregnancy category B. No well-controlled studies in pregnant women. Use only if potential benefits justify potential risks to fetus.
- Not recommended in breast-feeding due to limited data.

Oral Therapy

- **Gastrointestinal:** Abdominal pain, anorexia, diarrhea, dyspepsia, elevated LFTs, flatulence, nausea, hepatotoxicty, taste disturbances.
- **Hematologic:** Blood cell disorders.
- **Musculoskeletal:** Arthralgia, myalgia.
- **Nervous:** Dizziness, fatigue, headache, hypoesthesia, malaise, paresthesia.

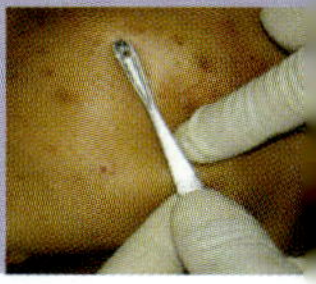

Table 24.6: Classification and mechanism of action of antifungal antibiotics

Class	*Representative drugs*	*Mechanism of action*	*Antifungal effects*
Polyenes	Nystatin	Interaction with ergosterol, formation of aqueous channels	Fungistatic and Fungicidal
	Amphotericin B	Increased membrane permeability and subsequent leakage of intracellular components	Fungicidal
Azoles		Inhibition of fungal lanosterol *14-a* demethylase resulting in depletion of ergosterol and accumulation of toxic sterols in the fungal cell membrane	Fungistatic
Imidazoles	Clotrimazole Econazole Ketoconazole Miconazole		
Triazoles	Fluconazole Itraconazole Voriconazole		*Candida:* time-dependent fungistatic *Aspergillus:* time-depend slow fungicidal
Allylamines	Naftine Terbinafine	Interferes with synthesis of ergosterol by inhibiting squalene 2,3-epoxidase that is responsible to convert squalene to squalene oxide	Dermatophytes: fungicidal *Candida:* fungistatic
Benzylamines	Butenafine		
Echinocandins	Caspofungin, Micafungin	Blocks I, 3-I3-D-glucan synthase resulting in depletion of cell wall glucan and osmotic instability	*Candida:* fungicidal Aspigillus: fungistatic
Hydroxypyridone	Ciclopirox	Inhibition of essential enzymes by creating a large polyvalent cation through chelation, thus interfering with mitochondrial electron transport processes and energy production	Fungicidal and fungistatic
Other antifungals	Griseofulvin	Inhibition of fungal cell mitosis and nucleic acid synthesis and interference with the function of spindles and cytoplasmic microtubules by binding to alpha and beta tubulin	Fungistatic

- **Skin:** Hair loss, photosensitivity, pruritis, rash, Stevens-Johnson syndrome, toxic epidermal necrolysis, urticaria.

Contraindications

- Hypersensitivity to terbinafine, or any other component.
- Pre-existing hepatic impairment with oral use, and potentially prolonged topical use.

2. Griseofulvin

Mechanism of Action

It inhibits fungal cell mitosis at *metaphase*; binds to human keratin making it resistant to fungal invasion.

Dosages

Adult

Microsize formulation

- **Oral:** 500-1000 mg once a day or in divided doses.
- **Treatment course:** Minimum of 4 months (fingernails); minimum of 6 months (toenails).

Ultramicrosize formulation

- **Oral:** 375-750 mg once a day or in divided doses.
- **Treatment course:** Minimum of 4 months (fingernails); minimum of 6 months (toenails).

Pediatric

Microsize formulation

- **Oral:** 10-15mg/kg/day.
- **Treatment course:** Minimum of 4 months (fingernails); minimum of 6 months (toenails); treat until nails become clinically normal.

Ultramicrosize formulation

- **Oral:** 5-10mg/kg/day.
- **Treatment course:** Minimum of 4 months (fingernails); minimum of 6 months (toenails); treat until nails become clinically normal.

Hepatic/Renal Impairment

Use with caution in hepatic impairment; contraindicated in severe **liver disease**.

Administration

Doses should be taken with or after food to minimize the incidence of gastrointestinal adverse effects.

Contraindications

- Hypersensitivity to griseofulvin, or any other component.
- Porphyria.
- Severe liver disease.

Monitor

- LFTs.
- Renal function.
- CBC.

Adverse Effects

- **Rare:** Photosensitivity, lupus erythematosus.

Interactions

- Alcohol (enhanced effect of alcohol).
- Cyclosporine (decreased serum cyclosporine level).
- Estrogens (reduced contraceptive effect).

Risks

- Use additional barrier contraceptive measures during treatment. Women should not try getting pregnant for at least one month after treatment has been completed, and men should not father children for at least 6 months after treatment completed as it may effect spermatogenesis.
- May cause lupus erythematosus, lupus-like syndromes, or exacerbation of existing lupus erythematosus.
- Pregnancy category C. Embryotoxic and teratogenic in animals. No adequate human studies. Chance of fetal harm, use only if potential benefits outweigh the potential risks to fetus.

3. Azoles

These inhibit sterol demethylase to reduce ergosterol synthesis, and include imidazoles (e.g. ketoconazole) and triazoles (e.g. itraconazole).

Itraconazole

Dose

Onychomycosis (toenails with or without fingernail involvement)

- **Adult oral:** 200 mg once daily.
- **Treatment course:** 12 consecutive weeks.

Onychomycosis (fingernails only)

- **Adult oral:** Two treatment pulses, each consisting of 200mg twice daily (400mg/day).
- **Treatment course:** One week.
- The pulses are separated by a 3-week period without itraconazole.

Contraindications

- Breast-feeding.

Fluconazole

- Fluconazole is an option in tinea pedis and tinea manuum infections, and as an alternative in tinea corporis infections.

Dose

Tinea pedis, tinea manuum, tinea corporis and tinea cruris:

- **Adult oral:** 150 mg once weekly.
- **Treatment course:** 3-4 weeks.

Tinea capitis:

- **Adult oral:** 50 mg once daily.
- **Treatment course:** 3 weeks.

Onychomycosis:

- **Adult oral:** 150 mg once weekly.
- **Treatment course:** 9 months.

Tinea versicolor:

- **Adult oral:** 400 mg once.
- **Treatment course:** Single dose.

Risks

- Safety and efficacy in pediatric patients under 6 months have not been established.
- Pregnancy category C. No adequate human studies. Chance of fetal harm, use only if potential benefits outweigh the potential risks to fetus.

ANTIHISTAMINES

Oral H-1 receptor antagonists antihistamines are widely used in dermatology.

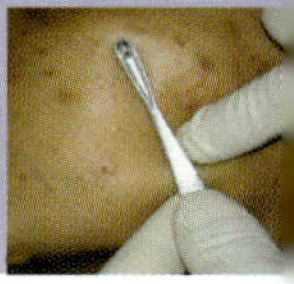

They include:

- **Conventional or first-generation 'sedating' antihistamines**, for example chlorpheniramine (chlorphenamine), cyproheptadine, hydroxyzine, and promethazine.
- **Second-generation 'non-sedating' antihistamines**, for example acrivastine, loratadine or desloratidine, cetirizine or levocetirizine, fexofenadine and mizolastine.

Other antihistaminic agents, such as cimetidine, work primarily at H_2 receptors causing inhibition of gastric secretion; still other experimental antihistamines act on presynaptic H_3 receptors.

1. Diphenhydramine hydrochloride

First-generation H_1 antagonist.

Dose

- **Adult:** 25-50 mg three times a day.
- **Child:** 5 mg/kg/24 hours.

Risks

- Use considerable caution in narrow-angle glaucoma, stenosing peptic ulcer, pyloroduodenal obstruction, symptomatic prostatic hypertrophy, bladder neck obstruction.
- Overdosage may cause hallucination, convulsion, or death, especially in infants and children.
- May diminish mental alertness, may produce excitation in young children.
- Risk of dizziness, sedation, and hypotension is greater in the elderly.
- May cause drowsiness.
- Use in pregnancy only if clearly needed (category B).

Side-Effects and Adverse Effects

- **Cardiovascular system:** Palpitations, tachycardia.
- **Central nervous system:** Sedation, dizziness, drowsiness.
- **Eyes, ears, nose and throat:** Blurred vision, dry nose and throat.
- **Gastrointestinal:** Constipation, nausea, vomiting, dry mouth.
- **Genitourinary:** Urinary difficulties.
- **Hematologic:** Bone marrow suppression, hemolytic anemia.
- **Respiratory:** Increased secretions, wheezing.

Interactions

May enhance central nervous effects of anticholinergics.

2. Chlorphenamine maleate (chlorpheniramine maleate)

First-generation H_1 antagonist.

Dose

- **Adult oral:** 2-8 mg three or four times daily; maximum 36 mg/day.
- **Child:** 6-12 years of age, Oral: 2 mg every 4-6 hours, maximum 12 mg/day.
- **Child:** 2-5 years of age, oral: 1mg four times a day, maximum 6 mg/day.

Risks

- May impair ability to drive or perform other potentially hazardous tasks. May have an additive effect with alcohol or other central nervous system depressants.
- Overdosage may produce convulsions and/or death, particularly in infants and children.
- May cause rebound nasal congestion and blockage.
- Use caution in epilepsy, raised intra-ocular pressure including glaucoma, prostatic hypertrophy, severe hypertension, cardiovascular disease, bronchitis, bronchiectasis and asthma, hepatic disease, thyrotoxicosis.

3. Hydroxyzine

Sedating antihistamine; competes with histamine for H_1-receptor sites on effector cells in the gastrointestinal tract, blood vessels and respiratory tract.

Indication

Relief of allergy symptoms (e.g. pruritus).

Dose and Dose Information

Adult

Oral:

- 25-50 mg three to four times a day, when required for itch.

Pediatric

Oral:

- 2mg/kg/day, given in divided doses every 6-8 hours, when required for itch.
- Pediatric patients are more susceptible to adverse effects.
- Contraindicated in neonates and premature infants.

Elderly

- Elderly patients are more susceptible to adverse effects including sedation and confusion.

Contraindications

Hypersensitivity to hydroxyzine, or any component.

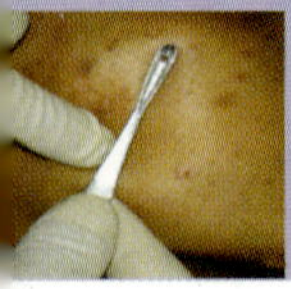

Adverse Effects

- **Common:** Dry mouth, blurred vision, urinary retention, gastrointestinal disturbances, headache, psychomotor impairment, sedation.
- **Rare:** Extrapyramidal effects, convulsions, respiratory depression, palpitations, arrhythmias, hypotension.

Interactions

- Alcohol (increased sedative effect).
- Anticholinergics (increased risk of anticholinergic effects).
- Anxiolytics and hypnotics (increased sedative effect).
- Tricyclic antidepressants (increased anticholinergic and sedative effects).

Pregnancy and Lactation

- Manufacturer states that hydroxyzine is contraindicated in first trimester of pregnancy.
- May cause neonatal withdrawal at high maternal doses.
- Can be used during labor to relieve anxiety.
- Other antihistamines are preferred in pregnancy.
- Not recommended in lactation due to limited data.

4. Cetirizine

Second-generation H_1 antihistamine.

Dose

Cetirizine:
- **Adult oral:** 10 mg once daily.
- **Children over 6 years of age, oral:** 5-10 mg once daily.
- **Children under 6 years of age, oral:** 2.5-5 mg once daily (or in two divided doses).

Levocetirizine:
Adult and child over 6 years of age: 5 mg once daily orally.

Benefits

- Suitable for use in children.
- Cetirizine nonsedating in 80% of patients.
- Levocetirizine appears to be free of this side-effect.

5. Fexofenadine

Second-generation antihistamine.

Dose

- **Adult:** 60 mg twice daily orally.
- **Child 12 years of age and over:** 60 mg twice daily orally.
- **Child 6-11 years of age:** 30 mg twice daily orally.
- **Renal impairment:** Adult 60 mg once daily, child 30 mg once daily.

Benefits

- Convenient twice-daily dosage.
- Low incidence of side-effects.

Side-Effects and Adverse Effects

- **Central nervous system:** Headache, dizziness, sedation, agitation, fatigue.
- **Gastrointestinal:** Dry mouth, dyspepsia, diarrhea, nausea.
- **Hypersensitivity:** Angioedema, wheezing, rash, flushing.
- H_2 antagonists may be useful in combination with H_1 antagonists in resistant cases.

6. Doxepin

Tricyclic antidepressant with potent and H_1 and H_2 blocking activity.

Dose

- **Adult:** 10-75 mg/day orally at bed time.

Efficacy

Can be very effective in individual patients.

Benefit

May be helpful where night-time pruritus is troublesome.

SYSTEMIC CORTICOSTEROIDS

Corticosteroids represent the complete immusuppressant, having an impact on all levels, including antigen presentation and activation of T cells, and an impact on effector processes as release of prostaglandins and activity of neutrophils. They inhibit:
- IL-2, inhibiting T-cell activation.
- Release of IL-I, IL-6, tumor necrosis factor (TNF)-α.
- Blockade of prostaglandin synthesis.
- Antigen processing.
- Inhibition of neutrophil adhesion.

Corticosteroids are the mainstay of treatment in **eczematous dermatoses** primarily because of their effect on **IL-2.** Once the activation of **T cells** is blocked, there is no secretion of **IL-4 and IL-5** to stimulate mast cells and **eosinophils,** which are at high levels in early and late stages of atopic dermatitis, respectively. In addition, inhibition of the actions of prostaglandins favorably impacts pruritus, erythema from vasodilation, and other components of the disease other than inflammation.

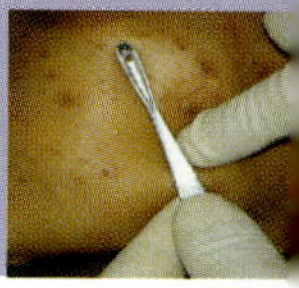

An unfortunate consequence of overuse of corticosteroids, aside from the well-known sequelae of cutaneous atrophy and striae, is the induction of a **"steroid addiction"**

A classification of steroids is given below (Table 24.7).

Situations in ***which systemic corticosteroids have a role include the following:***

Immunobullous disorders—Bullous pemphigoid, pemphigus, epidermolysis bullosa acquisita, etc.

Neutrophilic dermatoses and vasculitis—Sweet syndrome, pyoderma gangrenosum, Henoch–Schönlein purpura and other cutaneous small-vessel vasculitis, Wegener granulomatosis, etc.

Connective tissue diseases—Systemic lupus erythematosus and dermatomyositis.

Severe forms of common dermatoses—Pompholyx, contact dermatitis, drug eruptions, erythema multiforme, and acute urticaria

Other inflammatory diseases—Eosinophilic cellulitis or fasciitis, lichen planus (scarring, nail, or scalp), sarcoidosis and hemangiomas (with bleeding or functional impairment).

Corticosteroids may be combined with, or gradually substituted by, other agents such as cytotoxic drugs that have a steroid-sparing effect. In some cases, such as in bullous pemphigoid, corticosteroids may be used initially for their speed of action, but the dose can be reduced once a slower-acting drug such as azathioprine starts to work.

Guidelines for the Use of Systemic Corticosteroids

- Screen for tuberculosis.
- Monitor weight, temperature, pulse, blood pressure, blood sugar and electrolytes.
- Use in the morning between 8-9 a.m. after breakfast i.e. in accordance with circadian rhythm to decrease side-effects.
- Prefer alternate day therapy.
- Use adjuvant therapy to decrease duration and dose steroid therapy.
- Taper steroid slowly if used for > 3 weeks.
- Dietary salt restriction and potassium supplementation may be necessary.

Efficacy

Usually effective as a short-term measure.

Risk

- Patients on corticosteroid therapy require an increased dosage of rapidly acting corticosteroids before, during, and after unusual stress.
- Risk of masking of signs of infections or emergence of new infections.
- Risk of cataracts, glaucoma, and secondary ocular infections.
- Oral corticosteroids are generally contraindicated in active tuberculosis. Use with caution in latent tuberculosis or tuberculin reactivity: chemoprophylaxis should be used with prolonged therapy.
- Use with caution with strongyloides infestation.
- Do not administer live or live attenuated vaccines to patients receiving immunosuppressive doses of corticosteroids. Response to killed or inactive vaccines may be diminished.
- Caution in congestive heart failure, diabetes mellitus, renal disease, glaucoma and peptic ulcer.
- Risk of osteoporosis in pregnancy, nursing mothers, or women of child-bearing potential, possible benefits must be weighed against potential hazards to mother and fetus (**category B**). Infants born of mothers who

Table 24.7: A classification of steroids

Compound (mg)	*Equivalent Gluco-corticoid (GC) dose*	*Mineralocorticoid potency*	*Duration of action hours*
Short acting			
Cortisone	25	2+	8-12
Hydrocortisone	20	2+	8-12
Intermediate acting			
Prednisone	5	1+	24-36
Prednisolone	5	1+	24-36
Methylprednisolone	4	0	24-36
Triamcinolone	4	0	24-36
Long acting			
Dexamethasone	0.6	0	36-54
Betamethasone	0.75	0	36-54

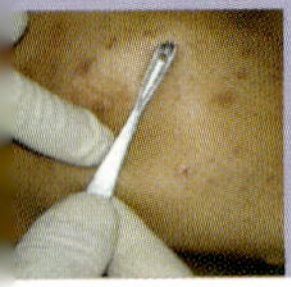

receive substantial doses of corticosteroid during pregnancy should be observed for signs of hypoadrenalism.

Side-Effects and Adverse Effects (Table 24.8)

- Side effects are minimized by short duration or alternate day therapy.
- ***Cardiovascular system:*** Hypertension, thromboembolism.
- ***Central nervous system:*** Insomnia, euphoria, depression, psychosis.
- ***Endocrine:*** Adrenal suppression, impaired glucose tolerance, growth suppression in children, Cushing's syndrome. Prednisone taken in doses higher than *7.5 mg for 3 weeks or longer may lead* to clinically relevant suppression of the pituitary-adrenal axis.
- ***Eyes:*** Cataract, glaucoma, blurred vision.
- **Gastrointestinal:** Dyspepsia, peptic ulceration, esophagitis, oral candidiasis, nausea, diarrhea.
- ***Musculoskeletal:*** Proximal myopathy, osteoporosis
- ***Skin:*** Delayed healing, acne, striae.

Interactions

- Adrenergic neuron blockers, alpha-blockers, beta-blockers, beta-2 agonists.
- Anticonvulsants (carbamazepine, phenytoin, barbiturates).
- Antidiabetics.
- Antidysrhythmics (calcium channel blockers, cardiac glycosides).
- Antifungals (amphotericin, ketoconazole).
- Antihypertensives (ACE inhibitors, loop and thiazide diuretics, acetazolamide; angiotensin II receptor antagonists, clonidine, diazoxide, hydralazine, methyldopa, minoxidil).

Table 24. 8: Effects of glucocorticoids during chronic therapy

Endocrine and Metabolic Suppression of HPA axis (adrenal suppression) Growth failure in children Hyperinsulinemia/Insulin resistance Abnormal gloucose tolerance test/Diabetes mellitus	**Immune System** Suppression of delayed (type IV) hypersensitivity (important with Mantoux testing for tuberculosis) Inhibition of leukocyte and tissue macrophage migration Inhibition of cytokine secretion/action Suppression of the primary antigen response
Cushingoid Features Moon facies (broad cheeks with temporal muscle wasting) facial plethora Generalized and truncal obesity (more marked in adults) Supraclavicular fat collection Posterior cervical fat deposition (**Dorsocervical hump**) Glucocorticoid-induced acne Thin and fragile skin, violaceous striae (occurring more commonly in adults) Impotence, menstrual irregularity Decreased TSH and T3 **Hypokalemia with very high cortisol levels or in the presence of potassium wasting diuretics), metabolic alkolosis**	**Musculoskeletal System** Osteoporosis, spontaneous fractures Avascular necrosis of femoral and humoral heads and other bones Myopathy (particularly of the proximal muscles) unable to comb hair or climb stairs **Ophthalmic** Posterior subcapsular cataracts (more common in children) Elevated intraocular pressure/glaucoma
Gastrointestinal System Gastric irritation, peptic ulcer Acute pancreatitis (secondary to insulin resistance and **hypertriglyceridemia**) Fatty infiltration of liver (hepatomegaly) (rare)	**Neuropsychiatric Disorders (CNS)** Sleep disturbances, insomnia (particularly with long acting glucocorticoids and nocturnal dosing) Euphoria, depression,mania, psychosis (more commonly seen in adults) Pseudotumor cerebri (benign increase of intracranial pressure)
Hemopoietic System Leukocytosis *Neutrophilia:* Increased recruitment from bone marrow, demargination, and decreased migration from blood vessels *Lymphopenia:* Migration from blood vessels to lymphoid tissue **Eosinopenia, Monocytopenia**	**Cardiovascular** Hypertension Congestive heart failure in predisposed patients

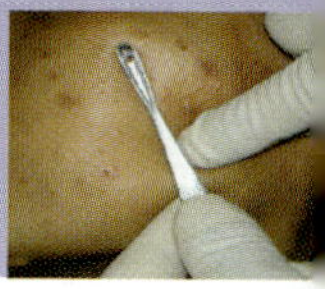

- Cyclosporine.
- Erythromycin.
- Methotrexate.
- NSAIDs.
- Oral contraceptives.
- Rifampicin.
- Ritonavir.
- Vaccines.

CONTRAINDICATION OF SYSTEMIC CORTICOSTEROIDS

Absolute

- Systemic fungal infection.
- Herpes simplex keratitis.
- Hypersensitivity reaction.

Relative

- Psychosis, severe depression.
- Glaucoma cataract.
- CHF, HT.
- Osteoporosis.
- DM.
- Active T.B. or positive tuberculin test.

DOSING OF STEROIDS

Usually prescribed as 40 mg/day for 5 days (single dose or 20 mg twice daily).

Dosage should be individualized. A tapered course may be preferred. A 6-day tapering prednisone course of 60-50-40-30-20-10 mg daily is often used, particularly for more severe cases.

DAILY DOSING OF STEROID

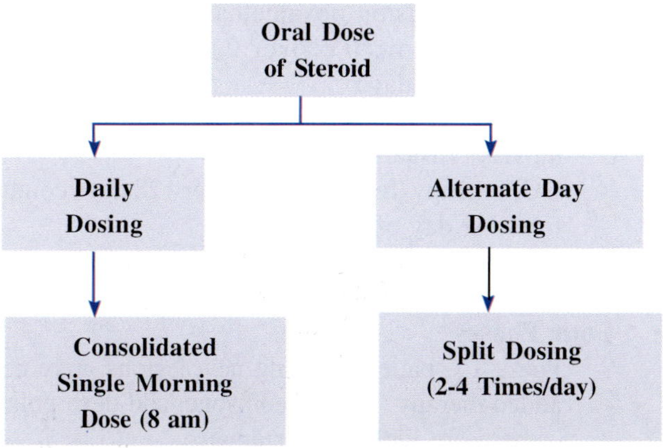

Rationale and Principle

For Initiation of Steroid Therapy

- Physiological cortisol secretion: Mirror ACTH pulses which are maximum at time of waking, and then decrease throughout the day.
- Divided dosing is more effective but causes more HPA axis suppression.
- Consolidating the split doses into a single morning dose.
- Tapering of steroids should be started as soon as adequate disease control is achieved.

ALTERNATE DAY DOSING

- There is a disassociation between the plasma and biological half life of glucocorticoids.
- Duration of action is determined not by the plasma ½ life, but by intracellular effects secondary to binding of steroid to cytoplasmic receptors.
- ACTH suppressing effect of glucocorticoid is shorter than its tissue effect.
- Alternate day provides 48 hours efficacy while only slightly blunting the HPA on the off day.
- Glucocorticoid chosen should be short to intermediate acting.
- Alternate day should be tried in any skin disease where therapy is for > 1 month.
- All common steroid side effect are diminished / eliminated except for osteoporosis and post subcapsular cataract.

Prerequisites for Alternate Day Dosing

- Complete/near complete disease control.
- Dose of prednisone 20 – 30 mg.
- Change to alternate day from consolidated dose only.

Strategies to Convert to Alternate Day Rx:

- *First aim to reach 40 mg od*: Taper by 20 mg/2 weeks till 60 mg, then by 10 mg/2 weeks till 40 mg od.
- 40 mg od 1st reduce 2nd day dose by 5 mg 40/35, 40/30, 40/25....40/10; 40/7.5...40/0.
- *Once 5 mg ALTERNATE DAY reached* – Assess need for maintenance Rx by 8 am serum cortisol levels 4 weeks later (cutoff 10 micrograms/dl).

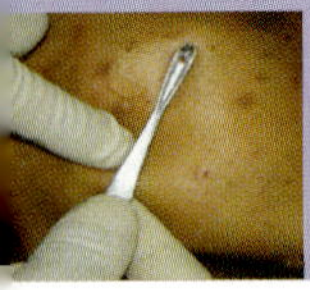

INTRAMUSCULAR STEROID RX

- **Advantages**
  - Better compliance – physician supervised.
  - Steady release of glucocorticoid from depot.
  - Better disease control.
- **Disadvantages**
  - More HPA axis suppression.
  - Less predictable absorption as compared to oral dosing.
  - Oral doses can be tapered more precisely.
  - ALTERNATE DAY Rx possible with oral dose.
  - Lipoatrophy at injection site – more with longer acting steroids.

PULSE STEROID THERAPY

- Supra pharmacological doses of glucocorticoids, usually high dose and usually by the parenteral route.
- **Regimens used vary widely.**
- Doses in each pulse:
  - Methylprednisolone – 10 to 20 mg/kg/day (250 to 1000 mg).
  - Dexamethasone – 2 to 5 mg/kg.
- Duration: 3 to 5 days.
- Similar doses may be given orally – similar efficacy.
- **Disadvantages of oral route**
  - Large no. of tablets to be swallowed.
  - Danger of patient self-medicating.
  - Long-term glucocorticoid sparing effects yet to be compared with the I/V route.
- **Principles**
  - Pharmacological effects of each dose last about 2 days.
  - Doubling the dose of glucocorticoid increases the time of action by one half life.
  - Some effects of Pulse Rx too rapid to be mediated by genomic glucocorticoid action.
  - Non genomic MOA may be important in pulse Rx.
  - Apoptosis of inflammatory cells, particularly peripheral blood CD4+ T cells, may occur only at pulse doses of glucocorticoids.
  - With prolonged daily glucocorticoid therapy: Glucocorticoid receptors down regulated, making glucocorticoids less effective –Pulse dosing avoids this.
  - HPA axis suppression short-lived – recovery in 2-3 days.

Oral Mini-Pulse Therapy

- Low to moderate (5 to 10 mg) doses of oral steroids (betamethasone/dexamethasone) given on one/two days per week as single morning dose.
- Used in *vitiligo vulgaris, lichen planus, hemangiomas.*
- May be used for longer periods with minimal side effects as compared to daily glucocorticoid therapy.
- Minor side effects: Weight gain, insomnia, acne, agitation, menstrual disturbance and hypertrichosis.

Adverse Effects of Pulse Therapy

- **Mild**
  - Acute psychosis
  - Depression
  - Reversible memory impairment
  - Metallic taste
  - Facial flushing
  - Hiccups
  - Arthralgias
  - Hyperglycemia.
- **Serious**

  Cardiovascular
  - Acute CVS side effects
  - Cardiac arrythmias
  - Congestive heart failure
  - Hypotension
  - Pulmonary edema
  - Ischemic heart disease.
- Electrolyte shifts.
- Anaphylaxis.
- Avascular necrosis.
- Renal crisis in scleroderma patients.

Dexamethasone–Cyclophoshamide Pulse Therapy

- **Regimen**
  - 100 mg infusion dexamethasone in 500 ml 5% dextrose, slow I/V over 2 hrs, repeated on 3 consecutive days.
  - 500 mg cyclophoshamide added to drip on one of the days (usually 2nd day).
  - DCP therapy repeated after every 28 days counted from 1st day of pulse.
  - Patient receives 50 mg daily oral dose of cyclophoshamide in between pulses.
- **Four Phases**
  - Phase 1 – patient getting new lesions, may need added therapy (daily prednisone, add dexa pulses) – these are withdrawn stepwise.

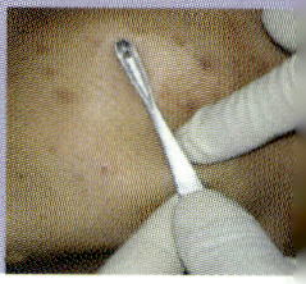

- Phase 2 – all skin and mucosal lesions healed. 9 more DCPs given.
- Phase 3 – DCPs stopped, 50 mg daily cyclophosphamide continued for 9 months.
- Phase 4 – Therapy completely stopped. Patient followed up for 10 years.

Indications

Bullous diseases
Pemphigus group.
Bullous pemphigoid.
Cicatricial pemphigoid.
Dermatits herpetiformis.
Chronic bullous disease of childhood.
Reiter's disease.
Collagen vascular diseases
PSS.
SLE.
Dermatomyositis.
Generalised morphoea.
Pyoderma gangrenosum.
Miscellaneous diseases
LP, vitiligo, alopecia areata, prurigo nodularis etc.

Contraindications

- Pregnancy.
- Lactation.
- Severe infection.
- Severe herpes simplex, zoster, chickenpox.

Side Effects of DCP Therapy

- Diffuse hair loss.
- Amenorrhea, azoospermia.
- Weakness and tiredness due to glucocorticoid withdrawal 2-3 days after pulse.
- Bad taste in the mouth.
- Loose motions.
- Recurrent hiccup.
- Cataract.
- Bone pains and aseptic necrosis.
- Bladder toxicity.
  - Hemorrhagic cystitis due to bolus dose of cyclophosphamide (CP), due to *acrolein.*
  - MESNA (sodium 2-mercaptoethane sulphonate) – given simultaneously, dose equivalent to dose of CP, given as 15-30 min infusions in 5 divided doses over 24 hours.
- Infections – bacterial, fungal.
- Reactivation of TB.
- Leukopenia, anemia, thrombocytopenia rarely.

General Principles to Reduce Side Effects of Systemic Steroids

- Use lowest effective dose for the shortest possible time.
- If dose > 30 mg x 3 weeks: Taper; do not stop abruptly.
- Wherever possible use topical steroid therapy first.
- After 1 month of daily dosing, alternate day dosing should be attempted if disease has been controlled.
- For severe dermatosis likely to require long term intermediate to high dose steroids consider I/V pulse therapy.
- Oral mini pulse for appropriate conditions.
- Use of steroid sparing agents (e.g. cyclophosphamide, azathioprine).
- Watch for drugs interacting with systemic steroids.

IMMUNOSUPPRESSANTS (Tables 24.9 and 24.10)

Azathioprine

This is a widely used drug in dermatology. It has a slow onset of action, and is therefore mainly used as a steroid-sparing agent rather than as initial therapy.

MOA

Antagonizes purine metabolism and inhibits synthesis of DNA, RNA and proteins.

- TPMT testing is done. Low-activity TMPT patients are at very high risk of azathioprine toxicity.
- Allopurinol causes azathoprine toxicity.

Uses

As a steroid sparing agent, for autoimmune blistering disorders, Connective tissue diseases, Vasculitis and Dermatitis.

- Causes bone marrow suppression and hepatotoxicity.
- Monitoring-Hemogram, liver and kidney function test.

Methotrexate

MOA

This is an antimetabolite that interferes with folate metabolism.

Its primary use is as a folic acid antagonist that inhibits DNA synthesis in tissues with high rates of turnover, such as psoriatic plaques.

Has immunosuppressive effect by acting on mononuclear cells in skin, blood and lymphatics.

Table 24.9: Pharmacology of the common immunosuppressants used in dermatology

Features	*Azathioprine*	*Cyclophosphamide*	*Methotrexate*	*Cyclosporine*	*MMF*
Mechanism of action	*Cell cycle-Specific* inhibition of neutrophil trafficking, inhibition of cellular cytotoxicity	*Non-cell cycle-specific* selective macrophage inhibition, Selective B-cell suppression	*Cell cycle-specific inhibition* of neutrophil chemotaxis, inhibition of IL-I, IL-6, and IL-8 release	Inhibition of *IL-2* induction in lymphocytes	Cell cycle-specific antimetabolite, *inhibition of T and B-cell proliferation*
Rate of onset of clinical immunosuppressant	Slow (4-8 weeks)	Moderately rapid (2-4 weeks)	Moderately rapid (2-4 weeks)	Rapid (1-2 weeks)	Slow (4-8 weeks)
Route of administration	**Per os**	**Per os**/IV	**Per os**/SC/intramuscular/IV	**Per os**	Per os
Route of elimination	Hepatic metabolism and renal excretion	Hepatic metabolism and renal excretion	Renal excretion by active tubular secretion	Hepatic metabolism	Hepatic metabolism and renal excretion
Dose modification in presence of:					
Renal insufficiency	Moderate decrease in dosage may be required	Moderate decrease in dosage may be required	Relatively contraindicated, significant Dose reduction necessary	No change in dosage necessary	Moderate decrease in dosage may be required
Hepatic insufficiency	No change in dose necessary	Moderate decrease in dosage may be required	Moderate decrease in dosage may Be required	Significant dose alteration needed	No change in dose necessary
Major potential drug interactions	Allopurinol, warfarin	Allopurinol	Probenecid, NSAIDs, **clotrimazole**	Multiple (see text)	Acyclovir, iron, antacids, cholestyramine
Major toxicity	Bone marrow depression, carcinogenesis	Bone marrow depression, hemorrhagic cystitis, carcinogenesis	Hepatotoxicity, bone marrow depression, carcinogenesis	Hypertension, nephrotoxicity, carcinogenecity	Bone marrow depression, carcinogenesis

For all immunosuppressants, lymph node examination, complete physical examination, stool guaiac, skin cancer examination and PAP smear every 6 months in females are recommended.

MMF = Mycophenolate mofetil.

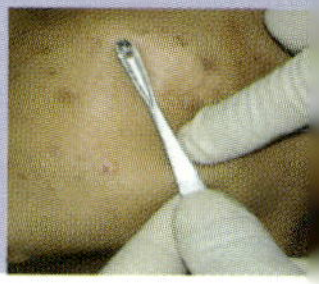

Table 24.10 : Monitoring guidelines for the use of immunosuppressant

Drug	*Monitoring tests*	*Frequency*	*Guidelines for dosage modification*
Azathioprine	CBC with differential WBC and platelets	Weekly x4, every 2 wk x2, then monthly	Decrease dose if WBC < 4000 platelets < 1 lakh, discontinue if WBC < **2,000**
Cyclophosphamide	CBC with differential WBC and platelets	Weekly x 8, then monthly	Decrease dose if WBC < 4000 platelets < 1 lakh, discontinue if WBC < **2,000**
	Renal function tests: BUN, creatinine	Monthly	
	Urinalysis	Weekly x8, then every 2 weeks, urine cytology when> 50 g total dose monthly is reached	Discontinue if hematuria
	Liver function tests	Monthly	
Methotrexate	CBC with differential WBC and platelets	Weekly x2, every 2 weeks x2, then monthly	Discontinue for 2-3 weeks if WBC < 3.500, discontinue if WBC < 25 00 or platelets < 1 lakh
	Renal function tests: BUN, creatinine	Every 3-4 months	
	Liver function tests	First time 1 week after last dose, then every 2-3 months	If persistently elevated, withhold for I - 2 weeks and repeat; if elevation persists tor 2 - 3 months perform Liver biopsy
	Liver biopsy	*If no risk factors*, at cumulative doses of 1.5 gm, 3 g, and 4 g. *If risk factors*, then first at 2-4 months of therapy, then at cumulative doses of 1- 1.5 g, 3 g, 4 g. After a cumulative dose of 4 g, biopsy every 1 -1.5 g	
Cyclosporine	CBC with differential WBC and platelets	Every month, then every 2-3 months	Decrease dose if creatinine increase is > 30% over baseline; if persistent over 2 evaluations, discontinue
	Renal function tests: BUN and creatinine (x3)	Biweekly X6, then monthly	
	Blood pressure	Biweekly x6, then monthly	
	Urinalysis	Biweekly x2, then monthly	
	Liver function tests	Biweekly x2, then monthly	

Contd.

Contd.

Cyclosporine	Potassium, uric acid, magnesium, cholesterol, triglycerides	Biweekly × 2 then monthly	
	Creatinine clearance	Not done routinely	
Mycophenolate mofetil (MMF)	CBC with differential WBC and platelets count	Weekly × 4, every 2 weeks × 4, then monthly	Decrease dose or discontinue if neutropenic

Abbreviations: BUN, blood urea nitrogen; CBC, complete blood (cell) count; WBC, white blood cell (count), IV, intravenous, SC, subcutaneous.

Uses

Psoriasis, connective tissue disease and vasculitis, bullous pemphigoid.

Treatment is usually commenced with a small test dose to identify patients with significant side effects, and is then increased with close monitoring of blood counts and liver function. It should not be used in patients with with known liver disease or heavy alcohol intake. **Liver biopsy is normally performed in the first few months as a baseline for assessment of the potential side effect of liver fibrosis.** Ongoing monitoring may include routine liver function tests, further liver biopsy, and/or serial measurements of the amino terminal peptide of type III procollagen (PIIINP), a serum marker of fibrosis.

Cyclosporine

MOA

Inhibits production of interleukin 2, the cytokine responsible for inducing T-cell proliferation.

Uses

- Severe psoriasis or eczema (especially atopic type in adults).
- Immunobullous disorders - usually as a steroid-sparing agent.
- Chronic urticaria - especially of proven autoimmune type.

Cyclophosphamide

MOA

An alkylating agent.

Uses

One of the first-line treatments for Wegener granulomatosis and is sometimes used in other vasculitides.

It is also used in severe immunobullous diseases, such as refractory pemphigus, or in sight-threatening mucous membrane pemphigoid or linear IgA disease.

Mycophenolate Mofetil

MOA

This is a newer agent that selectively inhibits lymphocyte proliferation.

Inhibits inosine monophosphate dehydrogenase and suppresses de novo purine synthesis by lymphocytes, thereby inhibiting their proliferation. Inhibits antibody production.

Uses

It is mainly used as a steroid-sparing drug.

RETINOIDS

Isotretinoin

Isotretinoin or *13-cis* retinoic acid, is a synthetic vitamin A (retinol) analog first approved by the US Food and Drug Administration (FDA) in 1982 for the treatment of severe recalcitrant nodulocystic acne. Although, initially developed for that purpose, isotretinoin has been used more recently for patients with moderate and moderately severe acne who are unresponsive to conventional therapies.

The half-life is 22 hours and the bioavailability, which can be increased by taking isotretinoin with **food, is 25%.**

Isotretinoin acts primarily by decreasing the size of the sebaceous glands and reducing sebum production by upto

90%, thereby inhibiting the growth of *P acnes* and subsequent inflammation. In addition, like topical retinoids, it inhibits comedone formation by normalizing follicular keratinization.

Mechanism of Action

Isotretinoin is the only oral retinoid known to have profound effect on sebaceous gland activity, although the exact mechanisms remain elusive. Evidence supports the fact that isotretinoin can influence each of the four factors involved in the pathogenesis of acne by influencing cell-cycle progression, cellular differentiation, cell survival and apoptosis.

Unlike tretinoin (*all-trans* retinoic acid [ATRA]), isotretinoin has little to no ability to bind to cellular retinol-binding proteins or the retinoic acid nuclear receptors (RARs and RXRs). Instead, it may act as a pro-drug that is converted **intracellularly to A-TRA and *9-cis* RA**, which are agonists for RAR nuclear receptors and both RAR and RXR nuclear receptors, respectively. It is well established, however, that isotretinoin is superior to either *9-cis* RA or ATRA for suppression of sebaceous gland activity and sebum production. Another proposed theory is that isotretinoin may act in a receptor independent manner, influencing cellular signaling pathways by either direct protein interactions, as demonstrated with other retinoids, or by enzyme inhibition.

The primary change within the sebaceous follicle in acne is an alteration in follicular keratinization; isotretinoin may decrease hyperkeratinization by 50%. Of all of the treatments available for acne, isotretinoin is the most potent inhibitor of sebum production. Histologically, a drastic decrease in the size, shape, and lipid content of sebaceous glands is seen **after 16 weeks** of isotretinoin therapy. It seems likely that the decrease in sebum production may be the net result of sebaceous gland involution in response to isotretinoin treatment.

Clinical Applications

In addition to its proven benefit in the treatment of nodulocystic acne, isotretinoin has been used successfully to treat, although sometimes only temporarily, other acneiform conditions, such as solid facial edema (Morbihan's disease), and gram-negative folliculitis, as well as disorders of cornification and as chemoprophylaxis of skin cancer in patients with defective DNA repair. This includes patients with basal cell nevus syndrome (Gorlin syndrome), xeroderma pigmentosum, and inhibiting eruptive keratoacanthomas. Interestingly, **isotretinoin's benefits** span most fields of medicine, including its successful use in treating renal cell cancer, prostate cancer, recurrent malignant gliomas, and spinal cord astrocytomas among other visceral malignancies.

Dosing

Traditionally, when being used for acne, isotretinoin has been prescribed at a dose of **0.5 to 1.0 mg/kg per day** for 4 to 6 months, to reach a cumulative dose of 120 mg/kg. Recently, **low dose isotretinoin at 20 mg per day for 6 months** has been used to treat patients with moderate acne with nearly 95% achieving significant improvement or complete remission. The relapse rate was between 4% and 6%, with a mean total dose of 66 to 70 mg/kg at the end of 6 months. The most common side effects in this study were mild cheilitis and xerosis.

Of all patients treated with isotretinoin, approximately **40%** of patients are acne free at the end of the treatment period, whereas another **40%** have a recurrence that responds to medications previously tried. The remaining **20%** will require a ***second course*** of isotretinoin.

Patients more likely to relapse include those younger than 16 years of age, adult females, and those with significant truncal involvement.

For the most severe cases, patients may initially be started at a dose of 0.5 mg/kg daily for the first month to prevent a significant acne flare and then increased over the next month to 1.0 mg/kg daily. In addition, simultaneous administration of prednisone may be helpful in cases of acne fulminans or in those with a severe initial flare.

Side Effects

Multiple mucocutaneous and systemic side effects have been described with isotretinoin use and the observed side effects are usually dose dependent and reversible. Many side effects are similar to those seen in hypervitaminosis A, since isotretinoin is a vitamin A analog. Cheilitis is by far the most common symptom, occurring in.

An overview of medication used in acne are given in Table 24.11.

Caution

Females of childbearing age must take effective contraception for 1 month before treatment is started, during treatment, and for 1 month after treatment is stopped; check pregnancy test(s) before starting treatment and monthly. Females should sign a consent form which states the dangers of teratogenicity. Before starting a course of isotretinoin, patients and their doctors should know about the risk of the appearance or worsening of depression. The drug should be stopped immediately if there is any concern on this score. Avoid in renal or hepatic impairment.

Table 24.11: Acne medications effecting sebum production		
Drug	*Dose*	*Side effects*
Oral retinoids		
Isotretinoin	0.5—1.0 mg/kg/day cumulative 120 mg/kg	Teratatogenicity, mood changes, elevated liver enzymes, hypertriglyceridemia, cheilitis, xerosis, visual disturbances, pseudotumor cerebri, arthralgias
Hormonal agents		
Spironolactone	50-200 mg daily	Menstrual irregularities, diuretic effect hyperkalemia, breast tenderness, decreased libido, feminization of male fetus
Cyproterone acetate	2-100 mg daily	Similar to spironolactone
Flutamide	250 mg twice daily	Severe hepatitis, teratogenicity, thromboembolism, migraine
Oral contraceptives	Daily	Menstrual irregularities

Acitretin

Severe psoriasis, resistant to other forms of treatment (may be used with PUVA), palmoplantar pustulosis, severe ichthyoses, Darier's disease, pityriasis rubra pilaris (0.2–1.0 mg/kg daily).

Acitretin is not recommended for children except under exceptional circumstances.

Bexarotene

A new agent, used in lymphomas.

SIDE EFFECTS

1. Mucocutaneous (Common)

Rough, scaly, dry-appearing skin and mucous membranes
Atrophy of skin and nails
Diffuse thinning of scalp and body hair
Curly hair
Exuberant granulation tissue
(especially toenail folds)
Disease Flare-up
Photosensitivity

2. Systemic

Teratogenesis
Diffuse interstitial skeletal hyperostosis
Arthralgia, myalgia and headache
Benign intracranial hypertension

3. Laboratory abnormalities

Haematology:
↓ White blood cells , ↑ Erythrocyte sedimentation rate

4. Liver function tests

Bilirubin ↑
↑ AST/ALT
↑ Alkaline phosphatase
(abnormal in 20% of patients)

5. Serum lipids

↑ Cholesterol
↑ Triglycerides
↓ High-density lipoprotein
(abnormal in 50% of patients)

Cautions

- All women of childbearing age must use effective oral contraception for 1 month before treatment, during treatment and for at least 1 month (Isotretinoin) and 2 years (Acitretin) after treatment.
- Patients should sign a consent form indicating that they know about the danger of teratogenicity.
- **Should not donate blood** during or for 1 year after stopping the treatment.

Regular screening should be carried out to exclude:

1. Abnormalities of liver function.
2. Hyperlipidaemia.

ANTIVIRAL AGENTS

Available Antiviral Therapies for Herpes Virus Infections

Acyclovir, Valacyclovir, Famciclovir, Penciclovir, Ganciclovir, Cidofovir, Fomivirsen, Foscarnet.

Nucleoside Antiviral Agents

1. **Acyclovir**
   The synthetic guanosine analog acyclovir is the most extensively used antiviral drug worldwide. It requires the herpesvirus **thymidine** kinase to phosphyralate **the drug.**

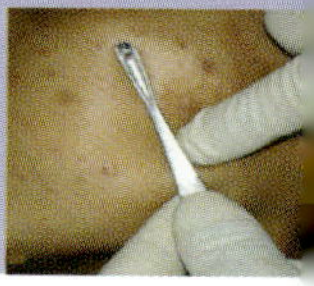

Uses

a. **Herpes labialis**
Although not specifically FDA-approved for this indication, ***oral acyclovir 400 mg five times daily for 5 days*** can be used for the treatment of herpes ***labialis***. This antiviral agent has clinical benefit, reducing duration of pain by 36% and time to loss of crust by 27%.

b. **Herpes genitalis 400 mg TDS – 5 days**

c. **Herpes zoster 800 mg 5 times/d – 7 days**

2. Valacyclovir

Valacyclovir is a prodrug of acyclovir (the L-valyl ester of acyclovir), and it seems to have a similar safety profile to acyclovir.

a. **Herpes genitalis**
Initial episode (1 gm twice daily for 10 d).

b. **Herpes labialis**
Initial episode (2 g, twice a day for 1 d).

c. **Herpes zoster**
Valacyclovir at a dosage of 1 g, 3 times daily for 7 days halps and in reducing time to crusting time to 50% healing, and the appearance of new zoster lesions. Further, the median duration of pain after healing is reduced from 60 days with acyclovir to 40 days with valacyclovir. Valacyclovir and famciclovir have similar efficacy in the reduction post herpetic neuralgia. Valacyclovir is more convenient more effective and as safe as acyclovir.

3. Famciclovir

Famciclovir is an acyclic guanosine analog that is metabolized into penciclovir, the active metabolite. It requires phosphorylation by viral thymidine kinase and cellular kinases and, once activated, inhibits DNA polymerase.

Famciclovir is effective against HSV-I, HSV-2, and VZV. patients.

4. Penciclovir

Another acyclic guanosine analog that has activity against HSV-l, HSV-2, and VZV is penciclovir, the metabolite of famciclovir. Because it has low oral bioavailability, it is an FDA-approved topical treatment for herpes labialis. Similar to acyclovir, penciclovir is phosphorylated by viral thymidine kinase and cellular kinases before it can inhibit viral DNA polymerase.

Topical penciclovir 1% is approved for first episodic therapy of herpes labialis and is applied every 2 hours during waking hours for 4 days. It has been found to speed healing and decrease pain.

5. Cidofovir

Cidofovir is an acyclic phosphonate nucleotide analog of deoxycytidine monophosphate and inhibits viral DNA synthesis.

Cidofovir is FDA-approved for the therapy for CMV retinitis in AIDS patients.

Recent studies have shown that topical cidofovir (1 % gel or cream) is effective in the treatment of recalcitrant and otherwise unmanageable viral lesions.

7. Fomivirsen

Fomivirsen is a 21-nucelotide phosphorothioate oligonuceotide that has a novel mechanism of action by inhibition of human virus replication through an antisense mechanism.

It has activity against cidofovir and ganciclovir-resistant strain. Fomivirsen is indicated for use in HIV patient, with CMV retinitis who are not responsive to or are unable to take cidofovir and ganciclovir. Fomivirsen is given by intravitreal injection.

8. Foscarnet

Foscarnet directly inhibits herpesvirus DNA polymerase, by reversibly blocking the pyrophosphate binding site of the viral polymerase.

Foscarnet is active against HSV, VZV, EBV, CMV, and human herpes virus **(HHV-8).** Foscarnet also has activity against acyclovir resistant HSV and-VZV strains, ganciclovir resistant. Foscarnet is approved for therapy for CMV retinitis in AIDS patients and in acyclovir-resistant HSV mucocutaneous infections.

For acyclovir-resistant mucocutaneous HSV infections, 40 mg/kg every 8 hours administered for 14 to 21 days.

Foscarnet toxicity includes mainly nephrotoxicity, metabolic and hematologic abnormalities, and CNS side effects. Patients may develop isolated or combined hypomagnesemia (15%-44%), hypocalcemia (15%-35%), hypokalemia (10%-16%), and hypophosphatemia CNS side effects include headache (25%), seizures (upto 10%), irritability, tremor, and hallucinations. Other reported side effects include fever, rash, painful genital ulcerations diarrhea, nausea and vomiting.

Experimental Therapy for Herpes Virus Infections

Helicase-Primase Inhibitors

A new type of drug, helicase-primase inhibitors, recently has been shown to be effective **in antiviral-resistant HSVs**. Both newly described drug classes are active orally

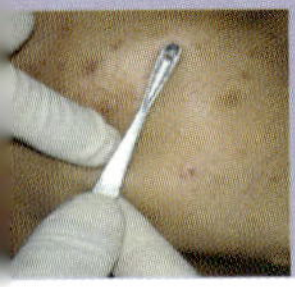

and show significant effectiveness in HSV-I and HSV-2 in the guinea pig, mouse and rat model. They also show great efficacy when given several hours or even days after the cutaneous lesions appear.

AVAILABLE THERAPIES FOR HUMAN PAPILLOMA VIRUS INFECTIONS

Most Commonly Used Therapies

Chemical Agents

- Trichloroacetic acid
- Podofilox
- Imiquimod
- Topical cidofovir
- Interferon.

Surgical Agents

- Surgical removal
- Cryotherapy
- Laser surgery.

Less Commonly Used Therapies

- Electrosurgery
- 5-Fluorouracil
- Retinoids
- Bleomycin (intralesional and systemic)
- Salicylic acid.

NEWER ANTIBIOTICS

Daptomycin

Mechanism of Action

Daptomycin is derived from the fermentation of *Streptomyces roseosporus*. Its mode of action is unique in that it rapidly kills **gram-positive bacteria** by disrupting many aspects of bacterial membrane function. Although gross morphologic changes occurred in both a methicillin-sensitive and a methicillin-resistant strain of *Staphylococcus aureus* and in a strain of *Enterococcus faecalis,* the bacteria were not lysed when observed under electron microscopy. Daptomycin is **bactericida**l, and bacterial killing is concentration-dependent.

Indications

Daptomycin is indicated for the treatment of complicated infections of skin and skin structures caused by susceptible strains of the gram-positive organisms *Staphylococcus aureus* (including methicillin-resistant strains), *Streptococcus pyogenes, Streptococcus agalactiae, Streptococcus dysgalactiae* subsp *equisimilis* and *Efaecalis.*

Linezolid

Mechanism of Action

The oxazolidinones have a unique mechanism of action: they stop the first step in which bacteria assemble ribosomes from their dissociated subunits by binding to a site on the 50S ribosomal subunit near its interface with the 30S unit, thus preventing the fornation of a 70S initiation complex.

Spectrum of Activity

Linezolid has excellent *in vitro* activity against all of the major **gram-positive** pathogens in humans, including activity against the **gram-negative bacteria** *Neisseria gonorrhoeae* and *N meningitidis.* It has only borderline activity against *Haemophilus influenzae* and is inactive against both *Enterobacteriaceae* and *Pseudomonas* species.

Linezolid has good activity against many **gram-positive anerobes**. Its activity against *Bacteroides fragilis* is borderline, but it provides bactericidal activity against these organisms. Linezolid exhibits relatively good *in vitro* activity against many strains of *M tuberculosis* and has activity against the *M avium* complex and several rapidly growing mycobacteria, including *M fortuitum, M chelonae,* and *M abscessus.* Linezolid also has excellent *in vitro* activity against *Nocardia* species (including *N asteroides, N farcinica, N brasiliensa,* and four other species).

Indications

Use for the treatment of complicated infections of skin and soft tissue caused by *Staphylococcus aureus* methicillin-resistant and susceptible strains), *Streptococcus pyogenes,* or *Streptococcus agalactiae* and for treating uncomplicated infections of skin and soft tissue caused by *Staphylococcus aureus* (methicillin-susceptible strains only) or *Streptococcus pyogenes*, vancomycin-resistant *Efaecium* infections (including cases with concurrent bacteremia), community-acquired pneumonia caused by *Streptococcus pneumoniae.*

Quinupristin-Dalfopristin

Quinupristin-dalfopristin has a short half-life (1 to 2 hours), but the prolonged postantibiotic effect and additional growth inhibition at sub-minimum inhibitory concentration levels suggest that dosing intervals of 8 or 12 hours will suffice.

Dosing

Dosage of quinupristin-dalfopristin should be 7.5 mg/kg every 8 hours. For complicated infections of skin and skin structures, the dosage should be 7.5 mg/kg every 12 hours. Dose adjustment in renal failure, hemodialysis, or peritoneal dialysis is not required.

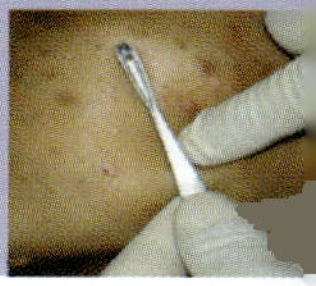

Third-Generation Fluoroquinolones: Gatifloxacin and Moxifloxacin

The third-generation fluoroquinolones bind to bacterial topoisomerase II **(DNA gyrase)** and IV, which impedes DNA replication, repair and transcription, thereby resulting in bacterial death. The ability to target both enzymes helps to prevent or delay resistance.

Indications

Both drugs inhibit gram-positive bacteria, most notably penicillin-susceptible and-resistant strains of *Staphylococcus pneumoniae*. Compared with ciprofloxacin, moxifloxacin and gatifloxacin have enhanced activity against ***Staphylococcus aureus*** but less activity against methicillin-resistant strains than against methicillin-susceptible strains.

Antibiotics in Development: Dalbavancin and Oritavancin

Two glycopeptide antibiotics may soon be available, dalbavancin, a novel semisynthetic glycopeptide with a half-life of 9 to 12 days, and oritavancin, another semisynthetic with a chemical structure that enhances better anchoring to bacterial cytoplasmic membranes. Both agents have the same mechanism of action, that is, the inhibition of cell-wall peptidoglycan cross-linking.

DAPSONE

Mechanism of action is similar to sulfonamides and it causes competitive antagonists of PABA prevent formation of folic acid, inhibiting bacterial growth.

Dapsone is used in treatment of the following:

1. Leprosy.
2. Prophylaxis of malaria and of *pneumocystis carinii* infection.
3. Immunobullous disorders—especially dermatitis herpetiformis, neutrophilic dermatoses and vasculitis.

The main toxicity of dapsone relates to its effects on hematopoiesis. Agranulocytosis hemolysis and methemoglobinemia occurs in all recipients; hemolysis occurs especially in patients with glucose-6-phosphate dehydrogenase deficiency. Headache is also common, probably due to methemoglobinemia. Monitoring includes regular blood counts.

Other side effects include a motor peripheral neuropathy, anorexia, and headache; if severe rash occurs with eosinophilia (dapsone syndrome), then treatment should be stopped, as there is a risk of progression to hepatitis, psychosis, and even death.

COLCHICINE

Colchicine affects microtubule function and probably produces its antiinflammatory effects mainly by interfering with polymorphonuclear leukocyte function. In dermatology it has a potential role in a number of vasculitic and neutrophilic disorders, Behçet disease (and other aphthous ulceration), occasionally in immunobullous diseases and amyloidosis.

The main side effects when used at doses traditionally applied for gout are gastrointestinal disturbance and diarrhea.

POTASSIUM IODIDE

This is an old agent that may be useful in the following conditions. Infections–sporotrichosis, panniculitis or vasculitis, neutrophilic disorders.

Potassium iodide has an unpleasant taste, and treatment may be limited by gastrointestinal disturbance. It can cause various rashes, including iododerma, and may cause hypothyroidism.

ANTIMALARIALS

Chloroquine phosphate: Inhibits chemotaxis of eosinophils and locomotion of neutrophils, and impairs complement-dependent antigen-antibody reactions. May also have photoprotective effect.

Uses include: Lupus erythematosus - especially discoid, subacute cutaneous LE, polymorphic light eruption, porphyria cutanea tarda.

Main side effect include ocular toxicity.

Dose: 250–500 mg daily, maintaining level at lowest effective dose. Must not exceed 3.5 mg/kg body weight/day (based on the ideal/lean body weight and not on the actual weight of the patient.

Hydroxychloroquine

Uses include: Systemic and discoid lupus erythematosus, polymorphic light eruption.

Dose: 200–400 mg daily, maintaining level at lowest effective dose. Must not exceed 6.5 mg/kg body weight/day (based on the ideal/lean body weight and not on the actual weight of the patient).

Side Effects

- Retinopathy which may cause permanent blindness.
- Corneal deposits.
- Headaches.
- Gut upsets, pruritus and rashes.

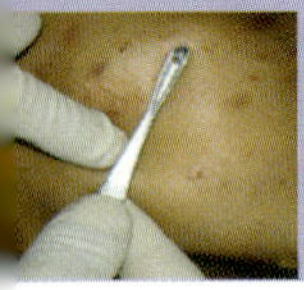

- Worsening of psoriasis.
- Vivid dreams.

Monitoring

During treatment, patients should be asked annually about visual symptoms and their visual acuity should be monitored using the standard reading chart.

Discontinue drug if any change occurs. Reduce dose with poor renal or liver function. Best avoided in the elderly and children.

Prefer intermittent short courses to continuous treatment if possible.

THALIDOMIDE

Immunomodulatory agent that may suppress activated lymphocytes or prevent their activation.

Thalidomide inhibits tumor necrosis factor (TNF) and various other cytokines, and decreases lymphocyte proliferation and neutrophil activity. It is not commonly used due to its potentially significant side effects, but it may be useful in the following.

1. Aphthous ulceration - Especially due to Behçet disease or in HIV infection.
2. Nodular prurigo.
3. Erythema nodosum leprosum.
4. Graft-versus-host disease.
5. Chronic discoid lupus erythematosus.
6. Pyoderma gangrenosum.

Side effects include the following:

1. Teratogenicity - Common and severe, so pregnancy must be avoided.
2. Neuropathy - Nerve conduction studies are a required part of monitoring.
3. Other common effects - Sedation, mood disturbance, nausea, decreased thyroid function and rashes.

Careful monitoring and application of precautions to avoid pregnancy are mandatory and reduce the usefulness of this agent. Perform pregnancy test within 24 hours prior to initiating therapy.

INTERFERONS

Interferons are cytokines that have antimicrobial, anti-tumor, and antiinflammatory actions. They are administered by subcutaneous injection.

The major uses in dermatology (although usually administered by oncologists) are:

1. Melanoma or cutaneous T-cell lymphoma.
2. HIV-related Kaposi sarcoma may also be treated.
3. Warts.
4. Hemangiomas.

Side effects of interferons include the following: General malaise, flu-like symptoms and gastrointestinal upset.

PHOTOTHERAPY

Initiated only in the presence of extensive and widespread disease. Resistance to topical treatment is another indication for phototherapy.

- **UVB irradiation (290-320 nm):** UVB therapy is usually combined with one or more topical treatments. The **Goeckerman regimen** uses coal tar followed by UVB exposure and has been shown to induce disease remission in more than 80% of patients. The **Ingram method** is based on anthralin application following a tar bath and UVB treatment.
- UVB phototherapy is extremely effective for treating moderate-to-severe plaque psoriasis.
- **Narrow-band UVB phototherapy** uses a fluorescent bulb with a narrow emission spectrum that peaks at 311 nm (UVB spectrum, 290-320 nm). This selective and relatively longer wavelength is more effective than broadband UVB for the treatment of plaque-type psoriasis.
- **PUVA photochemotherapy,** also known as PUVA, uses the photosensitizing drug methoxsalen (8-methoxypsoralens) in combination with UVA irradiation to treat patients with more extensive disease. UVA irradiation uses light with wavelengths of 320-400 nm. PUVA leads to a localized immunosuppression.
- More than 85% of patients report relief of disease symptoms with 20-30 treatments. Therapy is usually administered 2-3 times per week in an outpatient setting, with maintenance treatments every 2-4 weeks until remission.
- Adverse effects of PUVA therapy include nausea, pruritus, and a burning sensation. Long-term complications include increased risks of photo damage to the skin and (more importantly) skin cancer. PUVA has been combined with oral retinoid derivatives to decrease the cumulative dose of UVA radiation to the skin.

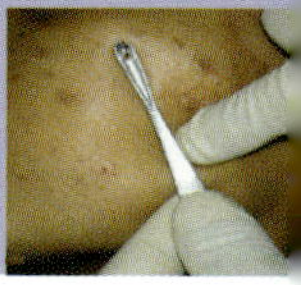

PUVA

8-Methoxypsoralen (methoxsalen)

Severe psoriasis, vitiligo, localized pustular psoriasis, cutaneous T-cell lymphoma rarely, lichen planus, atopic dermatitis.

Tablets: 0.6–0.8 mg/kg body weight taken as a single dose 1–2 hours before exposure to UVA.

Side Effects

- Nausea.
- Itching.
- Photoxicity.
- Cataracts.
- Lentigines.
- Ageing changes of skin.
- Hyperpigmentation.
- Cutaneous neoplasms.

Caution

The following should be checked before treatment:

- **Skin:** Examine for premalignant lesions and skin cancer.
- **Eyes:** Check for cataracts. Fundoscopic examination of retina.

Visual acuity

- **Blood:** Full blood count, liver and renal function tests and antinuclear factor test.
- Urine analysis.
- Eyes should be protected with appropriate lenses for 24 hours after taking the drug.
- Protective goggles must be worn during radiation. If feasible, shield face and genitalia during treatment.
- Patients must protect skin against additional sun exposure after ingestion.
- Monitor eyes for development of cataracts.
- Try to avoid maintenance treatment, more than 250 treatments and a cumulative dose of more than 1000 joules/cm^2 (skin cancer risk).

BIOLOGIC THERAPY

These relatively new systemic therapies provide selective, immunologically directed intervention at key steps in the pathogenesis of the disease. Similar to the systemic agents, these therapies are typically reserved for more severe and recalcitrant cases including psoriatic arthritis.

An overview is given in Table 24.12.

Efalizumab

Recombinant humanized monoclonal Anti-CD11a antibody.

Etanercept

Prevents excess TNF from binding to cell-bound receptors.

Infliximab

Monoclonal antibody that targets TNF and inhibits its activity.

REFERENCES

- Dermatological Therapy, Dermatology Clinics 2005.
- Arndt, K.A. (1995): Manual of Dermatologic Therapeutics, 5th edn., Little, Brown, Boston, MA.

Table 24. 12: Biologic therapy

Features	Alefacept	Efalizumab	Etanercept	Infliximab
Type of agent	Fusion protein	Humanized monoclonal antibody	Fusion protein	Monoclonal antibody TNF-α
Mechanism of action	Blocks T-cell action	Anti CD la blocks T-cell	TNF-α inhibitor	TNF-α inhibitor
Route of administration	1M 2nd line for psoriasis	IM Banned	IM Psoriatic arthritis	IV 2nd line for psoriasis

Surgical and Cosmetology

RELAXED SKIN TENSION LINES (RSTL) (Fig. 24.2)

Imaginary lines along which maximal forces are generated by the skin in conjunction with underlying muscle, collagen fibers and fibrous bands.

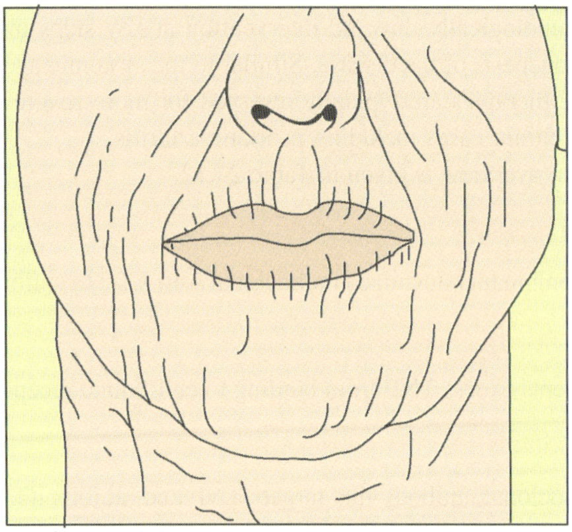

Fig. 24.2: Relaxed skin tension lines (RSTL)

- Excisions/incisions should be parallel to RSTL.
- Orientation of the RSTL:
  – Exercise test.
  – Pinch/compression test.
  – Punch biopsy test.

LOCAL ANAESTHESIA

Combination with vasoconstrictor (adrenaline):

- ↓ anaesthetic absorption.
- Prolonged duration of action.
- Less bleeding at the operative site.
- Lignocaine available in combination with adrenaline usually at a conc. of 1:1,00,000.
- For complete vasoconstriction 7-15 minutes.

Contraindications of Adrenaline

- **Absolute:** Severe hypertension, cardiac disease, hyperthyroidism, peripheral vascular disease, phaechromocytoma.
- **Relative:** Sites (distal extremities, lip, nose and penis), pregnancy (1st and 3rd trimester).
- Certain procedures like vitiligo grafting and non-healing ulcers.

Types of LA

Topical Anaesthesia

Skin: EMLA (eutectic mixture of LA) contains 2.5% lignocaine and 2.5% prilocaine. Apply 1 hour before procedure.

Mucosal agents: Lignocaine (2-5% jelly), Mucopaine.

Infiltration Anaesthesia

Anaesthetic drug directly placed at nerve endings present in the dermis and subcutaneous fat,via an I/D or S/C injection.

Tumescent LA

- Larger diluted amounts of lignocaine are inj. S/C to tumefy the area.
- Onset of this technique takes about 10-15 min.
- **Indications:** Liposuction, hair transplantation, dermabrasion.

Field Blocks (Ring Blocks)

Extension of infiltration anaesthesia where the entire operative field is anaesthetised by injecting from the periphery.

Indications: Biopsies, cyst excisions, therapeutic excision of skin malignancies, large area to be anaesthetised.

BIOPSY TECHNIQUE

Skin Biopsy

- Most common basic and essential diagnostic procedure carried out by dermatologist.
- Sites for biopsy.
  (i) **Lesional:** Routine biopsies.
  (ii) **Perilesional:** DIF in vesicobullous disorders.
  (iii) Clinically uninvolved skin-lupus band test.

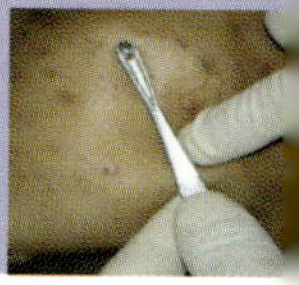

Types

- Shave (Fig. 24.3).
- Punch (Fig. 24.4).
- Excisional.
- Incisional.
- Others.

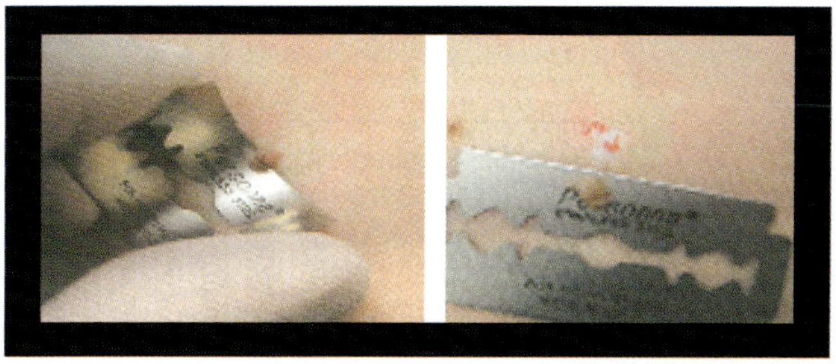

Fig. 24.3: Shave biopsy

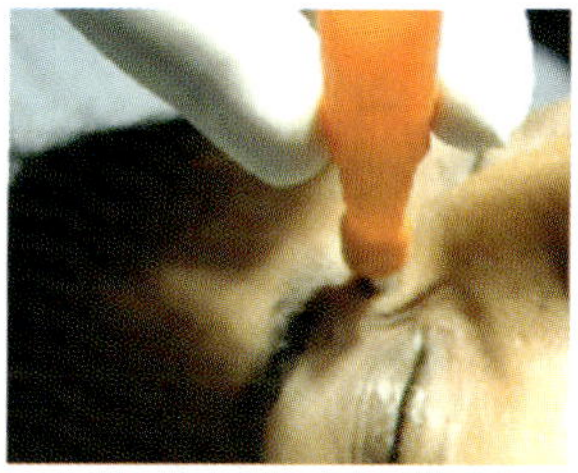

Fig. 24.4: Punch biopsy

Other Biopsy Techniques

- Clip biopsy–pedunculated lesions.
- Mucosal biopsy.

CURETTAGE

- **Curette:** A spoon or ring shaped instrument.
- **Indication:**
  - Small, firm, benign superficial tumors.
    (i) Seborrheic warts.
    (ii) Actinic (solar) keratosis:
    (iii) Solitary plantar wart.
- **Advantages:**
  - Simple, rapid technique.
  - No complicated equipment require.
- **Disadvantages:**
  - Heal with secondary infection.

INTRALESIONAL THERAPY (Fig. 24.5)

Mode of topical drug therapy whereby the barrier zone is bypassed by establishment of a subepidermal depot by intralesional (IL) injection.

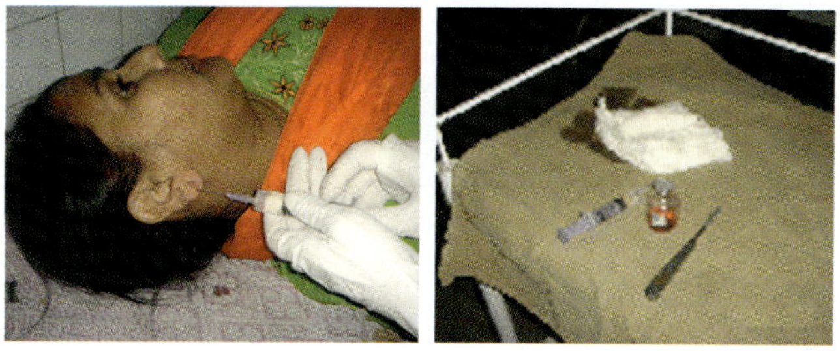

Fig. 24.5: Intralesional corticosteroids

Indications

- **Inflammatory:** Nodular and cystic acne, alopecia areata, DLE, LSC, prurigo nodularis, relapsing polychondritis.
- **Infiltrative lesions:** Keloids, hypertrophic scars.
- **Noninfectious granulomas:** GA, NLD, sarcoidosis.
- **Miscellaneous:** Vitiligo, LS et atrophicus, PHN.

  Triamcinolone acetonide most commonly used in conc.
- From 2 mg/ml - 40 mg/ml.
- Max. 1 mg/site, 30-40 mg/session.
- Use 26 G needle, the drug should be deposited in the dermis.

Intramatrix Steroid Injection

Indications:

- Nail dystrophy–Psoriasis, lichen planus.
- 26 G needle attached to insulin syringe, skin is penetrated at 45° angle near a point 2-2.5 mm proximal and lateral to the junction of proximal and lateral nail fold.
- **2–4 ml** steroid injected.

  S/E–Pain, subungual haematoma, secondary infection.

Complications:

Pain, atrophy, hyperpigmentation, hypo/depigmentation, telangiectasia, striae, hirsutism, secondary infection, HPA axis suppression.

Other Drugs

- Interferons–2b for genital warts.
- I/L Bleomycin for recalcitrant warts.
- I/L 5-florouracil for keloids.

CHEMICAL CAUTERIZATION

Agents used:

- Podophyllin.

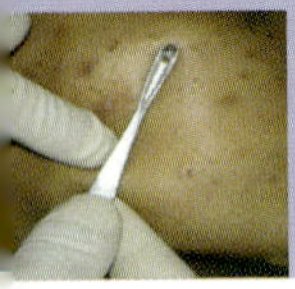

- Trichloroacetic acid.
- Silver nitrate.
- Phenol.

ELECTROSURGERY (Fig. 24.6)

Electrosurgery is a general term to describe all the different procedures employing electrically generated heat.

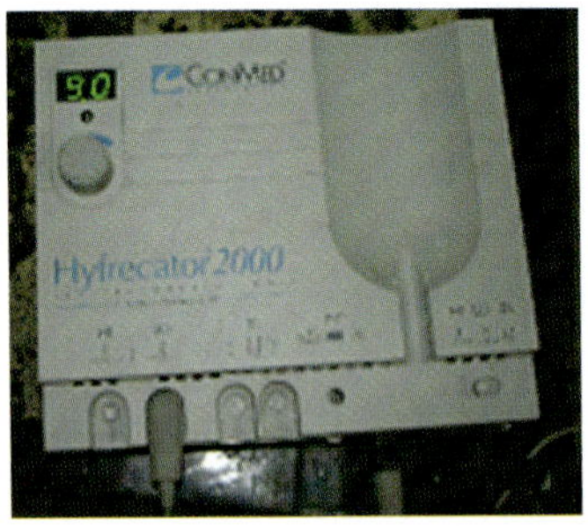

Fig. 24.6: Electrosurgery

Basic principle of electrosurgery is to boost the voltage and frequency while decreasing the amperage of AC from the standard wall outlet.

- Tissue resistance to the passage of high frequency alternating current converts electrical energy to heat, resulting in thermal tissue damage.

Types of Electric Surgery

- **Electrofulgration** (Fig. 24.7)
  - Monoterminal.
  - Damped sine waves. Low amp, high voltage current.
  - Electrode does not touch the tissue.
  - Superficial tissue is charred.
- **Electrodesiccation** (Fig. 24.8)
  - Monoterminal.
  - Damped sine waves. Low amp high voltage current.
  - The lesion is touched with the electrode.

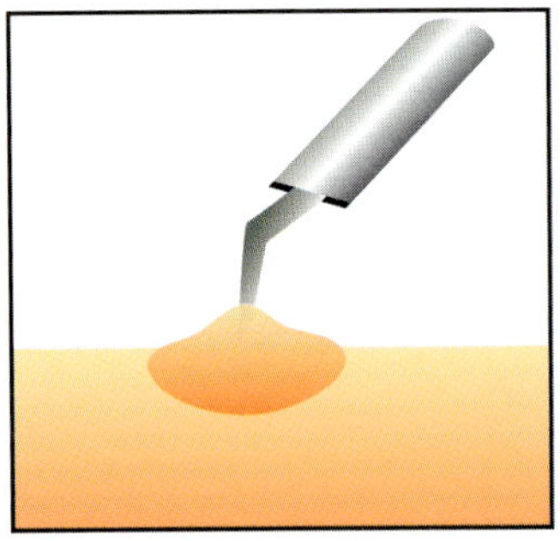

Fig. 24.7: Electrofulgration

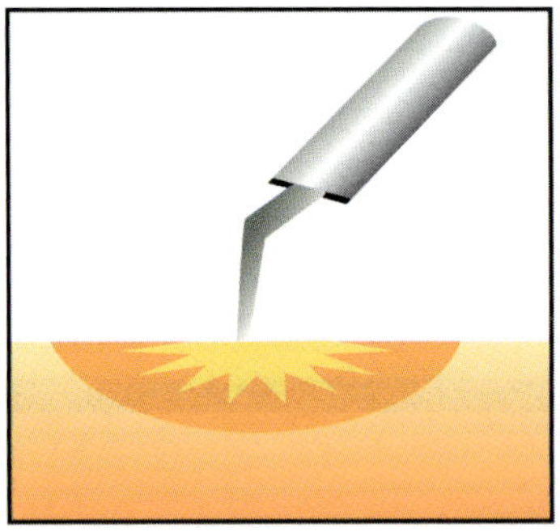

Fig. 24.8: Electrodessication

- **Electrocoagulation**
  - Biterminal with ground plate.
  - Partially rectified sine waves. Low voltage and high amperage.
  - Possible with the common electrosurgical unit used, pass current for longer period and give high intensity of current.
- **Electrosection**
  - Biterminal with ground plate.
  - Rectified sine waves.

Precautions and Preventions

- Avoid inflammable sterlization.
- Adequate exhaust facilities.
- Check all connections and wires face mask, gloves.

Local anaesthesia: In case of warts give perilesional.

Common Clinical Applications

- Warts.
- Acrochordons and **DPN**.
- Molluscum contagiosum and milia.
- Adnexal lesions–Acne, trichoepithelioma, syringoma, adenoma sebaceum.
- BCC and SCC.
- Vascular naevi.
- Pyogenic granuloma.
- Mucosal cysts.

Radiosurgery (Fig. 24.9)

Thermal tissue destruction with various waveforms of AC whose frequencies (ultrahigh) fall within the range of radiofrequency (RF 500-4000 khz).

Four types of waveforms are produced:

- Fully filtered and rectified (90% cutting and 10% coagulation).
- Fully rectified (50% cutting and 50% coagulation).

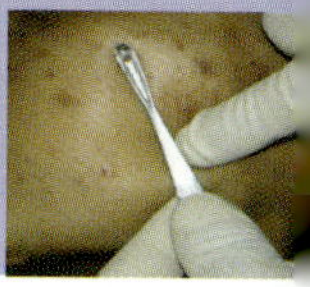

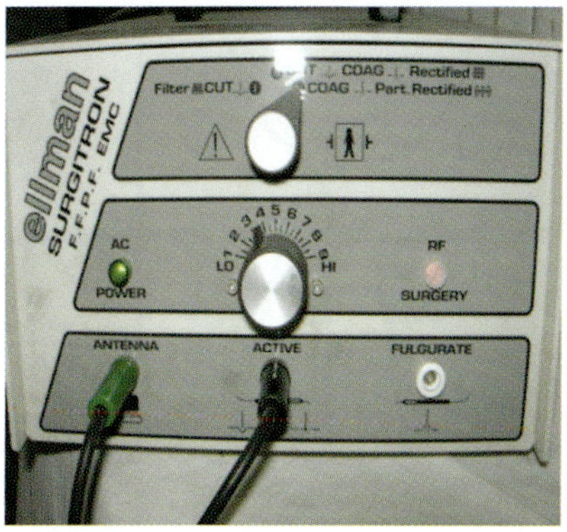

Fig. 24.9: Radiofrequency apparatus

- Partially rectified (90% coagulation and 10% cutting).
- Fulguration.

Clinical Applications

Electrosection.
Pure cutting – Biopsy, skin incisions, excison of cysts and tumors.
Cutting and coagulation: Skin tags, keloids, seborshoeic keratosis.

Advantages over Routine Electrosurgery

- Generates 3 types of energies, wider application.
- Less lateral heat spread.
- Better control and lesser side effects and complications.

Cryosurgery (Fig. 24.10)

- Use of local freezing for controlled destruction/removal of unwanted tissues.

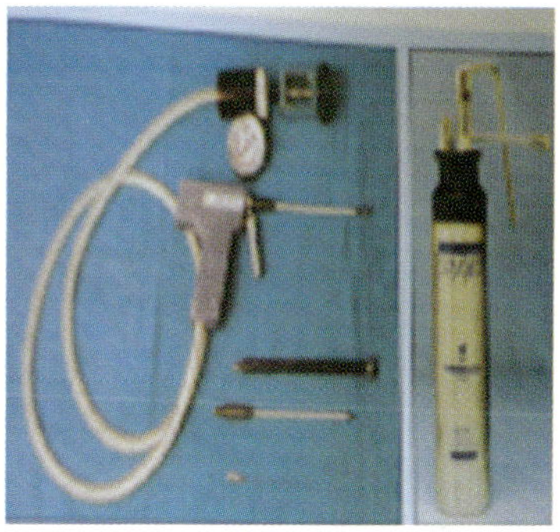

Fig. 24.10: Cryosurgery

- Rapid freezing, slow and complete thawing, single or repeat thaw cycles.
- Cryogen is a freezing substance used for withdrawal of heat in cryosurgery.
  Freon (-30°C), N_2O(-70°C), **LN_2 (-196°C)**.
- Can be used alone or combined e.g. with I/L steroids.

Mechanism of Action (Cryonecrosis)

- Cellular injury.
- Intracellular and extracellular ice formation.
- Osmolarity changes.
- Thermal shock.
- Denaturation of lipoprotein complexes.
- Vascular stasis.
- Immunological-freezing stimulates immune response which helps in destruction of tumour cells.

Differential Sensitivity of Cells

Melanocytes	-4°C to - 8°C
Keratinocytes	-20°C to -30°C
Dermal connective tissue and fibroblast	-30°C to -40°C

- **Freeze time:** Time duration from formation of ice till maintenance of ice field.
- **Freeze thaw cycle:** Period of freezing of tissue and thawing up till return to room temperature.
- Thaw time is usually double the freeze time.
  Rapid freezing and slow thawing is more destructive.

Indications

- **Benign lesions:** Warts, molluscum, keloid, skin tags, pyogenic granuloma, seb. warts, cystic acne.
- **Premalignant lesions:** Leukoplakia, Bowen's disease, Actinic keratosis.
- **Malignant:** BCC, SCC, lentigo maligna.

Contraindications

- Agammaglobulinemia, cold intolerance.
- Cold urticaria, cryoglobulinemia.
- Cryofibrinogenemia.
- Raynaud's disease, collagen vascular disease.

Common Conditions with Freeze Time

Benign	***Time (sec)***
Common warts	15-20
Keloid	20-30
Skin tags	5-10
Acne cysts, scars	2-7
Premalignant } Leukoplakia **Malignant**	25-30

Minimum of two 30 sec freeze thaw cycles with a 5 min thaw period between each freeze.

Complications and Side Effects

- **Immediate:** Pain, edema, blister formation, syncope.
- **Delayed:** Postoperative infection, pseudoepitheliomatous hyperplasia.

- **Prolonged:** Hypo or depigmentation, atrophy, cicatricial alopecia, milia etc.

ACNE SURGERY

- Adjuvant to the basic medical treatment.
- Shortens duration of the lesion, prevents additional infections.

Types of Surgical Procedures

- Comedone extraction (Fig. 24.11).
- Evacuation followed by incision and drainage.
- I/L corticosteriods (26G needle most non-dependent part).
- Electrodessication.
- Superficial chemical peeling.
- **LN_2** cryoroller, cryopeel.

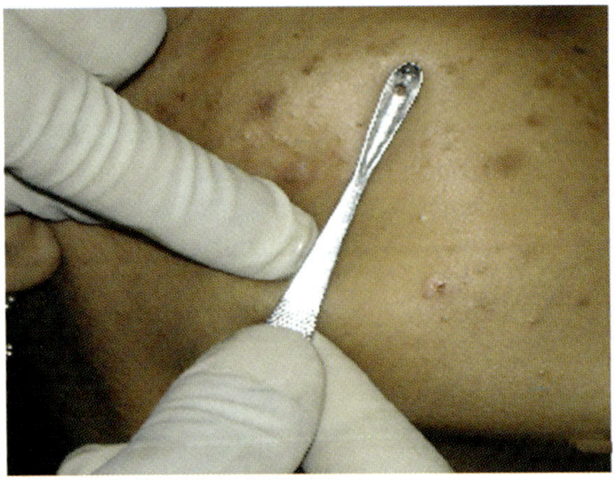

Fig. 24.11: Comedoe extraction

ACNE SCAR REVISION

Classification of Acne Scars (Fig. 24.12)

Icepick scars: Narrow (<2 mm), deep, taper down into dermis or S/C.

Rolling scars: Shallow usually wider than 4-5 mm. Occur due to dermal tethering of otherwise relatively normal looking skin.

Boxcar scars: Round or oval with sharply demarcated vertical edges. Shallow or deep.

Types of Techniques

- Local undermining (subcision) (Fig. 24.13) – uplifting the scar by cutting the S/C bands under the pits.
- Punch excision and closure.

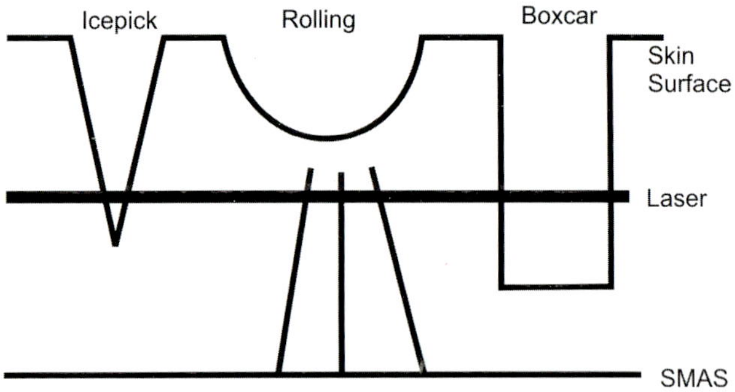

Fig. 24.12: Classification of scars

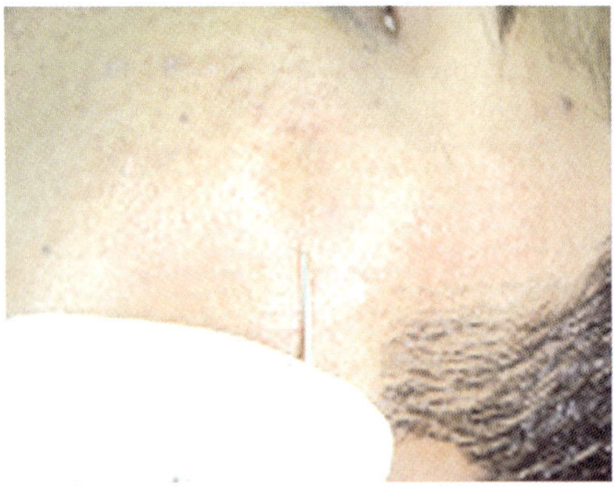

Fig. 24.13: Subcision

- Punch incision and elevation (Fig. 24.14).
- Punch excision and graft replacement.

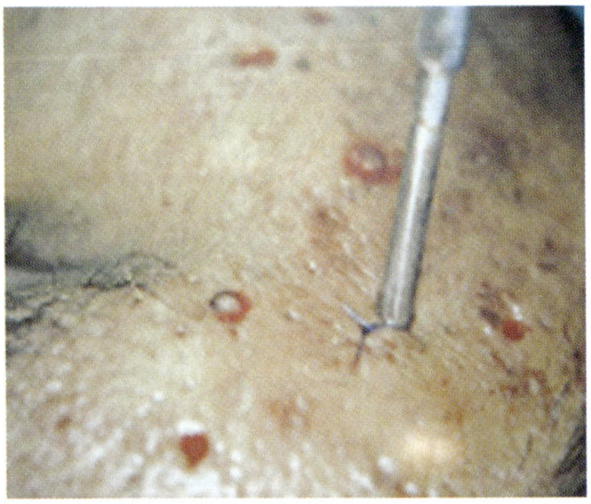

Fig. 24.14: Punch incision and elevation

NAIL SURGERY (Fig. 24.15)

General Principles for Nail Surgeries

- Proper case selection.
- LA: No adrenaline, Ring block, max. 8-10 ml.
- Strict hemostasis: Proper exsanguination followed by basal tourniquet.

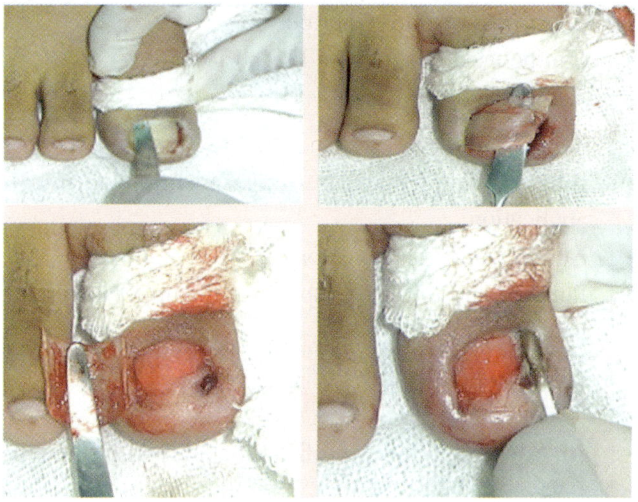

Fig. 24.15: Nail surgery

- Minimum/gentle manipulation of nail matrix to avoid trauma and dystrophic nail formation, post operative wound care.

Nail Avulsion

Distal Nail Avulsion: Total, partial.

Indications: Nail bed, Nail matrix biopsy, Onychomycosis, Ingrown toe nail, Sub-periungual warts, Subungual hematoma/abscess drainage, Onychodystrophy.

SKIN GRAFTING

Types of Grafts

- Split thickness Graft.
- Thin (thiersch).
- Intermediate.
- Thick.
- Full thickness graft.

Skin Graft use in Vitiligo

- Punch grafting.
- Split thickness grafting.
- Suction and blister grafting

TATTOING

Introduction of various dyes and pigments into the skin.

Indication:

- Localized stable vitiligo.
- Portwine stain.

HAIR TRANSPLANTATION (Fig. 24.16)

Follicular Unit (FU)

- Hair occurs in group of one, two or three hairs called follicular unit.
- Dissection of such units and then transplanting them is called follicular unit transplantation.
- The number of hairs a person has depends on the type of units and the type of density.

Indication

- Male pattern baldness (MPA).
- Female AA.
- Cicatricial alopecia.
- Reconstruction of eyebrow.
- **Side burns.**

Contraindication

- Large bald area.
- Small donor area.
- Low hair density.
- Bleeding disorder.
- Keloidal tendency.

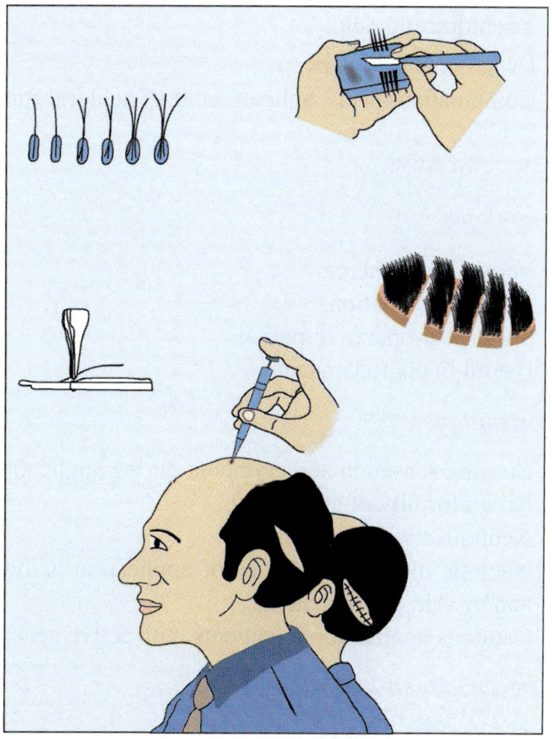

Fig. 24.16: Hair transplantation

- Systemic debiliting disease.
- Progressive MPA in young patient.

Other Methods

- Alopecia reduction.
- Transposition of scalp flap.
- Synthetic hair grafting.

CHEMICAL PEEL

Chemical peel produces a controlled partial thickness injury to the skin. Following the insult to the skin, a wound healing process ensues that can regenerate epidermis from surrounding epithelium and adnexal structures, decrease solar elastosis, and replace and reorient the new dermal connective tissue. The result is an improved clinical appearance of the skin, with fewer rhytides and decreased pigmentary dyschromia.

Peeling Agents

- Glycolic acid.
- Jessner's solution.
- Pyruvic acid.
- Resorcinol.
- Salicylic acid.
- Trichloracetic acid.
- Deep chemical peels.
- Combinations peels: Salicylic acid +Trichloracetic acid.

(i) Glycolic Acid

Advantages

- Very mild erythema.
- Mild desquamation.
- Short post-operative period.
- Useful in photodamage.

Disadvantages

- Burning sensation and erythema during application.
- No uniformity of application.
- Neutralization is mandatory.
- Necrotic ulcerations if time of application is too long and/or skin pH is reduced.
- Cautious application in patients with active acne.

(ii) Pyruvic Acid Advantages

- Very mild erythema.
- Mild desquamation.
- Short post-operative period.
- Can be used in skin type III and IV.

Disadvantages

- Intense stinging and burning sensation during the application.
- Neutralization is mandatory.
- Pungent and irritating vapors for the upper respiratory mucosa.

(iii) Salicylic Acid Advantages

- An established safety profile in patients with skin types I-VI.
- Excellent in patients with acne.
- Given the appearance of the white precipitate, uniformity of application is easily achieved.
- After several minutes the peel can induce an anesthetic effect whereby increasing patient tolerance.

Disadvantages

- Limited depth of peeling.
- Minimal efficacy in patients with significant photodamage.

(iv) Deep Chemical Peels

- Useful in patients with photodamage.
- Useful in patients with perioral wrinkles.
- Useful in patients with atrophic acne scars.
- Useful for facial skin rejuvenation.

(v) Combination Peels

Salicylic Acid + TCA

- Efficacy in all skin types.
- Well tolerated in darker racial/ethnic groups.
- Most beneficial in treating recalcitrant melasma and post-inflammatory hyperpigmentation.

Disadvantages

- Increased depth of superficial peeling.
- Increased desquamation in some patients lasting up to 7-10 days.
- Post-inflammatory hyperpigmentation more common than with salicylic acid peeling alone.

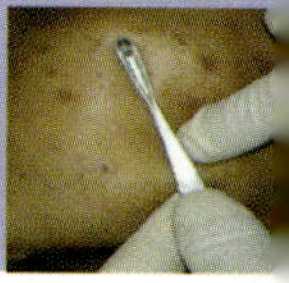

USE OF PEELS IN VARIOUS SKIN DISORDERS/SKIN TYPES

Acne

Comedonal acne	Salicylic acid 25%, Pyruvic acid 40-70% Jessner's solution, Unna Paste, Glycolic acid 70%
Mild/moderate inflammatory acne	Salicylic acid 25-30% Pyruvic acid 40-70%, Jessner's solution, Unna Paste Glycolic acid 70%
Severe nodulo-cystic acne	Pyruvic acid 40-60%
Superficial post-acne scars	Pyruvic acid 40-70% Trichloracetic acid>(25-50%) lotion Salicylic acid 25% +trichloracetic acid 25-30% gel
Medium-deep post-acne scars	Phenol 45-80% Trichloracetic acid> (40%) excision, elevation, subcision.

Dark Skin

- Salicylic acid 20-30%.
- Jessner's solution.
- Glycolic acid 20, 35, 50, 70%.
- Trichloracetic acid 10-30%.

Melasma

- Salicylic acid 25%.
- Salicylic acid 25% + trichloracetic acid 10% gel.
- Pyruvic acid 40-50%.
- Glycolic acid 50-70%.
- Trichloracetic acid 15-20%.
- Resorcinol.

Photoageing

• Mild to moderate	Glycolic acid 50-70% Trichloracetic acid 50%, Salicylic acid 20-30%, Salicylic acid 25% +trichloracetic acid >(25%) gel
• Extensive	Glycolic acid 70% + trichloracetic acid 35% Jessner's solution + trichloracetic acid 35% Pyruvic acid 60-70% Phenol 45-80%

Postinflammatory Pigmentation

- Salicylic acid 20-30%.
- Glycolic acid 70%.
- Jessner's solution.
- Pyruvic acid 40%

LASER SURGERY

- The Principle of Selective Photothermolysis was proposed in 1983 by Anderson and Parrish.
- Selective photothermolysis is the process in which transfer of laser energy is restricted to a particular site because of the selective absorption of a chromophore at that site.
- In other words, ***proper selection of the wavelength and exposure time damages only the desired target tissue***.

For selective photothermolysis to occur, the surgeon must choose:

- The appropriate **Wavelength** selectively absorbed by the target tissue.
- The appropriate **Exposure time** which should be less than the thermal relaxation time of the target tissue.
- The appropriate **Energy density**, or ***Fluence*** to produce the desired effect, such as vaporization, coagulation, or photodisruption.
- **Pulse duration:** The time during which the laser output pulse power remains continuously above half its maximum value.
- **Power Density, or *Irradiance*** refers to the power of the laser per unit area.
- **Energy Density, or *Fluence*** is the irradiance multiplied by the exposure time, measured in Joules/square centimeter.

Types of Lasers

- **Solid-state lasers** have lasing material distributed in a solid matrix (such as the ruby or neodymium:yttrium-aluminum garnet "Yag" lasers). The neodymium-Yag laser emits infrared light at 1064 nanometers (nm).
  - Nd: YAG laser.
  - Er: YAG laser.
  - Ti: Sapphire laser.
  - Holmium: YAG laser.
  - Alexandrite laser.
- **Gas lasers** (helium and helium-neon, HeNe, are the most common gas lasers) have a primary output of visible red light. CO_2 lasers emit energy in the far-infrared, and are used for cutting hard materials.
  - CO_2 laser.
  - Argon ion laser.
  - Kryptonion.
  - Copper vapor laser.
  - Excimer laser.
  - Nitrogen laser.
  - He-Ne laser.

- **Excimer lasers** (the name is derived from the terms excited and dimers).

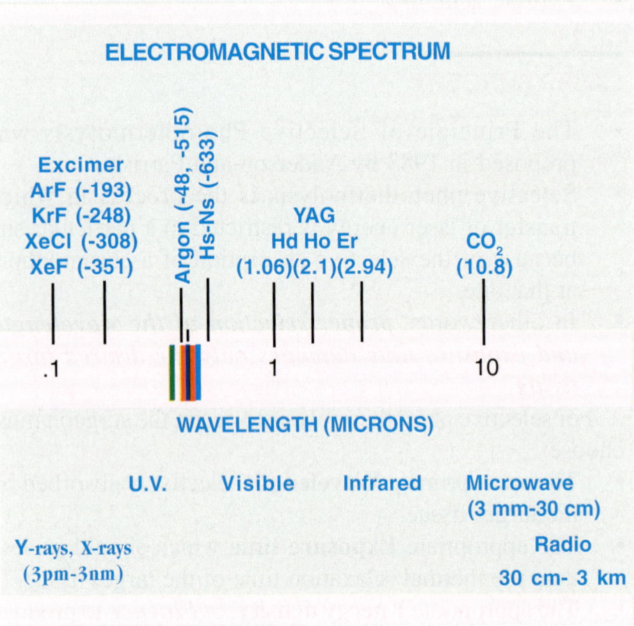

- **Semiconductor lasers,** sometimes called **diode lasers**, are not solid-state lasers. These electronic devices are generally very small and use low power.

LASER OUTPUT

- Pulsed
  - 10^{-6} seconds: Microseconds.
- Superpulsed
  - 10^{-3} seconds: Milliseconds, repetitive train pulses.
- Q-switched
  - 10^{-9} seconds: Nanoseconds.

LASER TISSUE INTERACTIONS

Laser: Type and Uses

Portwine stains	Flashlamp pulsed Dye Laser.
	Argon Laser, KTP Laser,IPL
Pigmentary disorder	Nd YAG
Cholasma	Tunable Dye Laser
Café au lait macules	Nd:YAG Laser
Lentigenes	Nd:YAG Laser
Tattoos	Q Switched Ruby Laser Alexandrite Laser Tunable Dye Laser
Hair removal	Diode, Nd:YAG, IPL

Type of Light	Primary Chromophore
Infrared	Water
Visible light	Hemoglobin
Ultraviolet	Melanin

- **Importance of wavelength**
  As the wavelength decreases toward the blue-violet, and ultraviolet, penetration of the light into the tissue decreases and scattering increases.
- **Thermal relaxation time**
  The time taken by a target structure to dissipate 50% of the energy absorbed to surrounding tissue, immediately after irradiation.
- **Thermal containment time**
  The time in which no heat (and hence no thermal effect) is dissipated to surrounding tissue, and is roughly *one-quarter* of the thermal relaxation time. This TCT defines the ideal pulse width for treating a given chromophore.

LASER HAIR REMOVAL (Fig. 24.17)

Hair removal lasers selectively target Melanin:

- There are two types of melanin in hair: *Eumelanin* (which gives hair brown or black color) and *pheomelanin* (which gives hair blonde or red color). Because of the selective absorption of photons of laser light, only black or brown hair can be removed.
- Laser is attracted to dark pigment and therefore works best with dark coarse hair. Light skin and dark hair are an ideal combination.
- Wavelengths between approximately 700 and 1000 nanometers (nm) are selectively absorbed by melanin; the competing chromophores (oxyhemoglobin and water) absorb less energy at these wavelengths.

Therefore, any light source that operates between 700 and 1000 nm is appropriate for targeting melanin in the hair shaft.

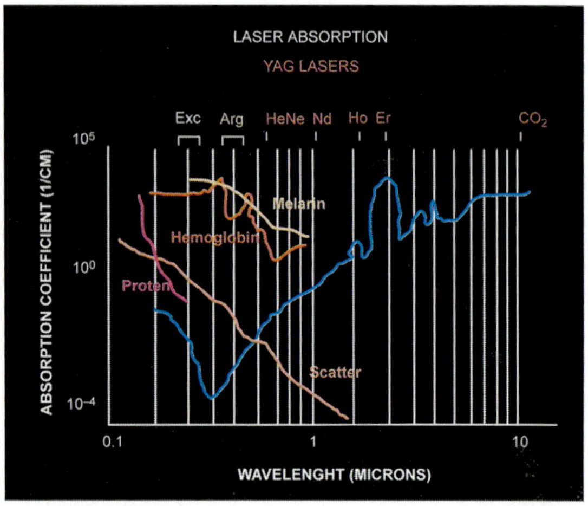

Fig. 24.17: Selective absorption of laser by target antigen

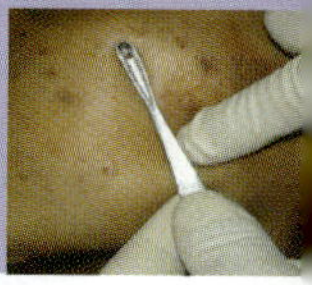

Table 24.13: Laser types and selective absorption

Laser	*Wavelength (nm)*	*Specific**	*Application*
• Er:YAG	2940	Water	Skin resurfacing
• Argon	488/514	Hb	Vascular lesions
• KTP:YAG	532	Hb	Vascular lesions
• Copper vapor	578	Hb	Vascular lesions
• FLPDL	585	Hb	Vascular lesions
• Nd: YAG Long pulse	595-600	Hb, Melanin	Leg veins
• Ruby, Q-switched	694	Hb, Pigment	Tattoo removal
• Long pulse	694	Hair removal	
• Nd:YAG	1064	Hb	Deep vascular
• Q-switched YAG	1064	Pigment	Tattoo removal
• CO_2	10600	Water	Coagulation/resurfacing

* Specific absorption for various skin constituents.

FLPDL: Flash lamp pump dye laser.

Table 24.14: Thermal relaxation time of some potential targets

Target	*Thermal relaxation time*
Erythrocyte	2 µs
200 µm hair follicle	40 ms
0.5 µm melanosome	0.25 µs
10 µm nevus call	0.1 ms
0.1 mm diameter vessel	10 ms
0.4 mm diameter vessel	80 ms
0.8 mm diameter vessel	300 ms

LASER TREATMENT OF VASCULAR LESIONS

- Portwine stains.
- Hemangiomas.
- Venous malformations.
- Lymphangiomas.

Acquired Lesions

- Telangiectasias.
- Cherry angiomas.
- Pyogenic granulomas.
- Venous lakes.
- Poikiloderma.
- Kaposi sarcoma.

FLASHLAMP-PUMPED PDL

Target chromophore	Oxy-Hemoglobin
Wavelength	585 nm
Pulse duration	1.5 ms

Argon Laser

Target	Oxy-Hemoglobin
Wavelength	488-514 nm
Spot size	0.1-1.0 mm
Tissue penetration depth	1-2 mm

- It emits blue-green light, 80% of emission in the 488- to 514 nm.
- Predominantly absorbed by oxyhemoglobin, to some extent by epidermal and dermal melanin because of its shorter wavelength.

KTP

KTP laser uses a 1064 nm Nd:YAG source passed through a KTP crystal to emit light that is frequency doubled with a wavelength of 532 nm.

The 568 nm krypton laser used for treatment of facial telangiectasias.

IPL devices are as a rule less effective at a given task than a laser dedicated to the purpose

Nd:YAG emits a near-infrared invisible light at 1064nm or 1320 nm.

ER: Yag Laser

- Referred to as the "Erbium" laser.
- It emits a mid-infrared beam at 2940 nm, which coincides with the absorption peak for water.

- Principal use is to ablate tissue for cosmetic *laser resurfacing* for wrinkles.
- The **Erbium** laser causes less redness, decreased side effects and rapid healing compared to the pulsed or scanned CO_2 laser, but does so by its limited penetration into tissue, which limits the results compared to the more versatile CO_2 laser.
- **Ruby laser** light is strongly absorbed by blue and black pigment, and by melanin in skin and hair.
- Current uses include:
  1. Treatment of tattoos (Q-Switched mode).
  2. Treatment of pigmented lesions including freckles, liver spots, Nevus of Ota, café-au-lait spots (Q-Switched mode).
  3. Laser hair removal (free-running mode).

Alexandrite Lasers

It contains a rod of synthetic chryso-beryl, a gemstone discovered in Russia in 1830 on Czar Alexander II's 13th birthday.

- It emits a deep red light at 755 nm, and has properties similar to the ruby laser. It's slightly longer wavelength permits slightly deeper penetration into skin, with slightly less absorption by melanin.
- Prinicipal uses include laser hair removal in millisecond-range pulsed mode, and tattoo removal in Q-Switched mode.

Excimer Lasers

Noble gas: Halide, Excimer Lasers, emit invisible ultraviolet (UV) light that triggers a photochemical reaction on the target tissue.

- This very short wavelength is capable of high resolution and microscopic surgery.
- The most common medical application is the Argon: Fluorine (Ar: F) laser at 193 nm, used for PRK and LASIK (Laser in-situ Keratomilieusis) vision correction.

CO_2

- Developed by Patel at Bell Laboratories in 1964. Often referred to as the "Surgical Laser".
- Strongly absorbed by water, which constitutes over 80% of soft tissue.
- **CO_2 laser** emits continuous wave (CW) or pulsed far infrared light at 10,600 nm, which can be focused into a thin beam and used to cut like a scalpel, or defocussed to vaporize, ablate, or shave soft tissue.

Used for cutting or volume ablation by means of tissue vaporization. This unique characteristic makes the CO_2 laser the most widely used medical laser today.

LASER TREATMENT OF PIGMENTED LESIONS

- Melanin or tattoo pigments absorb laser light at wavelengths from 400 to 1000 nm.
- The longer wavelengths like red and infrared light are able to penetrate deeper into the dermis and hence are used to treat dermal lesions.
- The shorter wavelengths of green light are used to treat epidermal lesions.

Epidermal Pigmented Lesions

- Lentigenes and freckles respond very well to laser. Any of the lasers emitting light of wavelength **510-694** are suitable. Generally the lesions are eliminated with one or two laser sessions at 6-8 weeks apart.
- Café-au-lait macules have variable response to laser treatment. They may clear with a few treatments, only after as many as 10 treatments, or they may be unresponsive to laser treatment. The recurrence rate is high.
- Becker's naevus is another epidermal pigmented lesion that responds poorly to laser treatment.

Dermal Pigmented Lesions

Naevus of Ota: The pigments are deep in the dermis and surgery will result in scarring.

- Laser treatment is able to clear the pigmentation without scarring.
- Multiple treatments (at least 5-6 treatments).
- The lasers emitting the longer infrared light e.g. Q-switched Nd: YAG are more suited for dermal pigmented lesions.
- Moles can also be treated with lasers. However there is the disadvantage of multiple treatments, misdiagnosis of a malignant melanoma and incomplete removal of naevus cells.

LASER FACIAL REJUVENATION

Choice of Laser

The Erbium Yag laser is selected for:

- Superficial to moderate facial wrinkles.
- Mild surface scars or discolorations.
- In areas where the skin is more delicate like those around the eyes, mouth, neck and hands.
- For patients with darker skin types.
- For those who cannot tolerate prolonged redness after the procedure.

The CO_2 laser is more effective for:

- Deeper facial wrinkles.
- Severe sun damage.

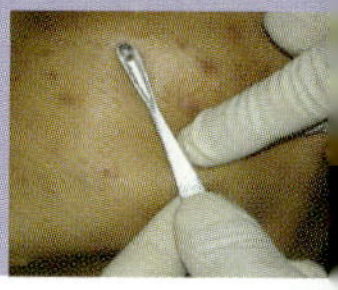

- Where patient can tolerate longer healing time and more prolonged redness.

ANTIAGEING TREATMENT MODALITIES

1. Botulinum toxin application.
2. Mesotherapy.
3. Liposuction.
4. Soft tissue augmentation (dermal filler substance).
5. Antiptosis suspension threads.
6. Hair restoration (medical and surgical).
7. Chemical peeling.
8. Dermabrasion.
9. Microdermabrasion.
10. Laser treatment for pigmented skin.
11. LED photomodulation.
12. Filling agents.

Filling Agents (Fig. 24.18)

Soft tissue augmentation (STA) techniques are minimally invasive surgical procedures in which filling agents (fillers) or surgical techniques alone are used to increase or replace local volume.

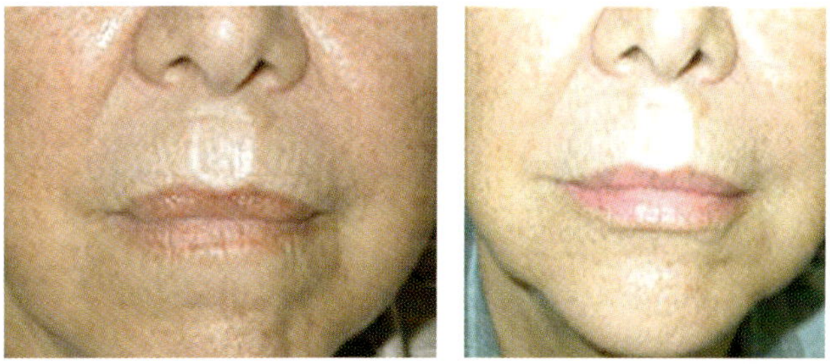

Fig. 24.18: Filling agents

2 months after for correction of nasolabial fold

Fillers can be used in combination with other medical or surgical treatments in the same or different treatment sessions. Fat grafting is recognized as the first STA technique used for cosmetic purposes.

Uses

Highly effective in the rejuvenation, aesthetic and functional restoration of face.

Replace volumes lost as a result of ageing or certain pathological conditions.

Indications

1. Lip augmentation.
2. Facial wrinkles and lines.
3. Asymmetries.
4. Subcutaneous facial defects.
5. Lost volume of the face is a new, modern and natural indication for fillers.

CLASSIFICATION OF FILLERS ACCORDING TO MATERIALS

Biological Fillers from Human Body

1. **Autologous**
   a. Autologous fat transplantation.
   b. Autologous dermal grafting.
   c. Blood/Subcision.
   d. Vein grafting.
   e. Autologen.
   f. Isolagen.
2. **Heterologous**
   a. Dermalogen.
   b. AlloDerm.
   c. Cymetra.
   d. Fascian.
   e. CosmoDerm.
   f. CosmoPlast.

Fillers from other Living Beings

Bovine Collagen

a. Zyderm I and II.
b. Zyplast.
c. Arteplast.
d. Artecoll.
e. Artefill.
f. Koken atelocollagen.
g. Resoplast .

Porcine Collagen

a. Fibrel.
b. Permacol.

Nonbiological or Inorganic Fillers

1. **Injectable Silicone**
   a. Liquid Injectable Silicone Sebbin, SilSkin, Silikon 1000
   b. Biopolimer III or Biocell Ultravital.
   c. PS-35.
   d. Bioplastique.
2. **Methacrylates**
   a. Arteplast.
   b. Artecoll.
   c. Artefill.
   d. Dermalive.
   e. Dermadeep.

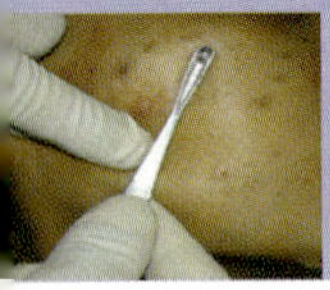

Botulinum Toxin (Fig. 24.19)

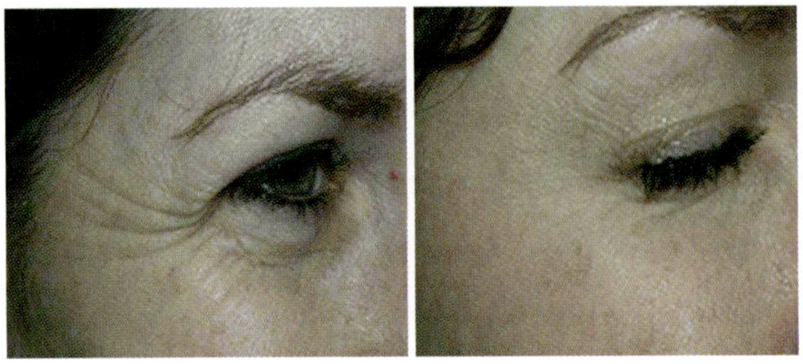

Preinjection   2 weeks after injection

Fig. 24.19: Botulinum toxin

Indications

- Treatment of facial lines and wrinkles.
- Most commonly treatment areas—Frown lines, "surprise" or forehead lines. Crows feet or "laugh lines". Occasionally lip lines and neck bands.

Preparation and Treatment

- BoNT/A Complex is supplied in 100 unit vials, must be kept frozen.
- After reconstitution with saline, the toxin be used within 4 hours, although activity remains upto 30 days if leftover solution is properly refrigerated.

INDEX

A

N

O